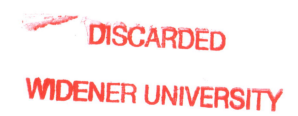

Pollock's Textbook of Cardiovascular Disease and Rehabilitation

J. Larry Durstine, PhD
University of South Carolina

Geoffrey E. Moore, MD
Healthy Living & Exercise Medicine Associates

Michael J. LaMonte, PhD
University at Buffalo

Barry A. Franklin, PhD
William Beaumont Hospital

Human Kinetics

Library of Congress Cataloging-in-Publication Data

Pollock's textbook of cardiovascular disease and rehabilitation / J. Larry Durstine, editor ... [et al.].
   p. ; cm.
   Based on: Heart disease and rehabilitation / Michael L. Pollock, Donald H. Schmidt, editors.
3rd ed. c1995.
   Includes bibliographical references and index.
   ISBN-13: 978-0-7360-5967-1 (hard cover)
   ISBN-10: 0-7360-5967-9 (hard cover)
   1. Heart--Diseases--Patients--Rehabilitation. I. Durstine, J. Larry. II. Pollock, Michael L. III.
Heart disease and rehabilitation. IV. Title: Textbook of cardiovascular disease and
rehabilitation.
   [DNLM: 1. Cardiovascular Diseases--rehabilitation. WG 120 P762 2008]
   RC682.P65 2008
   616.1'203--dc22

                        2007050866

ISBN-10: 0-7360-5967-9
ISBN-13: 978-0-7360-5967-1

The Web addresses cited in this text were current as of January 2008, unless otherwise noted.

Acquisitions Editor: Loarn D. Robertson, PhD; **Developmental Editor:** Maggie Schwarzentraub; **Assistant Editor:** Kyle G. Fritz; **Copyeditor:** Julie Anderson; **Proofreader:** Kathy Bennett; **Indexer:** Michael Ferreira; **Permission Manager:** Dalene Reeder; **Graphic Designer:** Bob Reuther; **Graphic Artist:** Dawn Sills; **Cover Designer:** Keith Blomberg; **Photographer (cover):** © PhotoDisc, Inc.; **Photo Office Assistant:** Jason Allen; **Art Manager:** Kelly Hendren; **Associate Art Manager:** Alan L. Wilborn; **Illustrators:** Figures 11.1 and 11.2, Cleveland Clinic medical illustration department; cover art, provided by author; all others, Tammy Page and Jennifer Gibas; **Printer:** Sheridan Books

Printed in the United States of America   10   9   8   7   6   5   4   3   2   1

Human Kinetics
Web site: www.HumanKinetics.com

United States: Human Kinetics
P.O. Box 5076
Champaign, IL 61825-5076
800-747-4457
e-mail: humank@hkusa.com

Canada: Human Kinetics
475 Devonshire Road Unit 100
Windsor, ON N8Y 2L5
800-465-7301 (in Canada only)
e-mail: info@hkcanada.com

Europe: Human Kinetics
107 Bradford Road
Stanningley
Leeds LS28 6AT, United Kingdom
+44 (0) 113 255 5665
e-mail: hk@hkeurope.com

Australia: Human Kinetics
57A Price Avenue
Lower Mitcham, South Australia 5062
08 8372 0999
e-mail: info@hkaustralia.com

New Zealand: Human Kinetics
Division of Sports Distributors NZ Ltd.
P.O. Box 300 226 Albany
North Shore City
Auckland
0064 9 448 1207
e-mail: info@humankinetics.co.nz

This book is dedicated to the memory of Dr. Michael L. Pollock, preeminent scientist, clinician, researcher, teacher, and friend, who collapsed and died from a cerebral aneurysm a few hours before he was scheduled to give a presentation at the 1998 American College of Sports Medicine (ACSM) Annual Meeting in Orlando, Florida.

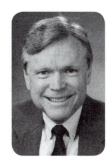

MICHAEL L. POLLOCK, PHD
(1936-1998)

Mike was a mentor and role model for so many of us in the fields of sports medicine, exercise science, and cardiopulmonary rehabilitation. He contributed immensely to our present state of knowledge through his prolific writing and seminal publications, articulate and informative presentations, outstanding annual conferences, and exemplary service to numerous professional organizations, including the ACSM, American Association of Cardiovascular and Pulmonary Rehabilitation (AACVPR), and American Heart Association (AHA).

To the end of his days, Mike carried an aura of curiosity, inquisitiveness, and anticipation—always asking why and looking forward. Indeed, I was fortunate enough to have dinner with him the night before he died. That evening, he told me that several of his graduate students were engaged in a series of exciting research studies and that he had just received a major NIH grant to revisit some of his earlier interests in exercise training. He also acknowledged how grateful and appreciative he was for the extraordinary professional and travel opportunities that he had had over the years, how fortunate he was to love his work, and how proud he was of his beautiful family (his wife, Rhonda, and three children, Jonathan, Lauren, and Elle).

An accomplished collegiate baseball player, Mike attended the University of Illinois, intending to become a coach. However, he soon developed a passion for scientific inquiry, with specific reference to cardiopulmonary exercise testing and training. When the field first emerged, several critics emphasized that there were a lot of enthusiasts but few scientists and good researchers. Mike and his fellow graduate students (whose names are a *Who's Who* of contemporary exercise science, e.g., Drs. William Haskell, Jim Skinner, Paul Ribisl), all trained by the legendary Dr. T.K. Cureton, soon changed that perception.

During his years at the University of Illinois, Mike developed the first signs and symptoms of ankylosing spondylitis, a degenerative inflammatory disease characterized by impaired mobility of the spinal column. In true fashion, Mike never let his health problems limit his tireless work ethic, his fitness regimen, or his enjoyment of life. Indeed, Dr. William Haskell, a good friend and an esteemed colleague, put it this way: "Mike's fight not to let a chronic medical condition turn into a chronic disability was conducted without complaints or the expectation that any less should be demanded of him. This fight was painful but inspirational to his many friends."

Mike's early work dealt with changes in cardiorespiratory fitness relative to the prescribed intensity, frequency, duration, and modes of exercise training. He also chronicled the associated incidence of musculoskeletal injury that resulted from varied exercise dosages and was one of the first to report on the salutary effects of brisk walking programs. Collectively, these studies led to the development of the concept of exercise prescription. Along with a handful of other prominent investigators (e.g., Fox, Hellerstein, Shephard, Balke, Cooper, Roskamm, Karvonen), Mike was among the first to attempt to provide a scientifically defensible answer to the question "How much exercise is enough?"

His career path included pioneering studies in body composition assessment and anthropometric measures and quantification of the cardiorespiratory fitness and training regimens of elite distance and champion masters runners, including a 20-year follow-up on the latter cohort. From a clinical perspective, Mike played a key role in the development of the contemporary model of cardiac rehabilitation, highlighting the role of β-blocker therapy and perceived exertion on submaximal and maximal exercise tolerance as well as the use of valuable surveillance data obtained during exercise rehabilitation, which were used to enhance medical management. A selection of his career contributions and awards are summarized here:

- Wrote more than 200 peer-reviewed publications as well as numerous book chapters and books, including *Heart Disease and Rehabilitation* (co-edited with Don Schmidt) and *Exercise in Health and Disease* (co-authored with Jack Wilmore)

- Chaired the writing group for the American College of Sports Medicine's first position stand on the quantity and quality of exercise in 1978 and co-authored its third revision 2 decades later

- Participated in professional organizations: Fellow of the ACSM, AACVPR, and the American College of Cardiology; President of ACSM (1982-1983); Founding Member of AACVPR

- Received the ACSM Citation Award (1994)

- Received the AACVPR Award of Excellence (1996)

- Served on the editorial board of numerous scientific and clinical journals, including *Medicine and Science in Sports and Exercise* and the *Journal of Cardiopulmonary Rehabilitation*

- Organized state-of-the-art annual conferences on cardiopulmonary rehabilitation

- Founded the *Journal of Cardiopulmonary Rehabilitation*; served as co-editor from 1979 to 1991

- Contributed to *ACSM's Guidelines for Exercise Testing and Prescription*

- Contributed to the development and implementation of ACSM's workshop and certification programs

- Gave hundreds of invited talks and presentations, nationally and internationally

- Received numerous funded research grants, including NIH support

- Conducted numerous landmark studies in body composition, cardiorespiratory fitness, exercise prescription, and cardiac rehabilitation

Perhaps even more noteworthy was the personal side of Mike Pollock. What impressed us about him? A number of fond memories immediately come to mind: his unwavering friendship; his dedication to his family; his religious fervor (he was deeply committed to his church); his tolerance for pain; his ability to laugh at the world and himself; his caring and compassion for others; his honesty and integrity; his unspoiled and unassuming humility; his enthusiasm regarding the success and achievements of others (as much as his own!); his unique ability to make friends and colleagues feel special about themselves; his willingness to help others, especially students and junior faculty; his delight in sharing special moments and experiences; his penchant for never saying a negative word about anyone; and his warm, contagious smile—a smile that he offered to everyone he met. Indeed, Mike exuded the tenets of appreciation and gratitude; he truly exemplified the eternal optimist.

With Mike's passing we lost an esteemed colleague, but it's difficult to say whether he will be remembered more as a scientist, a teacher, an author, a professional society leader, or simply a friend. Perhaps Dr. Carl Foster summed it up best in Mike's obituary, published in *Medicine and Science in Sports and Exercise:* "Those of us privileged to know him or work with him know that a wonderful soul is gone from among us." Foster went on to expound upon a description of the legendary long-distance runner Arthur Newton, reproduced in Tim Noakes' book *The Lore of Running*, which (in a different idiom) describes Mike perfectly:

"If one thing stands out above all others, it must be the honesty and trust of the man, the sheer goodness—it shows out in any photograph."

I vividly recall listening to a sermon by a member of our clergy several years ago. One of his comments was particularly relevant to this discussion. He said, "Small people talk about other people; average people talk about material things or themselves; and great people talk about ideas, concepts, and programs that benefit others." Clearly, Mike Pollock was one of the great people.

Sir Isaac Newton said, "If I have seen further . . . it is by standing upon the shoulders of giants." Michael Pollock provided such shoulders to a myriad of junior colleagues in exercise science, sports medicine, and cardiac rehabilitation. We (i.e., the co-editors of this textbook) were among these individuals.

Barry A. Franklin, PhD

Contents

CHAPTER 9   **Contemporary Approaches to Cardiovascular Disease Diagnosis** **83**

Peter H. Brubaker, PhD

CHAPTER 10   **Pharmacologic Management** **95**

Nina B. Radford, MD, John S. Ho, MD, and Larry W. Gibbons, MD

CHAPTER 11   **Surgical Management of Cardiovascular Disease** **109**

Sotiris C. Stamou, MD, and Tomislav Mihaljevic, MD

CHAPTER 12   **Cardiovascular Disease in Women** **119**

Nanette K. Wenger, MD

PART III Lifestyle Management of Cardiovascular Disease............ 129

PART V Rehabilitation of the Patient With Cardiovascular Disease.... 269

Contributors

James A. Blumenthal, PhD

Department of Psychiatry and Behavioral Sciences
Duke University Medical Center
Durham, North Carolina

Peter H. Brubaker, PhD

Professor, Department of Health and Exercise Science
Exective Director, Healthy Exercise & Lifestyle ProgramS
    (HELPS)
Wake Forest University
Winston-Salem, North Carolina

J. Larry Durstine, PhD

Distinguished Professor and Chair, Department of
    Exercise Science
Director of Clinical Exercise Programs
University of South Carolina
Columbia, South Carolina

Matt S. Feigenbaum, PhD

Associate Professor
Department of Health and Exercise Science
Furman University
Greenville, South Carolina

Daniel E. Forman, MD

Division of Cardiology
Brigham and Women's Hospital
GRECC, VAMC of Boston
Harvard Medical School
Boston, Massachusetts

Carl Foster, PhD

Department of Exercise and Sport Science
University of Wisconsin at La Crosse
La Crosse, Wisconsin

Barry A. Franklin, PhD

Director, Cardiac Rehabilitation and Exercise Laboratories
Division of Cardiology
William Beaumont Hospital
Royal Oak, Michigan

Victor F. Froelicher, MD

Director ECG/Exercise Laboratory
Professor of Medicine
VA Palo Alto Health Care System
Stanford University
Palo Alto, California

Larry W. Gibbons, MD

Cooper Clinic
Dallas, Texas

Neil F. Gordon, MD, PhD

Chief Medical and Science Officer,
Nationwide Better Health
Savannah, GA
Clinical Professor, Emory University School of Medicine,
Atlanta, GA

Amy E. Griel, PhD

Department of Nutritional Sciences
The Pennsylvania State University
University Park, Pennsylvania

Linda Hall, PhD

Retired

John S. Ho, MD

Director, Nuclear Cardiology
Cooper Clinic
Dallas, Texas

W. Guyton Hornsby, Jr., PhD

Division of Exercise Physiology, School of Medicine
West Virginia University
Morgantown, West Virginia

Terence Kavanagh, MD

Associate Professor, Faculty of Medicine
Professor, Graduate School of Exercise Science
University of Toronto
Toronto, Ontario, Canada

Mary Ann Kelly, PhD

Senior Research Psychologist
Translational Neuroscience Program
University of Pittsburgh Medical Center
Pittsburgh, Pennsylvania

Steven J. Keteyian, PhD

Division of Cardiovascular Medicine
Henry Ford Hospital
Detroit, Michigan

Christopher E. Kline, MS

Doctoral Student, Department of Exercise Science
Arnold School of Public Health
University of South Carolina
Columbia, South Carolina

Laurie A. Kopin, MS, RN

Associate Professor of Nursing
Senior Instructor of Medicine
University of Rochester
Rochester, New York

Penny M. Kris-Etherton, PhD

Distinguished Professor of Nutrition
Department of Nutritional Sciences
The Pennsylvania State University
University Park, Pennsylvania

Michael J. LaMonte, PhD

Department of Social and Preventive Medicine
University at Buffalo
Buffalo, New York

Alejandro Lucia, MD, PhD

European University of Madrid
Madrid, Spain

Gordon O. Matheson, MD, PhD

Division of Sports Medicine
Department of Orthopaedic Surgery
Stanford University School of Medicine
Stanford, California

Patrick E. McBride, MD

Professor of Medicine and Family Medicine, Associate
    Dean for Students, Co-Director Preventive Cardiology
    Program
University of Wisconsin School of Medicine and Public
    Health
Madison, Wisconsin

Peter A. McCullough, MD

Chief, Division of Nutrition and Preventive Medicine
Medical Director, Preventive Cardiology
Department of Medicine
Divisions of Cardiology, Nutrition, and Preventive
    Medicine
William Beaumont Hospital
Royal Oak, Michigan

Terri A. Merritt-Worden, MS

Vice President of Program Development
Preventive Medicine Research Institute
Sausalito, California

Tomislav Mihaljevic, MD

Staff Surgeon
Department of Thoracic and Cardovascular Surgery
Cleveland Clinic
Cleveland, Ohio

A. Lynn Millar, PhD

Professor of Physical Therapy
Department of Physical Therapy
Andrews University
Berrien Springs, Michigan

Henry S. Miller Jr., MD

Professor, Section on Internal Medicine (Cardiology)
Healthy Exercise & Lifestyle ProgramS (HELPS)
Wake Forest University School of Medicine
Winston-Salem, North Carolina

Wendy M. Miller, MD

Medical Director, Weight Control Center
Department of Medicine
Division of Nutrition and Preventive Medicine
William Beaumont Hospital
Royal Oak, Michigan

Geoffrey E. Moore, MD

Healthy Living and Exercise Medicine Associates
Ithaca, New York
Adjunct Assistant Professor
Department of Exercise Science
Syracuse University
Syracuse, NY

Jonathan Myers, PhD

Clinical Associate Professor of Medicine
VA Palo Alto Health Care System
Stanford University
Palo Alto, California

Cara Frances O'Connell-Edwards, PhD

Department of Physical Medicine and Rehabilitation
University of North Carolina at Chapel Hill School of
    Medicine
Chapel Hill, North Carolina

Thomas A. Pearson, MD, PhD

Albert D. Kaiser Professor of Community and Preventive
    Medicine
Senior Associate Dean for Clinical Research
University of Rochester
Rochester, New York

J. Brent Peel, MS

Department of Exercise Science
University of South Carolina
Columbia, South Carolina

Linda S. Pescatello, PhD

Professor
Department of Kinesiology
University of Connecticut
Storrs, Connecticut

John P. Porcari, PhD

Department of Exercise and Sport Science
University of Wisconsin at La Crosse
La Crosse, Wisconsin

Nina B. Radford, MD

Director, Cardiovascular Medicine
Director, Clinic Research
Cooper Clinic
Dallas, Texas

William Clifford Roberts, MD

Executive Director
Baylor Heart and Vascular Institute
Departments of Pathology and Internal Medicine
    (Division of Cardiology)
Baylor University Medical Center
Dallas, Texas

William O. Roberts, MD, MS

Professor
Department of Family Medicine and Community Health
University of Minnesota Medical School
Minneapolis, Minnesota

Richard J. Rodeheffer, MD

Professor of Medicine
Mayo Clinic
Rochester, Minnesota

Sunil Sharma, MD

Sleep-i
Sleep Diagnostics Center
West Columbia, South Carolina

Ian Shrier MD, PhD

Associate Professor (Family Medicine), Centre of Clinical
    Epidemiology and Community Studies
SMBD-Jewish General Hospital
McGill University
Montreal, Quebec, Canada

Sidney C. Smith, Jr., MD

Center for Cardiovascular Science and Medicine
University of North Carolina at Chapel Hill
Chapel Hill, North Carolina

Ray W. Squires, PhD

Professor of Medicine
Director, Cardiovascular Health and Rehabilitation
    Program
Division of Cardiovascular Diseases and Internal Medicine
Mayo Clinic
Rochester, Minnesota

Sotiris C. Stamou, MD

Cleveland Clinic
Cleveland, Ohio

Kerry J. Stewart, EdD

Professor of Medicine
Director of Clinical and Research Exercise Physiology
School of Medicine
Johns Hopkins University
Baltimore, Maryland

Justin E. Trivax, MD

Department of Medicine
William Beaumont Hospital
Royal Oak, Michigan

Irma H. Ullrich, MD

Louis A. Johnson Veterans Administration Medical Center
Clarksburg, West Virginia

Thomas E. Vanhecke, MD

Department of Medicine
William Beaumont Hospital
Royal Oak, Michigan

Kevin R. Vincent, MD, PhD

Department of Physical Medicine & Rehabilitation
University of Virginia
Charlottesville, Virginia

Stanley S. Wang, MD

Center for Cardiovascular Science and Medicine
University of North Carolina at Chapel Hill
Chapel Hill, North Carolina

William A. Webster, IV, PhD

Director of Cardiology Research
Greenville Hospital System
University Medical Center
Greenville, South Carolina

Nanette K. Wenger, MD

Professor of Medicine (Cardiology), Emory University
    School of Medicine
Chief of Cardiology, Grady Memorial Hospital
Consultant, Emory Heart & Vascular Center
Atlanta, Georgia

Philip K. Wilson, EdD

Professor Emeritus
Department of Exercise and Sport Science
University of Wisconsin at La Crosse
La Crosse, Wisconsin

Frank G. Yanowitz, MD

Professor of Medicine (Cardiology, Geriatrics)
University of Utah School of Medicine
Salt Lake City, Utah
Medical Director, The Intermountain Health & Fitness
    Institute

Emily York, PhD

Supervisor, Health Behavior Unit
Kaiser Permanente
Portland, OR

Shawn D. Youngstedt, PhD

Assistant Professor, Department of Exercise Science
Arnold School of Public Health
University of South Carolina
Research Scientist
Dorn VA Medical Center
Columbia, South Carolina

Foreword

I am honored to write the foreword for this text dedicated to the memory of Michael L. Pollock, PhD (1936-1998). Mike and I shared much throughout our careers: both growing up in southern California and serving in the U.S. Army before attending graduate school at the University of Illinois; rooming together; attending class and conducting research while earning our doctoral degrees. Our career-long interests in determining the role of physical activity in health and performance and our involvement in professional organizations such as the American College of Sports Medicine (ACSM), American Heart Association (AHA), and American College of Cardiology (ACC) were the natural outgrowth of this friendship. Mike was truly a great colleague and friend, and I benefited greatly from our association of 30 years.

With Mike, you got what you saw. His approach to his research and to the rest of his life was amazingly straightforward and honest. As a graduate student at Illinois, Mike was known as Mr. Clean, not only for his personal neatness but also for getting and keeping the facts straight. As a consummate scientist he just didn't want the truth: He wanted the exact truth. He wanted to know not only whether walking or jogging was good for cardiovascular health but, if so, how vigorous, long, and frequent the exercise needed to be. His inquisitive nature about such questions resulted in a series of studies that started with his doctoral dissertation. These studies were seminal contributions to the development of science-based exercise prescriptions and the concept of dose–response. This interest and the knowledge he gained from his research led to a major review on the quantification of endurance exercise training programs published in *Exercise and Sports Sciences Reviews* in 1973. This publication provided much of the scientific basis for the ACSM position statement on *The Recommended Quantity and Quality of Exercise for Developing and Maintaining Fitness in Healthy Adults* in 1978. This document was updated by ACSM in 1990 and again in 1998, with Mike playing a leadership role in the preparation of all three documents (the latter being published very shortly after his death).

After completing his doctorial work at Illinois, Mike went to Wake Forest University, where he teamed up with Henry Miller, MD. Together they developed an early, highly successful outpatient cardiac rehabilitation program that provided a great service to patients and a platform for conducting research on patients with coronary heart disease. Mike and Henry along with their students and colleagues at Wake Forest rapidly became one of the leading groups in the country to study cardiac rehabilitation, generating data to be used in developing endurance exercise-based rehabilitation for cardiac patients.

In 1973, Mike became director of research at the Institute for Aerobics Research in Dallas. Here he continued his research concerning how much exercise is enough for specific performance and health outcomes. Mike organized a comprehensive biological, psychological, and biomechanical evaluation of a number of world-class distance runners, the results of which were featured in the now-classic publication *The Marathon: Physiological, Medical, Epidemiological and Psychological Studies* (New York Academy of Sciences, 1977). During this period Mike also pursued the longitudinal evaluation of older (masters) distance runners, research that helped define the changes in endurance capacity with aging, which was a project he continued throughout much of his career. His research at the institute on both endurance and resistance training significantly contributed to the integration of resistance exercise into exercise programs designed to promote health and the development of circuit training regimens.

Mike continued his cardiac rehabilitation research later when he directed the cardiac rehabilitation and human performance laboratories at Mt. Sinai Hospital in Milwaukee. Working with Donald Schmidt, MD, Carl Foster, PhD, and colleagues, Mike contributed his exercise knowledge and scientific approach to the development and evaluation of inpatient as well as outpatient cardiac rehabilitation, involving new patient groups including those who had undergone coronary artery bypass surgery.

In 1986, Mike became the director of the Exercise Science Laboratory at the University of Florida and a professor in health and physical education with a joint appointment in cardiology. He continued with many of his previous research interests but also made major scientific contributions in resistance exercise evaluation and training, prevention and management of low back pain, and geriatric cardiology. His highly systematic approach to research and the interpretation of results added substantially to the standardization of resistance exercise recommendations in cardiac rehabilitation and for the general public.

Mike was not only a highly innovative and prolific scientist; he also was a highly productive communicator and educator. During his 35-year career he published more than 200 manuscripts in peer-reviewed journals, numerous reviews, book chapters, and books. He had a major presence as an invited speaker at numerous national and international scientific meetings over the years, and he was involved in or led many writing groups that produced exercise recommendations for the ACSM, AHA, ACC, and the NIH. Mike's legacy as an educator is ensured by the numerous scientists successfully conducting exercise research throughout the world who were substantially influenced by his teaching and research and the many persons who are more fit and in better health because of his research and sage advice.

Mike consistently advanced the professions of exercise science and sports medicine. He was a Fellow of ACSM, AHA, and ACC and one of the founders of the American Association of Cardiovascular and Pulmonary Rehabilitation; he was the first co-editor with Victor F. Froelicher, MD, of the *Journal of Cardiac Rehabilitation* in 1979 (now the *Journal of Cardiopulmonary Rehabilitation and Prevention*). In the ACSM he was a very active member or chair of various committees, especially those dealing with professional certification and guidelines for exercise testing and training, and was ACSM president in 1982-1983.

Over the years Mike was involved with a variety of committees or writing groups working under the auspices of the AHA preparing recommendations and educational materials for health and exercise professionals and the public regarding the cardiovascular benefits of exercise, the proper use of exercise testing, and effective exercise programming.

What Mike achieved both professionally and personally is even more impressive when you consider that he was in a day-to-day battle for much of his adult life with the debilitating chronic rheumatic disease of ankylosing spondylitis. Most people only knew that Mike appeared to have some low back stiffness as he moved about during work or play, but he never considered that he was disabled in any way. He was always very positive and looking ahead to the next project. Mike was a true inspiration to his family, friends, colleagues, and students. This book is one more recognition of his enormous contribution to exercise science, medicine, and mankind.

William L. Haskell, PhD
Stanford Prevention Research Center, Stanford University
School of Medicine

Preface

During the last 40 years, enormous advances have been made in the understanding and treatment of cardiovascular disease, including implantable left ventricular assist devices, new and emerging biomarkers, new medications such as A-II inhibitors and ezetimibe, smoking reduction, and risk factor education. These advances have led to a decline in the prevalence of several established cardiovascular risk factors, such as hypertension, hypercholesterolemia, and smoking, as well as the prevalence of coronary artery disease, and as a result cardiovascular survival rates have improved. Nonetheless, cardiovascular disease continues to inflict a sizeable economic and public health burden as the leading cause of death among U.S. adults.

A tremendous amount of knowledge and understanding have been gained regarding medical management of cardiovascular disease. In particular, we have learned the importance of therapeutic lifestyle changes. Regular physical activity, whether in the form of routine daily activities such as brisk walking or structured cardiac rehabilitation exercise participation are forms of therapeutic lifestyle change that can result in many functional and health benefits among apparently healthy individuals as well as people with cardiovascular disease. Endurance and resistance exercise training, other habits such as healthy dietary practices and stress management, and medical management provide the basis for primary prevention of cardiovascular disease, particularly among individuals with elevated disease risk, as well as secondary prevention of cardiovascular disease for people with established disease.

Many physicians and allied health professionals now accept the use of exercise for the prevention, diagnosis, and rehabilitation of various cardiovascular conditions. Assessments of body composition, muscular strength and endurance, flexibility, and cardiorespiratory endurance provide valuable information that enables exercise professionals to determine a patient's overall functional capability, prescribe individualized and safe exercise interventions, and track and evaluate the influence of an intervention on the targeted physiological adaptations or disease outcomes. Maximal or submaximal exercise testing provides a safe and noninvasive method of collecting hemodynamic, electrocardiographic, and pulmonary data that have prognostic value related to the morbidity and mortality associated with cardiovascular disease. The results from these exercise assessments provide information for exercise professionals to develop personalized exercise interventions, which result in fewer complications and more favorable outcomes than generic interventions.

This textbook has its conceptual origins in a textbook titled *Heart Disease and Rehabilitation*, first published by Michael L. Pollock, PhD, and Donald H. Schmidt, MD, in 1979, with second and third editions published in 1986 and 1995, respectively. This textbook has been the premier reference on the rehabilitation of the patient with coronary heart disease, not only presenting the latest concepts of cardiac rehabilitation but also establishing the foundation for managing other chronic diseases and disabilities.

The aim of this book is to present contemporary approaches to comprehensive rehabilitative strategies in the context of atherosclerotic cardiovascular disease and to provide topical coverage across the expanse of cardiovascular diseases as well. This textbook has several important aspects to acknowledge. First, this book is meant to honor the legacy of Dr. Michael L. Pollock by providing a view of cardiovascular disease rehabilitation as comprehensive as the vision that Dr. Pollock so passionately pursued in his research and clinical practice. A second major aspect of this book reflects the growth of the profession. *Pollock's Textbook of Cardiovascular Disease and Rehabilitation* opens the doors to studying all aspects of the cardiovascular system, not just those pertaining to coronary heart disease. We need to make this move, because the field must break out of the "cardiac rehabilitation" paradigm and form a broader base. Many patients don't meet the traditional entry criteria for cardiac rehabilitation but need our help nonetheless (e.g., patients with peripheral arterial disease).

A third aim of this book is the emphasis on the entire cardiovascular system rather than just the heart. As a result, chapters have been added to discuss the pathophysiology of these other problems (e.g., peripheral arterial disease and stroke), detailing the appropriate medical evaluation, exercise testing, medical and exercise management of these patients. The current approach to exercise prescription includes both endurance and resistance training activities, but few textbooks give the appropriate attention to resistance exercise training.

This textbook is organized into five parts containing 34 chapters and two appendixes. In part I, five chapters trace the history of the field, epidemiological evidence of cardiovascular disease, and the use of exercise as a medicine. Part I also summarizes evidence about interventions for multiple risk factors and clinical practice guidelines. Seven chapters are included in part II and describe the pathophysiology, diagnosis, and medical management for disease. Topics include the inflammatory process of atherosclerosis, surgical management of cardiovascular disease, and specific management strategies for women. The focus of part III is lifestyle management for cardiovascular disease, whereas part IV examines the common comorbidities and complicating circumstances of cardiovascular disease. Part V describes the rehabilitation process for patients with various cardiovascular diseases, ranging from coronary artery disease to thromboembolism. Finally, two appendixes provide information on commonly used drugs for cardiovascular disease and the physiologic effect of drugs on exercise performance.

The chapters of this book are laid out deliberately to cover epidemiology, pathophysiology, and medical and lifestyle management of cardiovascular disease. A review of medications, the mechanism of action, side effects, and exercise interactions is also provided.

Pollock's Textbook of Cardiovascular Disease and Rehabilitation is a comprehensive book based on science and clinical applications. The content information will assist any qualified clinician in providing safe and effective exercise testing and programming for clients with cardiovascular diseases. This textbook is essential for graduate student education and also is a key reference for all health professionals including physicians, physician assistants, nurses, physical and occupational therapists, and rehabilitation specialists who work with patients who have cardiovascular disease.

Perspectives of Cardiovascular Disease and Rehabilitation

This part presents an overview of the evolution and current state of cardiovascular disease and rehabilitation. Chapter 1 provides an historical perspective of cardiovascular rehabilitation, whereas chapter 2 discusses cardiovascular disease from an epidemiologic perspective. Chapter 3 focuses on the perspective that exercise is a type of medicine. Chapter 4 describes interventional strategies for multiple risk factors, and chapter 5 describes current clinical guidelines and target outcomes.

CHAPTER 1

History of Cardiovascular Rehabilitation

Philip K. Wilson, EdD

Terence Kavanagh, MD

The evolution of cardiovascular rehabilitation since the 1800s has been cautious and slow, and the development of services has varied around the world. In this chapter, the development of cardiovascular rehabilitation in Europe, Canada, and the Pacific region is presented by Dr. Kavanagh. Subsequently, Dr. Wilson discusses the development of cardiovascular rehabilitation in the United States.

Worldwide Perspective

Cardiovascular rehabilitation in Europe, Canada, and the Pacific region was first documented in the early 19th century. Numerous research studies and clinical experiences over the ensuing 200 years confirmed the benefits of formal rehabilitation programs. Today, organizations such as the World Health Organization and the World Heart Foundation are sharing knowledge at the international level and are turning their attention to developing countries.

Origins of Cardiovascular Rehabilitation

In 1802, the English physician William Heberden recorded the case of a patient suffering from angina "who set himself the task of sawing wood for half-an-hour every day and was nearly cured" (14).

Some 50 years later, the Irish physician William Stokes published his classic work, *The Diseases of the Heart and the Aorta*, in which he described his "pedestrian exercise" for the treatment of "fatty disease of the heart" (28). Over the ensuing years, Stokes' training regime was largely obscured by the teaching of English surgeon John Hilton, who advocated strict bed rest for patients with heart disease (16). Hilton's philosophy became the key ingredient of medical care throughout most of the English-speaking medical community, and seldom was it practiced more assiduously than after a myocardial infarction (MI). Almost 100 years passed before this practice was challenged, when in 1944, at the annual meeting of the American Medical Association, physicians for the first time collectively questioned the wisdom of prolonged bed rest.

In Germany, however, Stokes' teaching was not forgotten. In 1875, the Munich physician Oertel described his spa program, which combined Stokes' walking therapy with strict dieting to remove "superfluous

Address correspondence concerning this chapter to Philip Wilson, 423 N. 24th Street, La Crosse, Wisconsin 54601. E-mail: pkwilson@centurytel.net deposits of fat" (24). In the early 1900s the Schott brothers, continuing in the spa tradition, recommended mineral baths together with resistance exercises and hill walking (26).

In Sweden, gymnastics was the preferred exercise mode for patients with heart disease. A prominent exponent of this method, Zander, refined the approach by introducing various types of muscle-strengthening machines (9, 37). These practices were later improved upon by Herz, leading ultimately to such modern apparatuses as the cycle ergometer and the rowing machine (26).

Later Developments

The mid-20th century saw the height of the heart disease epidemic and the recognition that early mobilization followed by low-intensity exercise held the greatest promise of return to normality for the MI survivor. Later, with the discovery that the healed heart responds normally to a session of vigorous exercise, came the realization that asymptomatic survivors of MI could respond favorably to an aerobic training program (7). In 1968, Gottheiner in Israel published a comprehensive report of his experience in training some 100 patients over 4 years (11). Using a variety of vigorous aerobic activities such as brisk walking, jogging, cycling, swimming, and rowing, he was able to demonstrate that his methods were safe and effective. Other early proponents of fitness training included Kellerman and Brunner, also of Israel; Kentala and Kallio, of Finland; Wihelemson, of Sweden; and Carson, of the United Kingdom. In 1974, the pinnacle of this era seemed to be reached with the report of the successful completion of the Boston Marathon by seven Canadian post-MI patients—a medical first (18). In Ireland, Mulcahy and Mickey advocated a less formal training protocol, eschewing group exercise sessions in favor of individual counseling and home physical activities including daily walking, cycling, and golfing (23).

Early programs used exercise conditioning empirically, but developments in exercise testing permitted a more scientific approach not only to prescribing a training regimen but also to determining the prognosis in men and women referred for cardiac rehabilitation (6, 17).

By the late 1980s, exercise training had been established as the linchpin of cardiac rehabilitation but only as part of a comprehensive program that also involved smoking cessation, weight control, risk factor modification, dietary advice, drug treatment, and psychosocial counseling. By then the spectrum of potential candidates for cardiac rehabilitation had broadened to include patients who had undergone coronary artery bypass graft and percutaneous coronary intervention, heart transplant (19), compensated chronic heart failure (8), and valvular surgery.

Delivery of Cardiac Rehabilitation Services

The preferred approach to the delivery of cardiac rehabilitation in most countries is based on the U.S. model of a short inpatient program followed by formal group classes two or three times weekly for 8 to 12 weeks. Financing is usually through third-party insurance coverage. The very close relationship between Canadian and American health professionals results in similar approaches to cardiac rehabilitation in those countries, with considerable overlap in program core. Nevertheless, there are dissimilarities, driven largely by philosophical differences regarding health care funding. Health care funding in Canada allows greater latitude in determining program length, frequency of attendance, and choice of patients (e.g., patients with diabetes or chronic heart failure or other patients who are considered to be at high risk) than appears to be possible under the U.S. reimbursement system (12, 29).

Cardiac rehabilitation in Canada began in the 1960s, and there are 140 comprehensive multidisciplinary programs across the country. The province of Ontario is the most populated and has the largest number of programs. Of the remaining programs, the majority are in western Canada, with fewer in Quebec and the Maritime provinces. The need for a national body was realized in 1990 with the formation of the Canadian Association of Cardiac Rehabilitation (CACR). A guidelines document was published in 1998, with the second edition published in 2004 (29).

In parts of Europe, the traditional spalike residential four-week program retained its popularity, the main thrust being return to work. However, with the faltering economy in the 1980s, this approach began to decline in favor of the less costly outpatient movement. Nevertheless, the work of Mathes and Halhuber, of Germany, attested to the benefits accruing from the residential specialized center, which is still favored in eastern Europe, Switzerland, and various regions of Germany (21).

The growth of the European Union provided increasing opportunity and mounting enthusiasm for cooperation and exchange of information between the cardiac rehabilitation programs of various member states. A survey carried out by the European Association of Cardiac Rehabilitation in 1999 verified and evaluated 20 professional guidelines in nine languages across Europe (two of them Europe-wide) as well as most of the prominent programs (33).

In the Pacific region, apart from Australia and New Zealand, where hospital-based outpatient programs started in the 1970s, interest in cardiac rehabilitation was slower to develop. Formal outpatient programs began to appear in the 1980s and 1990s, and an important impetus was the workshops held throughout the region by the Australian physicians Alan Goble and Marion Worcester. The latter two, together with Dr. Michael Jelinek, can take much credit for the vibrant network of comprehensive programs that exist in Australia today. Elsewhere in the region, at last count there were 19 programs in the Philippines, 13 in Hong Kong, 5 in Thailand, 4 in Korea, and 3 in Singapore. Some of those who helped introduce and foster cardiac rehabilitation in Asia include Drs. Esguerra and Bellosillo and Ms. Pendon in the Philippines; Drs. Lau and Li in Hong Kong; Drs. Jitpraphai, Tanprasert, and Kantaratanakul in Thailand; and Dr. Oon in Singapore.

Growth of National and International Organizations

The World Health Organization first defined cardiac rehabilitation in 1964 and over the years has continued to develop expert committees and working groups to evaluate progress and make recommendations. Under the auspices of the International Federation and Society of Cardiology (presently the World Heart Foundation), knowledge is shared at the international level by means of the World Congress of Cardiac Rehabilitation, which first met in Hamburg, Germany, in 1977 and has met every 4 years since—in Israel, Venezuela, Australia, France, the Philippines, and Ireland. Similar meetings are held every 2 years by the Asian Pacific Congress of Cardiac Rehabilitation.

In 1985, the American Association of Cardiovascular and Pulmonary Rehabilitation (AACVPR) was formed, a multidisciplinary national organization designed to further the aims and aspirations of professionals working in the field. Its success is mirrored in the formation of similar bodies in Australia, Canada, the United Kingdom, Europe, the Pacific, Mexico, Cuba, and South America. An offspring of the AACVPR is the World Council for Cardiovascular and Pulmonary Rehabilitation (WCCPR), formed in 1995, with current membership of 15 countries.

Worldwide Need for Increased Services

In the past 150 years, cardiac rehabilitation has evolved from the empiric use of ambulation to an evidence-based, comprehensive, long-term treatment program of coronary artery disease in all of its many manifestations. Increasing urbanization and the adoption of the Western cardiotoxic lifestyle have brought a worldwide increase in the incidence of cardiovascular disease, with the need for greater efforts in primary and secondary prevention. The gradual spread of cardiac rehabilitation services beyond Europe and North America, although gratifying, highlights the need for more trials involving ethnically and culturally diverse populations. In a recent Cochrane Library meta-analysis of 48 cardiac rehabilitation randomized trials, 1 came from India, 2 from Australia, 15 from North America, and 30 from Europe (30). It seems inevitable that more countries will require cardiac rehabilitation services in the 21st century. How the challenge will be met remains to be seen, but the growth in the number of cardiac rehabilitation professionals, the enthusiasm of those professionals, and the attention being directed toward developing countries by the World Health Organization and the World Heart Foundation suggest that we are entitled to a high degree of optimism.

United States Perspective

Although the origins of cardiovascular rehabilitation can be traced to the early 19th century in England, physicians in the United States began prescribing rehabilitation in the mid-20th century.

First 3 Decades

The beginning of modern-day concepts of cardiac rehabilitation in the United States can be traced to Levine and Lown (20), who in 1952 described the use of armchair exercise for cardiac patients. Levine and Lown's report was followed by a report by Hellerstein and Goldstein in 1954 (15), who described work classification units with cardiac patients. The significance of Hellerstein and Goldstein's report was its advocacy of a complete evaluation of the patient, including cardiovascular fitness, emotional status, and the ability to return to work. Starting in the late 1950s and continuing into the 1970s, there were numerous reports on the value of cardiac rehabilitation and the management of inpatient and outpatient programs.

In the early to mid-1970s, cardiac rehabilitation gained recognition and was accepted by various professional associations. In 1972, the American Heart Association released *Exercise Testing and Training of Apparently Healthy Individuals: A Handbook for Physicians* (4). Although this book was specific to the "healthy individual," it was valuable to cardiac rehabilitation because it confirmed many of the concepts of exercise testing and exercise prescription. In 1975, the American College of Sports Medicine (ACSM) released the *Guidelines for Graded Exercise Testing and Prescription* (3), which became the authority on this topic. In conjunction with publishing this text, ACSM developed a certification program for personnel working in adult fitness and cardiac rehabilitation. This program began in 1975 and initially offered four levels of certification (22). The program has continued to be refined and developed to meet current needs and remains the gold standard for program personnel, and the ACSM guidelines book is currently in its seventh edition. In 1975, the American Heart Association released *Exercise Testing and Training of Individuals With Heart Disease or at High Risk for Its Development: A Handbook for Physicians* (5). This handbook verified many modern practices of cardiac rehabilitation and aided the medical profession's acceptance of this field.

However, concerns about the risk of exercise for the recovering cardiac patient continued until Haskell's report in 1978 titled "Cardiovascular Complications During Exercise Training of Cardiac Patients." Haskell gathered data from 30 programs with 13,570 participants, from 1960 to 1977, and showed there was very little risk to the participating cardiac patient. Risk for cardiac arrest was on the order of 1 event per 34,000 patient hours, and risk for exercise-related death was 1 per 116,000 patient hours (13). The low risk of exercise for cardiac patients was verified by other reports in the literature.

The 1950s and 1960s were a time of research and reports declaring the benefits of exercise and rehabilitation for the cardiac patient and the ill effects of bed rest and restricted physical activity. During the late 1960s and the 1970s, many more cardiac rehabilitation programs were started and their benefits reported. Unfortunately, during this period most programs used only exercise in the rehabilitation process, and few included other necessary services. Missing was the overall approach to cardiac rehabilitation, including patient education regarding primary and secondary cardiovascular risk factor modification.

The 1970s also saw an emphasis on the academic backgrounds and experience of program staff, as ACSM certification opportunities became available and university master's degree–level curricula specific to cardiac rehabilitation were established.

1980s

The first issue of the *Journal of Cardiac Rehabilitation (JCR)* was released in March 1981 with Victor Froelicher, MD, and Michael Pollock, PhD, as co-editors (10). In 1985, the AACVPR became the professional organization for cardiac and pulmonary rehabilitation personnel. In 1986, the *Journal of Cardiac Rehabilitation* became the official journal of the AACVPR and was renamed the *Journal of Cardiopulmonary Rehabilitation*. The 20-year anniversary of AACVPR was celebrated in 2005, and it remains the association for personnel involved in cardiac and pulmonary rehabilitation programs.

The 1980s saw acceptance of exercise-based cardiac rehabilitation, and by this point few in the medical community still believed that limited exercise for the patient was preferred. In addition, resistance to exercise physiologists on staff at hospital and medical clinic cardiac rehabilitation programs decreased. Many programs began to include patient education on nutrition, smoking cessation, lipid level reduction, and stress modification.

1990s

During the 1990s the profession of cardiac rehabilitation matured, beginning with the *Guidelines for Cardiac Rehabilitation Programs,* published in 1991 (1). In 1995, the results of a federally funded guidelines project were released, consisting of *Cardiac Rehabilitation, Clinical Practice Guideline* (34), a quick-reference document titled *Cardiac Rehabilitation as Secondary Prevention* (35), and a lay document titled *Recovering From Heart Disease Problems Through Cardiac Rehabilitation* (32). These three documents introduced the concept of cardiac rehabilitation as a secondary prevention program and emphasized that comprehensive cardiac rehabilitation involved cardiac risk factor management in addition to exercise therapy. This concept of secondary prevention for the cardiac patient involved education about a patient's risk factors, and as a result the AACVPR added to the association name the tag line "Promoting Health and Preventing Disease." The second and third editions of *Guidelines for Cardiac Rehabilitation Programs* were also published in the 1990s, with the title of the third edition being *Guidelines for Cardiac Rehabilitation and Secondary Prevention Programs.*

The 1990s also brought a concern with program objectives, outcomes, and, ultimately, quality control.

In 1994 Southard and others published their article "Core Competencies for Cardiac Rehabilitation" (27), and in 1995 Pashkow and others published their article "Outcome Measurement in Cardiac and Pulmonary Rehabilitation" (25). In 1996, the outcomes committee of AACVPR released the *AACVPR Tools Research Guide* (2). All of these reports focused on components of a high-quality program, as determined by evidence-based outcome measurements.

In 1998, after years of debate and an in-depth developmental process, the AACVPR unveiled a certification process for both cardiac and pulmonary rehabilitation programs, and 168 cardiac rehabilitation programs and 101 pulmonary rehabilitation programs were certified in the first year. Certification was for a 3-year period, with a recertification process available (36). AACVPR program certification now contributes to program quality control and updated professional program standards throughout the world.

Refinement and advancement of the profession occurred during the 1990s. However, by the late 1990s major concerns began regarding third-party reimbursement and the potential effect on services. Funding for programs decreased as reimbursement amounts per rehabilitation session and the number of sessions per patient decreased. Some programs were closed or had to reduce staff and services.

Availability and Funding

Cardiac rehabilitation services have continued to increase but are still unavailable in many U.S. locations. In 2005, Thomas and colleagues reported that only 2,621 cardiac rehabilitation programs were available in the United States (31). An additional major problem remains with the referral process of patients to cardiac rehabilitation. Of patients appropriate for referral, fewer than one half are actually referred. In addition, of patients who are referred, only one third actually enroll in a program. Finally, in exercise programs for presumably healthy participants, approximately two thirds of enrolled cardiac patients drop out before completing the program (31).

Funding for cardiac rehabilitation programs, which largely depends on third-party reimbursement, has continued to be problematic in the United States, especially concerning the duration of services and sessions. Because the availability of cardiac rehabilitation programs is related to reimbursement, the content and purpose of programs continue to be examined and redefined. Disease management, as a broader spectrum than cardiac rehabilitation, appears to offer significant program and professional growth. Disease management involves a multidisciplinary approach, including a staff of cardiac nurses, exercise physiologists, dieticians, and cardiologists. Staff focus on individual patient care, with an emphasis on measurement outcomes. Key to disease management is quality service that results in patient satisfaction and is offered in a cost-effective manner.

Summary

Cardiac rehabilitation is here to stay. The delivery and menu of services changed greatly from the mid-1970s to today, and the next 5 to 10 years will show many changes as well. Advancement of the profession, cost-effective programming, and a menu of extensive and necessary services will provide the patient the best care possible, at an appropriate and equitable cost.

CHAPTER 2

Epidemiology of Cardiovascular Disease

Michael J. LaMonte, PhD

Epidemiologic investigations have long contributed to our understanding of the distribution and etiology of cardiovascular diseases (CVD). Causal inferences between putative risk factors and CVD have been supported by the timing, strength, and consistency of observed associations and by biological plausibility in related experimental studies (16). From the epidemiological view of CVD emerged a portrait of the coronary disease–prone person that informed and guided clinical research on primary and secondary prevention strategies. In the third edition of Pollock and Schmidt's textbook *Heart Disease and Rehabilitation*, Dr. William Kannel provided an update on the epidemiology of CVD in the Framingham Heart Study. This chapter presents some recent findings in the area of CVD epidemiology that expand on those previously discussed by Kannel. The major sections of this chapter are the population burden of CVD, the contribution of the major CVD risk factors to CVD occurrence, and the role of physical activity and fitness in determining the risk of primary CVD events. The term *cardiovascular diseases* broadly encompasses several conditions of the heart and blood vessels, including coronary heart disease (CHD), hypertension, peripheral artery disease, stroke, heart failure, cardiomyopathy, valvular heart disease, and congenital heart disease. Atherothrombotic CVD, primarily CHD and stroke, is the principal contributor to the global burden of mortality and disability and thus is the primary focus of this chapter.

Lessons From Framingham

One of the most productive epidemiologic investigations on CVD has been the Framingham Heart Study, which was established in 1948 under the leadership of Dr. Thomas Dawber. The study set forth to prospectively relate antecedent biological and lifestyle factors with the occurrence of CVD in a population sample of 5,209 women and men who were 30 to 62 years of age and living in Framingham, Massachusetts (12). Early observation of a positive gradient in the rates of CHD events across incremental categories of total cholesterol provided epidemiologic evidence in support of the then largely speculative lipid hypothesis of atherothrombotic CVD (2, 12). Interestingly, the greatest burden of events derived from the middle of the cholesterol distribution, between 200 and 300 mg/dL, rather than from more extreme values. The Framingham study also established the importance of lipoprotein subfractions as primary predictors for CHD events. One of the more provocative findings was that greater levels of high-density lipoprotein cholesterol

I thank Dr. Joan Dorn for helpful editorial comments on early drafts of this manuscript.

Address correspondence concerning this chapter to Michael J. LaMonte, Department of Social and Preventive Medicine, 270 Farber Hall, University at Buffalo, Buffalo, NY 14214. E-mail: mlamonte@buffalo.edu

(HDL-C) favorably modified the adverse association between the atherogenic low-density lipoprotein cholesterol (LDL-C) subfraction and incident CHD events (figure 2.1). Higher HDL-C was associated with significantly lower CHD risk at any level of total or LDL cholesterol. In fact, so powerful was the near monotonic cardioprotective effect of HDL-C on CHD risk that

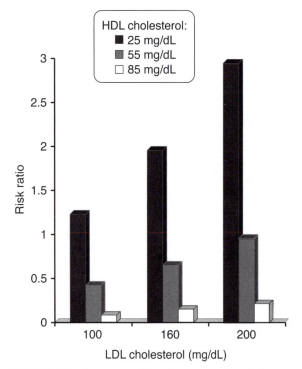

FIGURE 2.1 Four-year risk of coronary heart disease by low-density lipoprotein (LDL) and high-density lipoprotein (HDL) cholesterol in men—the Framingham Heart Study.

This figure was published in *American Heart Journal*, Vol 110, W.B. Kannell, "Lipids, diabetes, and coronary heart disease: Insights from the Framingham Study," pgs. 110-117, Copyright Elsevier, 1985.

the ratio of total to HDL cholesterol soon emerged as the single best lipid predictor of CHD occurrence in the Framingham experience (2).

Abnormal lipid concentrations were not the only consistently observed precursor of CVD events in Framingham. Other major risk factors identified in women and men included elevated blood pressure, cigarette smoking, left ventricular hypertrophy detected on the resting electrocardiogram, excessive relative body weight, impaired glucose tolerance, and sedentary living habits (2, 12). Coexistence of these and other atherogenic traits accelerated the clinical manifestations of CVD by fourfold or more compared with people who had only one prevalent risk factor. Excess CVD risk was seen even in people with multiple marginal risk factor abnormalities. On this basis, quantitative risk prediction models were developed using the entire distribution of major risk factors rather than arbitrary categorical thresholds. With the exception of electrocardiogram abnormalities, the previously mentioned risk predictors along with dyslipidemia remain today the six major independent modifiable risk factors identified by the American Heart Association as focal targets for primary CVD prevention (7).

The Framingham experience gave way to a paradigm shift from a single-etiology theory of CVD to a multifactorial CVD framework. The foundation of the *risk factor paradigm* consists of biological and lifestyle risk factors that interact with genetic and environmental influences to initiate and promote atherosclerotic plaque development, endothelial cell dysfunction, arterial stenosis, and other subclinical manifestations of atherothrombotic CVD and that eventually precipitate clinical events such as angina, myocardial infarction, stroke, and sudden death (figure 2.2). In Framingham,

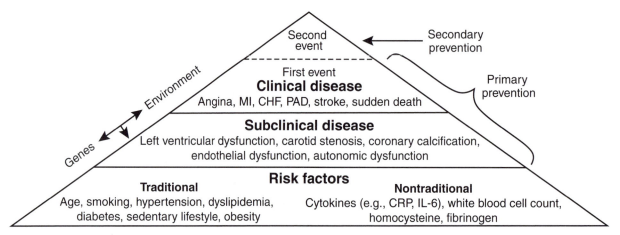

FIGURE 2.2 Multiple risk factor framework of cardiovascular disease. MI = myocardial infarction; CHF = congestive heart failure; PAD = peripheral artery disease; CRP = C-reactive protein.

Jurca R, LaMonte MJ, Durstine JL, Physical activity and nontraditional CHD risk factors: new pathways for primordial prevention of coronary heart disease. *President's Council on Physical Fitness and Sports Research Digest.* 2005; 6(4): 1-8.

approximately 33% of first myocardial infarctions occurred with unrecognized symptoms, and sudden death was the only clinical manifestation of CVD in 20% of victims (2, 12). Waiting for clinical signs or symptoms of CVD obviously is an ineffective approach to managing individual risk and preventing primary CVD events. The findings from Framingham and other epidemiological studies led to a departure from symptom-based medical management of CVD and to development of a prevention paradigm. The prevention paradigm is based on individual risk assessment to guide the initiation and intensity of clinical therapies aimed at risk factor management and risk-reducing lifestyle behavior modification. Atherothrombotic CVD soon was seen not simply as a natural consequence of aging but rather as a disease that selectively manifests in susceptible people. Coronary disease–prone people could probabilistically be identified in a population based on the presence and number of adverse CVD risk factors *before* clinical events occurred. Thus, the multifactorial model of CVD is the basis of contemporary approaches to individual CVD risk assessment and of strategies for primary and secondary CVD prevention (7), each of which is discussed in subsequent chapters.

Population Burden of CVD

CVD is the leading cause of death and disability among adults in industrialized countries (16, 38). In 1998, CVD accounted for the greatest proportion of total global mortality (30.9%) and disability-adjusted life-years (10.3%) compared with three other major noncommunicable diseases linked by common lifestyle underpinnings: total cancers (13.4% and 5.8%), diabetes (1.1% and 0.8%), and chronic obstructive pulmonary disease (4.2% and 2.1%) (38). Even in developing countries, the population disease burden gradually has shifted away from infectious disease and malnutrition to chronic degenerative diseases, primarily CVD (16, 38). The shift in that predominate underlying cause of morbidity and mortality within a population is referred to as an *epidemiologic transition* (table 2.1). Transitions can occur between disease types (e.g., from infectious diseases to degenerative diseases) and within a specific disease domain such as CVD (e.g., from rheumatic heart disease to obstructive coronary artery disease). Our genetic makeup generally has remained unchanged over the past 50,000 years. Thus, it is likely that an evolutionary mismatch in lifestyle habits between our

TABLE 2.1 Summary Characteristics of the Epidemiologic Transition of CVD

Period of epidemiologic transition	Percentage of total deaths attributed to CVD	Specific type of CVD	Major contributing risk factors	Global examples
Pestilence and famine	5-10	Rheumatic heart disease; infection and nutrition-related cardiomyopathy	Uncontrolled infections, malnutrition	Sub-Saharan Africa, rural India
Receding pandemics	10-35	Above plus hypertensive CVD, hemorrhagic stroke	High salt intake, smoking	China
Degenerative diseases	35-55	Hemorrhagic and ischemic stroke, ischemic CHD	High fat intake, sedentary habits, smoking, diabetes, obesity	Urban India, former socialist economies, aboriginal populations
Delayed degenerative disease	<50	Stroke and ischemic CHD at older ages	Population prevention strategies for lower risk factors	Western Europe, North America, Australia, New Zealand

CVD = cardiovascular disease; CHD = coronary heart disease.

Adapted from Labarthe 1998 and Yusuf et al. 2001.

hunter–gatherer ancestors and people living in modern industrialized societies underlies the global burden of chronic degenerative diseases such as CVD. Contemporary living environments in many geographic regions, developed and developing alike, are characterized by low daily energy expenditure, a calorie-dense food supply, tobacco use, and high levels of life stress, each of which contributes to CVD occurrence. Because the prevalence of CVD and associated mortality sharply increase with age (figure 2.3) and because the worldwide average life expectancy at birth increased from

46 to 66 years between 1950 and 2000 (38), a steady global escalation in the proportion of deaths and disability attributed to CVD can be expected in the early decades of the 21st century.

Mortality and Incidence Rates in the United States

CVD mortality rates have sharply declined in U.S. adults since peaking in the 1950s and 1960s (figure 2.4). Age-adjusted mortality rates have fallen by about

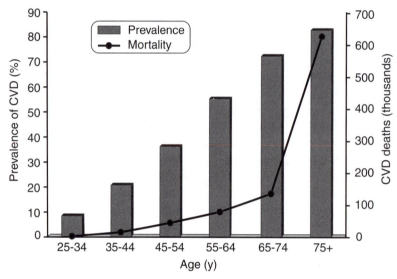

FIGURE 2.3 Prevalence of cardiovascular disease (CVD) and total CVD deaths by age in U.S. adults. Prevalence data are for the period 1999 to 2000, and mortality data are for 2003. Adapted from Thorn et al. 2003.

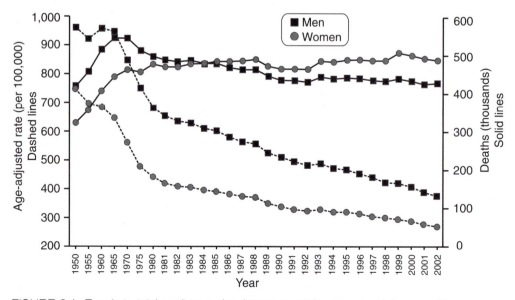

FIGURE 2.4 Trends in total cardiovascular disease mortality among adults ages 20 years and older by sex, U.S. 1950-2002. Dashed lines are age-adjusted rates (per 100,000 population) and solid lines are deaths (thousands). Data from National Center for Health Statistics (NCHS).

50% over the past 2 decades, with women experiencing a substantial advantage in the age-adjusted rate of CVD death compared with men. Despite the secular decline in CVD mortality rates, the absolute number of CVD deaths remains high in both genders. A small decline in the number of CVD deaths in men occurred between 1970 and 2002, whereas CVD deaths in women gradually increased during this time interval. The absolute number of CVD deaths has been higher in women than in men since the mid-1980s. This paradox between absolute and age-adjusted CVD mortality is consistent with an aging population, improved early detection and medical care of CVD, and an overall delay in clinically manifest CVD until the later years of life. Because women tend to live longer than men, the overall burden of CVD is becoming disproportionately higher in women than men. Declines in rates of CVD mortality and its major causes, CHD and stroke, also have occurred within the major racial–ethnic population subgroups (table 2.2). There is substantial variation in CHD and stroke mortality rates across racial–ethnic groups. Black people have the highest rates of CHD

and stroke. The lowest rates of CHD are in Asians and Pacific Islanders, and the lowest stroke rates are in Native Americans and Native Alaskans.

Trends in CVD incidence rates may not be as impressive as the reported declines in CVD mortality. For example, in the Minnesota Heart Survey between 1985 and 1995, the annualized rate of hospitalization for a first myocardial infarction declined, on average, by 1.2% in men and by 0.5% in women (24). In the Atherosclerosis Risk in Communities (ARIC) study between 1987 and 1997, the annual rate of first infarctions increased by 3% to 7% in black people and decreased only by 0.3% to 3% in white people (29). The annual 28-day case fatality rate among those hospitalized with an acute infarction declined both in Minnesota (4-5%) and in ARIC (3-12%). The 3-year case fatality in Minnesota declined by 25% to 47%. It is unclear whether the more subtle secular decline in incident first myocardial infarction compared with the greater declines in subsequent mortality and overall CVD mortality is related to better CVD risk factor profiles at the time of case presentation, better medical

TABLE 2.2 **Trends in Coronary Heart Disease (CHD) and Stroke Mortality Rates by Race–Ethnicity**

	Non-Hispanic white	Black	Native American or Native Alaskan	Asian or Pacific Islander	Hispanic
CHD					
1970	360.8	347.9	179.9	181.2	*
1980	347.6	334.5	173.6	168.2	*
1990	249.7	267.0	139.1	139.6	173.3
2000	185.6	218.3	129.1	109.6	153.2
2003	161.7	195.0	114.1	98.2	130.0
STROKE					
1970	143.5	197.1	66.4	78.6	*
1980	93.2	129.1	57.8	66.1	*
1990	62.8	91.6	40.7	56.9	45.2
2000	58.8	81.9	45.0	52.9	46.4
2003	51.4	74.3	34.6	45.2	40.5

Data are age-adjusted rates per 100,000; data from National Center for Health Statistics (NCHS).

*Data unavailable.

responsiveness and management of acute events, or both. In other words, there may be little change in the rate of incident events within the population; however, the severity of events and their acute and interim care may be sufficiently improved to result in overall declines in CVD mortality rates. This issue is difficult to sort out. Given the few ongoing population-based CVD registries, this question should be a focus of future epidemiologic investigations on CVD.

Impact of Various Forms of CVD

CVD continues to exact a large economic and public health toll as the leading cause of death in U.S. adults (figure 2.5*a*). Between 1993 and 2003, the estimated total costs of CVD rose from US$108 billion to US$368 billion. In 2003, CVD was prevalent in more than a third of U.S. adults and accounted for more than 1 in 3 adult deaths (33). Atherothrombotic CHD is the primary cause in greater than 50% of all CVD deaths (figure 2.5*b*). CHD is the single largest killer of U.S. adults and accounts for greater than 36% of the total economic costs associated with CVD. In 2003, CHD was responsible for approximately 653,000 of the more than 2 million deaths in U.S. adults, or about 1 in 4 deaths (33). Even though CHD events tend to lag by about 10 years in women compared with men, absolute deaths attributable to CHD are comparable. In 2003, there were 233,886 CHD deaths in women (49% of total CVD deaths), comparable to the 245,419 CHD deaths in men (55% of total CVD deaths). It is estimated that 1 in 3 women eventually will die from CHD or stroke compared with 1 in 30 who eventually will die of breast cancer. Yet there persists a misconception that CHD is not a major cause of mortality and disability in women. The lifetime risk of a primary CHD event after age 40 in men and women has been estimated to be 49% and 32%, respectively, and after age 70 the predicted risk is 35% and 24%, respectively (21). Greater than 1 in 3 new or recurrent myocardial infarctions occur in adults less than 65 years of age including 5% in those less than 45 years, presumably during their peak years of productivity (33). Women are 55% less likely than men to participate in cardiac rehabilitation following a CHD event, which partly may account for the greater rate of recurrent myocardial infarction in women (35%) than in men (18%) and the higher one-year mortality following a first myocardial infarction in women (38%) than in men (25%).

Stroke accounts for the second greatest proportion of CVD deaths. In 2003, 17% of CVD deaths in the United States were from strokes (figure 2.5*b*), of which the majority are of ischemic origin. The clinical manifestations of atherothrombotic cerebrovascular disease generally occur later in life (after age 65). Nonetheless, stroke accounted for 1 in 15 deaths during 2003, making stroke the third leading cause of death behind CHD and cancer (33). The lifetime risk of ischemic stroke in women and in men between the ages of 55 and 75 years is estimated to be 16% to 20% (30).

Other forms of CVD make smaller but nonetheless important contributions to the overall population burden of CVD morbidity and mortality. Subclassifications such as peripheral artery disease, chronic heart failure, and arrhythmia (e.g., atrial fibrillation) are becoming more onerous with an aging population. Information on the population distribution and impact of these forms of CVD is less available. Readers are referred elsewhere for more detailed discussions (16, 33).

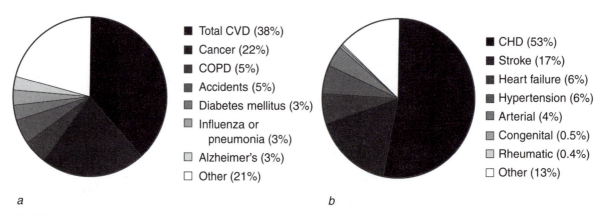

a   *b*

FIGURE 2.5   *(a)* Distribution of total deaths by underlying cause, U.S. 2003. *(b)* Distribution of CVD deaths, U.S. 2003. CVD = cardiovascular disease; COPD = chronic obstructive pulmonary disease. Data from NCHS 2006.

Significance of Major Risk Factors on CVD Occurrence

The major modifiable CVD risk factors are common in U.S. adults (table 2.3) and they account for a large proportion of clinical CVD events. Approximately 40% of U.S. adults who are without known CVD have at least one major CVD risk factor (33). Rates of CVD are four- to fivefold higher in people with at least one major risk factor than in those with no risk factors. Pooled analyses were conducted on data from 386,915 women and men who were age 18 to 59 years at baseline and were followed 21 to 30 years for CHD death in three large prospective cohorts (5). Exposure to at least one major risk factor (hypercholesterolemia, hypertension, diabetes, or smoking) ranged from 87% to 100% in those who experienced a fatal CHD event compared with 58% to 85% in those who remained event free. Likewise, in a post hoc analysis of data from 122,458 women and men who were 60 to 66 years of age and had established atherosclerotic CHD at entry

into 14 randomized trials, 81% to 85% of patients had at least one prevalent risk factor (same four risk factors mentioned previously), whereas only 15% to 19% of patients had no risk factors (13). In another pooled analysis on data from two large prospective cohorts, CVD rates were computed during 16 to 22 years of follow-up and were reported in participants defined as having low CVD risk (absence of the four risk factors) at baseline and in all others (31). Age-adjusted event rates (per 10,000 person-years) for total CVD, CHD, and stroke mortality in men 40 to 59 years of age were 6.7 to 15.8, 4.4 to 8.8, and 0.6 to 8.3 in the low-risk group and 27.5 to 53.1, 19.9 to 38.1, and 2.2 to 13.5 in those with one or more prevalent risk factors. Similar patterns of association were seen in women and in younger study participants (31). Less than 10% of the population sampled from each cohort met the definition of low risk. Clearly, a large proportion of the population occurrence of CVD is attributed to the presence of major CVD risk factors. Remarkably, these data may underestimate the actual attributable fraction of CVD events because people may have been

TABLE 2.3 **Prevalence* (%) of Major CVD Risk Factors by Sex Among U.S. Adults, 2003**

	Women	Men
Current smoker	18.5	23.4
Dyslipidemia		
Hypercholesterolemia†	24.1	24.9
Total cholesterol ≥240 mg/dL	17.8	16.3
LDL-C ≥130 mg/dL	35.8	43.1
HDL-C <40 mg/dL	12.6	33.6
Hypertension†	32.8	31.5
Sedentary habits†	26.4	22.0
Diabetes mellitus†	6.3	6.7
Obesity BMI ≥30 kg/m²	33.2	27.6
Abdominal obesity†	59.9	38.3

CVD = cardiovascular disease; LDL-C = low-density lipoprotein cholesterol; HDL-C = high-density lipoprotein cholesterol; BMI = body mass index.

*Crude prevalence defined as the proportion of the population with the condition.

†Hypercholesterolemia defined as total cholesterol ≥240 mg/dL or use of lipid-lowering medication; hypertension defined as resting systolic blood pressure ≥140 mmHg, diastolic blood pressure ≥90 mmHg, or use of antihypertensive medication; sedentary habits defined as reporting no leisure time physical activity during the previous month; diabetes mellitus defined as fasting plasma glucose ≥126 mg/dL or use of diabetes medication; abdominal obesity defined as waist circumference ≥102 cm in men and ≥88 cm in women.

Adapted from Thorn et al. 2006. Data on sedentary habit from Kruger et al. 2005.

unaware of or not diagnosed with prevalent risk factors at baseline and because other highly prevalent major risk factors (e.g., obesity, physical inactivity) were not included in the reported analyses.

Favorable temporal trends in the prevalence of some CVD risk factors may partly explain recent declines in CVD mortality. Data from five cross-sectional nationally representative surveys show that between 1960 and 2003 there was a marked decline in the prevalence of high total cholesterol, low HDL-C, hypertension, and smoking (figures 2.6 and 2.7). Not all risk factors show favorable changes. The prevalence of obesity and diabetes has risen steadily to an all-time high among U.S. adults. The prevalence of sedentary living habits

generally has remained at 20% to 30% (figure 2.8). A modest upward trend for higher total energy intake has occurred in women and in men (table 2.4). Although there has been a decline in the percentage of caloric intake from total and saturated fat, neither factor is at the recommended level of ≤30% and ≤7% of energy intake, respectively. Despite the availability of more effective pharmacological therapies for managing abnormalities in lipid, blood pressure, and glucose homeostasis, more effective widespread risk-reducing behavior modification is needed.

Additional discussion on the pathogenic role and management of selected risk factors is provided in other chapters of this textbook. Also to be found elsewhere in

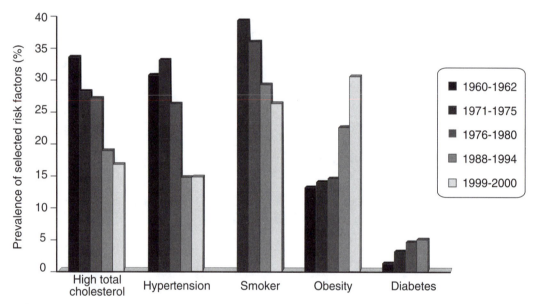

FIGURE 2.6 Trends in selected major CVD risk factors among U.S. adults ages 20 to 74 years. Adapted from Gregg et al. 2005. Obesity data from Flegal et al. 1998 and Ogden et al. 2006.

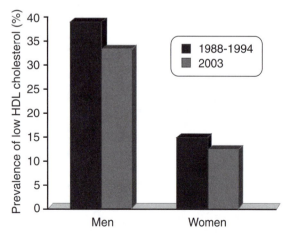

FIGURE 2.7 Trends in the prevalence of low high-density lipoprotein cholesterol (<40 mg/dL) in U.S. adults ages 20 years and older. Data from NCHS.

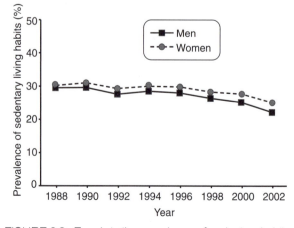

FIGURE 2.8 Trends in the prevalence of sedentary habits in U.S. adults ages 18 years and older. Adapted from Ham et al. 2004.

TABLE 2.4   Average Values of Total Energy and Macronutrient Intake Among U.S. Adults Ages 40 to 59 Years by Sex—National Health and Nutrition Examination Surveys (NHANES), 1971-2000

	1971-1974	1976-1980	1988-1994	1999-2000
MEN				
Energy intake, kcal	2,303	2,315	2,568	2,590
Carbohydrate intake, % kcal	41.6	41.5	47.8	47.5
Total fat intake, % kcal	36.9	37.3	34.2	33.4
Saturated fat intake, % kcal	13.5	13.5	11.3	11.1
Protein intake, % kcal	16.9	16.3	15.7	15.8
WOMEN				
Energy intake, kcal	1,510	1,473	1,736	1,828
Carbohydrate intake, % kcal	44.4	45.0	50.0	50.9
Total fat intake, % kcal	36.9	37.3	34.2	33.4
Saturated fat intake, % kcal	13.1	12.7	11.3	11.1
Protein intake, % kcal	17.3	16.3	15.6	15.2

Similar trends were reported in men and women aged 20 to 39 and 60 to 74 years.

Adapted from Wright et al. 2004.

this textbook is a discussion on subclinical CVD measures (e.g., ankle–brachial index, carotid intima–media thickness, coronary artery calcium scores) and markers of disease activity (e.g., C-reactive protein, fibrinogen) in relation to the occurrence of CVD events.

Physical Activity, Fitness, and Primary CVD

We now turn to a brief discussion of the epidemiology of physical activity and fitness in the context of primary CVD. Other chapters discuss the use of exercise testing in the clinical evaluation of CVD and exercise training in managing CVD risk factors and in secondary CVD prevention.

Physical Activity and Primary CVD Risk

Human evolution has depended on an active way of living. Thus, existence in a modern world where physical activity largely has been engineered out of daily life is an aberration from our evolutionary constitution (3). A sedentary lifestyle should logically be unhealthy to our species, and considerable evidence indicates that sedentary habits and low cardiorespiratory fitness are among the strongest predictors of CVD events and premature mortality (13, 17, 34, 35). In the seminal 1996 Report of the U.S. Surgeon General on Physical Activity and Health, experts evaluated epidemiologic evidence from 12 studies relating physical activity or fitness levels with total CVD risk, 41 studies on CHD risk, and 14 studies on stroke risk (35). Based on the strength and consistency of an inverse association, a conclusion of causality was made for total CVD and CHD outcomes; data were insufficient for such a conclusion on stroke. The risk of CHD events is at least twofold higher in sedentary compared with active people when summarized across studies. As is seen with other major CHD risk factors, the prevalence of sedentary habits is relatively high (table 2.3 on page 15) and the distribution worsens across CHD-prone population subgroups such as older adults, people who are obese or have diabetes, people with low educational and socioeconomic status, and members of racial–ethnic minority groups. Given the prevalence of sedentary living habits and their strong association with CHD risk, the population burden of CHD may be substantial in the physically inactive. Indeed, Hahn and colleagues (8) estimated that of the 593,111 total CHD deaths among U.S. adults in 1986, more than 205,000 deaths were attributed to physical inactivity, an attributable fraction second only to hypercholesterolemia (253,194 CHD deaths) when considered with other established CHD risk factors including hypertension, smoking, diabetes, and obesity.

Epidemiologic studies on physical activity in relation to primary CVD did not begin in earnest until the second half of the 20th century. Professors Jeremy Morris, Henry Taylor, and Ralph Paffenbarger, Jr., each made early significant contributions by reporting that people with higher levels of occupational physical activity had CHD rates that were half or less of those who had predominantly sedentary jobs (35). Classifying physical activity levels according to job title provides only a crude exposure because this approach assumes that all persons expend a similar amount of energy to perform a given job task, and it does not account for nonoccupational forms of activity-related energy expenditure that may contribute to lower CVD risk. With increasing mechanization and automation and the disappearance of human locomotion as a major form of transportation, epidemiologic studies were expanded to include leisure-time activity exposures (14, 35). In a landmark report by Ralph Paffenbarger on 16,936 male Harvard alumni (28), multivariable adjusted CVD death rates across incremental groups of leisure-time activity-related energy expenditure (<500, 500-1,999, ≥2,000 kcal/week) were 39.5, 30.8, and 21.4 per 10,000 person-years (trend $p < .001$). CVD risk was 45% lower ($p < .05$) among men who expended 2,000 kcal/week or more compared with men in the lowest activity group. The pioneering studies by Morris, Paffenbarger, and others are summarized in the Surgeon General's report on physical activity and health (35).

Since the 1996 Surgeon General's report, additional epidemiologic work has expanded the understanding of

physical activity and CVD risk, particularly in women and on stroke end points. Space limitations preclude an extensive review of all recently reported studies; however, selected findings are briefly discussed. Most of the studies considered in the Surgeon General's report included only men, and in studies on women and men, physical activity was assessed using questionnaires that had been developed to assess occupational and leisure-time activity habits of men. Thus, it is not surprising that physical activity was either not associated or only weakly associated with CVD risk in the few studies on women. The importance of accurate physical assessment in women is illustrated by a study on 6,620 Canadian women 30 years of age and older who completed a baseline physical activity questionnaire and then were followed for CVD mortality during the subsequent 7 years (36). Age-adjusted odds ratios (95% confidence interval) of CVD mortality were 1.0 (referent), 1.01 (0.68-1.51), 0.70 (0.44-1.11), and 0.51 (0.28-0.91) across incremental quartiles of total energy expenditure. However, further investigation revealed that of the 8.2 kcal/kg/day average daily total energy expenditure, only 1.2 kcal/kg/day (15%) was spent in sport and leisure activities, whereas 7.0 kcal/kg/day (85%) was spent in nonleisure activities (e.g., house and family care). CVD was not associated with leisure activity but was inversely associated with incremental quartiles of nonleisure activity: 1.0 (referent), 0.85 (0.56-1.28), 0.61 (0.39-0.96), and 0.49 (0.28-0.86). The physical activity questionnaire used in the Canadian study was based on an instrument originally developed and validated in men living in Minnesota. This led to an underestimation of activity-related energy expenditure in those women whose primary daily physical activity was house and family care. Thus, the true association between physical activity and CVD mortality in these women was biased and not detected until a nonleisure activity exposure was examined. This may partly explain why a significant inverse association between physical activity and CVD risk is less consistently observed in women than men and, when this association is observed, why the effect sizes tend to be smaller in women than in men (14, 35).

Two of the more recent and largest studies on leisure-time physical activity and CVD risk involved women participating in the Nurses Health Study (22) and in the Women's Health Initiative (23). In each study, more than 70,000 women ages 40 to 79 years at baseline were followed for primary CVD events during an average of 3 to 8 years. In both studies, multivariable analyses showed that compared with women in the lowest physical activity quintile, women in the upper four quintiles had a CVD risk that was 12%, 19%, 22%

to 26%, and 28% to 34% lower, respectively (trend $p \leq .002$). Significant inverse associations also were seen when women were categorized by race–ethnicity, smoking status, body mass index, and history of premature parental CVD. Perhaps the most provocative finding in these studies was that significant and similar CVD risk reduction was seen in walking activity or vigorous physical activities when energy expenditure was held constant. For example, the multivariable risk of CVD was, on average, 14% and 6% lower ($p < .05$ each) for each 5 MET-hour increment of energy expenditure in walking and vigorous activity, respectively (22). The benefits of walking on primary CVD risk also have been recently established in men. CVD rates have been 18% to 50% lower in men reporting higher levels of walking activity in the Honolulu Heart Study, the Health Professionals Follow-Up Study, the Finnish Health Studies, and the Zutphen Elderly Study. These studies in diverse population samples of women and men suggest that significant cardiovascular benefits are conferred from moderate amounts and intensities of physical activity, and the findings support current public health and clinical recommendations therein (34, 35).

In some studies, however, greater walking pace also has been associated with significant CVD risk reduction independent of total walking volume (22, 23, 32). For example, when men were grouped into walking pace categories of <2, 2 to 3, 3 to 4, and ≥4 mph and after adjustment for total amount of walking, CHD risk was 28%, 39%, and 49% lower (trend $p < .001$) in those in the upper three groups compared with the lowest group (32). Some of the apparent independent effect of walking pace on CHD risk may be attributable to misclassification bias from using reported walking speed. However, other recent cohort data suggest that physical activity intensity may be important to consider when examining associations with CVD (20). Additional research using objective measures of physical activity intensity and of total energy expenditure is needed to clarify this issue.

Specific physical activity types (e.g., cycling, swimming, racket sports) have been examined as CVD risk predictors, and it appears that the patterns of cardioprotective associations do not vary considerably by activity type providing the prevalence of the specific physical activity and the case distribution is adequate for analysis (32). There is growing interest in the potential cardiovascular benefit of resistance exercise. After adjustment for several CHD risk predictors and for reported aerobic activity levels, CHD risk was 23% lower ($p < .05$) in men who reported at least 30 min of weekly resistance exercise compared with those

reporting none (32). This observation is consistent with other recently published studies reporting significant inverse associations between skeletal muscle strength and CVD risk factor prevalence or chronic disease incidence, and it suggests that skeletal muscle fitness may confer metabolic and cardiovascular benefits that are to some extent independent of those associated with aerobic fitness. Resistance exercise training is covered in detail in chapter 16.

Since the 1996 Surgeon General's report, additional epidemiologic investigations have enhanced our understanding of physical activity and primary stroke risk (14, 19). Collectively, the reported data suggest a causal association between physical inactivity or low fitness and total and ischemic stroke risk; data are less consistent for hemorrhagic strokes. Differences in associations between activity and stroke subtype may partly reflect the difficulty in classifying strokes or simply may reflect a stronger biological relationship between activity and atherothrombotic CVD. A recent meta-analysis of 18 cohort and 5 case-control studies indicated that when compared with people in the lowest physical activity or fitness group, those in the middle and highest groups had a risk of total fatal and nonfatal stroke events that was 20% and 27% lower ($p < .001$ each), respectively (19). Protective associations generally were seen with both ischemic and hemorrhagic strokes among those in the high-activity or high-fitness groups. The meta-analysis did not address the dose–response characteristics of the activity or fitness and stroke association; published data are variable and include U-shaped, J-shaped, and near-linear associations. A study in Finnish women and men expanded on these findings by showing that walking and commuting activity were inversely associated with risk of total and ischemic, but not hemorrhagic, stroke incidence, even after accounting for other leisure-time physical activities (10).

The vast majority of studies, including those reviewed here, have related a single baseline physical activity exposure with CVD risk. Misclassification on exposure during follow-up can lead to biased estimates of association with this study design, although this bias would likely be toward the null. A stronger test for a causal relationship is to examine the association between a change in exposure and the subsequent risk of CVD. In other words, do people who are initially sedentary but who become physically active have a lower CVD risk than those who remain sedentary across two separate assessments? The first large epidemiological investigation on this issue was conducted by Dr. Ralph Paffenbarger in the Harvard Alumni Health Study (27). Physical activity questionnaires were completed in 1962 or 1966 and again in 1977 by 10,269 men who then were followed for CHD death during the subsequent 11 years. After the investigators accounted for differences in several health characteristics, initially sedentary men who took up physical activity of moderate or higher intensity had a 41% (p = .044) lower risk of CHD mortality than their peers who reported being sedentary on both questionnaires (27). In the Nurses Health Study, physical activity questionnaires were completed in 1980 and 1986, and then CHD events were ascertained during the subsequent 8 years (22). Compared with women who were sedentary on both questionnaires, women who were classified as having increased their activity levels into the upper four quintiles had a multivariable-adjusted CHD risk that was 15%, 21%, 33%, and 29% lower (trend p = .03), respectively.

Cardiorespiratory Fitness and Primary CVD Risk

Cardiorespiratory fitness (CRF) is an objective reproducible physiological measure that reflects the combined functional influences of physical activity habits, genetics, and disease status. This measure, therefore, may better reflect the adverse health consequences of a sedentary lifestyle than do self-reported physical activity exposures. However, the cost and administration burden of exercise testing have limited inclusion of CRF exposures in large-scale epidemiologic studies. Data on CRF and primary CVD risk were brought to the forefront of epidemiologic research by Dr. Steven Blair, who in 1989 reported on an 8-year mortality follow-up in 13,344 women and men enrolled in the Aerobics Center Longitudinal Study (ACLS) in Dallas, Texas (1). Low-, moderate-, and high-CRF groups were defined as the lowest fifth, middle two fifths, and upper two fifths of the distribution of age- and sex-standardized maximal treadmill exercise test duration. Age-adjusted CVD death rates (per 10,000 person-years) across incremental CRF groups were 24.6, 7.8, and 3.1 in men and 7.4, 2.9, and 0.8 in women, respectively. The multivariable-adjusted CVD risk was 58% higher in men and 94% higher in women with low CRF compared with their peers in the moderate and higher CRF groups combined. The asymptote of the dose–response curve between CRF and all-cause mortality was about 9 metabolic equivalents (METs) in women and 10 METs in men. Given that CVD accounted for the majority of deaths in the analysis, it is likely that these same MET levels of CRF would be reasonable targets in primary CVD prevention, although many people might obtain considerable cardiovascular benefits at even lower CRF

levels. Similar strong inverse associations between measures of CRF and CVD risk, independent of abnormal exercise electrocardiogram and heart rate responses, and the pretest probability of CVD have been reported in other well-characterized cohorts of women and men participating in the Lipid Research Clinics study, the Palo Alto VA study, the Framingham Heart Study, the Finnish health studies, and the Cleveland Clinic population (14, 18, 35).

The inverse gradient in CVD rates tends to be steeper across levels of CRF than self-reported physical activity, particularly in women (14, 35). CVD rate differences between the lowest and highest physical activity groups tend to be on an order of magnitude of two- to fourfold, but these differences are between five- and eightfold between low- and high-CRF groups. Possible explanations for the apparent stronger association between CVD and CRF may relate to the more objective and reliable measurement of CRF and thus better classification into CRF exposure groups than is possible with self-reported physical activity exposure classification. This may be particularly relevant in women, among whom questionnaire-based physical activity assessment is more problematic than in men. The etiological pathway between CRF and CVD also may be influenced by other biological or environmental factors independent of physical activity per se. Genetics influence the expression of CRF just as they influence other risk factors such as lipid concentrations, body size, blood pressure, and perhaps even disposition toward sedentary lifeways. Although physical activity is a major environmental factor that influences the degree to which bad genes express unfavorable phenotypes, CRF may be a better indicator of the combination of genetics and behavior and thus stronger than physical activity as a predictor of CVD outcomes. Therefore, the population burden of CVD may be considerable in those with low CRF. Epidemiologic data evaluating the proportion of CVD attributed to low CRF are sparse.

Recently, some initial computations were done to quantify the impact of low CRF on CVD mortality in the ACLS population. Table 2.5 shows the case prevalence of low CRF and five other established modifiable CVD risk factors along with their relative hazards and attributable fractions of CVD mortality. In men, low CRF carries the largest relative hazard for CVD mortality, and in women it carries the second largest relative hazard: a greater than 2.5-fold risk of CVD death in those with low compared with moderate and high CRF. Given this strong association and because low CRF is highly prevalent among decedents, the fraction of CVD deaths attributed to low CRF is high. This underscores the importance of low CRF in a public health context. If the association between CRF and CVD mortality is causal, and if all unfit people in the ACLS became fit, greater than 40% of CVD deaths might have been avoided in women and men each. Only hypertension accounted for a higher proportion of CVD deaths in the ACLS sample of women and men. These findings parallel those of Hahn and colleagues (8) on the fraction of CHD deaths attributed to sedentary habits. Clearly, low levels of physical activity and functional capacity account for a large portion of the population burden of CVD.

Prospective epidemiologic data also have been used recently to evaluate the potential role of functional capacity as a noninvasive cardiovascular measure that might be used to enhance individual risk assessment beyond that achieved by conventional office-based methods (18). Reported data from a small number of prospective studies suggest that measures of functional capacity significantly enhance CVD risk prediction over and above that based on multiple risk factor prediction models in women and men who are asymptomatic and without known CVD at the time of exercise testing. Such analyses were conducted in the ACLS on 41,708 men and 12,805 women who were followed an average of 17 years for primary CVD events (17). Maximal MET levels of CRF were assessed during maximal

treadmill exercise testing, and 10-year probabilities of coronary events were computed with the Framingham Risk Score (FRS) using measured risk factors. In the top portion of table 2.6, likelihood ratio tests indicate that CVD and CHD mortality prediction is significantly better when based on FRS and CRF jointly than when based on FRS alone. Based on the data shown in the bottom portion of the table, CVD risk assessment should not stop with stratification of a person's predicted probability of CVD based on multiple risk factor scoring. Lower CRF identifies people with significant CVD risk within each stratum of FRS. Each 1 MET decrement in CRF was, on average, associated with a 15% to 21% greater risk of CVD mortality in low-risk and high-risk participants alike, even after the investigators accounted for differences in other CVD risk predictors, including abnormal exercise electrocardiogram and chronotropic responses. These findings are consistent with other epidemiologic data demonstrating significant prognostic information from functional capacity measures over and above conventional CVD risk factor stratification in asymptomatic adults (18). Additional work is needed to develop and evaluate effective implementation strategies. Greater discussion on the clinical relevance of assessing functional capacity is provided in other chapters of this book.

TABLE 2.5 Hazard Ratios and Attributable Fractions of Cardiovascular Disease Mortality in Participants Who Were Followed for an Average of 17 Years in the Aerobics Center Longitudinal Study, 1970-2003

	MEN			WOMEN		
	P_c	HR (95% CI)	AF%	P_c	HR (95% CI)	AF%
Low CRF	42.9	2.78 (2.29-2.89)	29.9	41.2	3.32 (2.31-4.78)	28.8
Obesity	19.3	2.08 (1.81-2.39)	9.9	13.7	3.01 (1.82-4.97)	9.2
Smoking	25.5	1.51 (1.33-1.72)	8.6	19.1	1.61 (1.03-2.51)	7.2
Hypertension	56.9	2.23 (1.99-2.49)	31.4	50.4	3.24 (2.29-4.57)	34.8
High cholesterol	43.2	1.68 (1.51-1.88)	17.4	38.2	1.68 (1.18-2.39)	15.5
Diabetes	15.8	2.26 (1.94-2.62)	8.8	9.2	3.55 (1.96-6.44)	6.6

Participants were 40,872 men and 12,943 women ages 18 to 100 years. P_c = risk factor prevalence among cases; HR = hazard ratio; CI = confidence interval; AF% = attributable fraction expressed as the percentage of deaths that might have been avoided if participants had not been exposed to the risk factor; CRF = cardiorespiratory fitness. Hazard ratios, 95% CI, and AF% were adjusted for differences in age and baseline examination year. AF% was computed as $P_c(1 - 1/HR)$. There were 1,279 deaths in men and 131 deaths in women. Low CRF was defined as being in the lowest fifth of the age- and sex-specific distribution of maximal treadmill exercise duration. Obesity was defined as a body mass index ≥ 30 kg/m². Hypertension, high total cholesterol, and diabetes were defined as a history of physician diagnosis or measured phenotypes of $\geq 140/90$ mmHg, ≥ 240 mg/dL, or ≤ 126 mg/dL, respectively. The prevalence of each risk factor among all study participants, decedents and survivors (as ordered in the table), was 19.8%, 14.6%, 17.8%, 32.2%, 26.8%, and 4.9% in men and 15.9%, 6.9%, 10.5%, 10.5%, 21.2%, and 3.0% in women.

Data from S.N. Blair 2005 (principal investigator) and M.J. LaMonte.

TABLE 2.6   **Risk of CVD Death by Framingham Risk Score and Cardiorespiratory Fitness in 41,708 Men Followed an Average of 17 years—Aerobics Center Longitudinal Study, 1970-2003**

	CVD death (1,307 deaths)	CHD death (792 deaths)
FRS alone*		
FRS (per 1 unit increment)	1.06 (1.04-1.07)	1.06 (1.05-1.08)
FRS plus METs*		
FRS (per 1 unit increment)	1.03 (1.02-1.06)	1.02 (1.01-1.06)
METs (per 1 unit decrement)	1.24 (1.21-1.27)	1.27 (1.22-1.32)
Likelihood ratio†	214.6 p < .001	165.7 p < .001
	10-YEAR FRS		
	10% (low risk)	10-20% (intermediate risk)	≥20% (high risk)
CVD death			
METs (per 1 MET decrement)‡	1.21 (1.15-1.27)	1.15 (1.10-1.22)	1.18 (1.10-1.25)
CHD death			
METs (per 1 MET decrement)‡	1.21 (1.12-1.28)	1.22 (1.14-1.29)	1.16 (1.08-1.27)

Data are hazard ratio (95% confidence interval). CVD = cardiovascular disease; CHD = coronary heart disease; FRS = Framingham risk score; MET = metabolic equivalent.

*Model also includes age, examination year, and family history of CVD.

†The likelihood ratio test was used to determine whether risk prediction was improved with the addition of CRF (METs) to the model based on FRS alone.

‡Model also includes age, examination year, family history of CVD, FRS, abnormal exercise electrocardiogram responses, and chronotropic incompetence.

Adapted from LaMonte et al. 2005.

Summary

Atherothrombotic CVD is a major force of morbidity and mortality in the United States and elsewhere. Epidemiologic studies have elucidated the multifactorial nature of CVD, of which the clinical manifestations largely are explained by the major modifiable risk factors. Thus, the coronary disease–prone person is identifiable and CVD is preventable. Favorable secular trends in hypertension, smoking, and hypercholesterolemia have occurred among U.S. adults. However, the prevalence of obesity and diabetes continues to rise, and less than half of U.S. adults achieve recommended levels of physical activity. The role of physical inactivity and low functional capacity in predisposing primary CVD events has become more prominent in epidemiologic investigations. An even better understanding of the population disease burden associated with physical inactivity and low CRF will come through the use of objective surveillance measures (e.g., accelerometry, isokinetic strength assessment, and submaximal exercise testing) that recently have been included in the U.S. National Health and Nutrition Examination Studies. Epidemiologic data on the role that subclinical CVD measures and markers of disease activity have in assessing CVD risk and in monitoring interventions will inform future investigations on the efficacy of pharmacologic and nonpharmacologic therapies for primary CVD prevention. Against the backdrop of epidemiologic data briefly reviewed here, the clinical assessment and management of CVD are covered in subsequent chapters.

CHAPTER 3

Exercise as a Medicine

Geoffrey E. Moore, MD

Gordon O. Matheson, MD, PhD

This chapter reviews how physicians have perceived exercise as it relates to medicine from times of antiquity to the present day. Over the ages, physicians' views on the ways that exercise creates, maintains, and restores health have changed, although the trend has been to increasingly view exercise as providing medical benefit. Today, the scientific evidence is very strong as to how exercise can be used as a therapy. In the next few pages we review the seminal moments and advances and show how future physicians will almost surely regard exercise *as a medicine*.

Exercise From Antiquity to the Renaissance

Hippocrates was an early advocate of diet and exercise as a path to good health. This is hardly surprising, given that Hippocrates had much more limited and less potent pharmacopoeias than we have today. Hippocrates has been widely attributed with this quote: "If we could give every individual the right amount of nourishment and exercise, not too little and not too much, we would have found the safest way to health." Although this statement cannot be found in any of Hippocrates' writings (1), it is very likely that he would have wholeheartedly agreed with this statement. Much of his writing deals with the role of food and exercise in maintaining a healthy constitution and good musculoskeletal function.

Greek physicians, according to historians, fell into one of three categories: priest–physicians, philosophers, or gymnasts. The gymnasts pursued diet and exercise as a path to asceticism, or achieving a higher spiritual state through the melding of mind and body. Plato was not a gymnast but a philosopher, yet he too believed strongly that exercise was an integral component of mind–body health. In *The Republic*, Plato discussed the elements of education and their role in society and therein most eloquently summarized the concept of mind–body medicine (18):

> The ordinary athlete undergoes the rigors of training for the sake of muscular strength, but ours will do so rather with a view to stimulating the spirited element in their nature. So perhaps the purpose of the two established branches of education, i.e., philosophy and physical exercise, is not, as some suppose, the improvement of the mind in one case and of the body in the other. Both, it may be, aim chiefly at improving the soul.

It may well prove impossible for the modern mind to improve on that observation.

The Romans used exercise in spas for general well-being and in gladiatorial combat as displays of athleticism. Sidney Licht, a prominent American physiatrist in the 20th century and curator of the Physical Medicine Collection at the Yale Medical Library, noted that

Address correspondence concerning this chapter to Geoffrey E. Moore, Cayuga Center for Health Living, 310 Taughannock Boulevard, Ithaca, NY 14850. E-mail: gmoore@cayugamed.org many of the Roman concepts of therapeutic exercise were quite similar to modern notions (14). According to Licht, the greatest of Roman physicians, Galen, classified exercise by apparatus or body part, vigor, duration, and frequency. This seems very contemporary and consistent with present-day principles of exercise prescription: frequency, intensity, time, and type. Antyllus, who lived in the second century, cautioned against the use of rest in persons with chronic disease, advocating that bed rest only be prescribed during acute exacerbations of illness and that during intervening periods the patient should be more active. Philostratus believed that therapeutic exercise had its limitations and that gymnasts were insufficiently trained to manage many acute injuries such as lacerations, wounds, visual disturbances, and sprains; he believed such cases should be referred to physicians. Licht noted that Caelius Aurelianus gave very detailed descriptions of aquatic therapy, use of pulleys and suspension in maintaining range of motion, and use of assisted kinetic activities in patients with paralysis. Discovering ancient Roman medicine is much like seeing Roman ruins—it becomes readily apparent that their society was very much like ours today. Regrettably, the advanced medical concepts of ancient Roman physicians were lost for centuries. Licht noted that much of the athletic exercise in Roman coliseums was abuse inflicted on Christians, and the fall of Rome led to a rejection of all Roman ideals, including therapeutic exercise. The historical "darkness" of the Middle Ages was in part a reaction to longstanding persecution, and the Greco–Roman concept of exercising the mind and body was forgotten.

In contrast, Asian physicians have believed in diet and exercise since early Taoism and used *Cong Fou* as mind–body therapy dating back a millennium before Christ. Asian physicians have promoted lifestyle as a path to health through all of recorded history; in comparison, recent occidental recognition of mind–body therapy is many centuries belated. One can only wonder what path Western medicine might have followed if diet and exercise had been key components of the pharmacopoeia through medieval times and the Renaissance.

In medieval Europe, Catholic doctrine was that sloth and gluttony were two of the seven deadly sins. Of course, in the view of the Church this meant deadly to the spirit rather than to the body. Licht (14) credited the Arabs for maintaining the traditions of Greco–Roman medicine through the Middle Ages. The view of exercise as a pathway to health started its comeback in the 14th and 15th centuries and early Renaissance. Licht credited the first printed medical text about exercise as being *Libro del Exercicio*, by Christobal Mendez of Jaen,

published in 1553 and of which there are only three extant copies. Licht did not comment on the influence of Gutenberg's invention of the Western version of moveable typeset printing technology in 1447 (Bi Sheng is credited with inventing this in China, circa 1041), but it seems likely that the spread of knowledge prior to typesetting was limited by the unavailability of hand-copied texts and by the suppression of scientific knowledge by the Holy Roman Empire. Gutenberg is believed by many to be the most influential person of the 2nd millennium, and few medical students would question whether the ability to publish medical texts in large numbers has had a major influence on the progress of medical knowledge.

In the Renaissance, physicians who advocated exercise in various writings are a veritable *Who's Who* of anatomy and medicine: Malphighi, Sydenham, Cheyne, Stokes, Hoffman, Boerhaave, Tissot, and Hunter. Renaissance physicians progressively pushed the state-of-the-art of exercise in medicine, culminating with Nicolas Andry. Licht credited Andry with making an enormous advance in 1723, when he presented a paper to the Medical Faculty of Paris, titled "Is Exercise the Best Means of Preserving Health?" The answer to his question, strongly in the affirmative, awaited the research of epidemiologists nearly 300 years later. For most of that time, science was more observational and lacked the statistical rigor to evaluate this hypothesis. During the last 50 to 100 years, physicians became more consumed with molecular biology and inventing technological skills, while health promotion was shoved to the sidelines of medicine. It was, after all, epidemiologists and not physicians who recently brought health promotion to the forefront.

Exercise From the Renaissance to the 20th Century

In the 19th century, scholars of therapeutic exercise gradually diverged onto two paths—musculoskeletal and cardiovascular. Those in the musculoskeletal realm increasingly turned their attention to deformities like scoliosis and to chronic musculoskeletal maladies. The musculoskeletal protagonists were led by Pehr Henrik Ling and Gustav Zander. Ling emphasized agonist and antagonist muscle functions. Zander's teaching was very mechanical and advocated specific doses of exercise, limited by fatigue; his ideas were the basis of Lagrange's *La Medication par L'Exercice* (Medication by Exercise). This is perhaps an idea 100 years in advance of modern notions that exercise can be used *as a medicine*.

In the Napoleonic era and afterward, especially during the first and second world wars, therapeutic exercise became heavily oriented toward rehabilitation of soldiers wounded in battle. In North America, this model was advanced by R. Tait McKenzie, a graduate of McGill University and arguably the first modern physician to practice sports medicine. McKenzie's practice reflected the heritage of gymnastic physicians since ancient Greece, because he was both a physician and the chairman of the Department of Physical Education at the University of Pennsylvania. McKenzie's 1909 textbook, *Exercise in Education and Medicine*, was a seminal work in the founding of modern sports medicine, if for no other reason than its insight that exercise has a medicinal role (3). McKenzie, like his colleagues and many of their disciples in the 20th century, served in the medical corps and became devoted to rehabilitation of wounded soldiers. McKenzie was interested in all aspects of exercise and wrote about the role of exercise in longevity, health of the heart, and physical therapy for wounded soldiers. Perhaps more than any other factor, the world wars of the 20th century guided practitioners of therapeutic exercise toward the practice of what E.F. Cyriax called *orthopedic medicine* (4).

Origins of Therapeutic Exercise for the Heart

Physicians of antiquity had only rudimentary understandings of anatomy and physiology, including circulatory anatomy and physiology, fluid and electrolyte balance, and energy metabolism. Their advocacy of exercise was largely driven by personal anecdotal observations of individuals who did and did not exercise. Given that biological aspects of exercise are less obvious than musculoskeletal aspects, it is understandable that therapeutic exercise has historically emphasized musculoskeletal more than cardiovascular health. With time, however, it became clear that exercise is good cardiovascular medicine.

The first widely cited example of exercise being good for cardiovascular health was a case cited by William Heberden, in 1772, in his writings on angina pectoris (8):

> I knew of one case who set himself the task of sawing wood for half an hour each day, and was nearly cured.

Thus, Heberden unwittingly documented the first known example of cardiac rehabilitation. It is thought that this was completely unwitting, because the cause of angina pectoris remained a mystery to Heberden. He knew the cure without knowing the nature of the disease!

Exercise as cardiac rehabilitation was virtually unheard of until late in the 19th century. By 1884, William Stokes had become a supporter of exercise for persons with heart disease. By 1885, Oertal (in treating himself for what he was told was a weak heart) used hiking in the mountains as a treatment to rehabilitate himself and other patients with heart disease. And by about 1900, the Schotts had developed a therapy for heart disease that consisted of single-limb exercises and baths, which became known as the Schott treatment offered at a spa in Bad Nauheim, Germany. These examples were a rarity, however, because the medical mainstream, characterized by the view of William Osler, was that bed rest should be the mainstay of treatment for persons with heart disease (17).

During this period of the late 1800s, physicians became interested in the nature of cardiac hypertrophy. In particular, they were intrigued by the phenomenon called *soldier's heart* (today, more commonly known as *athlete's heart)*, and there was lively debate as to whether soldier's heart was good or bad. The nature of cardiac hypertrophy was not understood, and physicians sided pro and con about the merits of exercise. R. Tait McKenzie, as mentioned previously, became perhaps the foremost proponent of exercise as a method of rehabilitation.

In the early 1900s, physicians were divided about whether exercise was good for the heart. Sir James MacKenzie, a noted British cardiologist who invented the polygraph, met R. Tait McKenzie while they were serving in the medical corps during World War I. McKenzie and MacKenzie agreed that exercise was good for the heart (3), and both of them authored manuscripts on the phenomenon of soldier's (athlete's) heart. Louis F. Bishop, Sr., was also an advocate of exercise. Bishop graduated from the New York College of Physicians & Surgeons in 1890 and completed his internship at St. Luke's Hospital in New York. He became a prominent internist in New York City, where he specialized in heart diseases, and is regarded as the first cardiologist in the United States.

From 1908 to 1910, Bishop studied at the baths in Bad Nauheim, met Sir James MacKenzie , and learned how to use MacKenzie's polygraph, which recorded the cervical and radial artery pulses. Bishop embraced the concepts of specialization and pathophysiology and joined the clinical faculty at Fordham University School of Medicine in diseases of heart and circulation. Bishop advocated the use of technologies such as fluoroscopy, electrocardiography, sphygmomanometry, and polygraph, mostly out of a desire to increase practice revenues! Bishop believed in exercises for treatment of heart disease, and his son, Louis F. Bishop, Jr., who also became a cardiologist, was a founder of the American College of Sports Medicine (7).

Mainstream medical opinion, it must be reiterated, was mostly opposed to the view of exercise as a therapy, particularly so for persons with heart disease. William Osler (later knighted) is regarded by most as the founder of modern medicine; he recommended in the 1909 edition of his textbook *The Principles and Practice of Medicine* that the optimum treatment for heart disease was strict bedrest and Schott treatments (17). Paul Dudley White, who studied cardiology under James MacKenzie and then became the first cardiologist at Harvard University and the Massachusetts General Hospital, also believed that bedrest was the best therapy for heart disease (3, 7).

The early 1900s were thus a period during which an increasing understanding of the pathophysiology of heart disease led to the development of the field of cardiology. The medical mainstream, including William Osler and Paul Dudley White, was opposed to exercise in persons with heart disease. A few prominent physicians, all of whom had been athletic themselves, had a bias in favor of exercise—regardless of whether someone had heart disease. The sides of this debate can hardly be described as intellectual or scientific—they clearly were chosen by whether one liked to participate in sports!

During the first half of the 20th century, medical opinion about exercise in heart disease shifted away from, and then back toward, exercise as therapy for the heart. The bias *against* exercise after myocardial infarction gained strength in 1939, with the publication of an article that identified aneurysm formation, heart failure, left-ventricular rupture, dysrhythmias, and sudden death as complications of myocardial infarctions (15). It became feared that the hemodynamic stress of exercise would stretch the walls of the heart and create dilated cardiomyopathy. It was not long, however, before this view was challenged. In 1952, Levine and Lown published an article noting that patients who sat in an armchair did better than patients at strict bedrest (13). It would be difficult to convince anyone today that the orthostatic challenge of sitting constitutes exercise, but this article opened the door to the notion of putting cardiovascular demand on the heart after a myocardial infarction. By the late 1950s, even Paul Dudley White had become an advocate of cardiac rehabilitation (20). Finally, a notable physiologic study on five subjects who were put to 3 weeks of bedrest was published by Saltin and colleagues (19) in a landmark article that was the final blow, ending the widespread belief in therapeutic rest.

Thus, by the mid-1960s, scientists had shown that bedrest was physiologically detrimental and that exercise after a myocardial infarction was helpful. In addition, physicians from the medical corps were returning from the battlefield, and needing to create career opportunities they turned toward cardiac surgery. Vascular surgeons turned toward vascular surgery on the heart and created cardiac intensive care units. They applied the skills they had acquired on the battlefield to an American public that was having an epidemic of heart disease. Influenced by their experience in the military, where physiatrists and physical therapists aggressively advocated exercise, cardiac surgeons in the 1960s were very much in favor of cardiac rehabilitation.

In the latter 1960s and early 1970s, cardiac rehabilitation generated increased interest among scientists in the United States and the World Health Organization. In the United States, a multidisciplinary conference was convened in the mountains of West Virginia, a meeting now known as the *Airlie conference* (16). At this meeting, physicians, physiologists, psychologists, nutritionists, physical educators, lawyers, and economists developed the modern foundation for cardiac rehabilitation. Thus, modern cardiac rehabilitation has been multidisciplinary from its very inception.

During the 1970s and 1980s, numerous researchers studied exercise and comprehensive cardiac rehabilitation and demonstrated the efficacy and worthiness of this program, laying the foundation for cardiac rehabilitation:

1. Heberden (and subsequently others) showed that exercise was therapeutic for angina pectoris.

2. Many investigators showed the benefit of exercise for persons with myocardial infarction.

3. Surgeons supported postoperative exercise because they had seen its benefits in the military.

We were not able to trace the original Medicare ruling that these three conditions are the indications for cardiac rehabilitation, but numerous interviews indicate that they were chosen because these were the research interest, empiric findings, and biases of the proponents.

By the early 1990s, the Department of Health and Human Services ordered a review of cardiac rehabilitation, which was led by the cardiologist L. Kent Smith (2). This review confirmed the value of cardiac rehabilitation and held out promise that in the United States, the indications for cardiac rehabilitation might be expanded to include heart failure and that many other diseases could be considered for *cardiovascular rehabilitation*. In March 2006, the Centers for Medicare and Medicaid Services expanded the diagnoses eligible for cardiac rehabilitation to include valve replacement surgery, heart transplantation, and angioplasty.

Link Between Cardiovascular and Physical Rehabilitation

R. Tait McKenzie was unique, having published on both cardiovascular and musculoskeletal physiology and treatment. Being a physician and physical educator, he was in the center of the debate about athlete's heart. His background as a boxer and physical educator allowed him to see that wounded soldiers benefited from the same kinds of exercise training used by athletes in preparation for sports. McKenzie predated the era of specialization that would artificially divide rehabilitation by physiologic system. Physical therapy veered toward developing the concept of therapeutic exercise and focused primarily on the neuromusculoskeletal system, whereas physiologists studied the role of exercise in cardiovascular physiology. Eventually, these areas of study would reconverge, but for many decades physical rehabilitation and cardiac rehabilitation were separate. (Physical rehabilitators focused on cardiac rehabilitation, which has remained part of the physical medicine curriculum, but most cardiac rehabilitation programs ended up being run by cardiologists.)

Physical therapy and physiatry were both greatly affected by war in the 20th century. McKenzie himself was strongly influenced by his experience in the medical corps during World War I, in which there were many severe nonfatal casualties. It became clear that the twofold function of the medical corps was to return soldiers to active duty and rehabilitate soldiers with disabling wounds. Rehabilitation became a passion of McKenzie's and influenced the latter years of his career.

Subsequent wars—World War II, the Korean Conflict, Vietnam—created an environment that advanced the field of rehabilitation, although these wars indirectly favored the development of cardiac rehabilitation. In Korea, the medical corps first exploited the use of helicopters to evacuate wounded troops, and trauma surgeons honed their orthopedic and vascular surgery skills to save lives and limbs. After Korea and Vietnam, it was a natural evolution to use helicopters, urgent care systems, and vascular and trauma surgery to provide civilians with the many benefits learned by medical corps during combat.

From the standpoint of clinical services, cardiovascular and physical rehabilitation have been somewhat artificially divided by hospital divisions—vascular and orthopedics. The notion of integrated rehabilitation was suppressed, largely for administrative purposes and to divvy up clinical turf (5,10). The integrated view did exist, however (9). In 1949, Hans Kraus wrote *Principles and Practice of Therapeutic Exercise* and helped clarify models of muscle contraction, elasticity, coordination, goniometry, and passive, active, and assisted movement. Kraus noted that exercise prescriptions need to be specific (12):

> No physician merely prescribes "medicine"; he always specifies both drug and exact dosage.

Kraus believed in specifying (a) exercises for the whole body, upper and lower extremities, parts of the extremities, joints, muscles, and muscle groups; (b) components of stretching and relaxation; and (c) parameters of time, number of repetitions, and intensity. He applied exercise to specific conditions, including fractures, sprains, many varieties of nervous system disorders, and breathing disorders (such as polio, emphysema, and postoperative convalescence) as well as for general conditioning. He noted,

> Pre- and post-operative exercises before and after childbirth, exercises for cardiacs, etc., have yet to be accepted as an integral part of the treatment program.

Since the 1980s, more research articles and textbooks have been published on exercise in special populations, in which medically directed or therapeutic exercise is recommended for persons with a chronic disease or disability. These publications tend to focus either on cardiovascular or pulmonary diseases or on neuromusculoskeletal diseases. *ACSM's Exercise Management for Persons With Chronic Diseases and Disabilities* (6) departed from this trend by approaching exercise as a comprehensive activity that involves all physiologic systems and providing guidance for treatment of persons who have multiple chronic conditions—a common but rarely studied circumstance. This publication noted that exercise management increasingly involves a complex interaction of exercise physiology, pathophysiology of a disease, and medications that alter these interactions.

Next Era: Molecular Biology of Exercise

Since the 1990s, exercise research has increasingly become the domain of molecular biology. Every time someone exercises, his or her body has a multitude of physiologic responses—there is no physiologic system that is not affected by a bout of exercise. As we gain a better understanding of molecular biology, one can conceive of exercise in the traditional sense of frequency, intensity, time, and type, or one can begin to conceive of exercise as physiologic doses of endogenous compounds—self-medication, if you will. In such a view, exercise is a highly sophisticated form of physiologic polypharmacy of agonist and antagonist compounds. Unlike prescription medications, most of these compounds do not passively diffuse to their desired receptor but are delivered deliberately to receptors with appropriate timing and dosing in a pattern that is integrated with all the other compounds involved in physical activity.

Of the multitude of such compounds, an example is *nitric oxide* (NO), which the journal *Science* selected as the 1992 Molecule of the Year (11). In the 1990s, it became increasingly clear that NO mediates vasodilation in arterioles and thus has paramount importance in regulating skeletal muscle blood flow during exercise. Researchers have increasingly examined pharmacologic and exertional ways to manipulate NO biology to improve cardiovascular function.

This paradigm of delineating a molecule's physiologic significance, understanding how to use exercise to manipulate this molecule, and then learning to use pharmacotherapy to manipulate the molecule's response to exercise is destined to become a well-worn pathway. Researchers will increasingly use genomic and proteomic techniques to understand how exercise influences entire physiologic systems and how medications can be used to optimize physiologic responses to exercise. Today, we use target heart rates and measures of skeletal muscle fatigue to study physiologic responses to exercise but with a relatively crude understanding of the integrated biochemical response. Someday, instead of prescribing exercise empirically knowing a nominal response or adaptation rate, we will know why a given exercise dose yields a specific range of benefits. Geneticists anticipate that we will understand why some people respond better to exercise than do others. Perhaps we will be able to improve the exercise response in people who are nonresponders, by coupling an exercise prescription with pharmacologic therapy designed to improve the patient's ability to adapt to training.

In the molecular view, exercise may well be increasingly used as a medicine—and a very sophisticated medicine at that. A physician can prescribe a potion or a tablet or an injection, but all of those prescriptions are mainly a pathway to bathing all cells in the medication, with the hope that some of the medicine will get to the right place at the right time and that not too much of it will go where it isn't wanted to go. The idea of exercise is to make the compound go exactly to the tissue of interest and minimize how much of the active compound goes where it is not needed. There is no intensive care unit in the world capable of accurately mimicking the response to exercise. A very real challenge for exercise scientists of the 21st century is finding specific ways to overcome the broad generalities of exercise prescription (frequency, intensity, time, and type), to invent disease-specific exercise therapies that are based on the findings of molecular biology. If we fail to do this, physicians may never fully view exercise *as a medicine*, although history shows us that exercise has always been the best pathway to health.

Summary

In antiquity, a few physicians regarded exercise as a medicine. Because of advances in medical therapy, we have gradually learned more about how exercise can be applied to achieve medical benefit. During the Renaissance and preindustrial era, physicians did not have a clear view about the merits of exercise as a therapy. The 20th century brought an awakening on the clinical merits of exercise. Much of the insight on how to use exercise was gained through military medicine, as physicians learned how to save and rehabilitate wounded soldiers. Cardiovascular physicians were slower to perceive the value of exercise but ultimately found that convalescing with rest is a very bad idea. Despite the artificial division of therapeutic exercise into largely neuromusculoskeletal and cardiovascular domains, we gradually realized that exercise involves integrated biology and that exercise as therapy should involve all physiologic systems. The next task is to increase our understanding and use of exercise as a pharmacologic therapy. Modern research has begun to explain exercise at a molecular level, such that we are beginning to think of frequency, intensity, time, and type of exercise as constituting treatment with endogenous drugs. It seems that after 2,500 years of debate, we are coming to the conclusion that exercise really is a medicine. We can hope that it will not take so long to confirm Nicolas Andry's notion that exercise might be the *best* medicine.

CHAPTER 4

Multifactorial Risk Factor Intervention

Thomas A. Pearson, MD, PhD

Laurie A. Kopin, MS, RN

The term *risk factor* is widely used to describe conditions and behaviors that are thought to be causally related to the development of disease. The risk factor concept originated from the early longitudinal cohort studies of predictors of cardiovascular disease (CVD) and stroke (21). The risk factor concept was then logically extended to the prediction, prevention, and prognostication of CVD. This chapter discusses the risk factor concept as the dominant paradigm in cardiovascular disease prevention. This includes frequent misidentification of conditions as risk factors when in fact they are not etiologically linked to cardiovascular disease (so-called risk markers) or lack proof that they are etiologically linked to disease (so-called emerging risk factors). Many of the individual established risk factors are described in detail in part IV of this book.

Unfortunately, most patients do not have a single risk factor. The typical patient admitted to the coronary care unit has two or more, presenting a seemingly insurmountable challenge to practitioners. This chapter focuses on patients with multiple risk factors and discusses the diagnostic and therapeutic challenges presented by these patients. The nonrandom clustering of risk factors in patients and the multiplicative effect of this clustering on risk are important issues in screening for risk factors and assessing risk. To assist care providers, equations are available that take into account the contribution and interactions of multiple risk factors in a global risk score. Patients with multiple risk factors are frequently at high risk for CVD events, and the prospect of intervening on several risk factors at the same time is daunting to clinicians. Our discussion of therapeutic approaches to these patients emphasizes the optimal reduction in risk, rather than simply the control of risk factors, as the therapeutic goal. This chapter provides the clinician with an approach to the assessment and management of the patient with multiple risk factors.

The Risk Factor Concept

The identification of a condition or behavior as a risk factor for CVD implies a causal role for that condition or behavior in the pathogenesis of CVD (figure 4.1*a*) (1, 16). Indeed, a major objective of cardiovascular research is to define mechanisms by which these conditions or

Address correspondence concerning this chapter to Thomas A. Pearson, University of Rochester, Community & Preventive Medicine, 601 Elmwood Avenue, Box 644, Rochester, NY 14642. E-mail: Thomas_Pearson@urmc.Rochester.edu behaviors cause disease. In some instances, the conditions or behaviors can be modified in the setting of a human experiment (e.g., randomized clinical trial). In other cases, observational studies must be used to define the relation between exposure and disease. The evidence can then be assembled, as proposed by the U.S. Surgeon General's guidelines (27), to support or refute causality. Evidence, as considered strong to weak, includes the temporal relationship between exposures and disease, the strengths of the association, the presence of a dose–response relationship, the reproducibility of findings, the biologic plausibility of the relationship, consideration of alternate explanations, reduction of risk with cessation of exposure, and specificity of the association. If the scientific literature contains evidence fulfilling many of these criteria, the condition may be considered to be causal of CVD. Causal factors can be deleterious (risk factors) or beneficial (protective factors). Although many risk factors have a linear deleterious or beneficial dose–response relationship with CVD, other relationships may exist between a risk factor and disease, such as the U- or J-shaped relationship between alcohol consumption and total mortality (12).

The risk factor concept is frequently misinterpreted by clinicians. One source of confusion is that the *association* of a condition with CVD does not always mean causality (figure 4.1*b*) (16). Such conditions or behaviors are often called risk markers and they indeed can be useful in identifying a person at high risk. However, risk markers are frequently measures of the disease itself (e.g., coronary artery calcium) or byproducts of the atherosclerotic disease process (e.g.,

inflammatory markers). A key distinction is that if a risk factor is modified, the chain of causality is broken, thereby reducing risk. Conversely, an intervention to directly lower the level of a risk marker may not disrupt the disease process and potentially could delude the clinician into believing that risk has been reduced (16).

A second source of confusion among clinicians is the distinction between association and prediction. Association studies identify factors that occur more frequently than expected in persons with disease compared with those free of disease. Depending on the size of the case–control or cohort study, the statistical likelihood of a chance association may be very low. In general, the strength of a causal association is also expected to be large, with a relative risk of two or more generally accepted as consistent with a causal association. Although such data support the epidemiologist's claim that the risk factor may be causal, the clinician frequently is interested in whether the risk factor is a strong predictor of later CVD. The positive likelihood ratios for many of the emerging risk factors turn out to be quite poor, for example, with a relative risk of 1.5 to 2.0 between the upper and lower tertiles of high-sensitivity C-reactive protein levels (16). An ongoing controversy involves the best methods to describe the predictiveness of a risk factor or a risk marker. Both the relative risk or odds ratio and the C statistic (from receiver operating characteristic curves) present advantages and disadvantages as means to quantify and prioritize potential predictors of disease (7, 20).

A third source of confusion about risk factors is the difference between relative and absolute risks. Rela-

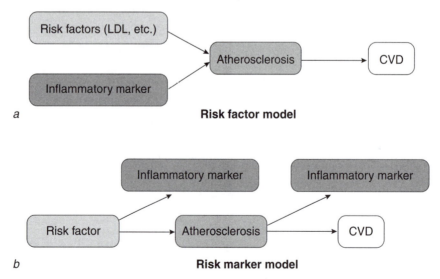

FIGURE 4.1 Alternative models by which a trait or state may be related to cardiovascular disease as *(a)* a risk factor or *(b)* a risk marker. LDL = low-density lipoprotein; CVD = cardiovascular disease.

Adapted, by permission, from T.A. Pearson et al., 2003, "Markers of Inflammation and Cardiovascular Disease. Application to Clinical and Public Health Practice," *Circulation* 107: 499-511.

tive risk, the ratio of incidences of persons *with* versus *without* the risk factor, is a measure of association. Frequently, of more utility to clinicians is the absolute risk, which is the difference in incidences of persons *with* versus *without* the risk factor, as a measure of the potential number of disease outcomes prevented in those at risk through modification of the risk factor. The reciprocal of the absolute risk reduction is an estimate of the number of persons needed to treat to prevent one case of the disease. For example, an intervention may halve the risk of a disease (relative risk of 0.5 for the intervention group), but given the low incidence of disease in the population, only a small absolute risk reduction is brought about and a large number of persons need to be treated to prevent one case. Conversely, clinicians are frequently unenthusiastic about interventions in high-risk groups with a rather small relative risk reduction. They may fail to recognize that frequently large absolute risk reductions and relatively small numbers of persons needed to be treated to prevent a case. This frequently occurs with interventions in elderly persons, with high rates of CVD in both exposed and unexposed persons resulting in small relative risks but often large absolute risk differences.

Established Risk Factors for Cardiovascular Disease

More than 50 years of cardiovascular epidemiologic research has identified a number of conditions and behaviors believed to be causally related to cardiovascular disease (figure 4.2) (17). Risk factors may then be classified into one of three categories: nonmodifiable, behavioral, or physiological. Nonmodifiable risk factors include age, sex, and positive family history (or other genetic determinants of risk). Although not targets for intervention, these factors remain powerful determinants of risk and are considered physiological risk factors. A number of behaviors are causally related to CVD, including tobacco exposure; sedentary lifestyles; diets containing high saturated fats and cholesterol, high sodium, or excess calories; and heavy alcohol consumption. Behavioral risk factors should be targets for modification in individual patients through counseling aimed at lifestyle change as well as targets for population-wide programs of environmental change. Another feature of behavioral risk factors illustrated in figure 4.2 is their role in chains of causation mediated through

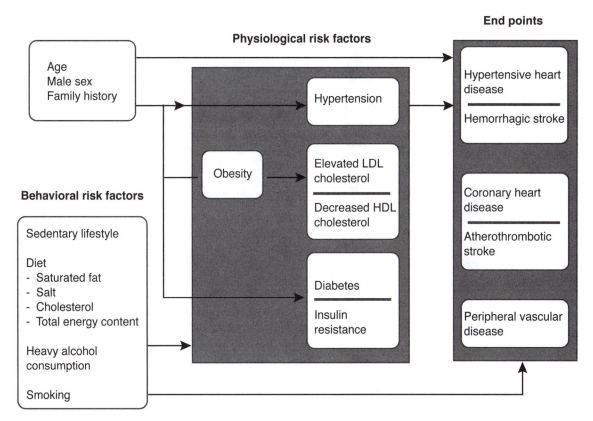

FIGURE 4.2 Established risk factors for cardiovascular disease and their interrelationships. LDL = low-density lipoprotein; HDL = high-density lipoprotein.

Adapted from T.A. Pearson, D.T. Jamison, and J. Trejo-Gutierrez, 1993, Cardiovascular disease. In *Disease centered priorities in developing countries*, edited by D.T. Jamison et al. (New York, Oxford University Press), 577-594. By permission of Oxford University Press, Inc.

physiological risk factors. For example, tobacco exposure may directly affect CVD risk, but it is also is related to reduced high-density lipoprotein cholesterol (HDL-C); a high-fat diet raises serum cholesterol and body weight. Physiological risk factors are those that frequently require measurement in a clinical setting (e.g., blood pressure, serum glucose, blood lipids). To target these risk factors, the health care provider frequently combines pharmaceutical interventions and behavioral modifications.

Figure 4.2 provides a simplified model of the chains of causality that lead to CVD. Coronary disease and atherothrombotic stroke clearly have multiple risk factors causing the disease. The presence of multiple risk factors for CVD makes its prevention much more complex; thus, consideration must be given to the interactions between risk factors in the causation of CVD. Multiple risk factors are additive or even multiplicative of the risk from a single risk factor. For example, the morbidity ratio increases in a stepwise fashion with the increase in the number of risk factors (figure 4.3).

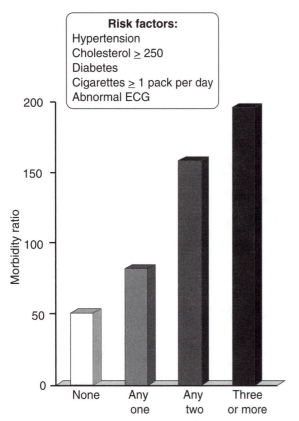

FIGURE 4.3 Morbidity ratios versus the number of risk factors (hypertension, cholesterol ≥250 mg/dL, cigarettes ≥1 pack per day, and abnormal electrocardiogram [ECG]) from the Pooling Project. Morbidity ratio of 100 is average.

Adapted from *Journal of Chronic Diseases* Vol. 31, The Pooling Project Research Group, "Relationship of blood pressure, serum cholesterol, smoking habit, relative weight, and ECG abnormalities to incidence of major coronary events: Final report of the pooling project," p. 202-206, Copyright 1978, with permission from Elsevier.

Individual risk factors have specific quantitative contributions to risk alone and through interactions with other risk factors.

Another consideration is whether a risk factor is necessary or sufficient. For example, because non-smokers develop CVD, smoking is not necessary for the development of CVD. A more interesting risk factor is blood low-density lipoprotein cholesterol (LDL-C). Cultures in East Asia and Africa have exceptionally high levels of hypertension, diabetes, and smoking but very low rates of coronary disease (14). These populations are characterized by very low total and LDL-C levels. This could be interpreted as evidence for a threshold of LDL-C that may be necessary before other risk factors can become important, thereby identifying a potentially unique and central role for lipid management in CVD prevention.

Another cautionary note involves the interpretation of studies that use statistical adjustment to account for the presence of multiple risk factors. Frequently, the association between a risk factor and disease may disappear after adjustment for other risk factors, leading some to incorrectly infer a lack of importance of that particular risk factor. For example, obesity frequently drops out as a risk factor after adjustment for diabetes, hypertension, and low HDL-C. The conclusion that obesity is not important is incorrect, however. Rather, adjustment may have taken into account those factors in a causal pathway through which obesity acts, such as diabetes, low HDL-C, or hypertension.

The final conclusion to be derived from figure 4.2 is the propensity of risk factors to cluster, that is, to coexist in frequency in excess of that expected by chance. Figure 4.2 illustrates several mechanisms by which this could occur. Multiple physiologic risk factors are related to age. A single genetic condition may predispose a person to several physiologic abnormalities. A single behavior, such as sedentary lifestyle, may cause a number of risk factors, such as obesity, hypertension, low HDL-C, and diabetes. Finally, obesity, as a physiological risk factor, likely manifests its risk through other physiologic risk factors, such as hypertension, diabetes, low HDL-C, and high LDL-C. Therefore, the patient admitted with an acute coronary syndrome or stroke with zero or one risk factor can be expected to be the exception, not the rule. Preventive cardiology is therefore a multifactorial risk reduction endeavor.

The aggregation of abdominal obesity, low HDL-C, high triglycerides, elevated blood glucose, and elevated blood pressure in the same patient has long been recognized to exceed that predicted by chance. This has been given multiple terms such as familial *dyslipidemic hypertension*, *Syndrome X*, and the *deadly quartet*. The National Cholesterol Education Program (NCEP) has termed this *metabolic syndrome* and has set down criteria for its definition, requiring abnormal levels of three of the preceding five risk conditions (table 4.1) (5). Frequently, patients have all five. The prevalence of metabolic syndrome in U.S. adults is approximately one in four; prevalence increases with age and is greater in Hispanic men and women and African American women (6). The metabolic syndrome is not a new concept; the nuance is the ability to diagnose patients with these aggregating risk factors by using this working definition. The pathophysiology linking the risk factors is thought to be insulin resistance, and indeed the most immediate risk of the metabolic syndrome is for the onset of type 2 diabetes mellitus, with CVD being a later manifestation. The metabolic syndrome is one of the major diagnostic and treatment issues confronting the clinician in the management of the patient with multiple, coexisting risk factors.

Cardiovascular Risk Assessment in Patients With Multiple Risk Factors

The American Heart Association recommends assessment of risk factors in adults beginning at the age of 20 years (18). Children with first-degree relatives

TABLE 4.1   Five Risk Conditions That Define Metabolic Syndrome

Risk factor	Defining characteristics
Abdominal obesity Men Women	Waist circumference 102 cm (>40 in.) >88 cm (>35 in.)
Triglycerides	≥150 mg/dL
HDL-C Men Women	 <40 mg/dL <50 mg/dL
Blood pressure	≥130/≥85 mmHg
Fasting blood glucose	≥110 mg/dL*

Metabolic syndrome is defined as a clustering of multiple CVD risk factors that increase the risk of diabetes mellitus and cardiovascular disease. Metabolic syndrome is identified when adult patients present with any three of the five risk factors.

*Some experts have recommended a fasting blood glucose of ≥100 mg/dL.

Reprinted from Expert Panel on Detection, Evaluation and Treatment of High Blood Cholesterol in Adults, 2001, Executive summary of the third report of the expert panel on detection, evaluation, and treatment of high blood cholesterol (Adult Treatment Panel III)," *Journal of American Medical Association* 285: 2486-2487.

who have experienced early-onset CVD or known familial risk factors may also benefit from screening. Risk factors measured at age 20 and at least every 5 years thereafter (or more frequently if risk factors are present) are listed in table 4.2. For assessments such as fasting lipid profile and blood glucose levels, some professional organizations have recommended waiting until the coronary-prone years (age ≥45 in men, ≥55 in women), based on randomized trials of interventions showing efficacy in those age groups. However, the American Heart Association rationale for the assessment of risk factors in young adults is

TABLE 4.2   Risk Factor Measurements Recommended for Assessment of Cardiovascular Risk in Adults ≥20 Years

Risk factor measurement	Recommendation
Family history of CVD	Update regularly
Smoking status	Assess at every routine visit
Diet	Assess at every routine visit
Alcohol intake	Assess at every routine visit
Physical activity	Assess at every routine visit
Blood pressure	Assess every 2 years or at each visit
Body mass index (height and weight)	Assess every 2 years or at each visit
Waist circumference	Assess every 2 years or at each visit
Pulse (atrial fibrillation screening)	Assess every 2 years or at each visit
Fasting serum lipoprotein profile*	Assess at least every 5 years
Fasting blood glucose*	Assess at least every 5 years

CVD = cardiovascular disease.

*Assess every 2 years if risk factors are present for diabetes and hyperlipidemia is elevated.

Reprinted, by permission, from T.A. Pearson, S.N. Blair, et al. 2002, "AHA guidelines for primary prevention of cardiovascular disease and stroke: 2002," Update, *Circulation* 106: 388-391.

to initiate changes in exercise, diet, and tobacco use in young adulthood. Moreover, community trials of population-wide screening have shown that persons screening positive for elevated blood cholesterol, for example, subsequently changed their behavior related to purchasing food and reading labels (15).

Assessment of Global Risk

The American Heart Association also recommends an assessment of global risk score in adults older than 40 years (6). Global risk is also referred to as absolute risk and is the estimated incidence of CVD for a person over the next 10 years. Assessment of global risk begins with determination of whether the patient already has symptomatic CVD, including histories of myocardial infarction, angina pectoris, and coronary revascularization (19). Numerous longitudinal studies have documented that such persons have at least a 20% chance of a myocardial infarction or cardiac death in the next 10 years. Such persons are considered high risk, regardless of their cardiovascular risk factors, although their risk factors may drive their actual risk even higher.

A second group of patients included in the high-risk group are those with so-called coronary heart disease (CHD) risk equivalents. These include patients with peripheral arterial disease (claudication, aortic aneurysm, ankle–brachial blood pressure index <0.9), cerebrovascular disease (stroke, transit ischemic attack, carotid stenosis >70% on Doppler ultrasound), and diabetes mellitus. The CHD equivalent concept stems from longitudinal studies that have documented a >20% risk of MI or CHD death per 10 years in these patient subgroups, similar to the rates in patients with symptomatic coronary disease (5). Again, risk factor assessment is essential in these patient groups as a prelude to aggressive risk factor intervention.

In patients without CHD, CHD equivalents, or diabetes, the challenge is to estimate global risk in patients of different age and sex with various numbers of risk factors and levels of risk factors. In the United States and Europe, this entails use of a global risk score that uses risk equations developed from the Framingham Heart Study (5, 8, 19) or other longitudinal studies. These equations have been developed to provide the best predictive ability with the simplest multiple risk equation. Risk factors used in global risk assessment include age, sex, current smoking status (yes/no), systolic blood pressure (mmHg), total cholesterol (mg/dL), and HDL-C (mg/dL). The Framingham risk equations are available on Web sites, on hand-held personal assistant devices, in color-coded tables, or on worksheets (19). They provide an estimate of a person's cardiovascular risk over the next 10 years for the development of MI or CHD death.

The global risk scores are generally used to classify persons at low, moderate, or high risk. Several issues deserve comment. First, the risk of the onset of CVD may actually be higher than the score indicates, because the absolute risk does not include risks of angina pectoris, stroke, or peripheral arterial disease. Again, the global risk is an *estimate* that is used to place patients in risk categories. Second, the global risk score can replace levels of individual risk factors as the primary target for intervention. Frequently, a patient at high risk is referred for management of a moderately elevated total cholesterol level with coexistent smoking or hypertension. If the goal of care is risk reduction, a cost-effective approach might include focusing on the other risk factors in addition to the one eliciting the referral. Third, a number of risk factors such as sedentary lifestyle, high-fat diet, and obesity are not included in the equation. These factors are important links in the causal chain but may not add predictive power to the equation. A likely exception is family history, which recently has provided additional predictive power above and beyond that of the risk equation. In such instances, a clinician can factor a positive family history into the risk assessment when deciding whether and how aggressively to intervene on risk factors. Finally, risk factors may have additive or multiplicative effects when they coexist. The quantitative risk equations generally incorporate these relationships. In many instances, a person's global risk can be affected as markedly by moderate elevations of several risk factors as by a high elevation of a single risk factor. The global risk scores therefore emphasize multifactorial risk factor intervention, with the target being global risk rather than levels of risk factors.

Definitions of Low, Moderate, High, and Very High Risk

Risk assessment has attempted to place patients in one of three strata of absolute risk for CVD (10). High risk denotes persons at >20% risk of MI or CHD death over the next 10 years and includes people with CHD, CHD risk equivalents, and multiple risk factors with high global risk scores. Moderate risk identifies persons at 10% to 20% risk. Low risk identifies persons at <10% risk. Some experts expand the moderate risk group to 6% to 20% risk, defining low risk as <6% risk. More recently, a very high risk group has been proposed (9), consisting of patients with established coronary heart disease *and* multiple major risk factors, severe and poorly controlled risk factors (e.g., cigarette smoking), the metabolic syndrome, or acute coronary syndromes.

Risk strata are then used for thresholds and goals for lipid-lowering interventions (5) and use of aspirin in primary prevention (10, 18).

Cardiovascular Risk Markers and Noninvasive Testing

Multiple strategies are being evaluated to improve the risk prediction provided by the multiple risk equations (24). One category of approaches includes new tests that measure serum factors that have been associated with CVD (table 4.3). The discussion of each of these approaches is beyond the scope of this chapter. Some of these might be considered better ways to measure currently established risk factors (e.g., lipoprotein number and particle size). Others might be considered emerging risk factors that have biologically plausible mechanisms of action and, with further evidence, may become established targets for intervention, such as lipoprotein (a), serum triglycerides, and fibrinogen. Others are risk markers that measure atherosclerotic disease activity, including the markers of inflammation and microalbinuria. The confident use of these markers in practice is hindered by lack of data demonstrating the cost-effectiveness of their use when added to the recommended multiple risk factor screening and absolute risk score (7, 16, 26).

A similar situation exists with a second approach, namely noninvasive testing for the presence and extent of atherosclerotic CVD (table 4.4) (24). Because atherosclerosis is a systemic disease, evidence for atherosclerotic disease in a person without prior symptoms should predict an increased risk. Several comments should be made. First, evaluation of these tests and technologies should be performed *in addition to* calculation of absolute risk. Of these tests, ankle–brachial blood pressure index has the best evidence for incremental benefit (18). In studies of some imaging modalities, testing has not added to the risk prediction of the absolute risk score. Suffice it to say that appropriate evaluation of these noninvasive tests should begin with the global risk score and should demonstrate incremental predictive value, preferably in several studies. If there is additive benefit, a multiplier may be used to adjust the global risk estimate. Second, the utility of these tests may be more than just risk estimation. For example, exercise ECG testing is recommended for moderate- to high-risk patients who intend to initiate a vigorous exercise program so the clinician can write a safe exercise prescription. Third, few studies have estimated the cost-effectiveness of this approach. Namely, does the risk estimation from a test allow better selection of patients needing treatment in order to justify the costs of the testing? Fourth, vascular imaging should be approached

TABLE 4.3   New Approaches to Cardiovascular Disease Risk Prediction for CVD

Serum risk markers	Noninvasive tests
Serum lipids and lipoproteins	Fasting triglyceride levels
	Lipoprotein (a)
	Lipoprotein size
	Lipoprotein number
	Apolipoprotein B and A1*
	Directly measured particle number*
Inflammatory markers	Soluble adhesion molecules (e.g., selectins)
	Cytokines (interleukins, tumor necrosis factor)
	Acute phase reactants (hsCRP, serum amyloid A)
	White blood cell count
	Lp-PLA$_2$
Other	Homocysteine
	Microalbuminuria
Prothrombotic factors	Fibrinogen (also an acute phase reactant)
	Plasminogen activator inhibitor

hsCRP = high-sensitivity C-reactive protein; Lp-PLA$_2$ = Lipoprotein-associated phospholipase A$_2$.

*Data from Pearson 2002.

TABLE 4.4   **Noninvasive Tests to Assess the Presence of Atherosclerotic Cardiovascular Disease**

Modalities	Noninvasive tests
Cardiodiagnostic	Exercise electrocardiography
	Electron beam computed tomography
	Magnetic resource coronary angiography
	Positron emission tomography
Peripheral arterial diagnostic	Ankle–brachial blood pressure index testing
	B-mode ultrasound for intima media
	Thickness of carotid, aorta, or femoral arteries*

*Data from Pearson 2002.

in a disciplined fashion, to avoid the slippery slope of coronary diagnostic testing and intervention. That is, a test considered indicative of disease should elicit aggressive intervention on multiple risk factors rather than invasive tests and vascular interventions. Little evidence exists to support the cost-effectiveness of revascularization in asymptomatic patients, whereas there is an evidence base supporting the cost-effectiveness of multiple risk factor modification.

Maximizing CVD Risk Reduction Through Multifactorial Risk Intervention

The dominant paradigms in preventive cardiology are to reduce the risk of cardiovascular events (e.g., myocardial infarction, stroke) or CVD death by reducing risk factors or using pharmacologic agents proven to reduce risk independent of risk factor levels (e.g., β-blockers, angiotensin-converting enzyme [ACE] inhibitors, antiplatelet agents). Guidelines for intervention on individual risk factors have been published by governmental agencies, professional societies, and voluntary health associations, and these have been synthesized into multifactorial guidelines by the American Heart Association for primary prevention (patients without evidence of CVD) (18) and secondary prevention (patients with diagnosed CVD) (24).

For the secondary prevention guidelines, for example, the inclusion of each intervention is based on a strong evidence base (24). This evidence base usually consists of multiple randomized trials of an individual intervention versus placebo. Far less evidence exists, however, for interventions used in the presence of multiple other interventions. For example, older studies established a role for β-blockers in protecting MI patients from recurrent coronary events. One might

ask whether β-blockers still add benefit when patients are also receiving ACE inhibitors, statins, antiplatelet agents, and cardiac rehabilitation. Conversely, might an ACE inhibitor replace the β-blockers (or vice versa)? Might the risk of recurrent coronary disease be so low with aggressive lipid management that the incremental benefit of a β-blocker is too small to be cost-effective? These questions are unlikely to be answered directly. Current recommendations nonetheless advise that all the interventions be used.

In this setting of multiple interventions in the patient with multiple risk factors, the opportunity exists for interactions between interventions that have either synergistic or antagonistic effects. A synergistic effect between risk factor interventions has been observed (table 4.5). For example, weight reduction is the cornerstone of management of the metabolic syndrome, because obesity-related insulin resistance is thought to be a common cause for all its components. Similarly, both the DASH (Dietary Approaches to Stop Hypertension) diet and the Mediterranean-type diet reduce not only LDL-C levels but also blood pressure levels (23). There is a growing body of evidence that ACE inhibitors may protect against development of diabetes mellitus in patients who are prescribed these agents for hypertension or post-MI prophylaxis (4). Finally, aspirin, when used with a statin such as pravastatin, provides risk reduction in excess of that predicted if aspirin and pravastatin were used separately (11). These beneficial interactions should encourage the use of these combinations of interventions as part of a multiple risk factor intervention program.

Some risk factor modifications may have deleterious effects on other risk factors, raising the possibility of no true risk reduction or, possibly, an increase in risk (table 4.6). Frequently, these require monitoring of

TABLE 4.5 Examples of Beneficial Effects of Interventions on Several Risk Factors

Intervention	Benefits on risk or risk factors
Weight reduction with caloric restriction and increased physical activity	Improves the control of elevated blood pressure, abnormal blood glucose, elevated LDL-C and triglycerides, reduced HDL-C, and the metabolic syndrome.
Diet high in fruits, vegetables, grains, low-fat dietary products, fish, legumes, poultry, and lean meats (e.g., DASH diet)	Multiple health benefits include reduction in LDL-C and blood pressure.
ACE inhibitor	Multiple studies suggest ability to prevent diabetes as well as control hypertension and provide cardioprotection.
Antiplatelet agent	Studies of aspirin and statins suggest a synergistic effect with reduction in CVD events greater than the sum of individual drug effects.

ACE = angiotensin-converting enzyme; LDL-C = low-density lipoprotein cholesterol; HDL-C = high-density lipoprotein cholesterol; CVD = cardiovascular disease.

TABLE 4.6 Examples of Detrimental Effects of Risk Factor Interventions on Other Risk Factors

Intervention	Deleterious effect on risk or risk factors
Smoking cessation	Weight gain with consequent effects on lipid, glucose, and blood pressure levels
Low-fat diet	Reduced HDL-C levels and increased triglyceride levels with high-carbohydrate diets
β-blockers and thiazides	Increased triglycerides and reduced HDL-C
Niacin at lipid-lowering doses	Increased fasting glucose levels in person with glucose intolerance and type 2 diabetes mellitus; increase incidence of hyperuricemia and gout

HDL-C = high-density lipoprotein cholesterol.

the adversely affected risk factor. Weight gain, often in the 5 to 10 lb (2.3-4.5 kg) range, is frequently seen after smoking cessation, suggesting that a smoking cessation program should include a dietary intervention featuring caloric intake reduction and a physical activity program featuring caloric expenditure increase. Very low fat diets had been very popular in coronary patients, but the replacement of saturated fat calories with carbohydrates increases serum triglycerides and reduces HDL-C levels, despite LDL-C reductions. This prompted the NCEP Adult Treatment Panel III (ATP III) to recommend therapeutic lifestyle changes that increase total fat in the diet up to 35% (previously recommended at <30% of calories), do not increase carbohydrates (50-60% of calories), include complex

carbohydrates, and increase monounsaturated fats (up to 20% of calories) (5). β-blockers and thiazide diuretics are known to increase fasting triglyceride levels and reduce HDL-C levels. The impact of these metabolic side effects was recently examined in the ASCOT-BPLA (Anglo-Scandinavian Cardiac Outcomes Trial, Blood Pressure-Lowering Arm) study, which randomized 19,257 patients with hypertension and three other risk factors to receive either amlodipine and perindopril (calcium channel blocker and ACE inhibitor) or atenolol and bendroflumethiazide (β-blocker and thiazide) (3). Patients in the calcium channel blocker and ACE inhibitor arm had 23% fewer strokes, 16% fewer CVD events, and 30% fewer cases of diabetes. Blood pressure was better controlled with the amlodipine and perindopril regimen and accounted for about half the CVD events, but differences in HDL-C, glucose, and triglycerides were also significant between the arms and appeared to account for some of the benefits of amlodipine and perindopril on coronary events (22). This study suggests that effects of antihypertensive agents on factors other than blood pressure enhance their ability to reduce CVD risk. Finally, niacin is well known to increase glucose intolerance in patients with borderline or abnormal fasting blood glucose levels. Although this is not a contraindication to using niacin in diabetic patients, niacin is usually avoided in diabetic patients with poor control. In other patients, blood sugar levels are monitored more regularly, along with uric acid levels.

Multifaceted Management of the Metabolic Syndrome and the Challenge of Controlling Multiple Risk Factors

The cluster of risk factors known as the metabolic syndrome can be explained by their association with a single pathophysiology, namely insulin resistance induced by genetic susceptibility, caloric imbalance, and a sedentary lifestyle with or without obesity. The insulin resistance and consequent hyperinsulinemia then affect a variety of organs and pathways. Metabolic syndrome can be viewed as a sequence of events, beginning with abdominal obesity from an imbalance of caloric intake and expenditure. Relatively early on, elevations in systolic and diastolic blood pressure and elevations in triglycerides with reduced HDL-C levels are observed. These coincide with abnormalities of platelet function and markers of inflammation. Glucose intolerance and diabetes develop later, often after years of hypertension and dyslipidemia. Finally, CVD (including coronary disease and stroke) is a rather late phenomenon.

This knowledge of the pathophysiology of metabolic syndrome provides several insights. First, the primary care provider may be faced with a patient for whom multiple treatments are recommended (e.g., treatment for obesity, hypertension, dyslipidemia, glucose intolerance or diabetes, or symptomatic CVD). Such a complex patient usually requires treatments for individual risk factors in the form of prescription drugs. Second, the individual risk factor–directed drug therapies have an important limitation in addition to cost and potential side effects: reduced efficacy in the setting of continued weight gain. Thus, the primary care provider will need to accelerate the number and potency of drugs unless the underlying pathophysiology (insulin resistance) is addressed. Therefore, any therapeutic regimen to treat the metabolic syndrome must have a lifestyle intervention (calorie-restricted diet, effective physical activity program) to avoid an expensive and ineffective pharmacologic regimen.

The need for this attention to upstream issues was demonstrated in diabetes prevention trials in which patients at risk for diabetes were randomized to lifestyle interventions, drug regimens such as metformin (an insulin sensitizing agent), or usual care (13, 25). In the Diabetes Prevention Trial, intervention with lifestyle modification emphasizing regular physical activity resulted in a lower incidence of diabetes than did intervention with metformin, which in turn showed a lower incidence of diabetes than usual care (13). Most of the glucose-intolerant patients in this trial would meet the criteria for metabolic syndrome.

The management of metabolic syndrome stresses lifestyle modification more than do most interventions for chronic diseases (table 4.7). Weight management and exercise prescription are frequently given lip service by both care provider and patient. In the metabolic syndrome, this is a serious error, derailing expensive pharmacologic regimens and allowing diabetes and CVD to develop. One often necessary approach is enrollment in structured weight management and physical activity programs. Phase III cardiac rehabilitation programs may be such a venue. Although patients with metabolic syndrome may not have symptomatic vascular disease, they certainly are at increased risk and may benefit from a regular program of exercise with appropriate intensity and duration to support weight maintenance if not beneficial weight reduction. The nonlipid risk factors should not be overlooked in the metabolic syndrome patient. Hypertension is one of the most common components of the metabolic syndrome, and a recent meta-analysis suggested that diabetes can be prevented with the use of ACE inhibitors or angiotensin receptor blockers, whereas patients treated with β-blockers and thiazide diuretics have an excess of diabetes compared with placebo (4). Because patients generally have a global risk of >10%, aspirin (81 mg/day) is recommended to manage the prothrombotic state created by the metabolic syndrome. Hyperuricemia and gout have long been associated with this syndrome, and measurement of uric acid and pharmacologic prevention of gout attacks in hyperuricemic or gouty patients should be considered. Insulin-sensitizing agents such as metformin or a glitazone might be considered in patients with glucose intolerance. Metformin appears to prevent the onset of diabetes (13). The use of glitazones is more controversial and awaits the results of ongoing clinical trials. The Diabetes Prevention Trial, in which diet and exercise outperformed metformin, emphasizes the

TABLE 4.7   Recommendations for Management of the Metabolic Syndrome

Intervention	Recommendation
Manage the underlying causes: overweight and obesity, physical inactivity.	Manage weight with structured program or under supervision of registered dietitian. Increase physical activity, with a structured program as required to induce weight loss.
Treat nonlipid risk factors.	Treat hypertension, preferably with ACE inhibitors, ARBs, or calcium channel blockers rather than β-blockers or thiazides. Use aspirin (81 mg/day) to reduce prothrombotic state. Measure uric acid and treat or prevent gout. Consider insulin-sensitizing agent (e.g., metformin).
Treat elevated serum triglycerides (≥200 mg/dL) after LDL-C goal is reached.	Use non–HDL-C values as treatment goals (non–HDL-C goals = LDL-C goals + 30 mg/dL). Treat to non–HDL-C goal by intensifying lipid-lowering drug (e.g., statin) or adding niacin or fibrate. Treat low HDL-C (<40 mg/dL) after reaching LDL and non–HDL-C goals with lifestyle modification and, if high-risk or CHD patient, consider niacin or fibrate to correct isolated low HDL-C.

LDL-C = low-density lipoprotein cholesterol; ACE = angiotensin-converting enzyme; ARBs = angiotensin receptor blockers; HDL-C = high-density lipoprotein cholesterol.

Adapted from Expert Panel on Detection, Evaluation and Treatment of High Blood Cholesterol in Adults, 2001, "Executive summary of the third report of the expert panel on detection, evaluation, and treatment of high blood cholesterol (Adult Treatment Panel III)." *Journal of American Medical Association* 285: 2486-2487.

importance of lifestyle over drug therapy. Treatment of triglyceride elevations and HDL-C reductions commonly seen in metabolic syndrome follows treatment of elevated LDL-C levels (5). Non-HDL-C levels are used when triglycerides exceed 200 mg/dL and are calculated simply by total cholesterol minus HDL-C. This provides a sum of atherogenic forms of cholesterol in the blood, and targets set by the NCEP ATP III Adult Treatment Guidelines are 30 mg/dL higher than those for LDL-C (5). If non–HDL-C remains elevated after diet, exercise, and weight reduction, intensification of LDL-C-lowering therapy might be entertained (e.g., statin therapy). Otherwise, niacin (e.g., extended release titrated up to 1,000-2,000 mg/day) or fibrates at standard doses can be considered. Fibrates are a useful substitute for niacin when patients are unable to tolerate the niacin because of flushing, hyperuricemia, or glucose intolerance. Likewise, niacin or fibrates might be used if HDL-C levels are reduced (<40 mg/dL), although no therapeutic target for HDL-C has been set by the NCEP ATP III (10).

Finally, the metabolic syndrome has several characteristics to which our health care system attends poorly. It is a chronic condition without symptoms; lifestyles notoriously difficult to change are key to successful treatment; multiple, expensive drug regimens may be required; and long-term compliance and adherence are major concerns. For these reasons, a systems approach may be required to effectively manage the metabolic syndrome. The chronic care model constitutes such an approach (2) with a reengineering of the health care system away from acute episodic care to long-term chronic care. In this model, care is provided by non-physician professionals with decision support tools and improved clinical information systems. Community resources (e.g., improved venues for exercise, healthful food) support the patient's treatment. Self-management tools are made available for patients and family members to use. The metabolic syndrome may epitomize the conditions that would benefit from this revamping of our health care system.

Summary

Cardiovascular diseases have a multifactorial etiology necessitating attention to multiple risk factors in the same patient. The patient with multiple risk factors is the rule, not the exception. The contribution of several risk factors to the patient's cardiovascular risk can be easily estimated in the form of a global coronary risk score, allowing categorization of the patient into one of several risk strata. Other modalities such as new risk markers or imaging techniques may add to these risk estimates. The goal of intervention is to lower CVD risk, not just to lower risk factors. Treatment of the patient with multiple risk factors requires knowledge of interventions that may have multiple benefits. Lifestyle modifications including supervised exercise programs have such an effect. Likewise, interventions on one risk factor may deleteriously affect another risk factor, negating any real risk reduction. A comprehensive approach to CVD risk reduction is increasingly difficult for the primary care provider and may require reorganization of care to support lifestyle behavior change and use of increasingly complex drug regimens to provide comprehensive risk reduction.

CHAPTER 5

Clinical Practice Guidelines and Target Outcomes

Bridging the Gap

Matt S. Feigenbaum, PhD

Patrick E. McBride, MD

William A. Webster, IV, PhD

The increasing social and economic costs of chronic diseases, particularly preventable cardiovascular diseases and diabetes mellitus, are enormous. The medical care costs alone accounted for more than 75% of the United States' $1 trillion medical care expenditures in 2005. Cardiovascular disease is the leading chronic disease for morbidity and mortality in the United States and is responsible for more than 1 million deaths annually, costing more than US$400 billion in 2006. In the same year, the direct and indirect medical costs associated with the primary lifestyle-related risk factors including hypertension, diabetes, smoking, and physical inactivity were US$47 billion, US$132 billion, US$68 billion, and US$76 billion, respectively (21).

Given the magnitude of the problem, the need to close the treatment gap between clinical practices and established guidelines for improving patient care and target outcomes is evident. During the past decade, key professional and government organizations have focused increased attention on chronic disease target outcomes, such as blood pressure <140/90 mmHg, low-density lipoprotein cholesterol (LDL-C) <100 mg/dL, and hemoglobin A_{1c} (HbA_{1c}) <7%, and have established evidence-based clinical practice guidelines. The development of new guidelines has been spurred by a growing realization that chronic disease management initiatives may be able to achieve a rapid and

Address correspondence concerning this chapter to Matt S. Feigenbaum, Department of Health and Exercise Science, Furman University, Greenville, SC 29613. E-mail: Matt.Feigenbaum@Furman.edu significant return on investment (e.g., by targeting clinical practices or patient behaviors that can reduce hospitalization risk).

The American Heart Association (AHA), the American College of Cardiology (ACC), the American Diabetes Association, and other organizations have issued clinical practice guidelines for improving physician awareness and treatment effectiveness. Chronic diseases including heart disease and diabetes have also drawn considerable attention from health care provider groups, managed care organizations, employers, and other private organizations concerned about the growing economic burden. Some organizations have taken a disease management approach, using individualized education, treatment planning, and resource coordination for each patient. Others have used quality improvement initiatives aimed at hospital and clinic-based care with significant success. Some programs are more population-based and include education initiatives aimed at patients and clinicians. In all cases, evidence-based clinical practice guidelines involve engaging patients in their health care, rather than having them passively accept treatment programs. Health care programs perform best when patients are aware of their health conditions and how they change with time, their treatment and lifestyle options, and the prevention and rehabilitation services that are available and how to access them. No better example exists than the evidence-based guidelines for the management of cardiovascular disease and diabetes, each dependent on the lifestyle choices of the individual patient as much as the treatment strategies used by the health care practitioner.

AHA–ACC Guidelines for Secondary Prevention

The AHA and the ACC have developed an aggressive multifaceted strategy to improve patient care (20). The AHA–ACC guidelines are evidence-based and were written in the spirit of recommending diagnostic and therapeutic interventions for patients in *most* circumstances. Accordingly, clinicians must use their judgment to adapt the guidelines to care for individual patients but also must recognize that the evidence supporting the guidelines is so strong that failure to perform such actions reduces the likelihood that optimal patient outcomes will be achieved. The AHA–ACC guidelines outlined in table 5.1 arise from a multitude of clinical trials that support the merits of aggressive risk-reduction therapies for patients with established

coronary and other atherosclerotic vascular disease. This growing body of evidence confirms that aggressive comprehensive risk factor management improves survival, reduces recurrent events and the need for interventional procedures, and improves quality of life for these patients.

Current evidence provides a strong rationale for the long-term aggressive control of multiple coronary heart disease (CHD) risk factors as an essential strategy to normalize coronary artery endothelial function; halt or slow the progression of coronary atherosclerosis; prevent the instability, rupture, and thrombosis of atherosclerotic plaques; and reduce the mortality, recurrent hospitalization, and the ongoing cost of medical care (10). The AHA–ACC guidelines outlined in table 5.1 address the major CHD risk factors and incorporate the recommendations from the National Heart, Lung, and Blood Institute's (NHLBI) Adult Treatment Panel (ATP) III report (11).

Lipid management is at the forefront of the AHA–ACC strategy to control atherosclerotic plaque formation and progression. Findings from lipid reduction trials involving more than 50,000 patients resulted in new optional therapeutic targets, which were outlined in the 2004 update of the NHLBI ATP III report (11) and were incorporated into the 2006 update of the AHA–ACC guidelines (20). These changes defined optional lower target cholesterol levels for very high risk CHD patients, especially those with acute coronary syndromes, and expanded indications for drug treatment. These new trials allow for alterations in guidelines, such that low-density lipoprotein cholesterol (LDL-C) should be <100 mg/dL for all patients with CHD and other clinical forms of atherosclerotic disease, but it is reasonable to treat to LDL-C <70 mg/dL if patients with cardiovascular disease have an additional major risk factor. When the <70 mg/dL target is chosen, increasing statin therapy in a graded fashion is prudent to determine a patient's response and tolerance. Furthermore, if it is not possible to attain LDL-C <70 mg/dL because of a high baseline LDL-C or non–high-density lipoprotein cholesterol (HDL-C), it generally is possible to achieve LDL-C reductions of >50% with either statins or LDL-C-lowering drug combinations. In addition, for patients with total triglycerides >200 mg/dL or low HDL-C, combination drug therapy is recommended (11). Moreover, this guideline for patients with atherosclerotic disease does not modify the recommendations of the 2004 ATP III update for patients without atherosclerotic disease who have diabetes or multiple risk factors and a 10-year risk level for CHD >20%.

TABLE 5.1 AHA-ACC Guidelines for Secondary Prevention for Patients With Coronary and Other Atherosclerotic Vascular Disease

Goals	Intervention recommendations
Smoking: Complete cessation. No exposure to environmental tobacco smoke.	■ Ask about tobacco use at every visit. ■ Advise every tobacco user to quit. ■ Assess the tobacco user's willingness to quit. ■ Assist by counseling and developing a plan for quitting. ■ Arrange follow-up, referral to special programs, or pharmacotherapy (including nicotine replacement and bupropion). ■ Urge avoidance of exposure to environmental tobacco smoke at work and home.
Blood pressure control: <140/90 mmHg or <130/80 mmHg if patient has diabetes or chronic kidney disease.	For all patients: Initiate or maintain lifestyle modification: weight control; increased physical activity; alcohol moderation; sodium reduction; and emphasis on increased consumption of fresh fruits, vegetables, and low-fat dairy products. For patients with blood pressure ≥140/90 mmHg (or ≥130/80 mmHg for patients with chronic kidney disease or diabetes): As tolerated, add blood pressure medication, treating initially with β-blockers or ACE inhibitors, with addition of other drugs such as thiazides as needed to achieve goal blood pressure. [For compelling indications for individual drug classes in specific vascular diseases, see Seventh Report of the Joint National Committee on Prevention, Detection, Evaluation, and Treatment of High Blood Pressure (5).]
Lipid management: LDL-C <100 mg/dL. If triglycerides are ≥200 mg/dL, non–HDL-C should be <130 mg/dL.*	For all patients: ■ Start dietary therapy. Reduce intake of saturated fats (to <7% of total calories), trans fatty acids, and cholesterol (to <200 mg/day). ■ Add plant stanol/sterols (2 g/day) and viscous fiber (>10 g/day) to further lower LDL-C. ■ Promote daily physical activity and weight management. ■ Encourage increased consumption of omega-3 fatty acids in the form of fish† or in capsule form (1 g/day) for risk reduction. For treatment of elevated triglycerides, higher doses are usually necessary for risk reduction. For lipid management: Assess fasting lipid profile in all patients and within 24 hr of hospitalization for those with an acute cardiovascular or coronary event. For hospitalized patients, initiate lipid-lowering medication as recommended below before discharge according to the following schedule. ■ LDL-C should be <100 mg/dL. ■ Further reduction of LDL-C to <70 mg/dL is reasonable. ■ If baseline LDL-C is ≥100 mg/dL, initiate LDL-C-lowering drug therapy.‡ ■ If on-treatment LDL-C is ≥100 mg/dL, intensify LDL-lowering drug therapy (may require LDL-C-lowering drug combination§). ■ If baseline LDL-C is 70-100 mg/dL, it is reasonable to treat LDL-C <70 mg/dL. ■ If triglycerides are 200-499 mg/dL, non–HDL-C should be <130 mg/dL. ■ Further reduction of non–HDL-C to <100 mg/dL is reasonable. ■ Therapeutic options to reduce non–HDL-C: more intense LDL-C-lowering therapy; or niacin# (after LDL-C-lowering therapy); or fibrate# therapy (after LDL-C-lowering therapy). ■ If triglycerides are ≥500 mg/dL,** therapeutic options to prevent pancreatitis are fibrate# or niacin# before LDL-lowering therapy; treat LDL-C to goal after triglyceride-lowering therapy. Achieve non–HDL-C <130 mg/dL if possible.
Physical activity: 30 min, 7 days/week (minimum 5 days/week).	■ For all patients, assess risk with a physical activity history or exercise test, to guide prescription. ■ For all patients, encourage 30-60 min of moderate-intensity aerobic activity, such as brisk walking, on most, preferably all, days of the week, supplemented by an increase in daily lifestyle activities (e.g., walking breaks at work, gardening, household work). ■ Encourage resistance training 2 days/week. ■ Advise medically supervised programs for high-risk patients (e.g., recent acute coronary syndrome or revascularization, heart failure).
Weight management: body mass index 18.5-24.9 kg/m². Waist circumference: men <40 in. (101.6 cm), women <35 in. (88.9 cm).	■ Assess body mass index or waist circumference on each visit and consistently encourage weight management or reduction through an appropriate balance of physical activity, caloric intake, and formal behavioral programs when indicated to maintain and achieve a body mass index between 18.5 and 24.9 kg/m². ■ If waist circumference (measured horizontally at the iliac crest) is ≥35 in. (88.9 cm) in women and ≥40 in. (101.6 cm) in men, initiate lifestyle changes and consider treatment strategies for metabolic syndrome. ■ Urge patient to reduce body weight by approximately 10% from baseline. With success, further weight loss can be attempted if indicated through further assessment.

(continued)

Table 5.1 (continued)

Goals	Intervention recommendations
Diabetes management: HbA$_{1c}$ <7%	■ Initiate lifestyle and pharmacotherapy to achieve near-normal HbA$_{1c}$. ■ Begin vigorous modification of other risk factors (e.g., physical activity, weight management, blood pressure control, and cholesterol management as recommended above). ■ Coordinate diabetic care with patient's primary care physician or endocrinologist.
Antiplatelet agents and anticoagulants	■ Start aspirin 75-162 mg/day and continue indefinitely unless contraindicated. Patients undergoing coronary artery bypass grafting should start aspirin within 48 hr after surgery to reduce saphenous vein graft closure. Dosing regimens ranging from 100 to 325 mg/day appear to be efficacious. Doses >162 mg/day can be continued up to 1 year. ■ Start and continue clopidogrel 75 mg/day in combination with aspirin for up to 12 months in patients after acute coronary syndrome or percutaneous coronary intervention with stent placement (≥1 month for bare metal stent, ≥3 months for sirolimus-eluting stent, ≥6 months for paclitaxel-eluting stent). Patients who have undergone percutaneous coronary intervention with stent placement should initially receive higher dose aspirin: 325 mg/day for 1 month for bare metal stent, 3 months for sirolimus-eluting stent, and 6 months for paclitaxel-eluting stent. ■ Manage warfarin to international normalized ratio = 2.0-3.0 for paroxysmal or chronic atrial fibrillation or flutter and in postmyocardial infarction patients when clinically indicated (e.g., atrial fibrillation, left ventricular thrombus). ■ Closely monitor use of warfarin in conjunction with aspirin or clopidogrel, because this is associated with increased risk of bleeding.
Renin–angiotensin–aldosterone system blockers	ACE inhibitors ■ Start and continue indefinitely in all patients with left ventricular ejection fraction ≤40% and in those with hypertension, diabetes, or chronic kidney disease, unless contraindicated. ■ Consider for all other patients. ■ Assess low-risk patients with normal left ventricular ejection fraction in whom cardiovascular risk factors are well controlled and revascularization has been performed; use of ACE inhibitors in these patients is optional. Angiotensin receptor blockers ■ Use in patients who are intolerant of ACE inhibitors and have heart failure or have had a myocardial infarction with left ventricular ejection fraction ≤40%. ■ Consider in other patients who are ACE inhibitor intolerant. ■ Consider use in combination with ACE inhibitors in systolic-dysfunction heart failure. Aldosterone blockade ■ Use in postmyocardial infarction patients without significant renal dysfunction[††] or hyperkalemia[‡‡] who are already receiving therapeutic doses of ACE inhibitor and β-blocker, have a left ventricular ejection fraction <40%, and either are diabetic or have heart failure.
β-blockers	■ Start and continue indefinitely in all patients who have had myocardial infarction, acute coronary syndrome, or left ventricular dysfunction with or without heart failure symptoms, unless contraindicated. ■ Consider chronic therapy for all other patients with coronary or other vascular diseases or diabetes unless contraindicated.
Influenza vaccination	Advise patients with cardiovascular disease to have an influenza vaccination.

Patients covered by these guidelines include those with established coronary and other atherosclerotic vascular disease, including peripheral arterial disease, atherosclerotic aortic disease, and carotid artery disease. Treatment of patients whose only manifestation of cardiovascular risk is diabetes will be the topic of a separate AHA scientific statement. LDL-C = low-density lipoprotein cholesterol; HDL-C = high-density lipoprotein cholesterol; HbA$_{1c}$ = hemoglobin A$_{1c}$; ACE - angiotensin-converting enzyme.

*Non–HDL-C = total cholesterol minus HDL-C.

†Pregnant and lactating women should limit their intake of fish to minimize exposure to methylmercury.

‡When LDL-C-lowering medications are used, obtain at least 30-40% reduction in LDL-C levels. If LDL-C <70 mg/dL is the chosen target, consider drug titration to achieve this level to minimize side effects and cost. When LDL-C <70 mg/dL is not achievable because of high baseline LDL-C levels, it generally is possible to achieve reductions of >50% in LDL-C levels by either statins or LDL-C-lowering drug combinations.

§Standard dose of statin with ezetimibe, bile acid sequestrant, or niacin.

‖The combination of high-dose statin and fibrate can increase risk for severe myopathy. Statin doses should be kept relatively low with this combination. Dietary supplement niacin must not be used as a substitute for prescription niacin.

**Patients with very high triglycerides should not consume alcohol. The use of bile acid sequestrant is relatively contraindicated when triglycerides are >200 mg/dL.

††Creatinine should be <2.5 mg/dL in men and <2.0 mg/dL in women.

‡‡Potassium should be <5.0 mEq/L.

Data from Smith et al. 2006.

American Diabetes Association Standards of Care

The American Diabetes Association (ADA) published the updated standards of care in January 2006 (2). The goal of diabetes mellitus (DM) care is to provide for ongoing patient self-management to prevent acute complications and to reduce the risk of long-term complications, particularly vascular disease events.

Diabetes care involves many factors and addresses substantially more than glycemic control (table 5.2). Often, by the time diabetes is diagnosed, complications have already developed. Therefore, screening is recommended for prediabetes in people less than age 45 if they are obese or have risk factors for diabetes (see Criteria for Testing for Diabetes in Asymptomatic Adults on page 46), and screening is recommended by the ADA in all adults greater than 45, particularly with obesity present. The fasting plasma glucose test is the recommended screening test because it is more

reproducible, more convenient, and less costly than other tests (2).

The patient with diabetes (type 1 or 2) is considered to have a "CHD risk equivalent" by the National Cholesterol Education Program (7). This is attributable to evidence demonstrating that 7 to 10 years of diabetes gives individuals the same risk for a subsequent CHD event as those who were previously diagnosed with CHD alone (2, 7). Those with DM and a history of atherosclerosis are at particularly high risk for a CHD event and should be followed to reduce subsequent risk (7). Therefore, quality improvement programs that monitor and systematically treat patients with DM, CHD, and other risk factors can make a significant difference in patient outcomes.

Glycemic control and diabetes treatment have been demonstrated to reduce coronary disease outcomes with the use of metformin, acarbose, and pioglitazone. Blood pressure control is vital in reducing the progression to chronic kidney failure or reducing risk for stroke and cardiovascular complications. The goal blood

TABLE 5.2 Summary of Recommendations for Adults With Diabetes

Measure	Recommended outcome
Glycemic control	
HbA$_{1c}$	<7.0%*
Preprandial capillary plasma glucose	90-130 mg/dL (5.0-7.2 mmol/L)
Peak postprandial capillary plasma glucose[†]	<180 mg/dL (<10.0 mmol/L)
Blood pressure	<130/80 mmHg
Lipids[‡]	
LDL-C	<100 mg/dL (<2.6 mmol/L)
Triglycerides	<150 mg/dL (<1.7 mmol/L)
HDL-C	>40 mg/dL (>1.1 mmol/L)§

Key concepts in setting glycemic goals:
- HbA$_{1c}$ is the primary target for glycemic control.
- Goals should be individualized.
- Certain populations (children, pregnant women, and elderly people) require special considerations.
- More stringent glycemic goals (i.e., normal HbA$_{1c}$ <6%) may further reduce complications at the cost of increased risk of hypoglycemia.
- Less intensive glycemic goals may be indicated in patients with severe or frequent hypoglycemia.
- Postprandial glucose may be targeted if HbA$_{1c}$ goals are not met despite reaching preprandial glucose goals.

HbA$_{1c}$ = hemoglobin A$_{1c}$; LDL-C = low-density lipoprotein cholesterol; HDL-C, high-density lipoprotein cholesterol.

*Referenced to a nondiabetic range of 4.0-6.0% using a Diabetes Control and Complications Trial–based assay.

[†]Postprandial glucose measurements should be made 1-2 hr after the beginning of a meal, generally peak levels in patients with diabetes.

[‡]Current NCEP/ATP III guidelines suggest that in patients with triglycerides ≥200 mg/dL, the non–HDL-C (total cholesterol minus HDL-C) be used. The goal is ≤130 mg/dL.

§For women, it has been suggested that the HDL-C goal be increased by 10 mg/dL.

Data from ADA Position Statement: Standards of Medical Care in Diabetes 2006.

■ Criteria for Testing for Diabetes in Asymptomatic Adults

- ■ Testing for diabetes should be considered in all people 45 and older, particularly those with a body mass index (BMI) $\geq$25 kg/m²*; if results are normal, testing should be repeated at 3-year intervals.

- ■ Testing should be considered at a younger age or be carried out more frequently in people who are overweight ($\geq$BMI 25 kg/m²*) and have additional risk factors:
  - Are habitually physically inactive
  - Have a first-degree relative with diabetes
  - Are members of a high-risk ethnic population (e.g., African American, Latino, Native American, Asian American, Pacific Islander)
  - Have delivered a baby weighing >9 lb (>4.08 kg) or have been diagnosed with gestational diabetes mellitus (GDM)
  - Are hypertensive ($\geq$140/90 mmHg)
  - Have an HDL-C level <35 mg/dL (0.90 mmol/L) or a triglyceride level >250 mg/dL (2.82 mmol/L)
  - Have polycystic ovarian syndrome
  - On previous testing, had impaired fasting glucose or impaired glucose tolerance
  - Have other clinical conditions associated with insulin resistance (e.g., polycystic ovarian syndrome or acanthosis nigricans)
  - Have a history of vascular disease

*May not be correct for all ethnic groups. Data from ADA Position Statement: Standards of Medical Care in Diabetes 2006.

pressure for those with diabetes is <130/80, attributable to evidence showing less progression at this lower blood pressure, and the preferred agents for blood pressure treatment are ACE inhibitors or angiotensin receptor blockers. Other agents that reduce events in the diabetic population are diuretics, β-blockers, and calcium channel blockers (2).

Diabetic patients must have aggressive treatment of cholesterol levels, because a large amount of evidence demonstrates reduced morbidity and mortality for diabetic patients treated with cholesterol medications, particularly statins. Lifestyle modification, including nutritional changes to reduce saturated fats, trans fats, cholesterol, and calories and increased physical activity, has proven beneficial for those with DM (2). Patients with DM should have individualized and family medical nutritional therapy to achieve goals. In persons without overt cardiovascular disease but who have DM, the LDL-C goal is <100 mg/dL. For those with known cardiovascular disease and DM, a statin to lower LDL at least 30% to 40% and to achieve an LDL-C <70 mg/dL is an option (7). Triglyceride levels should be <150 mg/dL (better if <100 mg/dL) and HDL-C $\geq$40 mg/dL. Combination therapy of a statin and other cholesterol medication may be needed to achieve these goals (7).

Identifying and tracking patients with DM are important, especially those with other CHD risk factors, given not only their high-risk status but also the benefit of treating these other CHD risk factors. Meticulous care and follow-up can significantly reduce poor outcomes. Self-management education is vital to help patients optimize metabolic control, prevent complications, and maximize quality of life. Cardiac rehabilitation professionals should target DM as a significant added risk, a treatment goal, and an area of additional need for patient education. By working together with dieticians and other health professionals, these high-risk patients can reduce risk significantly while recovering from cardiovascular events.

National Cholesterol Education Program Guidelines

The National Cholesterol Education Program (NCEP) guidelines have been available for almost 2 decades (7). Recent randomized clinical trials in CHD patients suggest that more aggressive treatment of LDL-C and other lipid parameters is associated with reduced recurrent cardiac events. Because of the results from those trials, the NCEP recently updated its guidelines to provide evidence-based treatment recommendations for patients with cardiovascular disease (11).

With the NCEP guidelines directing evidence-based treatment, progress has been made in improving adherence in the treatment of cholesterol, although a considerable treatment gap remains (9, 17). A National Health and Nutrition Examination Survey of high-risk adult patients showed that only 22% had an LDL-C <100 mg/dL and >60% were >10% above their LDL-C goal (17). In the Multi-Ethnic Study of Atherosclerosis, approximately 25% of high-risk patients had an LDL-C <100 mg/dL (9).

The reasons that patients do not achieve NCEP-recommended treatment goals are many and can be categorized as patient, physician, payor, pharmaceutical, or practice factors. Patients often do not adhere to therapy because of cost, concerns about medications, side effects, and health habits (6). Physicians are often unaware of or disagree with guidelines or do not have the time to address this issue with patients, or there may be very important health system barriers such as lack of insurance or access to care (6). In a recent survey, family physicians reported that patient factors accounted for 74% of the barriers to treatment, system factors 23% of the barriers, and physician factors only 3% of barriers (6). These gaps provide a critical opportunity for systematic approaches to improving care, such as hospital discharge treatment and cardiac rehabilitation systems for achieving treatment goals. At the University of Wisconsin Hospital and Clinics, only 31% of the patients entering outpatient cardiac rehabilitation program in 1996 were on lipid-lowering therapy. The development of a routine inpatient cardiac rehabilitation consultation for all myocardial infarction patients with a goal of getting all patients discharged on therapy, and routine discharge orders for all CHD patients, resulted in more than 90% of the post–myocardial infarction patients receiving cholesterol therapy before discharge. Follow-up systems to ensure that patients achieve NCEP LDL-C and other risk factor goals are in place through outpatient cardiac rehabilitation and electronic record databases.

Meis and colleagues (14) demonstrated the effectiveness of a cardiac rehabilitation program in implementing national guidelines. Using systems to test and follow cholesterol levels throughout cardiac rehabilitation and to communicate with the patient's cardiologist and primary care physician, the investigators found that patients in the intervention group had significantly greater reductions in total cholesterol and LDL-C compared with the control group, were more likely to achieve LDL-C goals (67% vs. 43%), and were more likely to have a lipid medication change. Cardiac rehabilitation is the ideal situation in which to create systems to identify and monitor cholesterol levels, provide education on treatment goals and lifestyle and medication, and coordinate care. The diagnosis of CHD or a surgical intervention is a significant teachable moment for the patient and the health care team.

The inclusion of systematic approaches and physician and patient education is important to improve adherence to national guidelines and risk factor control. The Extensive Lifestyle Management Intervention (ELMI) after cardiac rehabilitation study was a 4-year randomized, controlled trial of risk factor and lifestyle management after cardiac rehabilitation. The results from this study demonstrated that a systematic intervention (exercise sessions, telephone follow-ups, counseling sessions, and reports to the patient's primary care physician) improved patients' lipids, blood pressure, and Framingham Risk Score (13). A recent trial of improving blood pressure control found that including patient education with provider education and practice system changes improved patient blood pressures (18).

Closing the Treatment Gap With the HeartCare Partnership Model

Administrators of a disease management program must understand the status of the population that the management plan aims to benefit. An essential step is identification of the gaps between health care practices within a given community and clinical practice guidelines. These gaps define the opportunities for improving patient health and reducing the cost of care. Unfortunately, relatively few population data studies have used a randomized design, beyond the basic statistics on prevalence, morbidity, and mortality. To guide improvements in CHD management and raise awareness among practitioners, baseline data are needed within each medical community on the use of medications, achievement of target outcomes, patients' preventive and rehabilitative health care activities, and the impact of CHD on their employment and quality of life.

In recent years, the AHA has implemented the Get With the Guidelines (GWTG) program for CHD, stroke, and heart failure. GWTG identifies clinicians (champions) to develop, lead, and mobilize teams of health care specialists to implement treatment and discharge guidelines for patients in acute care hospitals. The program begins with an assessment of the participating hospital's acute treatment and discharge protocols to develop a baseline and then undertakes continuous quality improvement to ensure that patients are treated and discharged in accordance with the AHA–ACC guidelines (table 5.1 on pages 43-44). GWTG tracks target outcomes with particular emphasis placed on smoking cessation; physical activity counseling; and the use of aspirin, β-blockers, angiotensin-converting enzyme inhibitors, and lipid-lowering agents (12). This program has proven outstanding in helping close the treatment gap between the AHA–ACC guidelines and the inpatient standard of care as demonstrated in numerous studies that have documented GWTG target outcomes. The next opportunity to close the treatment gap and improve the standard of cardiac care lies in the outpatient domain.

Cardiac rehabilitation programs can serve a pivotal role in reducing a patient's cardiovascular disease risk following hospital discharge (table 5.3). Although cardiac rehabilitation programs were originally implemented when randomized controlled trials demonstrated a strong exercise-related mortality benefit (15, 16), the benefits of comprehensive multiple risk factor modification on clinical outcomes, as superbly demonstrated in the Stanford Coronary Risk Intervention Project (SCRIP) (10), have taken precedence during the past decade. The concept of cardiac rehabilitation as the site for comprehensive risk reduction was embraced by the *Cardiac Rehabilitation Clinical Practice Guidelines* (22) under the topic Cardiac Rehabilitation as Secondary Prevention, and *Core Components of Cardiac Rehabilitation/Secondary Prevention* was promoted and published jointly by AHA and the American Association of Cardiovascular and Pulmonary Rehabilitation (AACVPR) (3, 4). Despite having the support of the AHA–ACC and AACVPR outcomes and holding an ideal position in which to take a leadership role, many rehabilitation programs remain largely isolated from their medical communities.

The Greenville HeartCare Partnership (HCP) was initiated by the HeartLife Cardiac Rehabilitation Program of the Greenville Hospital System and designed as an interactive comprehensive risk reduction approach to CHD management in upstate South Carolina (8). The Greenville HCP strove to effect long-term behavioral change, for both patients and clinicians, through intense focus on published clinical practice guidelines and patient management strategies within the physician practice, hospital, and cardiac rehabilitation settings.

The goal of the project was to close the treatment gap between practice patterns in upstate South Carolina and the AHA–ACC and ADA guidelines for chronic disease (risk factor) management.

Directed by the HeartLife program, the Greenville HCP included hundreds of clinicians from hospitals, physician practices, and rehabilitation programs working collaboratively to bridge the treatment gap between clinical practice and AHA–ACC guidelines for improving patient care and target outcomes. Over a 3-year period, investigators randomly selected 3,174 diverse patients with documented CHD (from a database of more than 60,000 patients) to assess outcomes for CHD management. Patient charts were selected to represent progress toward target outcomes following hospital discharge (at three hospitals), standard of care at physician practices (five family practice, five internal medicine, four cardiology), and completion of comprehensive cardiac rehabilitation (three programs). Physicians involved in the partnership gained an increased focus on risk factor management that had applications to all of their patients. The patient management strategies were implemented through chart reviews, outcome measures, and interactive educational sessions. During these sessions, physicians and staff reviewed performance, identified barriers and solutions for implementing secondary prevention strategies, and developed educational materials.

Figure 5.1 depicts the percentage of patients achieving the nine target outcomes. The data indicate that patients referred to cardiac rehabilitation were more likely to achieve the AHA–ACC guidelines for patient care and CHD target outcomes. The model implemented in the Greenville HCP demonstrates that multidisciplinary management of CHD target outcomes can narrow the treatment gap and that the more aggressively patients are managed, the closer they will come to achieving treatment goals (8).

Comprehensive cardiovascular rehabilitation programs face increasing demands to demonstrate accountability in clinical and economic outcomes in disease management. This spotlight on evidence-based guidelines and comprehensive risk reduction is a valuable opportunity for the cardiac rehabilitation profession. Focusing on patient outcomes, patient satisfaction, and the increased need to incorporate secondary prevention clinical practice guidelines into daily program operations is a path to achieving this goal. Program directors need to carefully and thoughtfully develop risk factor modules and practice ongoing quality improvement by collecting target outcome data with colleagues within their medical communities.

TABLE 5.3 Summary of Patient Assessment and Outcomes Evaluation in Cardiac Rehabilitation and Secondary Prevention Programs

Core component	Assessment and outcome evaluation
Patient assessment	■ Review medical history: diagnoses, interventional procedures, comorbidities, test results, symptoms, risk factors, medications. ■ Assess vital signs and clinical status; administer a battery of standardized measurement tools to assess status in each component of care. ■ Goal: Develop a goal-directed treatment plan with short- and long-term goals for cardiovascular risk reduction and improvement in health-related quality of life.
Lipid management	■ Assess lipid profile, current treatment, and compliance. ■ Goal: LDL-C <100 mg/dL; secondary goals: HDL-C >40 mg/dL, triglycerides <150 mg/dL.
Hypertension management	■ Assess resting BP, current treatment strategies, and patient adherence. ■ Goal: BP <130 mmHg systolic and <80 mmHg diastolic.
Diabetes management	■ Assess presence of diabetes, HbA_{1c} and FBG, current treatment strategies, and patient adherence. ■ Goal: HbA_{1c} <7.0; FBG 80-110 mg/dL.
Weight management	■ Assess weight and height, calculate BMI, determine risk (obese ≥30 kg/m^2; overweight ≥25-29.9 kg/m^2). ■ Goal: If weight risk identified, have patient maintain energy deficit of 500-1,000 kcal/day with diet and exercise to reduce weight by at least 10% (1-2 lb [0.45-0.90 kg] per week).
Psychosocial management	■ Assess psychological distress (depression, anxiety, hostility); refer patient with clinically significant distress to appropriate mental health specialist for further evaluation and treatment. ■ Goal: Reduce psychological distress; enhance coping and stress management skills. Address issues affecting health-related quality of life.
Exercise training	■ Assess functional capacity (maximal or submaximal) and physiological responses to exercise. ■ Goal: Individualized exercise prescription defining frequency (times/week), intensity (training heart rate range, rating of perceived exertion, MET level), duration (minutes), and modality to achieve aerobic, muscular, flexibility, and energy expenditure goals.
Physical activity counseling	■ Assess current (past 7 days) physical activity behavior: include leisure and usual activities (occupational, domestic). Specify time (min/day), frequency (days/week), and intensity (e.g., moderate or vigorous). ■ Goal: 30 min/day on most (at least 5) days of the week for moderate (3-5 MET level); 20 min/day for 3-4 days/week for vigorous (6+ MET level). Promote adherence.
Nutritional counseling	■ Assess dietary behavior: dietary content of fat, cholesterol, sodium, caloric intake; eating and drinking habits. ■ Goal: Individualized prescribed diet based on needs assessed. Promote diet adherence.
Smoking cessation	■ Assess smoking status: current, recent (quit <6 months), former, never. ■ Goal: Abstinence from smoking and use of all tobacco products.

LDL-C = low-density lipoprotein cholesterol; HDL-C = high-density lipoprotein cholesterol; BP = blood pressure; HbA_{1c} = hemoglobin A_{1c}; FBG = fasting blood glucose; BMI = body mass index; MET = metabolic equivalent.

Data from Balady et al. 2000.

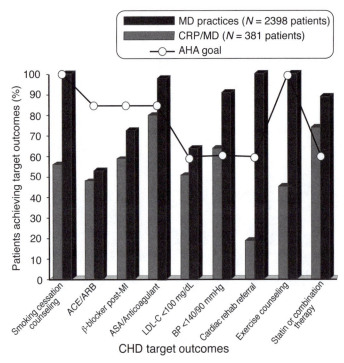

FIGURE 5.1 Closing the treatment gap in upstate South Carolina with the Greenville HeartCare Partnership. This figure depicts the percentage of patients for nine American Heart Association (AHA) target outcomes for coronary heart disease (CHD) as managed by physician practices alone (MD practices) or by cardiac rehabilitation programs in conjunction with physicians (CRP–MD). ACE = angiotensin-converting enzyme; ARB = angiotensin receptor blocker; MI = myocardial infarction; ASA = acetylsalicylic acid (aspirin); LDL-C = low-density lipoprotein cholesterol; BP = blood pressure. Adapted from Feigenbaum et al. 2003.

Summary

Approaching clinical care for patients with cardiovascular disease through existing programs can help to ensure that patients receive vital therapies. Each health care organization must assess baseline clinical data and determine methods to optimize clinical outcomes. Routine discharge orders, critical care pathways, standards of care, and routine cardiac rehabilitation referrals are just a few of the proven methods to improve the care of the patient with CVD.

Pathophysiology, Diagnosis, and Medical Management of Cardiovascular Disease

Part II discusses the pathophysiology and diagnosis of cardiovascular disease and reviews current medical management strategies. Chapters 6 and 7 discuss the atherosclerotic process from two different perspectives. Chapters 8 and 9 provide an overview of diagnostic techniques including exercise testing and more contemporary approaches such as the use of calcium scoring and angiographs. Chapter 10 reviews many of the pharmacologic strategies and chapter 11 the surgical techniques used in cardiovascular disease management. Because women present with specific concerns and cardiovascular complications, chapter 12 describes elements that physicians and health practitioners must consider in the management of heart disease in women.

CHAPTER 6

Morphologic Features of Arteries With Atherosclerotic Plaque

William Clifford Roberts, MD

Atherosclerosis is the most common condition, other than dental caries, affecting adults residing in the Western world. Atherosclerosis is rarely of genetic origin: Only 1 in 500 persons has the genetic variety, heterozygous familial hypercholesterolemia, and only 1 in 1,000,000 has the homozygous familial variety (1). The cause of atherosclerosis is now well established: cholesterol (14). Adults having serum total cholesterol levels >150 mg/dL, low-density lipoprotein levels >70 mg/dL, or serum high-density lipoprotein levels <20 mg/dL are candidates for this disease. Cigarette smoking, systemic hypertension, aging, hyperglycemia, hypercalcemia, overweight, and inactivity when associated with hypercholesterolemia worsen the problem, but none by themselves causes atherosclerosis.

At least four factors indicate that hypercholesterolemia causes atherosclerosis (14):

1. Hypercholesterolemia easily is produced experimentally by giving diets high in cholesterol (e.g., egg yolks) or saturated fat (e.g., bovine or porcine fat) to herbivores (e.g., rabbits, monkeys, human beings).

2. Cholesterol is present in experimentally produced plaques and in plaques of human beings.

3. Compared with groups of people with low levels of serum cholesterol, populations with high serum cholesterol levels have a much higher frequency of atherosclerotic events, a much higher frequency of dying from those events, and a much higher quantity of plaque in their arteries (plaque burden).

4. Lowering serum low-density lipoprotein cholesterol and lowering non-high-density lipoprotein cholesterol decreases atherosclerotic events and their complications and decreases the quantity of plaque (reversibility).

This chapter summarizes morphologic findings in the four major epicardial coronary arteries in patients with fatal coronary events and in those who have

Address correspondence concerning this chapter to William Clifford Roberts, 621 North Hall Street, Suite H030, Dallas, TX 75226. E-mail: wc.roberts@baylorhealth.edu endarterectomy of the right coronary artery at the time of coronary artery bypass grafting. In addition, this chapter discusses the state of the aorta and peripheral arteries in patients with transient ischemic attacks, aortic aneurysm, and leg ischemia or infarction.

Coronary Arteries

Most recent publications have indicated that coronary events are the result of rupture of coronary plaques, and most cardiologists believe that many coronary events are attributable to rupture of atherosclerotic plaques (2, 3, 25). Much research has been focused on detecting the vulnerable plaque, the one that has the potential to rupture and therefore precipitate a coronary event. But does rupture of a plaque cause sudden coronary death, the first episode of angina pectoris, or the conversion from stable to unstable angina pectoris? Most would answer no. Rupture of plaque is important in 70% of cases of acute myocardial infarction, and in the other 30% of cases no rupture of a plaque with superimposed thrombus is found at necropsy (7, 21). These latter cases do have a thrombus superimposed on a plaque, but the underlying plaque is not ruptured.

Findings at Necropsy

One reason coronary events occur is because the quantity of plaque present in the coronary arteries is enormous (15). Although a thrombus may be present in a coronary artery in patients with sudden coronary death or unstable angina pectoris, the thrombus is minute and too small to affect coronary flow (16, 17, 24). Furthermore, these minute, so-called mural thrombi are present at necropsy in no more than 20% of patients who suffer sudden coronary death or have unstable angina pectoris (a rare occurrence) (7). These minute thrombi are often present in our coronary arteries, and their organization may play a role in the development of the plaque. Indeed, they have been observed in the coronary arteries of patients dying from noncardiac conditions.

If rupture of a plaque is not the cause of sudden coronary death or unstable angina pectoris, what is? The answer is unclear, but the quantity of coronary plaque present (i.e., the plaque burden) is enormous (15). Several studies examining each 5 mm segment of the four major epicardial coronary arteries in these patients have demonstrated that plaque is present in

every 5 mm segment and that more than a third of these segments (an average of 18 of the 54 segments per patient) are narrowed >75% in cross-sectional area (15). Small changes in coronary flow precipitated by emotional or traumatic events or dreams, among other things, appear to have the potential to set off a malignant ventricular arrhythmia or chest pain without infarction.

The quantity of atherosclerotic plaque present in each 5 mm segment of the four major epicardial coronary arteries is similar in patients with fatal acute myocardial infarction, in those with healed myocardial infarcts dying from either cardiac or noncardiac conditions, in patients with sudden coronary death, and in those with stable angina pectoris dying from noncardiac conditions (15). Patients dying during periods of unstable angina pectoris tend to have the most severe quantity of plaque in their epicardial coronary arteries compared with patients who experience any of the other types of coronary events (15).

Examination of each 5 mm segment of the four major coronary arteries in this circumstance has disclosed that approximately 70% of the plaque is fibrous tissue, about 10% lipid, about 10% calcium, and about 10% other types of tissue (4-6, 8-13). Of course, these percentages vary with individual patients, but among groups of patients these percentages hold. The more lipids present in the plaque, the greater the potential for reversibility. It is unlikely that the fibrous and calcific portion of plaques can be reversed.

Findings at Endarterectomy

Endarterectomy of the right coronary artery at the time of coronary bypass provides the means of examining this artery in a living patient in the same manner that this artery can be examined at necropsy in patients with fatal coronary artery disease. Examination of each 5 mm cross section of the endarterectomy specimen has disclosed at least as much plaque in the lumen of these specimens as observed in the same artery at necropsy (23). In both specimens, more than a third of the length of the artery is narrowed >75% in cross-sectional area by plaque. In nearly all of the endarterectomy specimens, the internal elastic membrane is well preserved and its presence allows the endarterectomy and necropsy specimens to be compared similarly. In other words, the entire plaque is excised in the endarterectomy specimens because each contains a portion of media.

Carotid Artery

Carotid endarterectomy is the second most commonly performed cardiovascular operation. The average specimen weighs about 1.5 g and consists of the most distal portion of the common carotid artery and the most proximal portions of the internal and external carotid arteries. The lumen of the common carotid artery is in nearly all cases wide open, the lumen of the internal carotid is severely narrowed (>75% narrowed in cross-sectioned area), and the lumen of the external carotid most commonly is widely patent but occasionally is severely narrowed (22). The plaque in the internal carotid artery is usually complex, consisting of pultaceous debris (lipid), calcific deposits, and some fibrous tissue. These plaques tend to contain a higher volume of lipid than do the coronary plaques. These specimens contain a longitudinal continuous incision in both the common carotid and internal carotid arteries. In contrast to the coronary arteries, which have muscular media, the media of these arteries contain many elastic fibers (elastic arteries).

Abdominal Aorta

The diameter of the adult abdominal aorta just cephalad to the bifurcation into the common iliac arteries is <2 cm. Abdominal aortic aneurysm (AAA) is usually considered to be present if the maximal diameter is 3 cm, and resection or percutaneous intervention is usually considered appropriate if the maximal diameter is ≥5 cm. An AAA contains an intra-aneurysmal thrombus, which consists entirely of fibrin; in other words, the intra-aneurysmal thrombus never organizes (18, 20).

The aorta at the site of the AAA contains atherosclerotic plaque in every square millimeter of its wall. The media in the wall of the aneurysm is usually atrophic, presumably the consequence of pressure from the overlying atherosclerotic plaque and, of course, the intraluminal pressure. Systemic hypertension is usually present in patients with AAA, and their hearts virtually always have a large mass (>350 g in women; >400 g in men). Thus, one view is that AAA is a combination of hypercholesterolemia (serum total cholesterol >150, low-density lipoprotein cholesterol >100 mg/dL) and systemic hypertension (peak systolic blood pressure >140 or diastolic pressure >90 mmHg).

Peripheral Arteries

Atherosclerosis is always a systemic disease, meaning that persons with plaques in one arterial system always have plaques in other arterial systems (19). One system, however, may produce clinical consequences of the luminal narrowing without clinical consequences of the narrowing in the other arterial systems. Nevertheless, most patients with carotid arterial disease, AAA, or peripheral arterial disease in the legs usually die as a consequence of coronary artery disease. Why one system becomes symptomatic before another is unclear, because the same cholesterol level is present in all the arterial systems. (The peripheral arteries and aorta, however, are exposed to a systolic pressure, whereas the coronary arteries are exposed only to a diastolic pressure.) Of patients with disease in the arteries of the legs, the degree of stenosis resulting from the plaques is always >75% in cross-sectional area and usually >90%. The plaques in the leg arteries of patients with claudication or obvious ischemia or with infarction (gangrene) usually contain large amounts of calcium, which aids enormously in the identification by radiography during life. The quantity of calcium in these peripheral arteries is much greater than in the coronary or carotid arteries.

Summary

The connection between cholesterol elevation and atherosclerotic plaques is clear and well established. It appears that atherosclerosis is a cholesterol problem. Additional risk factors amplify the cholesterol damage, but these risk factors by themselves do not produce arterial plaque.

CHAPTER 7

Role of the Inflammatory Process in Atherosclerosis and Vascular Disease

Stanley S. Wang, MD

Sidney C. Smith, Jr., MD

The atherosclerotic process, described in detail in chapter 6, depends heavily on a complicated network of inflammatory pathways. Ongoing research has demonstrated that atherosclerosis on a molecular level is an inflammatory reaction to cardiovascular risk factors (76). Chronic inflammation is a crucial component of the atherosclerotic process and includes a wide array of processes including oxidation of low-density lipoprotein (LDL) particles responsible for transporting cholesterol, activation of macrophages and other leukocytes, and the local and systemic release of various cytokines and other inflammatory mediators (96). Acute inflammation is thought to account for the finding that acute coronary syndromes frequently occur in patients who have only minimal preexisting substrate or plaque that is detectable by current clinical approaches.

In this chapter, we discuss risk factors for inflammation, chemical and cellular markers and mediators of inflammation from vascular and extravascular sources, noninvasive and invasive assessment of inflammation, and potential diagnostic and therapeutic implications.

Proinflammatory Risk Factors

Endothelial injury, whether caused by mechanical, biochemical, or immune-mediated damage, including the deposition and oxidation of LDL, appears to be multifactorial and leads to the release of mediators that trigger, propagate, and amplify the inflammatory cascade (figure 7.1). Proinflammatory risk factors that may result in endothelial injury include well-established risk factors for clinical cardiovascular disease such as dyslipidemia, cigarette smoking, hypertension, and

Address correspondence concerning this chapter to Sidney C. Smith, Jr., CB 7075, Division of Cardiology, University of North Carolina School of Medicine, 099 Manning Dr., Chapel Hill, NC 27599.

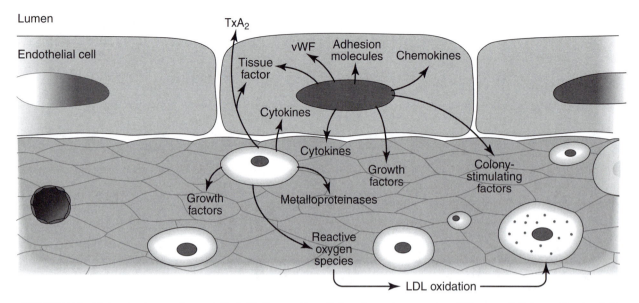

FIGURE 7.1 Molecular bases for endothelial inflammation. TxA$_2$ = thromboxane A$_2$; vWF = von Willebrand factor; LDL = low-density lipoprotein.

Reprinted from *Journal of American College of Cardiology*, Vol. 46, K.K. Koh, S.H. Han, and M.J. Quon, "Inflammatory markers and the metabolic syndrome," pgs. 1978-1985, Copyright 2005, with permission of Elsevier.

diabetes mellitus, as well as factors that have been the subject of recent interest such as visceral adiposity and cocaine use. Each of these factors has been the subject of intense mechanistic research.

Dyslipidemia is a particularly important risk factor for atherosclerosis, because oxidized LDL appears to be the primary triggering factor for the inflammatory cascade. On a clinical level, the risk of coronary events appears to increase in direct proportion to plasma cholesterol levels (86). A number of research findings implicate the molecular primacy of LDL. Quantitative and qualitative analyses of fatty streaks in fetal aortas demonstrate that native LDL uptake in the intima precedes LDL oxidation, which then leads to endothelial activation and monocyte recruitment (61). Oxidized LDL has been shown to increase endothelial expression of cellular adhesion molecules (CAMs), to attract monocytes and promote their differentiation into macrophages, and to play an essential role in stimulating macrophage release of proinflammatory cytokines.

Cigarette smoking promotes coronary artery disease through at least four pathophysiological pathways (49), including the induction of a hypercoagulable state attributable to increased plasma levels of factor VII and thromboxane A$_2$, reduction in oxygen delivery attributable to the generation of carbon monoxide, vasoconstriction of the coronary arteries (at least partially mediated by α-adrenergic stimulation), and direct hemodynamic effects of nicotine including a higher rate–pressure product.

Systemic hypertension appears to enhance monocyte preactivation, increase production of interleukin (IL)-1 and tumor necrosis factor-α (TNF-α) (27), and raise circulating levels of CAMs (12). The causative association between inflammation and hypertension is underscored by studies showing a clear relationship between elevated high-sensitivity C-reactive protein (CRP) levels in normotensive patients and risk of developing incident hypertension (82).

Diabetes mellitus is itself thought to result from inflammation, which may explain its well-known relationship to atherosclerosis. Evidence suggests that adipose tissue and macrophages recruited into adipose tissue release cytokines, including IL-1, IL-6, and TNF-α, which act on the liver, to promote dyslipidemia and dysfibrinogenemia; adipose tissue, to stimulate leptin secretion; and the pituitary gland, to increase secretion of adrenocorticotropic hormone (ACTH) (72). Moreover, serum levels of various inflammatory markers and mediators (including CRP, IL-6, fibrinogen, plasminogen activator inhibitor-1 [PAI-1], and serum amyloid A) correlate with the degree of hyperglycemia (84).

Visceral adiposity is another emerging atherosclerotic risk factor. Evidence suggests that adipose tissue acts as a metabolically active and dynamic endocrine organ with proinflammatory actions. Among the cytokines secreted by fat (sometimes referred to as *adipokines)* are IL-6, PAI-1, TNF-α, leptin, resistin, and angiotensinogen (figure 7.2). Although adipokine levels vary in proportion to overall adiposity, visceral adipose tissue appears to contribute to inflammation to a greater degree than does subcutaneous fat (29).

Plasma levels of the anti-inflammatory adipocyte-derived protein adiponectin are inversely related to visceral adiposity (20). Decreased adiponectin levels are associated with diabetes mellitus and reduced insulin sensitivity (4) as well as endothelial dysfunction, increased inflammation, and clinically significant atherosclerotic events including myocardial infarction (73).

Cocaine use is another risk factor for atherosclerosis, and emerging evidence implicates an inflammatory mechanism. Mouse studies suggest that cocaine increases the expression of CAMs and results in increased neutrophil adhesion to the coronary endothelium (19). In a study involving human neuronal progenitor cells, cocaine exposure led to increased expression of genes coding for a number of inflammatory markers including IL-1, IL-6, and TNF-α (21).

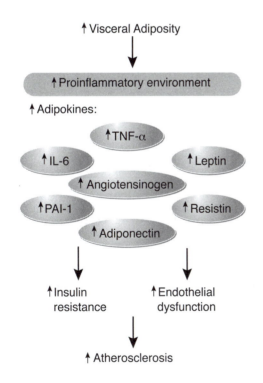

FIGURE 7.2 The inflammatory mediators through which adiposity contributes to atherosclerosis. PAI-1 = plasminogen activator inhibitor-1; IL-8 = interleukin-8; TNF-α = tumor necrosis factor-α; NF-κβ = nuclear factor-κβ.

Adapted from Lyon, Law, and Hsueh 2003.

Vascular and Extravascular Sources

The endothelium plays a central role in inflammation and atherosclerosis. In addition to secreting vasoactive substances, including endothelin, nitric oxide (NO), and prostacyclin, the endothelium reacts to atherosclerotic risk factors by increasing production and activation of protein kinase C and transcription factor κβ (92). Consequently, there is up-regulated production of angiotensin II and endothelial CAMs with resultant endothelial dysfunction.

The vasculature's role in inflammation includes the secretion of adhesion molecules, chemokines, interleukins, and growth factors by smooth muscle cells. The immune system plays a critical role by supplying leukocytes, including monocytes and macrophages, and mast cells. Additional sources of inflammatory mediators include the liver, which produces acute phase reactants such as CRP and serum amyloid A.

Mechanical endothelial injury appears to contribute to the inflammatory process. Secretion of CAMs appears to be greater at arterial branch points, presumably attributable to increased turbulence, and a number of other cytokines and mediators of endothelial function are altered at sites of high shear stress (22). Even in vein grafts, wall shear appears to affect the levels of proinflammatory cytokines (37).

Cellular and Chemical Mediators of Inflammation

A number of cellular and chemical mediators of inflammation are being studied. Early in the atherosclerotic process, monocytes are recruited into the arterial wall through the use of CAMs. Selectins and late antigens on the leukocyte surface induce rolling (92). Firm adhesion, arrest of motion, and migration across the endothelium ensue when endothelial CAMs—particularly vascular cell adhesion molecule-1 (VCAM-1) and intercellular adhesion molecule-1 (ICAM-1)—interact with leukocyte integrins (7). With subendothelial localization, monocytes become macrophages and secrete a wide array of cytokines, complement factors, proteases, and matrix metalloproteinases.

More than 50 cytokines (or *protein cell regulators*) (6) have been studied and categorized into classes including chemokines, colony stimulating factors, interferons, interleukins, transforming growth factors, and tumor necrosis factors. Some are proinflammatory (IL-1, IL-12, IL-18, interferon-γ, TNF-α); others are anti-inflammatory (IL-4, IL-10, IL-13, transforming growth factor-β) (figure 7.3).

A number of proinflammatory cytokines stimulate the NF-κβ pathway (figure 7.4), leading to the up-regulation of CAMs, chemokines, growth factors, and inducible enzymes including cyclooxygenases and nitric oxide synthase (26). Activated NF-κβ has been found

in a number of cellular mediators of atherosclerosis, including macrophages, endothelial cells, and smooth muscle cells, where enhanced activity of NF-κβ has been found to correlate with increased levels of pro-inflammatory cytokines and elevated risk of developing atherosclerotic lesions.

Another proinflammatory signaling pathway is the c-Jun NH₂-terminal kinase–activator protein-1 system, which regulates the action of cyclooxygenase 2,

Proinflammatory cytokines	IL-1, IL-2, IL-4, IL-6, IL-12, IL-18, TNF-α, CD40L/sCD40L, MCP-1, NF-κβ, MPO, MMP-3, MMP9
Anti-inflammatory cytokines	IL1ra, IL-6, IL-9, IL-10, IL18-BP, TGF-β

FIGURE 7.3 Pro- and anti-inflammatory cytokines. IL = interleukin; TNF-α = tumor necrosis factor-α; CD40L/sCD40L = CD40 ligand/soluble CD40 ligand; MCP-1 = monocyte chemotactic protein-1; NF-κβ = nuclear factor-κβ; CRP = C-reactive protein; MPO = myeloperoxidase; MMP = matrix metalloproteinase; TGF-β = tumor growth factor-β. Adapted from Tedgui and Mallat 2006.

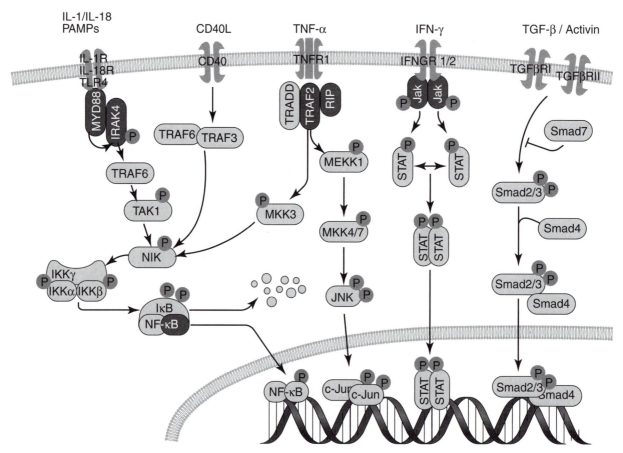

FIGURE 7.4 Primary intracellular signaling pathways in atherosclerosis. IL = interleukin; PAMP = pathogen-associated molecular pattern; CD40L = CD40 ligand; TNF-α = tumor necrosis factor-α; IFN-γ = interferon-γ; TGF-β = tumor growth factor-β; IL-1R = interleukin-1 receptor; IL-18R = interleukin-18 receptor; TLR-4 = Toll-like receptor-4; MYD88 = conduit between TLR or IL-1R receptors and downstream signaling kinases; IRAK = interleukin-1 receptor-associated kinase; TRAF = TNF receptor-associated factor; TAK1 = ubiquitin-dependent kinase of MKK and IKK; NIK = NFκ-inducible kinase; IKK = IκB kinase; NF-κβ = nuclear factor-κβ; MKK = mitogen-activated protein kinase kinase; TRADD = TNF receptor 1-associated protein; RIP = receptor interacting protein; MEKK = mitogen-activated protein kinase/extracellular signal-regulated protein kinase kinase; JNK = c-Jun NH₂-terminal kinase; JAK = Janus kinase; STAT = signal transducers and activators of transcription; Smad = genes encoding proteins that transducer signals from the TGF-β family of cytokines.

Reprinted from A. Tedgui and S. Mallat, 2006. "Cytokines in atherosclerosis: pathogenic and regulatory pathways," *Psychological Review* 86:515-81. Used with permission from American Physiological Society.

E-selectin, IL-2, IL-6, ICAM-1, VCAM-1, monocyte chemotactic protein-1, several matrix metalloproteinases (MMPs), and, perhaps most important, TNF-α. Finally, interferon-γ, IL-6, and IL-12 exert their effects on the Janus kinase-signal transducers and activators of transcription (JAK–STAT) pathways. Notably, there is significant crossover action between these signaling cascades (figure 7.5).

Several cytokines, especially IL-1 and transforming growth factor-β, stimulate proliferation of smooth muscle cells (63), leading to the formation of fibrous plaques. IL-1 and TNF-α attract inflammatory cells early in the process. They also activate the release of cellular adhesion molecules (such as ICAM-1), selectins, and heat shock proteins that have further vasoactive effects. MMPs destabilize the fibrous cap and lead to plaque degeneration and vulnerability to rupture (45).

CRP is an acute phase reactant that is synthesized in the liver. There is considerable evidence that CRP is an inflammatory marker (discussed subsequently), and CRP also appears to be a participant in the inflammatory process. CRP stimulates the uptake of LDL by macrophages as they become foam cells, activates the complement cascade, and promotes expression of endothelial CAMs (92).

Subendothelial macrophages, in addition to secreting chemical mediators, accumulate and oxidize LDL and eventually become the foam cells that presage fatty streaks and atherosclerotic lesions.

T lymphocytes may also participate in inflammation. Activated T lymphocytes can be found in the vessel wall at the earliest stages of atherogenesis, prior to the arrival of monocytes (39). Subsequent studies have suggested that these T lymphocytes may serve as memory cells (88). In addition, functional CD154 (previously known as CD40L) has been found on non-T-lymphocyte cells in atherosclerotic lesions and imply the presence of a T-lymphocyte-independent signaling pathway in the activation of inflammation (51).

Some cytokines inhibit atherosclerosis. For example, IL-10 is thought to induce antiatherogenic effects through the JAK1–STAT3 pathway (see figure 7.5 below). Adiponectin exerts antiatherosclerotic and anti-inflammatory actions, as described previously.

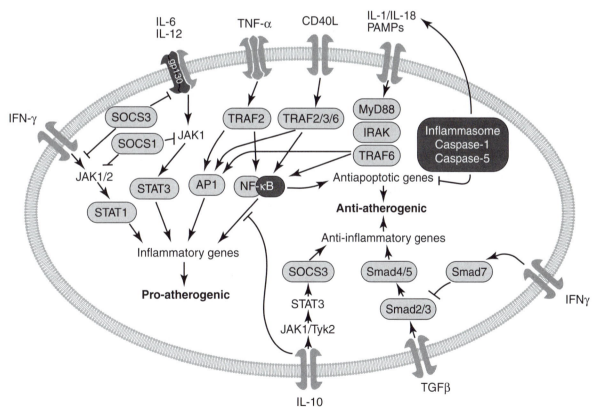

FIGURE 7.5 Crossover between selected signaling pathways. IL = interleukin; PAMP = pathogen-associated molecular pattern; CD40L = CD40 ligand; TNF-α = tumor necrosis factor-α; IFN-γ = interferon-γ; SOCS = suppressor of cytokine signaling; AP-1 = activator protein-1; MYD88 = conduit between TLR or IL-1R receptors and downstream signaling kinases; TGF-β = tumor growth factor-β; IRAK = interleukin-1 receptor-associated kinase; TRAF = TNF receptor-associated factor; NF-κβ = nuclear factor-κβ; JAK = Janus kinase; STAT = signal transducers and activators of transcription; Smad = genes encoding proteins that transducer signals from the TGF-β family of cytokines.

Reprinted, by permission, from A. Tedgui and S. Mallat, 2006, "Cytokines in atherosclerosis: pathogenic and regulatory pathways," *Physiological Review* 86: 515-81. Used with permission from American Physiological Society.

Markers of Inflammation and Their Predictive Value

CRP is a sensitive marker of inflammation that has attracted interest for use in establishing risk in specific clinical scenarios. Increased levels of CRP portend adverse clinical outcomes. Because acute elevation of CRP may be seen with many noncardiovascular conditions, repeat measurement is recommended in patients who are acutely ill or have evolving coronary syndromes (70).

Despite the statistical correlation of CRP with coronary artery disease, its clinical utility remains debatable. Incorporation of CRP into risk assessment may enhance the predictive accuracy of classic risk factors (41). However, a report from the ongoing Atherosclerosis Risk in Communities (ARIC) study, which includes varied ethnic groups, suggested that the routine measurement of CRP provides little if any additional risk stratification beyond that which can be obtained from assessment of established risk factors (33).

Lipoprotein-associated phospholipase A$_2$ (Lp-PLA$_2$) is another emerging inflammatory marker that may be more specific for vascular inflammation than CRP. Lp-PLA$_2$ is an enzyme that is secreted by monocytes–macrophages and T lymphocytes, binds to LDL through apolipoprotein B, and hydrolyzes phospholipids, producing proinflammatory mediators (52). Several studies have suggested that Lp-PLA$_2$ has significant independent prognostic value for future cardiovascular events (43). In addition, in a population-based cohort study, Lp-PLA$_2$ was independently associated with incident heart failure (94).

Fibrinogen is the precursor of fibrin and, as a mediator of inflammation, is also a proven marker of inflammation (24). A number of studies and meta-analyses (31) have demonstrated an association between fibrinogen and cardiovascular (91), cerebrovascular, and peripheral arterial disease (78).

IL-6, an early proinflammatory cytokine, has been studied as a potential marker for coronary artery disease. In addition to being strongly associated with an increased risk of developing type 2 diabetes mellitus (74), elevated IL-6 levels predict mortality risk in patients with unstable coronary syndromes (47). Another interleukin, IL-1, is both an inflammatory marker and a critical mediator of atherosclerosis in the coronary and peripheral arterial beds (44).

Serum amyloid A approaches CRP in its ability to predict cardiovascular events (66). In a study of female patients, serum amyloid A also appeared to have modest predictive value for angiographic coronary artery disease, whereas CRP did not (38).

Soluble CD40 ligand (sCD40L), produced predominantly by activated platelets, is found in higher concentrations in the blood in a wide variety of inflammatory conditions ranging from multiple sclerosis to inflammatory bowel disease. However, in the acute stages of the atherosclerotic cascade, sCD40L is proinflammatory and probably triggers the release of MMPs with consequent plaque destabilization (95). Measurement of sCD40L is emerging as a promising method for predicting the relative risk of cardiovascular events (48).

Homocysteine, previously shown to be modestly associated with the risk of ischemic heart disease (35), has uncertain value for prognosticating and guiding preventive and therapeutic interventions for atherosclerosis. Treatments that reduce homocysteine levels, including folic acid and vitamins B$_6$ and B$_{12}$ supplementation, may improve endothelial function and reduce carotid atherosclerosis, but these effects are not clearly mediated by lower homocysteine levels. Moreover, the lowering of homocysteine levels does not appear to affect the levels of other inflammatory mediators and markers including LDL and CRP (28). Finally, therapy to lower elevated homocysteine levels has not been correlated with improved cardiovascular outcomes (11, 90).

Myeloperoxidase (MPO), an enzyme found within neutrophils and macrophages that catalyzes the conversion of chloride and hydrogen peroxide to hypochlorite, is another inflammatory marker that is associated with coronary artery disease (100). Like CRP, MPO may be a mediator of inflammation, because it appears to participate in the oxidation of LDL (55). In patients with acute coronary syndromes, elevated MPO was found to be associated with a significantly increased risk of death and MI (5). Among patients presenting with chest pain, MPO was used to stratify patients into quartiles of progressive risk for major adverse events (13). Of note, however, MPO is released in a number of other infectious and infiltrative conditions and thus is not likely to be specific to cardiovascular etiologies (3).

Abnormal adiponectin levels may be found in acute coronary syndromes (60), and lower levels are associated with increased coronary lesion complexity, suggesting a potential role in plaque vulnerability (68). Paradoxically, acutely elevated adiponectin levels may independently predict the risks of death or cardiovascular events in patients who present with chest pain (17), but the strength of adiponectin's association with cardiovascular disease remains controversial (81). Of note, adiponectin concentration has been found to be inversely proportional to the severity of peripheral arterial occlusive disease (36).

Many more markers of inflammation have been shown to have predictive value. For example, MMP-3 (97), MMP-9 (10), and tissue inhibitor of metalloproteinase 1 (18) all appear to be related to likelihood of cardiovascular events in selected patient populations. Caspase-1 levels and polymorphisms of the caspase-1 gene also correlate with cardiovascular risk (9). Baseline levels of osteopontin, a calcium-binding glycophosphoprotein, may independently risk stratify patients with chronic stable angina (56). Lipoprotein(a) has a well-established association with cardiovascular and cerebrovascular disease (25). Pregnancy-associated plasma protein appears to have independent prognostic value in patients with angina (30). Neutrophil-activating peptide-2 levels are higher in acute coronary syndromes and may be related to platelet activation (85). Even the total white blood cell count has been shown to predict angiographic coronary artery disease (16) and to be inversely related to event-free survival in patients with heart disease (53).

Noninvasive Assessment of Inflammation

In addition to the multiple laboratory findings and markers of inflammation detailed here, a variety of noninvasive methods are evolving for the assessment of atherosclerosis. Computed tomography (CT) scanning of the coronary arteries has emerged as a valuable noninvasive means of determining the presence of atherosclerosis and estimating the risk of future cardiovascular events. Without intravenous contrast agents, CT can be used to assess the degree of coronary artery calcification, the presence of which has been shown to predict subsequent cardiac events (83). The use of intravenous contrast enables imaging of obstructive coronary lesions with high (>90%) sensitivity and specificity compared with invasive coronary angiography, at least in the proximal or larger diameter segments of the coronary arteries (58). Limited evidence is available to suggest a relationship between CT-derived coronary artery calcium scores and markers of inflammation, such as homocysteine and soluble IL-2.

B-mode ultrasound assessment of carotid intima media thickness is another noninvasive method of estimating inflammation and atherosclerosis. Intima media thickness is predictive of advanced vascular disease and risk of future events (67). In addition, a number of studies have demonstrated that increased intima media thickness correlates with diabetes and other atherosclerotic risk factors as well as inflammatory markers such as fibrinogen levels (71).

Contrast-enhanced ultrasound relies on ultrasonographic detection of microbubble intravascular contrast agents that couple to particles that target CAMs and other inflammatory mediators (46). More recent work involves the use of microbubbles targeted to P-selectins with potential implications for clinical applications in risk stratifying chest pain patients (8).

Magnetic resonance imaging (MRI) techniques are being refined for use in imaging inflammation and atherosclerosis. A growing body of preclinical studies has shown that MRI can be used to assess plaque composition and stability with promising levels of accuracy compared with histologic studies (14). Although clinicians await further study of the practical clinical utility of MRI, MRI-based assessment of atherosclerotic lesions is being used increasingly as a surrogate measure of the efficacy of various drugs, including statins (99).

Invasive Assessment of Inflammation

Invasive techniques for assessing inflammation also are emerging, although their clinical utility remains to be determined. Intravascular ultrasound (IVUS) is the most well-established of these techniques. This procedure is used to determine the presence and extent of vascular wall remodeling and outward expansion in the early phases of atheroma accumulation, before lesions encroach on the vascular lumen (62). In patients with acute coronary syndromes, IVUS can detect clinically significant atherosclerosis, even within angiographically unremarkable coronary arteries (57). The use of IVUS-based plaque characteristics as a surrogate marker of the efficacy of various antiatherosclerotic therapies is increasing, as evidenced by recent statin trials (including the REVERSAL and ASTEROID studies, discussed later). Thus, IVUS technology serves an important function in assessing the extent of chronic and acute coronary inflammation.

Catheter-based thermography to detect unstable, acutely inflamed atherosclerotic plaques was introduced in 1996. Subsequent studies showed variable degrees of correlation between increased heat production in atherosclerotic lesions and elevation of inflammatory markers (87). However, this technology remains unproven, and further studies are needed before its role in clinical practice can be determined (54).

Similarly, studies with Raman spectroscopy, which involves the use of a catheter-mounted laser technology to assess the composition of endovascular plaques, have provided interesting preclinical data, but considerably more trials are necessary before the technology can be of practical utility (93).

Treatment of Inflammation

Therapy to reduce inflammation has many theoretical bases (figure 7.6). Substantial evidence shows that a number of anti-inflammatory therapies can produce important clinical benefits; however, more evidence is needed to clarify the benefit of anti-inflammatory treatment beyond currently accepted approaches to maximal risk factor modification.

Aspirin has a number of anti-inflammatory effects; it is associated with improved clinical cardiovascular outcomes and inhibits the oxidation- and reduction-sensitive transcription factor NF-κβ. This, as discussed earlier, is an important proinflammatory signaling protein (26).

In addition to lowering LDL cholesterol (LDL-C), the 3-hydroxy-3-methylglutaryl coenzyme A reductase inhibitors (i.e., statins) have been shown to exert anti-inflammatory effects including the reduction of numerous inflammatory markers, including CRP (32), Lp-PLA$_2$ (2), MMP-9 (98), and CD40L (80). Two recent clinical trials provide evidence that these anti-inflammatory effects produce clinically meaningful benefit. The Pravastatin or Atorvastatin Evaluation and Infection Therapy–Thrombolysis in Myocardial Infarction 22 (PROVE IT-TIMI 22) (15) and Reversal of Atherosclerosis With Aggressive Lipid Lowering (REVERSAL) (65) trials found that patients with acute coronary syndromes who were treated with intensive statin therapy experienced fewer cardiovascular events. In PROVE IT, the greatest improvement in outcomes was seen in patients whose LDL-C and CRP levels both were lower on therapy. Outcomes for those with reduced CRP but no significant reduction in LDL-C were similar to those whose LDL-C was reduced but CRP remained elevated. These findings suggest a possible dual effect of statin therapy wherein a beneficial anti-inflammatory effect

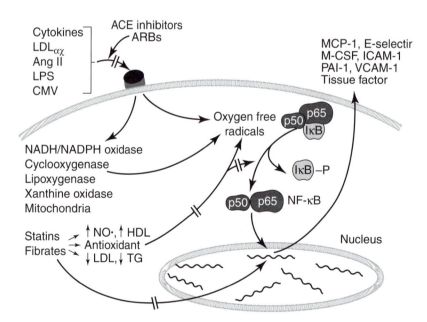

FIGURE 7.6 Established and theoretical molecular sites of action of anti-inflammatory therapies. LDL = low-density lipoprotein; CRP = C-reactive protein; Ang II = angiotensin II; LPS = lipopolysaccharide; CMV = cytomegalovirus; ACE = angiotensin-converting enzyme; NADH = nicotinamide adenine dinucleotide (reduced form); NADPH = nicotinamide adenine dinucleotide phosphate; NO = nitric oxide; HDL = high-density lipoprotein; TG = triglycerides; ARB = angiotensin receptor blocker; MCP-1 = monocyte chemotactic protein-1; M-CSF = macrophage colony-stimulating factor; ICAM-1 = intercellular adhesion molecule-1; PAI-1 = plasminogen activator inhibitor-1; VCAM-1 = vascular cell adhesion molecule-1; NF-κβ = nuclear factor-κβ.

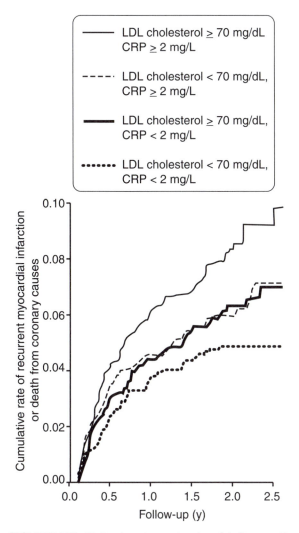

FIGURE 7.7 Patients whose levels of inflammation decreased, as defined by CRP levels, appear to have improved outcomes regardless of LDL levels. LDL = low-density lipoprotein; CRP = C-reactive protein.

occurs beyond that associated with LDL-C lowering (figure 7.7) (77).

Another statin study provided additional evidence to suggest that intensive LDL-C lowering may lead to plaque regression as assessed by IVUS techniques. In A Study to Evaluate the Effect of Rosuvastatin on Intravascular Ultrasound-Derived Coronary Atheroma Burden (ASTEROID), patients receiving relatively high doses of potent statin therapy had a mean on-treatment calculated LDL-C of 61 mg/dL (64). Among the 349 patients who underwent serial IVUS measure-ments, significant reductions were found in multiple IVUS measures of coronary artery disease burden, including percentage atheroma volume.

The benefit of combining statin therapy with fibrate therapy to reduce inflammation has not been proven. Although simvastatin and fenofibrate each reduced CRP and Lp-PLA$_2$, their use together did not produce a significantly greater inflammation reduction (59).

Moderate alcohol consumption (up to 2 drinks per day) appears to reduce inflammation and is associated with lower levels of CRP (1). A similar association has been found with other inflammatory markers, includ-ing IL-6 and soluble TNF-α receptor levels (69). Mild to moderate consumption of alcoholic beverages is associated with a lower risk of adverse cardiovascular outcomes (79).

As discussed previously, therapy to reduce homo-cysteine levels consists of folate and vitamin B$_6$ and B$_{12}$ supplementation. Although these interventions may improve endothelial function and surrogate markers of atherosclerosis and inflammation, they have not been shown to reduce clinical cardiovascular risk and may actually increase it.

Weight loss appears to reduce the contribution of adipocytes to inflammation by lowering levels of various adipokines, including TNF-α (23). Weight reduction also improves endothelial function (98). Early studies of surgical treatments of obesity suggested efficacy in reducing fibrinogen and PAI-1 (75).

Physical activity may reduce levels of several pro-inflammatory markers and mediators and increase plasma concentrations of the anti-inflammatory adi-pokine adiponectin (40). However, reductions in levels of fibrinogen, CRP, and sCD40L were not seen with fitness training in women who smoked (34).

Summary

Complex molecular cascades underlie acute and chronic inflammation and mediate atherosclerosis. Many inflammatory mediators and markers have been identi-fied, several of which may have important clinical value in prognostication. Noninvasive and invasive technolo-gies are under development, whereas some modalities are now available for clinical use. Both drug therapies and lifestyle interventions appear to hold promise for reducing inflammation and, thus, improving clinical outcomes for patients with atherosclerosis.

CHAPTER 8

Clinical Exercise Testing

Jonathan Myers, PhD

Victor F. Froelicher, MD

Despite the many recent advances in technology, the standard exercise test continues to be widely used to provide diagnostic, prognostic, and functional information for a wide spectrum of patients. The test is commonly used to evaluate the efficacy of medical therapy and assess interventions. It is a first-choice diagnostic tool in patients with suspected coronary artery disease (CAD), a role in which it functions as a gatekeeper to more expensive and invasive procedures. Although the exercise test originally was developed as a diagnostic tool, recent studies have confirmed its role in the selection of patients for cardiac transplantation, risk stratification, and the assessment of disability.

The exercise test has numerous indications. The most common reason patients are referred for exercise testing is to evaluate chest pain or, more generally, to assess signs and symptoms of coronary disease. However, there are many other clinical objectives for the test, including the following:

- Physiologic response of post-MI and postrevascularization patients to exercise
- Functional capacity for the purpose of exercise prescription
- Exercise capacity for the purpose of work classification (disability evaluation) and risk stratification (prognosis)
- The efficacy of medical, surgical, or pharmacologic treatment
- The presence and severity of arrhythmias

- Preoperative physiologic status
- Intermittent claudication

Because of the need to standardize the implementation and interpretation of the exercise test, professional organizations such as the American Heart Association (AHA), the American College of Cardiology (ACC) (15), the American College of Sports Medicine (ACSM) (1), and the American Thoracic Society (2) have developed guidelines designed to optimize the test's safety, methodology, and objectives. This chapter describes the applications, methodology, and principles of exercise testing and the professional standards for exercise testing described in the aforementioned guidelines.

Approach to the Patient

The highest information yield is obtained from the exercise test when it is accompanied by a physical examination and a detailed history. Historical information as part of the pretest assessment makes a critical contribution to the development of diagnostic and prognostic probabilities (see later section on multivariate scores). The clinician should calculate and consider these probabilities before beginning the test, because they not only influence the posttest risk of disease and prognosis

Address correspondence concerning this chapter to Jonathan Myers, VA Palo Alto Health Care System, Cardiology 111-C, 3801 Miranda Ave., Palo Alto, CA 94304. E-mail: drj993@aol.com but, in rare instances, can preclude performing the test. If the reason the patient was referred for the test is unclear, the clinician should postpone the test until this is clarified. The medical history should include any remote or recent medical problems, symptoms, medication use, and findings from previous examinations and tests. Major CAD risk factors and signs and symptoms suggesting cardiopulmonary disease should be identified. The clinician should assess physical activity patterns, vocational requirements, and family history of cardiopulmonary and metabolic disorders. If absolute contraindications are identified, the clinician should cancel the test and refer the patient to his or her primary physician for further medical management. Patients with relative contraindications should be tested only after careful evaluation of the risk–benefit ratio.

See Contraindictions to Exercise Testing below for lists of absolute and relative contraindications.

The clinician who will perform the test should provide detailed verbal and written instructions to the patient in advance, including a request that the patient refrain from ingesting food, alcohol, and caffeine and using tobacco products within 3 hr of testing. Patients should be well rested and should avoid vigorous activity the day of the test, and they should wear comfortable clothing that provides freedom of movement and allows access for electrode and blood pressure cuff placement. The clinician must thoroughly explain the potential risks and discomforts associated with exercise testing. Written informed consent has important ethical and legal implications and ensures that the patient knows and understands the purposes and risks of the exercise

■ Contraindications to Exercise Testing

Absolute

- A recent change in the resting electrocardiogram suggesting infarction or other acute cardiac event
- Recent complicated myocardial infarction
- Unstable angina
- Uncontrolled ventricular arrhythmia
- Uncontrolled atrial arrhythmia that compromises cardiac function
- Third-degree atrioventricular heart block without pacemaker
- Acute congestive heart failure
- Severe aortic stenosis
- Suspected or known dissecting aneurysm
- Active or suspected myocarditis or pericarditis
- Thrombophlebitis or intracardiac thrombi
- Recent systemic or pulmonary embolus
- Acute infections
- Significant emotional distress (psychosis)

Relative

- Resting diastolic blood pressure >115 mmHg or resting systolic blood pressure >200 mmHg
- Moderate valvular heart disease
- Known electrolyte abnormalities (hypokalemia, hypomagnesemia)
- Fixed-rate pacemaker
- Frequent or complex ectopy
- Ventricular aneurysm
- Uncontrolled metabolic disease (e.g., diabetes, thyrotoxicosis, or myxedema)
- Chronic infectious disease (e.g., mononucleosis or myxedema)
- Neuromuscular, musculoskeletal, or rheumatoid disorders exacerbated by exercise
- Advanced or complicated pregnancy

Reprinted, by permission, from American College of Sports Medicine, 2005, *Guidelines for exercise testing and exercise prescription*, 7th ed. (Baltimore, PA: Lippincott, Williams & Wilkins), 50.

test. There is significant legal precedent to indicate that informed consent should always be obtained before beginning a test, although this issue has been debated (19). The clinician or technician must show the patient how to get on and off the testing apparatus, describe what is expected of the patient (reporting of symptoms, level of exertion, testing end points), and answer any questions the patient has.

Whether patients should remain on all cardiovascular medicines for exercise testing has been the source of some debate. Many commonly used drugs can influence hemodynamic and electrocardiographic responses to exercise (particularly β-blockers and digoxin), but removing patients from their usual medicines can cause instability of symptoms, rhythm, and blood pressure and other problems. The aforementioned exercise testing guidelines suggest that most patients can remain on their medical regimen for testing without greatly compromising the diagnostic performance of the test (1, 2, 15). Tapering β-blockers or discontinuing antianginal or antihypertensive medications for several days before testing should be reserved for particular patients in whom diagnostic sensitivity is paramount, and the tapering process should be carefully supervised.

Safety, Personnel, and Supervision

Provided that contraindications to exercise testing are considered and patients who undergo exercise testing are appropriate, the exercise test is extremely safe. Widely cited data from the Cooper Clinic in Dallas suggest that an event serious enough to require hospitalization (e.g., sustained arrhythmia, heart attack, or death) occurs at a rate of 0.8 per 10,000 tests (16). This was confirmed in the year 2000 in a survey of 71 medical centers within the Veterans Affairs Health Care System, in which an event rate of 1.2 per 10,000 tests was reported (38). Surveys conducted in the 1970s suggested a somewhat higher event rate, ranging in the order of 1 to 4 per 10,000. It has been suggested that the apparent improvement in the safety of the test reflected in the more recent surveys is attributable to a significantly better understanding of when to perform and when to terminate the test and better preparation for emergencies that may arise (11, 15).

Clinical judgment is the most important consideration when deciding which patients should undergo exercise testing. Contraindications to testing (see page 68) usually describe conditions of cardiovascular insta-

bility, such as acute coronary syndrome, uncontrolled heart failure, and arrhythmias.

In the past, professional guidelines suggested that physician supervision was necessary for all exercise testing in the clinical setting. Given the remarkable safety record of exercise testing, particularly in recent years, there is now some debate regarding the need for physician supervision (11, 15, 16, 38). Although the recent AHA–ACC guidelines (15) recommend physician supervision when testing patients with heart disease in a clinical setting, the guidelines also state that "exercise testing in selected patients can be safely performed by properly trained nurses, exercise physiologists, physical therapists, or medical technicians working directly under the supervision of a physician, who should be in the immediate vicinity and available for emergencies." The physiologist or technician conducting the test should have a comprehensive knowledge of the indications, contraindications, equipment, physiologic responses to exercise; and clinical condition of the patient to optimize the information yield and conduct the test safely.

A joint statement by the American College of Physicians, the ACC, and the AHA regarding clinical competence in exercise testing outlined the cognitive skills needed to perform exercise testing (41). These include knowledge of indications and contraindications to testing, basic exercise physiology, principles of interpretation, and emergency procedures. The committee suggested that at least 50 exercise tests were required during training to achieve these skills. ACSM certification is widely used to establish competency for technicians, nurses, or physiologists who oversee exercise testing and training (1).

Modality and Protocol Considerations

The purpose of the test, the health and fitness of the patient, the exercise modality, and the exercise protocol are fundamental considerations when selecting a test for a given patient. In many exercise laboratories, these issues are determined by custom and the availability of equipment, but each can have a profound effect on the response to the exercise test. For example, a treadmill test may be inappropriate for a patient who has difficulty with balance or gait, such as someone who has had a stroke or is otherwise neurologically impaired, or someone who has severe peripheral vascular disease that prevents him or her from walking. A bicycle ergometer would be a more appropriate choice for such patients. Test specificity should also be considered. For example, it would be appropriate to use a cycle ergometer to assess physiologic responses to a cycling program.

Exercise Mode

An ideal exercise mode increases total body and myocardial oxygen demand to its highest level safely and in moderate, continuous, and equal increments. This requires a dynamic exercise device that uses major muscle groups, permitting large increases in cardiac output, oxygen delivery, and gas exchange. The bicycle ergometer and the treadmill are the most commonly used dynamic exercise devices. Bicycle ergometer testing is more commonly used in Europe, whereas the treadmill is more often used in the United States. The bicycle is usually less expensive, occupies less space, and is quieter. Upper-body motion is decreased, making blood pressure and electrocardiographic recordings easier. The workload administered by simple, mechanically braked bicycle ergometers is not always accurate and depends on pedaling speed, causing variations in the work performed. These have largely been replaced by electronically braked bicycle ergometers, which maintain the workload at a specified level over a wide range of pedaling speeds and are therefore more accurate.

The treadmill is usually more expensive than the cycle ergometer, is relatively immobile, and makes more noise. Studies comparing treadmill and bicycle ergometer exercise tests have reported maximal oxygen uptake to be roughly 10% to 20% higher and maximal heart rate 5% to 20% higher on the treadmill (34). Significant ST-segment changes are reported more frequently and angina is elicited more frequently during treadmill testing compared with cycle ergometer testing (34). In addition, exercise-induced myocardial ischemia by thallium scintigraphy has been reported to be greater after treadmill testing than ergometer testing (18). Although most of these differences are minor, if assessing the patient's functional limits and eliciting subjective or objective signs of ischemia are goals of the test, the treadmill may be preferable.

Protocols

The purpose of the test and the person tested are important considerations in selecting the protocol. Exercise testing may be performed for diagnostic purposes, for functional assessment, or for risk stratification. An often ignored but nevertheless consistent recommendation in the recent exercise testing guidelines is that the protocol be individualized for the patient being tested. For example, a maximal, symptom-limited test on a relatively demanding protocol would not be appropriate (or very informative) for a severely limited patient. Likewise, a very gradual protocol might not be useful for an apparently healthy, active person. The clinician should consider the person being tested and the goals of the test before determining use of submaximal testing, gas exchange techniques, the presence of a physician, and the exercise mode and protocol.

The most suitable protocols for clinical testing include a low-intensity warm-up phase followed by progressive, continuous exercise in which the demand is elevated to a patient's maximal level within a total duration of 8 to 12 min (1, 2, 15, 34, 36). In the absence of gas exchange techniques, the clinician should report exercise capacity in METs rather than exercise time, so that exercise capacity can be compared uniformly between protocols. METs can be estimated from any protocol using standardized equations (1, 15, 33). In general, 1 MET represents an increment on the treadmill of approximately 1 mph or 2.5% grade. On a cycle ergometer, 1 MET represents an increment of roughly 20 W (120 kpm/min) for a 70 kg person. The assumptions necessary for predicting MET levels from treadmill or cycle ergometer work rates—including that the subject is not holding the handrails, that oxygen uptake is constant (i.e., steady-state exercise is performed), that the subject is healthy, and that all people are similar in their walking efficiency—raise uncertainties as to the accuracy of estimating the work performed for an individual patient. For example, the steady-state requirement is rarely met for most patients on most exercise protocols; most clinical testing is performed among patients with varying degrees of cardiovascular or pulmonary disease; and people vary widely in their walking efficiency (33).

Ramp Testing

An approach to exercise testing that has gained interest in recent years is the ramp protocol, in which work increases constantly and continuously. The ramp protocol uses a constant and continuous increase in metabolic demand that replaces the staging used in conventional exercise tests. The uniform increase in work allows for a steady increase in cardiopulmonary responses and permits a more accurate estimation of oxygen uptake (35, 37). The ramp approach seems to optimize exercise testing, because large work increments are avoided and increases in work rate are individualized, permitting test duration to be targeted (1, 2, 15). Because there are no stages per se, the errors associated with predicting exercise capacity are lessened (1, 2, 9, 11).

Submaximal Testing

Maximal, symptom-limited tests usually are not considered appropriate until patients are more than 1 month post-MI or postsurgery. Thus, submaximal exercise testing has an important clinical role for pre-discharge, post-MI, or postbypass surgery evaluations. Submaximal tests have been shown to be important in risk stratification (i.e., for making appropriate activity recommendations); submaximal tests also can indicate the need to modify the medical regimen or undertake further interventions in patients who have sustained a cardiac event (13, 15). In addition, submaximal testing is appropriate for patients with a high probability of serious arrhythmias. The testing end points for submaximal testing have traditionally been arbitrary but should always be based on clinical judgment. A heart rate limit of 140 beats/min and a MET level of 7 are often used for patients younger than 40 years of age, and a limit of 130 beats/min and a MET level of 5 are often used for patients older than 40 years. For patients taking β-blockers, a Borg rating of perceived exertion level in the range of 7 to 8 (1-10 scale) or 15 to 16 (6-20 scale) is a conservative end point. The initial onset of symptoms, including fatigue, shortness of breath, or angina, is also an indication to stop the test. A low-level protocol should be used, that is, one that uses no more than 1 MET increment per stage.

Electrocardiographic Monitoring

The electrocardiographic response is the diagnostic cornerstone of the clinical exercise test. Thus, reliable test interpretation and patient safety mandate a high-quality exercise electrocardiogram.

Critical to obtaining a high-quality electrocardiogram tracing are proper skin preparation and precise electrode placement. The Mason–Likar limb lead placement is the standard configuration clinically because it provides a 12-lead electrocardiogram with less artifact and less restriction to movement than the standard limb placement (29). However, the Mason–Likar placement can result in differences in electrocardiographic amplitude and axis compared with the standard limb placement. Because these shifts may be misinterpreted as diagnostic changes, it is often recommended that a resting supine electrocardiogram be recorded using the standard limb lead placement.

Position changes may alter the electrocardiogram. For this reason, diagnostic ST-segment changes should always be made relative to the resting baseline position (i.e., upright rather than supine for treadmill and cycle ergometry).

Interpretation of Exercise Test Responses

The important exercise test responses that should be monitored and recorded are heart rate, blood pressure, electrocardiographic changes, exercise capacity, and subjective responses, including chest discomfort, undue fatigue, shortness of breath, leg pain, and rating of perceived exertion. Each of these responses should be described in a comprehensive test report. Useful programs have been developed that automatically summarize the test responses and apply published regression equations that report pretest and posttest risks of coronary disease, and some of these programs provide mortality estimates (12).

Heart Rate

Heart rate increases linearly with oxygen uptake during exercise. Of the two major components of cardiac output, heart rate and stroke volume, heart rate is responsible for most of the increase in cardiac output during exercise, particularly at higher levels. Thus, maximal heart rate achieved is a major determinant of exercise capacity. The inability to appropriately increase heart rate during exercise (chronotropic incompetence) has been associated with the presence of heart disease and a worse prognosis (13, 25). Although maximal heart rate has been difficult to explain physiologically, it is affected by age, gender, health, type of exercise, body position, blood volume, and environment (17). Of these factors, age is the most important. There is an inverse relationship between maximal heart rate and age, with correlation coefficients typically in the order of –.40. However, the scatter around the regression line is quite large, with standard deviations ranging from 10 to 15 beats/min (figure 8.1). Thus, age-predicted target maximal heart rate is a limited measurement for clinical purposes and should not be used as an end point for exercise testing (1, 2, 13, 15).

Blood Pressure

Assessment of systolic and diastolic blood pressure at rest and during the exercise test is important to ensure safety and can provide important diagnostic and prognostic information. Properly trained personnel

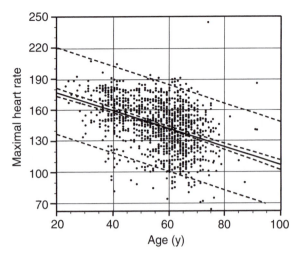

FIGURE 8.1 Relationship between maximal heart rate and age among patients referred for exercise testing. Inner lines represent the standard error; outer lines represent 95% confidence limits.

This figure was published in *Journal of American College of Cardiology*, Vol. 22, Morris et al., "Nomogram based on metabolic equivalents and age for assessing aerobic exercise capacity in men," pgs. 175-182. Copyright Elsevier 1994.

can obtain accurate and reliable blood pressures using noninvasive ausculatory techniques, and guidelines have been developed for this purpose (20). Blood pressure should be measured at rest before the test in both the supine and standing positions. Resting blood pressure, when measured before an exercise test, may be elevated compared with normal resting conditions because of pretest anxiety. Uncontrolled hypertension is a relative contraindication to exercise testing (1, 2, 15). However, if blood pressure is elevated because of anxiety, it is not uncommon or of concern to observe a slight decrease in blood pressure during the initial stage of an exercise test when the workload is light.

The increase in systolic blood pressure during exercise reflects the inotropic reserve of the left ventricle as well as the dynamic matching between changes in cardiac output and peripheral vascular control. Therefore, an abnormal systolic blood pressure response to exercise (either an excessive increase or a failure to increase appropriately) reflects an impairment in the matching between cardiac output and peripheral vascular function. Systolic and diastolic blood pressure should be assessed during the last minute of each exercise stage and more frequently if hypotensive or hypertensive responses are observed. Normally, systolic blood pressure increases in parallel with an increase in work rate, and it is not uncommon in healthy people to exceed 200 mmHg. A systolic blood pressure greater than 250 mmHg is an indication to terminate the exercise test (1, 2, 15). Diastolic pressure normally stays the same or increases slightly during exercise. The fifth Korotkov sound, however, can frequently be heard all

the way to zero in a young, healthy person. A diastolic blood pressure exceeding 115 mmHg is an indication to terminate the exercise test. A decrease in systolic blood pressure with progressive exercise suggests that cardiac output is unable to increase in accordance with the work rate and usually reflects severe ischemia. If systolic blood pressure appears to decrease the clinician should remeasure it immediately, and if the drop is confirmed, the test should be terminated. The clinical consequences of abnormal blood pressure responses to exercise range from modest to severe; for the latter, decreases in systolic blood pressure have been associated with ventricular fibrillation (1, 10, 15). Some investigators have observed that systolic blood pressure must drop below the standing resting value to be prognostically meaningful, whereas others have suggested that more modest decreases, in the order of 10 to 20 mmHg, are associated with severe ischemia, left ventricular impairment, a high incidence of future cardiac events, or all three (13).

Exercise Capacity

Exercise capacity has implications concerning the efficacy of current therapies, the assessment of disability, and risk stratification. A patient's exercise capacity says a great deal about overall cardiovascular health. The most accurate method of measuring exercise capacity is by using ventilatory gas exchange techniques, but this requires specialized equipment and is not available in many clinical laboratories. Thus, exercise capacity is usually expressed as exercise duration, watts achieved (on a bicycle ergometer), maximal exercise stage, or METs. In the absence of gas exchange techniques, it is preferable to express exercise capacity in METs rather than exercise time. This is because a MET value can be ascribed to any speed and grade on a treadmill or workload achieved on a cycle ergometer, so exercise capacity can be compared uniformly between protocols.

As mentioned previously in the discussion on protocols, there can be a great deal of uncertainty in predicting a person's energy cost from the treadmill or cycle ergometer workload. How accurately a MET level predicts a person's true oxygen uptake depends on several factors. For most patients with cardiovascular or pulmonary disease, there is a substantial overprediction of the MET level (1, 2, 33). The error associated with this prediction is accentuated when rapidly incremented protocols are used, when patients are unaccustomed to walking on a treadmill or pedaling a cycle ergometer, and when patients are allowed to use handrail support.

Exercise capacity should be expressed as both an absolute value and a relative percentage of normal for age and gender. The latter can be important because exercise capacity declines with increasing age and higher values are observed in men. Thus, when measuring or estimating oxygen uptake, the clinician should have reference values for comparison. Normal reference values can facilitate communication with patients and between physicians regarding levels of exercise capacity in relation to a given patient's peers. Numerous regression equations are available to determine normal reference values, but all of these are population specific. Numerous factors affect a person's exercise tolerance in addition to age and gender, including height, weight, body composition, activity status, smoking history, heart disease, and medications, and the mode of exercise used has an influence as well (1, 2, 33).

Electrocardiographic Responses

Exercise can cause an imbalance between myocardial oxygen supply and demand in patients with CAD, resulting in ST depression; this is the cornerstone of the exercise test clinically. Since electrocardiographic changes were first associated with myocardial ischemia in the 1920s, the diagnostic ECG criteria and leads that exhibit abnormalities during exercise have been the source of significant debate. Numerous ECG criteria, including complex mathematical constructs, combined scores, and ST areas during exercise and recovery, have been proposed to optimally diagnose the presence of CAD. Some of these are illustrated in figure 8.2. Few of these studies, however, have followed accepted rules for evaluating a diagnostic test (40). Exercise testing guidelines have continued to recommend the application of 1.0 mm or greater ST-segment depression that is horizontal or downsloping 60 to 80 ms after the J-point to represent a positive response. ST-segment depression greater than 1.0 mm that is downsloping is generally indicative of more severe CAD. Most (approximately 80-90%) ischemic ST changes occur in the lateral precordial leads (13, 15).

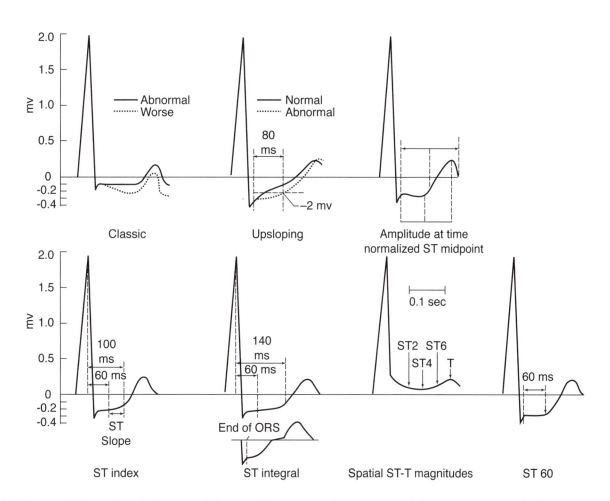

FIGURE 8.2 Normal and abnormal ST-segment responses to exercise and the various criteria for ST-segment depression.

The significance of exercise-induced ST-segment elevation depends on the presence or absence of Q waves. When ST elevation occurs in the presence of a normal resting electrocardiogram, it usually indicates severe transmural ischemia, it can be arrhythmogenic, and it localizes the ischemia. Conversely, exercise-induced ST-segment elevation occurring in leads with Q waves is more common and is related to the presence of dyskinetic areas. This response is relatively common in patients after an MI and is of much less concern. Examples of these two responses are illustrated in figure 8.3.

Several important nuances are involved in the proper measurement of exercise-induced ST-segment changes. ST-segment depression is measured as a change from the isoelectric line (PR segment) and is considered abnormal if the next 60 to 80 ms after the J-point is flat or downsloping. However, in patients who exhibit ST-segment depression at rest, exercise-induced ST depression is measured from the baseline (resting) level. In contrast, ST-segment elevation is measured from the level at which the ST segment starts, and slope is not considered. Examples of these are illustrated

in figure 8.4. The significance of upsloping or horizontal ST-segment depression with T-wave inversion has been debated. Infarction, ventricular aneurysm, bundle-branch block, hypokalemia, ventricular hypertrophy, abnormal oxygen-carrying capacity of blood attributable to anemia, pulmonary disease, and drugs such as digoxin and quinidine may all influence the ST-segment response; these and other conditions may cause exercise-induced ST-segment depression that is not attributable to CAD (see section on False-Positive and False-Negative Responses).

Arrhythmias During Exercise Testing

Arrhythmias can occur during the exercise test or recovery period and can range in severity from life-threatening to benign. There has been a great deal of debate about the importance of arrhythmias during exercise. The occurrence of serious arrhythmias during exercise, although rare, is an indication to terminate the exercise test. Arrhythmias may be overt, such as ventricular tachycardia, or more subtle, such as unifocal premature ventricular complexes (PVCs) increasing in

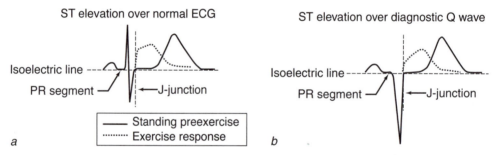

FIGURE 8.3 Example of exercise-induced ST-segment elevation when (a) the resting electrocardiogram is normal and (b) the resting electrocardiograph (ECG) has a diagnostic Q wave.

Reprinted from *Exercise and the Heart*, 5th ed., V.F. Froelicher and J. Myers, pg. 139, Copyright Elsevier 2006.

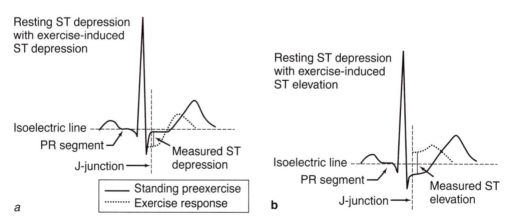

FIGURE 8.4 Example of how exercise-induced ST-segment (a) depression and (b) elevation are measured when the electrocardiogram shows ST depression at rest.

Reprinted from *Exercise and the Heart*, 5th ed., V.F. Froelicher and J. Myers, pg. 148, Copyright Elsevier 2006.

frequency or a period of supraventricular tachycardia. Arrhythmias for which there should be no debate about stopping the test include second- or third-degree heart block and ventricular tachycardia of any duration. Other arrhythmias that have been generally classified as significant or complex include R-on-T PVCs, frequent unifocal or multifocal PVCs (constituting 30% or more of the total heart beats), and coupling of PVCs (1, 5, 15). On rare occasion, any of these complex arrhythmias can be a precursor to a life-threatening sustained rhythm disturbance. When there is doubt as to the nature or origin of the arrhythmia, the test should be stopped.

The prognostic significance of exercise-induced PVCs, even when they occur frequently, has varied widely in the literature. This variation is most likely attributable to differences in how exercise-induced arrhythmias have been defined. Some studies have demonstrated that the occurrence of PVCs during an exercise test has minimal prognostic impact and should be interpreted in the context of "the company they keep" (e.g., considering the patient's history and hemodynamic stability and whether the arrhythmias are accompanied by symptoms during the test). Other studies have shown a clear association between PVCs that occurred during exercise, recovery, or both and increased mortality (1, 5, 10, 15). Short runs (approximately 3 beats) of ventricular tachycardia are not associated with increased mortality, whereas ventricular fibrillation and ventricular tachycardia carry a worse prognosis when they occur in either an apparently healthy person or those undergoing exercise testing for clinical indications (5).

Subjective Responses

Assessment of symptoms and perception of effort during the exercise test is important not only to maximize safety but also to provide valuable diagnostic information. Accurately assessing subjective measures during the exercise test requires the clinician to tell the patient what is expected of him or her and how to communicate these responses during the test. Angina and dyspnea are the most common cardiopulmonary symptoms elicited during exercise, and each is typically evaluated using a 4-point scale (table 8.1). Patients should be encouraged to report all symptoms during exercise (1, 35).

Clinicians must be able to distinguish between typical and atypical angina because they have quite different diagnostic implications. Typical angina tends to be consistent in its presentation and location (and is substernal), is brought on by physical or emotional

TABLE 8.1 Angina and Dyspnea Scales

Grade	Description of symptoms
ANGINA SCALE	
1	Onset of discomfort
2	Moderate, bothersome
3	Moderately severe*
4	Severe; most pain ever experienced
DYSPNEA SCALE	
1	Mild, noticeable to patient but not observer
2	Mild, some difficulty, noticeable to observer
3	Moderate difficulty but can continue
4	Severe difficulty, patient cannot continue

*Level at which patient would stop normal activities, take a sublingual nitroglycerin pill, or both.

stress, and is relieved by rest or nitroglycerin. Atypical angina presents as pain that has a location other than substernal, a prolonged duration, or inconsistent precipitating factors that are unresponsive to nitroglycerin. Exercise-induced chest discomfort that has the characteristics of stable, typical angina provides better confirmation of the presence of significant CAD than any other test response. A middle-aged male exhibiting the combination of typical angina and an abnormal ST response has a 98% probability of having significant CAD. An important indication to stop the exercise test is moderately severe angina (level 3 on a scale of 1-4; table 8.1), which should correspond with pain that would normally cause the patient to stop daily activities or take a sublingual nitroglycerin pill (1, 35).

Dyspnea may be the predominant symptom in some patients with CAD, but it is more often associated with reduced left ventricular function or chronic obstructive pulmonary disease. In both conditions, dyspnea may be the predominant factor causing poor exercise capacity. Dyspnea is also commonly quantified using a scale of 1 to 4 (table 8.1). Claudication is indicative of peripheral vascular disease. If peripheral vascular disease is known or suspected, pretest determination of the presence and strength of peripheral pulses should be made so that posttest comparisons are possible. Leg fatigue not related to claudication is often experienced at maximum exercise; a careful distinction should be made between these two symptoms.

Dizziness and lightheadedness commonly occur as a result of hyperventilation, but on rare occasions these symptoms may also reflect cerebral hypoxia that coincides with a feeling of exhaustion at maximum exercise. Lightheadedness can also be a sign of left ventricular dysfunction or hypotension. Dizziness may be accompanied by signs of gray or ashen pallor, diaphoresis, ataxic gait, dyspnea, and strained appearance as blood is shunted to the exercising muscles. Trained observers should be able to recognize these responses and determine when the test should be stopped.

Testing End Points

The usual goal of the exercise test in patients with known or suspected disease is to achieve a maximal level of exertion. This permits the greatest information yield from the test. However, achieving a maximal effort should be superseded by any of the clinical indications to stop the test (see Indications for Stopping an Exercise Test below), by clinical judgment, or by the patient's request to stop. The reason for stopping the test should be carefully recorded, because the symptoms or signs manifested by exercise often relate to the mechanism of impairment.

Determining the end point of an exercise test can be problematic. It requires integration of objective physiologic responses and termination criteria with subjective judgment based on clinical experience. Some patients may be unable or unwilling to exercise to an adequate level. In patients with suspected coronary disease, a symptom-limited, maximal test is usually more diagnostic. Thus, patients should be instructed to exercise to the point at which they can no longer continue because of fatigue, dyspnea, or other symptoms. Inability to fully monitor the patient's responses

■ Indications for Stopping an Exercise Test

Absolute

- Decrease in systolic blood pressure of >10 mmHg from baseline despite an increase in workload, when accompanied by other evidence of ischemia
- Moderate to severe angina
- Increasing nervous system symptoms (e.g., ataxia, dizziness, or syncope)
- Signs of poor perfusion (cyanosis or pallor)
- Technical difficulties in monitoring electrocardiogram or systolic blood pressure
- Subject's desire to stop
- Sustained ventricular tachycardia
- ST elevation ($\geq$1.0 mm) in leads without diagnostic Q waves (other than V_1 or aVR)

Relative

- Decrease in systolic blood pressure $\geq$10 mmHg from baseline blood pressure despite an increase in workload, in the absence of other evidence of ischemia

- ST or QRS changes such as excessive ST-segment depression (>2 mm of horizontal or downsloping ST-segment depression) or marked axis shift
- Arrhythmias other than sustained ventricular tachycardia, including multifocal PVCs, triplets of PVCs, supraventricular tachycardia, heart block, or bradyarrhythmias
- Fatigue, shortness of breath, wheezing, leg cramps, or claudication
- Development of bundle-branch block or intraventricular conduction delay that cannot be distinguished from ventricular tachycardia
- Increasing chest pain
- Hypertensive response (In the absence of definitive evidence, the ACC/AHA Committee on Exercise Testing suggests systolic blood pressure of >250 mmHg or a diastolic blood pressure of 115 mmHg.)

because of technical difficulties should result in immediate termination of the test.

Although many efforts have been made to objectify maximal effort, such as age-predicted maximal heart rate, a plateau in oxygen uptake, exceeding the ventilatory threshold, or a respiratory exchange ratio greater than unity, all have considerable measurement error and intersubject variability (15, 33). This variability occurs regardless of the population tested. The 95% confidence limits for maximal heart rate based on age, for example, range considerably (see figure 8.1 on page 72); therefore, this end point is maximal for some and submaximal for others (13, 15). The classic index of cardiopulmonary limits, a plateau in oxygen uptake, is not observed in many patients, is poorly reproducible, and has been confused by the many different criteria applied (33, 37, 39). Although subjective, the Borg rating of perceived exertion scale (figure 8.5) is helpful for assessing exercise effort (6). Good judgment on the part of the physician remains the most effective criterion for terminating exercise.

Recovery Period

Some debate exists as to whether the postexercise recovery period should be an active or passive process. This decision should be made based on the purpose of the exercise test. If the test is performed for diagnostic purposes, it appears to be of value to place the patient in the supine position immediately after stopping exercise.

6	No exertion at all
7	
8	Extremely light
9	Very light
10	
11	Light
12	
13	Somewhat hard
14	
15	Hard (heavy)
16	
17	Very hard
18	
19	Extremely hard
20	Maximal exertion

Borg RPE scale
© Gunnar Borg, 1970, 1985, 1994, 1998

FIGURE 8.5 The Borg rating of perceived exertion scale.

Reprinted, by permission, from G. Borg, 1998, *Borg's perceived exertion and pain scales* (Champaign, IL: Human Kinetics), 47.

The increase in venous return observed in the supine position results in increases in ventricular volume, wall stress, and consequently myocardial oxygen demand. Several studies have shown that ST-segment abnormalities are enhanced in the supine position and that an active recovery may attenuate the magnitude of these changes (13, 15, 24). Once thought to be false-positive responses, ST-segment changes 2 to 4 min into recovery are now known to be particularly important for the detection of ischemia. Patients with symptom-limiting angina or dyspnea may become more uncomfortable in the supine position and should recover in a seated upright or semirecumbent position. If the test is performed for nondiagnostic purposes such as for a fitness evaluation in a healthy or athletic person, an active recovery is usually safer and more comfortable. Regardless of the method of recovery, patients should be monitored for at least 6 to 8 min postexercise. The recovery period should be extended as long as necessary to resolve symptoms and stabilize hemodynamic and electrocardiographic responses.

Assessment of Test Accuracy

All diagnostic tests misclassify patients a certain percentage of the time. In the context of the exercise test, this is not a trivial issue, because people who are inaccurately identified as having disease may be subjected unnecessarily to invasive and costly procedures. When the test is performed properly, it identifies those who should or should not undergo these additional procedures. On the other hand, a patient with significant CAD who is incorrectly classified as normal may not receive appropriate medical therapy. How accurately the exercise test distinguishes those with disease from those without disease depends on the population tested, the definition of disease, and the criteria used for an abnormal test.

The common terms used to describe test accuracy are *sensitivity* and *specificity*. Sensitivity is the percentage of times a test correctly identifies those with CAD. Specificity is the percentage of times a test correctly identifies those without cardiovascular disease. Sensitivity and specificity are inversely related and are affected by the choice of discriminant value for abnormal, the definition of disease, and, most important, the prevalence of disease in the population tested. Although prevalence of disease in the population tested will not *increase* sensitivity, it will increase the predictive value of a positive response (i.e., the test accuracy).

Meta-analysis of the exercise testing literature indicates that the exercise test has, on average, a sensitivity of approximately 68% and a specificity of approximately 77% (14). However, these values range widely in the various studies; sensitivity can be as low as 40% among patients with single-vessel disease but greater than 90% among those with triple-vessel disease. Conversely, the specificity of the test is usually quite low (i.e., 50-60%) in patients who have more severe CAD but is quite high in populations that are relatively healthy. These values and the inverse relationship between sensitivity and specificity underscore the importance of considering the patient's pretest characteristics (chest pain and CAD risk factors) before beginning the test. No test result can be interpreted accurately without considering the patient in the context of his or her pretest characteristics.

Another important term that helps define the diagnostic value of a test is the *predictive value*. The predictive value of an abnormal test (positive predictive value) is the percentage of individuals with an abnormal test result who have disease. Conversely, the predictive value of a normal test (negative predictive value) is the percentage of individuals with a normal test result who do not have disease. The predictive value of a test cannot be determined directly from the sensitivity and specificity but is strongly associated with the prevalence of disease in the population tested. The calculations used to determine sensitivity, specificity, and predictive value are presented in table 8.2.

False-Positive and False-Negative Responses

The factors associated with false-positive or false-negative responses should also be considered before the test. A false-positive response is defined as an abnormal exercise test response in a person *without* significant heart disease and decreases the specificity of the test. A false-negative response occurs when the test is normal in a person *with* disease and decreases the sensitivity of the test. Factors associated with false-positive and false-negative responses are listed in Causes of False-Positive and False-Negative Test Results below. In people whom the probability of a false-positive or

---

■ **Causes of False-Positive and False-Negative Test Results**

False-Positive

- Resting repolarization abnormalities (e.g., left bundle-branch block)
- Accelerated conduction defects (e.g., Wolfe–Parkinson–White syndrome)
- Cardiac hypertrophy
- Digoxin
- Nonischemic cardiomyopathy
- Hypokalemia
- Vasoregulatory abnormalities
- Mitral valve prolapse
- Pericardial disease
- Coronary spasm in absence of coronary artery disease
- Anemia
- Female gender

False-Negative

- Failure to reach ischemic threshold secondary to medications (e.g., β-blockers)
- Monitoring an insufficient number of leads to detect electrocardiographic changes
- Angiographically significant disease compensated by collateral circulation
- Musculoskeletal limitations preceding cardiac abnormalities

---

TABLE 8.2 **Terms Used to Demonstrate the Diagnostic Value of a Test**

Term	Calculation
Sensitivity	(TP/TP + FN) × 100
Specificity	(TN/TN + FP) × 100
Positive predictive value	(TP/TP + FP) × 100
Negative predictive value	(TN/TN + FN) × 100

TP = true positives, those with abnormal test results and with disease; FN = false-negatives, those with normal test results with disease; FP = false-positives, those with abnormal test results and no disease; TN = true negatives, those with normal test results and no disease.

false-negative test is high, an alternative procedure (exercise or pharmacologic echocardiogram or radionuclide test) may be appropriate.

Application of the Exercise Test for Estimating Prognosis

The exercise test has been shown to be of value for estimating prognosis in patients with a wide range of severity of cardiovascular diseases (8, 13, 15, 25, 27). One of the most important clinical applications of the exercise test is to identify low-risk patients in whom catheterization (and revascularization) can be safely deferred. There are several reasons why accurately establishing prognosis is important. An estimate of prognosis indicates the probable outcome of a person's illness, which may be useful to the patient in planning return to work or making decisions regarding disability, recreational activities, and finances. A second reason to estimate prognosis is to identify patients for whom interventions might improve outcome. Combining clinical and exercise test information into scores has been shown to improve the estimation risk among men and women undergoing exercise testing (4, 8, 13, 15, 27).

Although many exercise test variables are valuable for estimating prognosis, including exercise capacity, maximal heart rate, a hypotensive response, ST depression, and symptoms, the most powerful predictor of risk appears to be exercise capacity. Recent studies from Duke University, the Mayo Clinic, the Cleveland Clinic, the Veterans Administration, and elsewhere have confirmed the value of including exercise capacity in the risk paradigm among patients referred for exercise testing (13). It has also been recently demonstrated that both an impaired heart rate response to an exercise test (termed *chronotropic incompetence)* and an impaired (slowed) heart rate in recovery from exercise are powerful factors in estimating prognosis (25).

Multivariate Scores for Diagnosis and Prognosis

Improved exercise test characteristics can be obtained by considering the many pretest variables associated with risk along with exercise responses in addition to the ST response. Validated statistical techniques that select, weigh, and combine variables to provide the best possible test accuracy have been used for many years in various areas of medicine, but recently there has been particular interest in applying these techniques, in the form of scores, to exercise testing. The use of scores has improved diagnostic and prognostic accuracy of the exercise test, and the AHA guidelines now recommend using these scores to improve test accuracy. The most widely used approach is the Duke score (24, 27). Although the Duke score was originally developed for prognosis, it has diagnostic applications as well. Other simplified scores have been derived from multivariate equations to determine the probability of disease and prognosis and have been validated in men and women and in different populations (4, 13). Recent studies have shown that multivariate scores perform as well for diagnosis of CAD as the best of the imaging technologies (4, 15).

Ancillary Methods for the Detection of Coronary Artery Disease

Several ancillary imaging techniques provide a valuable complement to exercise electrocardiography for the evaluation of patients with known or suspected CAD. These techniques are particularly helpful among patients with equivocal exercise ECGs or those likely to exhibit false-positive or false-negative responses. These techniques are frequently used to clarify abnormal ST-segment responses in asymptomatic individuals, those in whom the cause of chest discomfort remains uncertain, or those who cannot perform exercise. Combining exercise electrocardiography and an imaging technique when testing patients with an intermediate probability for CAD enhances diagnostic and prognostic accuracy (22, 23). The major imaging procedures are myocardial perfusion studies using radionuclides and exercise echocardiography. Inducing stress with pharmacologic agents can be used with echocardiography and nuclear perfusion for patients unable to exercise.

Myocardial Perfusion Imaging

The first radioactive substance to evaluate myocardial perfusion was thallium-201, an isotope of potassium. Like potassium, thallium-201 is taken up by viable tissue. It is injected intravenously at maximal exercise, and serial images are recorded using a scintillation camera. If a defect in the myocardium is noted immediately after exercise that fills in later, ischemia is present. If the defect remains, scar is present. Thallium emits X rays, has a limited shelf life, and must be obtained from a nuclear reactor. Technetium-99m ($_{99m}$TC) is an isotope with different, more convenient attributes, but it must be tagged to active substances for imaging. At one time, ventricular function studies were performed with $_{99m}$TC tagged to the patient's own red cells and gated to image the blood in the heart; it was also tagged $_{99m}$TC to pyrophosphate for myocardial infarct imaging. However, its most common use in cardiology currently is by tagging to a class of compounds called isonitriles. These are large enough to lodge in myocardial capillaries and permit imaging of the heart. They require two injections at separate times, once at rest and again during exercise, because they do not wash out quickly. When these tagged agents are injected intravenously at maximal exercise, they are rapidly extracted from the blood by living cells in the myocardium. Radiologic images are then taken, which reveal areas of absent, poor, or moderately poor uptake of the radionuclide. When exercise images are compared with rest images, the differences in uptake indicate areas of decreased blood flow. If areas absent of uptake are observed at rest, it can be assumed that this represents areas of myocardial scarring and not ischemia with exercise. This information, along with the exercise test, can be definitive in determining of the extent and localization of ischemia.

Sestamibi is the preferred radiopharmaceutical for obtaining tomographic images of the heart using single-photon emission computed tomography (SPECT). SPECT images are obtained with a gamma camera, which rotates 180° around the patient, stopping at preset angles to record the image. Cardiac images are then displayed in slices from three different axes to allow visualization of the heart in three dimensions. Thus, multiple myocardial segments can be viewed individually, without the overlap of segments that occurs with planar imaging. In addition, ECG gating allows for an estimation of ejection fraction.

An extensive review of the literature reported that the average sensitivity and specificity of exercise scintigraphic imaging for detecting coronary disease were 84% and 87%, respectively (23). Nuclear perfusion imaging is especially helpful in patients with equivocal exercise electrocardiograms, those taking digoxin, or those with left bundle-branch block or more than 1 mm of resting ST depression, in whom the interpretation of ST changes is problematic (13, 15, 22).

The limitations of nuclear imaging include their higher cost, the need for injections, and exposure of the patient to ionizing radiation. Additional equipment and personnel are also required for image acquisition and interpretation, including a nuclear technician to administer the radioactive isotope and acquire the images, the personnel and equipment to handle radioactive substances, and a physician trained in nuclear medicine to reconstruct and interpret the images.

Exercise Echocardiographic Imaging

Echocardiographic imaging of the heart is being used increasingly with either exercise or pharmacologic stress. Typically, a resting two-dimensional image is taken, and repeat images are obtained at peak exercise or immediately afterward. Rest and stress images are compared side by side in a cine-loop display that is gated during systole from the QRS complex. Myocardial contractility normally increases with exercise, whereas ischemia causes hypokinesis, akinesis, and dyskinesis of the affected segments. Therefore, a test is considered positive if wall motion abnormalities develop in previously normal territories with exercise or worsen in an already abnormal segment.

Some advantages of exercise echocardiography over nuclear imaging include the absence of exposure to ionizing radiation and a shorter amount of time required for testing and interpretation. Like other techniques, echocardiography has a diagnostic accuracy that depends primarily on the methodology used and the pretest probability of CAD in the subjects tested. The accuracy of echocardiographic testing also depends on observer experience. Reviews of studies published since the advent of exercise echocardiography in the early 1980s suggest that the average sensitivity and specificity of this technique for detecting coronary disease are both approximately 85% (3). The limitations of exercise echocardiography include dependence on the operator for obtaining adequate, timely images and variation in image interpretation. In addition, as many as 20% of patients have inadequate echocardiographic windows secondary to body habitus or lung interference.

Pharmacologic Stress Techniques

Pharmacologic stress is appropriate for patients who are unable to exercise on a treadmill or cycle ergometer to an adequate level. These include patients who have orthopedic limitations, peripheral vascular disease, and chronic obstructive pulmonary disease or other limiting pulmonary diseases; elderly patients with low functional capacity; diabetic patients with severe neuropathy; and patients with neuromuscular conditions.

Two types of pharmacologic stress agents have been used: those that increase coronary blood flow through coronary vasodilation and those that increase myocardial oxygen demand by increasing heart rate. The commonly used coronary vasodilators are adenosine and dipyridamole (Persantine), whereas dobutamine or arbutamine are used to increase myocardial oxygen demand. The vasodilators dilate normal coronary arteries but not in stenotic segments, causing a steal phenomenon, whereas dobutamine can create an imbalance between myocardial oxygen supply and demand by increasing heart rate and contractility. These drugs are given intravenously and, when used with one of the imaging techniques previously described, can provide important information about coronary artery occlusion. Comparisons between dipyridamole and standard exercise testing have demonstrated them to be comparable diagnostically (42). The disadvantages of dipyridamole and adenosine testing include side effects (40-50% of patients have minor side effects) and lack of cardiovascular response (approximately 10% of patients). Bronchospasm can be a problem in pulmonary patients with Persantine, and ischemia can be induced with the pressor agents.

Ventilatory Gas Exchange Techniques

Because of the inaccuracies associated with estimating oxygen uptake from work rate (i.e., speed and grade on the treadmill or watts on the cycle ergometer), the direct measurement of expired gases is useful in many situations. The measurement of gas exchange and ventilatory responses provides an added dimension to the exercise test by increasing the information obtained concerning a patient's cardiopulmonary function. The direct measurement of $\dot{V}O_2$ has been shown to be more reliable and reproducible than estimated values from treadmill or cycle ergometer work rate (33). Peak $\dot{V}O_2$ is the most accurate measurement of functional capacity and is a useful reflection of overall cardiopulmonary health. Heart and lung diseases frequently manifest themselves through gas exchange abnormalities during exercise, and the information obtained is increasingly used in clinical trials to objectively assess the response to interventions. Moreover, a growing body of literature suggests that exercise capacity and other cardiopulmonary responses (e.g., the slope of increase of ventilation relative to carbon dioxide production) provide superior prognostic information relative to exercise time or estimated METs (32). Situations in which gas exchange measurements are appropriate include the following (1, 2, 15):

- To provide a precise response to a therapeutic intervention for a particular patient
- To address a research question
- To determine the etiology of exercise limitation or dyspnea
- To evaluate exercise capacity in patients with heart failure to estimate prognosis and assess the need for transplantation
- To assist in the development of an appropriate exercise prescription for cardiac rehabilitation

The use of these techniques, however, requires added attention to detail and knowledge of the equipment and basic physiology. This is particularly important given advances in automation for the collection and calculation of cardiopulmonary responses.

Exercise Testing in Special Populations

Although the vast majority of studies on the diagnostic and prognostic performance of the exercise test have been conducted in middle-aged men, the use of the test has expanded across a more diverse spectrum of patients and indications. Clinicians must consider differences in how the test is applied and interpreted in particular populations, such as women, elderly persons, and cardiac transplant recipients.

Women

The interpretation of exercise testing results in women is more challenging than that in men (15, 28). Exercise-induced ST-segment depression is less sensitive among women compared with men (15, 30). Test specificity is also thought to be lower among women, although the reported studies vary widely (15). Some of these differences may be explained by differences in the meaning of chest pain presentation between men and women; although typical angina is as meaningful in women older than 60 years as it is in men, nearly half the women with anginal symptoms in the Coronary Artery Surgery Study (CASS) (who were younger than 65 years) had normal coronary arteries (21). Other possible explanations for the lower test accuracy in women include lower disease prevalence, higher incidence of mitral valve prolapse and syndrome X (chest pain without coronary disease), differences in microvascular function, and hormonal differences (7, 15).

The accuracy of diagnosing CAD in women is improved by the use of multivariate statistics and the addition of nuclear or echocardiographic imaging techniques. When exercise testing is performed in women, factors that may affect test accuracy should be carefully considered; if the exercise test results are uncertain or when otherwise appropriate, a radionuclide imaging procedure should be considered. The optimal strategy for circumventing false-positive test results in women remains to be defined. Nevertheless, AHA–ACC guidelines suggest that there are insufficient data to justify routine radionuclide imaging procedures as the initial test for CAD in women (15).

Elderly Persons

The prevalence of CAD increases with age, and the exercise test can be an extremely useful tool for diagnosing CAD in elderly persons. However, exercise testing in elderly persons can be problematic given their frequently compromised ability to adequately perform exercise. The occurrence of fatigue and lightheadedness attributable to muscle weakness and deconditioning, vasoregulatory abnormalities, and difficulties with gait are important concerns in these patients. Thus, a test modality and protocol should be chosen that provide the highest degree of safety. For instance, cycle ergometry may be more appropriate for elderly patients who have a residual deficit from a cerebral vascular accident. In addition, the testing protocol should be modified considering the expected levels of exercise tolerance. Gradually incremented protocols, such as the Balke, ramp, or Naughton, are usually suitable for elderly patients. Elderly patients are more likely to present with more complex medication regimens, more comorbidities, and increased prevalence of valvular disease, in addition to more severe CAD, compared with younger people. For these reasons, elderly persons require particularly close evaluation before clearance for exercise testing, a modified testing protocol, and particular attention to appropriate end points (15, 28).

Interpretation of the exercise test in elderly persons can also differ significantly from that in younger people. Resting electrocardiographic abnormalities, including prior MI, left ventricular hypertrophy, and intraventricular conduction delays, may compromise the diagnostic accuracy of the exercise test. Nevertheless, the application of standard ST-segment criteria among elderly subjects has been shown to have similar diagnostic characteristics as in younger subjects. No doubt because of the higher prevalence of CAD in elderly persons compared with younger people, test sensitivity is comparatively higher among elderly persons (84%), although specificity is somewhat lower when compared with younger populations (70%) (28).

Transplant Recipients

Over the last 3 decades, transplantation has become a widely used and successful treatment option for patients with end-stage heart failure. The 1-year survival rate for patients who undergo this procedure is now approximately 90%, compared with only 50% to 60% in patients with severe heart failure who receive medical treatment. The hemodynamic response to exercise in patients who have undergone cardiac transplantation has been characterized since the early 1970s. Because the heart is denervated, some intriguing hemodynamic responses are observed (26). The heart is not responsive to the normal actions of the parasympathetic and sympathetic nervous systems. The absence of vagal tone underlies the high resting heart rates in these patients (100-110 beats/min) and the relatively slow adaptation of the heart to a given amount of submaximal work. This slows the delivery of oxygen to the working tissue, contributing to an earlier than normal metabolic acidosis and hyperventilation during exercise. Although transplantation significantly improves the hemodynamic and ventilatory response to exercise, the transplanted patient still exhibits many of the responses typical of the patient with chronic heart failure. These include heightened ventilatory responses attributable to uneven matching of ventilation to perfusion and an increase in physiologic dead space. Maximal heart rate is lower in transplant recipients compared with normal subjects, which contributes to a reduction in cardiac output and peak $\dot{V}O_2$; the arteriovenous oxygen difference widens as a compensatory mechanism.

The exercise test in patients who have undergone cardiac transplantation is less a diagnostic and more a functional tool. In the latter role, the test is useful for assessing and modifying therapy in these patients in addition to evaluating the appropriateness of daily activities and return to work. Although rare cases of chest pain associated with accelerated graft atherosclerosis have been reported in transplant recipients, decentralization of the myocardium usually eliminates anginal symptoms. Exercise electrocardiography is also inadequate in terms of assessing ischemia, as evidenced by its low sensitivity (21% or less) (9). Thus, radionuclide testing may be more useful for assessing ischemia in these patients.

Summary

Although technologies for diagnosing CAD have advanced, the numerous applications and widespread availability of the exercise test make it one of the most important tools in cardiovascular medicine. An understanding of methodology, conduct, indications, and the physiology related to exercise testing is critical to properly applying the information gained from the exercise test to patients with various cardiovascular conditions. In addition to having diagnostic and prognostic applications, this information aids in the assessment of therapy, exercise prescription, and medical and surgical management decisions.

CHAPTER 9

Contemporary Approaches to Cardiovascular Disease Diagnosis

Peter H. Brubaker, PhD

Since the early 20th century, cardiovascular disease (CVD) has been the primary cause of death and disability in the United States. In 2005, nearly 2,600 Americans died from CVD each day, an average of 1 death every 34 s. CVD claims as many lives each year as the next 5 leading causes of death (cancer, chronic respiratory diseases, accidents, diabetes mellitus, and influenza and pneumonia) combined (9). During the past 3 decades, the number of Americans discharged from short-stay hospitals with CVD as the primary diagnosis increased by 30%, and in 2002 CVD ranked highest among all disease categories in hospital discharges. Consequently, in 2005 the estimated direct and indirect cost of CVD was US$393.5 billion (9). Much of the expense associated with CVD is from the plethora of diagnostic procedures available to evaluate CVD conditions. Although there are many established, cost-effective approaches for evaluating and managing CVD conditions, there has also been a rapid increase in the number and complexity of emerging diagnostic procedures whose role and cost-effectiveness have not been established. Consequently, the purpose of this chapter is to describe the process used to determine the presence and severity of CVD and to describe the most widely used diagnostic procedures as well as the emerging technologies for assessing CVD. It is essential that those working in CVD prevention and rehabilitation settings understand the rationale for selecting specific procedures, the information that is generated by each procedure, and the limitations and risks of these procedures.

First Step: History and Physical Examination

Before a clinician can decide which diagnostic procedures to use, he or she must obtain a thorough medical history of the patient. The details of conducting a physical examination lie beyond the scope of this book, but suffice it to say that people working in preventive and rehabilitative exercise must understand the role of the physical examination in evaluating the presence

Address correspondence concerning this chapter to Peter H. Brubaker, Departments of Medicine and Health and Exercise Science, Box 7628, Wake Forest University, Winston-Salem, NC 27109. E-mail: brubaker@wfu.edu of CVD. The key components of the medical history (summarized below) include diagnosis of previous medical conditions, including cardiac procedures; findings from a physical examination; presence of symptoms, particularly those related to the heart (i.e., discomfort, irregular heartbeat); recent illness or hospitalization; orthopedic problems; medication use and drug allergies; other habits (caffeine, alcohol, tobacco, and recreational drug use); exercise and physical activity habits; work history and requirements; and family history of disease. Careful history taking may reveal important clues about the presence of CVD, which may be valuable for making decisions regarding further evaluation and treatment. Determination of the location, type, and

---

▪ Key Components of the Medical History

Diagnosis of cardiovascular disease begins with a review of the patient's medical history and physical examination.

Medical Diagnosis

Cardiovascular Diseases and Conditions

- Coronary artery disease (myocardial infarction, revascularization procedures, angina)
- Valvular heart disease
- Congenital heart defects
- Arrhythmia and conduction defects
- Left ventricular dysfunction (systolic or diastolic heart failure)
- Peripheral and cerebral vascular disease

Noncardiovascular Diseases and Conditions

- Musculoskeletal or orthopedic problems
- Gastrointestinal disorders
- Pulmonary disease
- Metabolic and hematologic disorders
- Renal or hepatic disease
- Cancer
- Pregnancy

Physical Exam and Laboratory Findings

- Height, weight, body mass index, waist circumference
- Blood pressure and pulse rate
- Heart sounds (S1-S4)

- Peripheral pulses (presence of bruits)
- Peripheral or central edema
- Pulmonary findings (i.e., breath sounds and pulmonary function studies)
- Chest X ray
- Electrocardiogram
- Blood and urine glucose
- Blood lipids and lipoproteins

History of Symptoms

- Chest pain or discomfort
- Dyspnea
- Palpitations
- Dizziness, lightheadedness, or fainting (syncope)
- Transient loss of vision or speech
- Numbness and weakness
- Fatigue

Medication, Drug, and Supplement Use

- Cardiovascular and noncardiovascular medications
- Illicit drugs
- Vitamins, herbs

Other

- Family history of cardiovascular, metabolic, and pulmonary diseases
- Lifestyle habits

Adapted, by permission, from P. Brubaker, L. Kaminsky, and M. Whaley, 2002, *Coronary artery disease: essentials of prevention and rehabilitation program* (Champaign, IL: Human Kinetics, Inc.), 58-59.

intensity of pain or discomfort (angina), can accurately diagnose the presence or absence of coronary disease in about 80% of the cases (16). A feeling of pressure in the midchest, neck, shoulders, arms, and upper abdomen associated with or without sweating during physical activity, meals, emotional stress, or cold weather should be considered myocardial ischemia (angina) until ruled out by diagnostic testing.

Myocardial ischemia is not always the cause of chest pain or angina-like symptoms. The differential diagnosis of chest pain is a significant issue in medical management, because failing to recognize myocardial ischemia or infarction could result in disastrous consequences (i.e., death and disability). In contrast, hospitalizing all patients with chest pain can be very costly, not to mention inconvenient to the patient. Many medical centers have created specific chest pain centers to better diagnose and triage patients presenting with these often confusing symptoms. Common noncardiac causes of angina-like symptoms include esophageal disorders (reflux or spasm), biliary or cystic duct obstructions, costosternal syndromes, degenerative changes of the cervical or thoracic vertebrae leading to impingement of nerves or blood vessels, and anxiety disorders (5). A careful history, physical exam, and risk factor assessment can often distinguish these noncardiac conditions from those caused by myocardial ischemia.

A significant number of patients will have "silent" myocardial ischemia or infarction (MI). Population studies have observed that 20% to 60% of patients who had electrocardiographic evidence of a previous myocardial infarction never experienced an anginal symptom (5). Patients with silent myocardial ischemia are of particular concern in the exercise setting, because they do not have an intrinsic mechanism to monitor myocardial ischemia (i.e., they lack symptoms), which may allow them to exercise at levels that provoke myocardial ischemia.

Another important component of the physical exam is cardiac auscultation, which involves using a stethoscope to listen to the sounds made during the phases of the cardiac cycle. Heart sounds are relatively brief, discrete auditory vibrations of varying intensity (loudness), frequency (pitch), and quality (timbre). The first heart sound identifies the onset of ventricular systole, and the second heart sound identifies the onset of diastole. These two auscultatory events establish a framework within which other heart sounds and murmurs can be placed. The basic heart sounds are the first (S1), second (S2), third (S3), and fourth (S4). Although the first and second occur in most people, the third and fourth sounds do not occur in healthy adults. Most other heart sounds, with few exceptions, are abnormal.

A detailed description of heart sounds was provided by the American Heart Association (3).

Evaluating the peripheral pulses is another valuable component of the physical examination and can indicate the presence of atherosclerotic disease in noncoronary vessels. However, vascular disease rarely occurs in an isolated artery but rather usually appears in multiple arterial systems (coronary, cerebral, iliac, and femoral arteries) simultaneously. Systematic bilateral palpation (i.e., feeling with fingers) of the common carotid, brachial, radial, femoral, popliteal, dorsal pedis, and posterior tibial arteries, as well as palpation of the abdominal aorta, should be conducted by a trained clinician on any patient suspected of having CVD. Absent or weak peripheral pulses usually signify obstruction in that artery. When the lumen of the artery is reduced by approximately 50%, a soft bruit can often be auscultated. As the obstruction becomes more severe, the bruit becomes high-pitched, louder, and longer. Bruits in the carotid arteries suggest the presence of cerebrovascular disease and an increased risk for a transient ischemic attack or a cerebrovascular accident. Other important signs and symptoms of cerebrovascular disease include headaches, blurred vision or loss of vision, paralysis of one side of the face or one arm or leg, loss of motor skills, and an inability to speak or express thoughts.

Palpation of leg pulses during the physical exam can indicate the presence of peripheral arterial disease (PAD). Diminished or absent pulse waves in the femoral, popliteal, doral pedis, and posterior tibial arteries generally indicate obstruction in that artery. Blood pressure assessment in the lower limb can also help determine the presence of PAD. Changes to the pulse waves and pressures at these locations in the lower limb may become more obvious during physical exertion. Patients with PAD are likely to describe discomfort (burning or cramping) in the lower extremity, particularly during exertion, that is known as intermittent claudication (from the Latin word *claudicare*, meaning "to limp"). Although commonly used to confirm the presence of PAD, the ankle–brachial index also has potential to provide precise estimates of future risk for CVD events in both high-risk and diseased populations (9).

Acquiring More Information With General Laboratory Tests

Depending on the medical history and outcome of the physical examination, a series of laboratory tests may be indicated to evaluate the presence of CVD, including a chest X ray, 12-lead electrocardiogram (ECG), and blood tests. The chest X ray is used to identify the presence of cardiomegaly (enlarged heart) and evidence of pulmonary edema, both associated with left ventricular dysfunction.

The resting ECG can be used to identify a number of cardiac abnormalities, including acute MI and potentially lethal cardiac arrhythmias. When a patient presents to the hospital or physician's office with signs and symptoms suggestive of CVD, the ECG is routinely used to confirm or rule out an MI. Damage to the myocardial tissue often leads to profound changes on the ECG (i.e., ST-segment elevation in a transmural MI and ST-segment depression in a nontransmural or subendocardial MI). Old or previous MIs may result in abnormal or pathologic Q waves or persistent ST-segment depression. Surprisingly, approximately 50% of patients presenting with acute MI do not exhibit characteristic ECG changes (ST elevation or Q waves) with their myocardial injury (13). Often, patients suffering from an MI will experience ventricular arrhythmias, heart blocks, conduction defects, or bradyarrhythmias that can be detected on the ECG.

In light of the limited diagnostic value of patient symptoms and ECG changes, a great deal of importance is placed on measuring blood serum cardiac enzymes in a patient suspected of having an MI. These markers are used to determine whether heart muscle necrosis versus transient, reversible myocardial ischemia has occurred or whether another noncardiac event has caused the symptoms. Persistent inadequate blood flow to the myocardial tissue disrupts the cardiac cell membrane, which allows the cell constituents, including enzymes, to leak into the extracellular fluid and eventually into the venous blood. Four main enzymes are commonly used to identify myocardial damage (i.e., confirm an MI): aspartate transaminase (AST), lactic dehydrogenase (LDH), creatine kinase (CK), and the creatine kinase-MB (CK-MB) isoenzyme (5). Although three isoenzymes of CK have been identified (MM, BB, and MB), CK-MB is the most reflective of damage to cardiac muscle tissue. When the CK-MB increases to more than 5% of the total CK, the diagnosis of MI is made (13). Clinicians do not rely on measurements of CK or CK-MB at a single point in time but instead evaluate the temporal rise and fall of serially obtained measures. The time course of the common serum cardiac enzymes (LDH, total CK, CK-MB) and the biomarkers myoglobin and troponin I are shown in figure 9.1. Advantages of myoglobin and troponin I include shortened time to diagnosis and greater cardiac specificity, which have important implications in terms of cost containment. Rapidly responding biomarkers

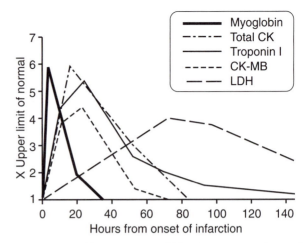

FIGURE 9.1 Time course of blood serum markers of acute myocardial infarction. The figure summarizes the relative timing, rate of increase, peak values, and duration of elevation above the upper limits of normal for traditional markers: lactic dehydrogenase (LDH), total creatine kinase (CK), creatine kinase-MB fraction (CK-MB), and other biomarkers—myoglobin and troponin I.

Reprinted, by permission, from P. Brubaker, L. Kaminsky, and M. Whaley, 2002, *Coronary artery disease: essentials of prevention and rehabilitation program* (Champaign, IL: Human Kinetics, Inc.), 64.

allow for shorter hospital stays for patients in whom MI is eventually ruled out as well as rapid and focused treatment for those confirmed as having an acute MI (5). Surprisingly, among patients admitted to the hospital with a chest pain syndrome, fewer than 20% are subsequently diagnosed with an MI (15).

Another approach to confirm or rule out an MI in patients who present to an emergency room with chest pain is to conduct a low-level graded exercise test (GXT). The GXT, using 12-lead electrocardiography, has been used for more than 30 years to diagnose the presence of coronary disease in nonemergent conditions. Using the GXT in the emergency department is a safe and cost-effective method to manage chest pain syndromes. Critical pathways have been developed that involve emergency department observation and exercise testing for the management of patients with chest pain who are at low risk for heart disease. Application of these pathways, with exercise testing as the first decision step, has been shown to save substantial money: 17% fewer hospital admissions and 11% fewer hospital days were reported on one study (19).

Using More Cardiac-Specific Diagnostic Tests

The information obtained from the patient's medical history, physical examination, laboratory tests, and calculated risk for cardiac events (i.e., Framingham

Risk Score) is considered when determining the need for further and specific diagnostic procedures. (See chapter 2 for further discussion of the Framingham Risk Score.) The number and variety of cardiovascular diagnostic procedures available to the clinician have increased exponentially over the last few decades. The judicious and appropriate use of these tests in evaluating patients for CVD requires a balance of clinical judgment along with a clear understanding of the indications and limitations of each procedure. The cost of the procedure must also be considered. To assist with this often difficult decision-making process, the American College of Cardiology and the American Heart Association have developed practice guidelines that describe a range of generally acceptable approaches for the diagnosis, management, and prevention of cardiovascular disease (1, 2). Diagnosing the presence of CVD usually begins with the least costly and least invasive procedures. Abnormal or inconclusive findings from a procedure lead to the decision to move to the next level of testing. Although each level of diagnostic testing potentially increases the diagnostic accuracy, it also increases the expense. Furthermore, as the testing becomes more invasive, the risk of complications often increases.

Noninvasive Approaches

Evaluating the presence or severity of coronary artery disease and subsequent myocardial ischemia is one of the most important objectives in CVD management.

Myocardial ischemia is simply an imbalance between myocardial oxygen supply and demand. Coronary artery disease leads to epicardial coronary artery stenoses, which can limit coronary flow. Although an obstructive lesion in a coronary artery may not be a problem at rest, when the demand for oxygen is low, any increase in metabolic activity of the myocardial tissue (increased heart rate or blood pressure) will increase the myocardial demand. When the demand for oxygen exceeds the supply to the tissue, ischemia ensues. The temporally related sequence of events leading from myocardial oxygen supply–demand mismatch to the clinical marker of angina has been described as the ischemic cascade (18). As shown in figure 9.2, this cascade of ischemic events progresses from subtle cellular changes (e.g., metabolic abnormalities in tissue) to mechanical changes in ventricular function, including diastolic and systolic dysfunction (inappropriate relaxation and diminished contractile response, respectively); alterations in electrical conduction through the cardiac tissue (e.g., ECG changes); and ultimately overt symptoms (e.g., angina). Numerous diagnostic techniques are available, each designed to identify a specific event in the ischemic cascade. Tests commonly used to detect these ischemic events are described in the following sections. A brief discussion of the traditional diagnostic procedures routinely used in most hospitals and medical offices is provided as well as some discussion, where appropriate, of new procedures and technology being used to evaluate the presence and severity of coronary disease.

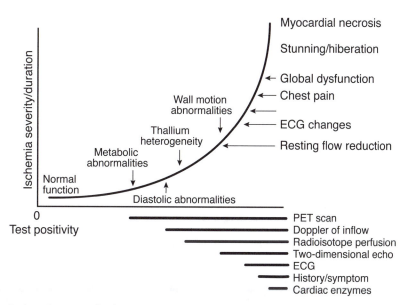

FIGURE 9.2 The ischemic cascade demonstrates the relationship between the severity of myocardial ischemia and the specific diagnostic tests. The earliest metabolic abnormalities associated with myocardial ischemia can be detected with positron emission tomography (PET) scan, whereas other diagnostic tests such as electrocardiography (ECG) do not reveal ischemia until much later.

Exercise stress testing is one of the most widely used tests in cardiology and, when performed appropriately, can yield valuable diagnostic, prognostic, functional, and therapeutic information at a relatively low cost and with minimal risk to the subject (1, 2). Details on exercise stress testing are provided in chapter 8. Although it is widely accepted that exercise provides the best stress to provoke myocardial ischemia, it has been estimated that a significant number (21%) of patients are physically unable perform an exercise test and another 20% fail to achieve adequate levels of exertion (i.e., submaximal or nondiagnostic levels) (16). Patients in these two categories often have orthopedic, neurologic, pulmonary, or peripheral vascular disease or lack adequate motivation. Furthermore, a fairly large number of patients (24%) will have an exercise electrocardiogram that is classified as uninterpretable for myocardial ischemia. Consequently, exercise testing, as a means of provoking and identifying myocardial ischemia, may only be appropriate for 35% of patients referred for diagnostic testing (16). Therefore, pharmacologic stress tests (commonly called nonexercise stress tests) are a reasonable alternative to elicit myocardial ischemia for those who cannot exercise adequately. Myocardial ischemia during a pharmacologic stress test is provoked by coronary artery vasodilation (through administration of intravenous dipyridamole or adenosine) or increasing myocardial oxygen demand (through intravenous dobutamine infusion). Pharmacologic stress testing via either mechanism is generally used in combination with a diagnostic technique other than electrocardiography. The mechanism of action of the vasodilators generally favors their use in combination with myocardial perfusion studies (discussed later). In contrast, the increased myocardial oxygen requirements in response to dobutamine or arbutamine favor their use with echocardiography (also discussed in the sections to follow).

Electrocardiography

The graded exercise test with simultaneous recording of the 12-lead ECG is often the first test used to diagnose the presence of coronary artery disease (CAD), primarily because of the relative safety and low cost of this procedure. Conventional exercise testing uses exercise-induced ST-segment changes on the ECG to identify myocardial ischemia. As discussed in greater detail in chapter 8, exercise testing with ECG measurement alone yields a surprisingly low sensitivity and specificity (68% and 77%, respectively) for detecting CAD (11). The sensitivity of the exercise ECG appears to increase with the number of diseased coronary arteries. In other words, the exercise ECG has only a 40% sensitivity for single-vessel CAD, whereas the sensitivity of this type

of testing improves to nearly 90% when three-vessel CAD is present. Furthermore, inclusion of other clinical variables obtained during the exercise test, including blood pressure response and symptoms, improves the sensitivity of this diagnostic approach. Although the sensitivity for exercise ECG is considerably lower than that of other diagnostic procedures yet to be discussed (particularly in subgroups such as women and recipients of heart transplants), the specificity of this technique is acceptable and is similar to that of other diagnostic procedures. The sensitivity of the exercise ECG can be improved by decreasing the number of false-negative tests, whereas the specificity can be improved by decreasing the number of false-positive tests. The ECG usually is *not* used in combination with a pharmacologic stress test because of the low sensitivity for detecting myocardial ischemia (16).

Echocardiography

Echocardiography refers to a group of tests that use ultrasound to examine the heart and record information in the form of echoes, that is, reflected sonic waves. Ultrasonic waves are generated from a source applied to the chest wall (transthoracic echocardiography) or from within the esophagus (transesophageal echocardiography). The standard echocardiographic examination encompasses M-mode, two-dimensional, conventional, and color-flow Doppler imaging. Additional applications include contrast echocardiography and stress (exercise or pharmacologic) echocardiography. The M-mode is a one-dimensional view of the heart that is useful when determining chamber dimensions, wall thickness, and valve movement. Two-dimensional echocardiography can be used to obtain multiple two-dimensional images of the heart and can identify the presence of ischemia by evaluating left ventricular wall motion during systole. Two-dimensional echocardiographic assessments are made before and after exercise or pharmacologic stress (e.g., stress echo). Rest and stress images of left ventricular function are compared side by side in a cine-loop display that is gated during systole from the ECG. Myocardial contractility normally increases with exercise, whereas myocardial ischemia causes hypokinetic, dyskinetic, or akinetic wall motion to develop or worsen in the ischemic segments (1). The sensitivity for detecting a significantly obstructed coronary artery (decrease in the lumen of >50%) is significantly higher with stress echocardiography than exercise electrocardiography (average of 86% vs. 66%, respectively). However, the average specificity of exercise echocardiography, 81%, is only slightly higher than the average exercise ECG specificity, 77% (4). Obtaining this valuable information via echocardiography requires very little additional time and effort during a standard graded exercise test. When used with pharmacologic stress agents (dobutamine and arbutamine are preferred over the vasodilators), echocardiographic images are obtained before and during the drug infusion. Approximately 5% of patients have a poor echocardiographic window because of lung interference (e.g., obstructive pulmonary disease or central obesity). Sonicated contrast agents can sometimes enhance endocardial definitions in these conditions (4).

Whereas M-mode echocardiography and two-dimensional echocardiography create ultrasonic images of the heart, Doppler echocardiography uses ultrasound to record blood flow within the cardiovascular system. Doppler echocardiography can detect changes in left ventricular diastolic function (e.g., filling patterns) that also occur early in the ischemic cascade of events. Recently, tissue Doppler imaging has been used to evaluate velocity of change in myocardial length and is very useful for assessing left ventricular diastolic (i.e., filling) function (10). Color flow Doppler can be used to identify the directional movement of blood within the two-dimensional or M-mode recording and is very helpful for identifying valvular abnormalities such as stenosis and regurgitation. Furthermore, contrast echocardiograms (after intravenous injection of agitated saline solution) can detect cardiac shunts and define chamber dimensions. Finally, echocardiograms that are oriented in a three-dimensional space have become available and are rapidly moving into clinical practice.

Nuclear Perfusion Imaging

The acquisition and display of nuclear images of the heart results from the detection of radiation emitted from the patient following the administration of a radionuclide (also called radioisotope). In nuclear perfusion imaging, the radionuclides are extracted by active myocardial cells but not ischemic or necrotic tissue. Over the past several years, single-photon emission computed tomography (SPECT) has become the preferred imaging technique for nuclear perfusion imaging. With SPECT, a series of planar images are obtained over a 180° arc around the patient's thorax to form several images (short axis, horizontal, and vertical long axis). Myocardial perfusion imaging requires an intravenous injection of a radionuclide that is extracted only by normal cardiac cells. The images of the heart, obtained as described earlier, appear bright (or lit up) in areas that extract the radionuclide but do not light up in areas where myocardial cells are ischemic. Nuclear perfusion imaging yields a sensitivity and specificity of 88% and 62%, respectively, when a clinician is testing for myocardial ischemia (1). Thus, SPECT imaging has

a sensitivity similar to that of stress echocardiography but has a lower specificity, likely associated with a greater occurrence of false-positive tests with nuclear imaging. The limitations of nuclear imaging include exposure to low-level ionizing radiation and the additional equipment and personnel required to conduct these studies.

Positron Emission Tomography

PET scanning, once viewed primarily as a research imaging modality, is becoming an increasingly valuable technique for evaluating coronary disease. PET perfusion imaging studies are recommended to identify myocardial viability (i.e., myocardial tissue that could resume function with improved perfusion secondary to revascularization) in patients with established coronary disease (7). Myocardial blood flow and myocardial viability can be assessed with PET through infusion of [^{18}F]-deoxyglucose or [^{13}N]-ammonia. These tracers provide an index of myocardial cell metabolism and, thus, cell viability. The initial capital cost of approximately US$1 million and the cost of maintaining PET technology have limited its availability. PET imaging may become more common as the clinical indications for this technique increase and as the price for the technology declines.

Computed Tomography

Computed tomography (CT) is a generic term that can apply to several methods used to evaluate cardiovascular diseases. *Electron beam computed tomography* (EBCT) is being used increasingly to screen asymptomatic people and people at high risk for developing coronary artery disease. Although unable to detect myocardial ischemia, this technology is highly sensitive for detecting coronary artery calcium, a measure that appears to be closely related to the degree of coronary atherosclerosis. Although highly promoted in the lay media and relatively inexpensive, EBCT has not produced results superior to other diagnostic procedures and is therefore not recommended for screening asymptomatic or high-risk people (20).

Cardiac CT has recently emerged as a potential alternative to invasive coronary angiography with the development of multislice spiral computed tomography (MSCT), which is able to noninvasively image native coronary vessels as well as bypass grafts (8). One of the difficulties in imaging coronary vessels stems from the constant motion of the heart, but current scanners allow for 64-slice images to be obtained in 10 to 15 s with minimal radiation. With reconstructed images, coronary arteries can be inspected for obstructive lesions, and right and left ventricular function (i.e., ejection fraction) can be determined with good accuracy (e.g., within 10% of magnetic resonance measures) via MSCT. Furthermore, MSCT can provide information regarding wall motion, myocardial infarction–induced wall thinning, and other structures in the chest cavity (aorta, pulmonary arteries and veins, lungs). The drawbacks of MSCT include radiation exposure and use of contrast agents.

Coronary Magnetic Resonance Angiography

Coronary magnetic resonance angiography (MRA) is a noninvasive way to depict major epicardial coronary arteries in most subjects with injection of contrast medium or radiation exposure. Although the spatial resolution of MRA has improved, breathing, cardiac motion, tortuosity, and small vessels make it difficult to accurately determine the severity of coronary stenosis. Most institutions use cardiac magnetic resonance imaging (MRI) for analysis of structure, function, and anatomy of the heart and great vessels but do not routinely use MRA for direct imaging of coronary arteries.

Invasive Diagnostic Procedures

Cardiac catheterization, the procedure used to obtain coronary angiograms (i.e., fluoroscopic images) of the coronary arterial tree, is generally accomplished through the femoral artery. Injection of contrast agents into the coronary artery ostia provides visualization of the coronary vessels and aids in determining the location and severity of any obstructive lesion. Although diagnostic procedures continue to evolve and improve, coronary angiography is the gold standard for evaluating patients with known or suspected coronary artery disease. Although more than 2 million coronary angiograms are made per year in North America alone, this procedure is relatively expensive and carries a relatively high level of risk attributable to the invasiveness of the procedure. Although conventional coronary angiography can indicate the degree and location of fixed coronary artery lesions, it cannot evaluate the nature of the lesion (large lipid core, calcified) or determine the functional consequence (i.e., level of ischemia) caused by this obstruction. Recent technologic advances allow for direct internal visualization of the lumen of the coronary arteries through ultrasonic transducers placed at the tip of the coronary catheter (referred to as *intravascular ultrasound*). A series of tomographic images are obtained as the catheter is slowly pulled back. The transducer provides a 360° cross-sectional picture of the artery and provides excellent images of the arterial wall. These images can be used to better describe the characteristics of the coronary lesion (stable vs.

unstable) and overall plaque burden. Modern devices can perform three-dimensional reconstructions online that provide information about the length, volume, and reference landmarks of plaque (12). Coronary angiography, potentially complemented with intravascular ultrasound, is the final procedure performed when clinicians are considering medical management versus revascularization for patients with obstructive coronary disease.

In addition to coronary angiograms, left ventriculograms are obtained during injection of a larger amount (40-50 ml) of the contrast agent through a catheter that has been advanced into the left ventricle. The left ventriculogram is used to assess systolic and diastolic wall motion, which allows for estimation of the ejection fraction. Furthermore, this technique is used to identify hypokinetic (decreased movement), akinetic (no movement), dyskinetic, or aneurysmal (movement in opposite direction) myocardial segments that can be the result of myocardial ischemia or infarction.

Right heart catheterization can be performed with venous access (usually the femoral vein) to measure pressures within the heart (e.g., pulmonary artery, right atrium, right ventricle, and pulmonary capillary wedge pressures) as well as pressure gradients across the pulmonic semilunar and atrioventricular valves. Blood sampled at various places in the heart can be analyzed for oxygen saturation, a technique helpful in identifying intracardiac shunts that cause mixing of arterial and venous blood. Finally, the cardiac output can be calculated with several different techniques during the right heart catheterization.

Choosing a Diagnostic Procedure

Rapid technological advances and new applications have led to explosive growth in cardiovascular imaging. In the United States, diagnostic imaging services reimbursement increased more rapidly than any other type of physician service from 1999 to 2003 (14). Although these advances present new opportunities for physicians to use noninvasive techniques, these tests are relatively expensive. To help clinicians select an appropriate diagnostic test, the ACC/AHA jointly developed an algorithm to assist with the decision-making process (figure 9.3). Furthermore, the AHA recently produced a scientific statement titled "Role of Noninvasive Testing in the Clinical Evaluation of Women With Suspected Coronary Artery Disease" (17) and a very useful decision-making algorithm specific for women (figure 9.4 and table 9.1).

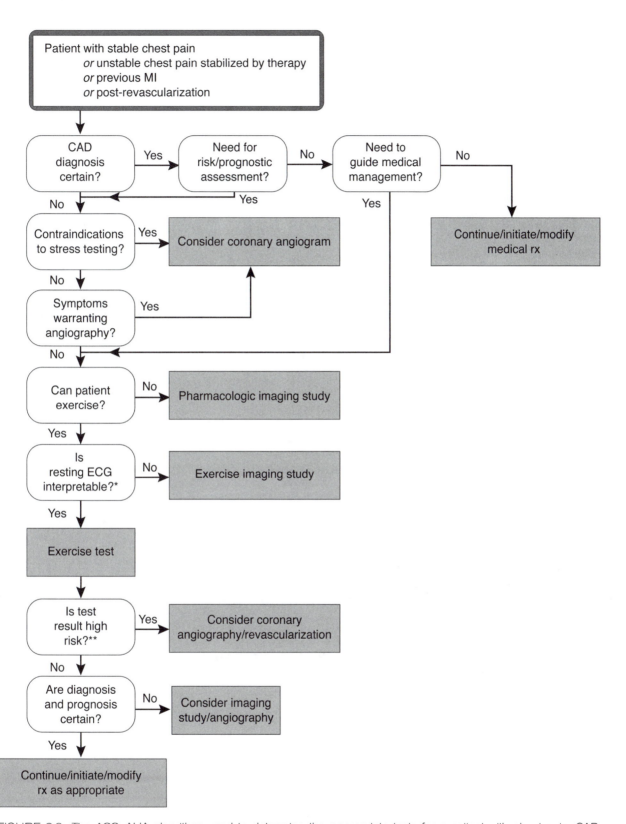

FIGURE 9.3 The ACC–AHA algorithm used to determine the appropriate tests for a patient with chest pain. CAD = coronary artery disease; ECG = electrocardiogram; MI = myocardial infarction; rx = treatment. *Electrocardiogram interpretable unless there is preexcitation, electronically paced rhythm, left bundle-branch block, or resting ST-segment depression >1 mm. **For example, a test is considered high risk if the Duke treadmill score predicts average annual cardiovascular mortality >3%.

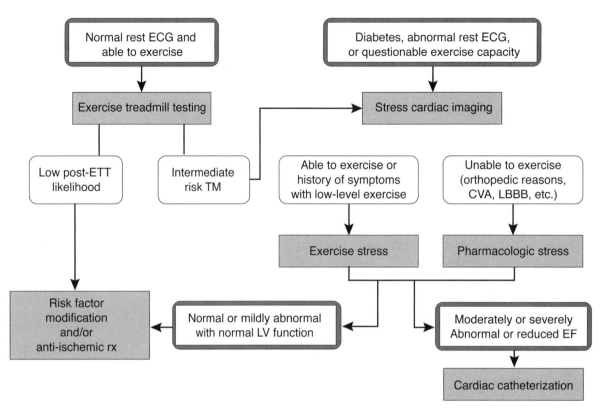

FIGURE 9.4 Algorithm that can be used to evaluate symptomatic (intermediate to high likelihood) women using exercise electrocardiography (ECG) or cardiac imaging. Refer to table 9.1 for determination of high, intermediate, low, and very low likelihood of coronary artery disease. ETT = exercise tolerance test; TM = treadmill; CVA = cerebrovascular accident; LBBB = left bundle-branch block; EF = ejection fraction; LV = left ventricle; rx = treatment.

Reprinted, by permission, from J.H. Mieres et al., 2005, "Role of non-invasion testing in clinical evaluation of women with suspected coronary artery disease," *Circulation* 111: 682-696.

TABLE 9.1 ACC–AHA Practice Guidelines on Exercise Testing: Pretest Probability of Coronary Artery Disease by Age, Sex, and Symptoms

Age, years	Typical or definite angina pectoris	Atypical or probable angina pectoris	Nonanginal chest pain	Asymptomatic
30-39	Intermediate	Very low	Very low	Very low
40-49	Intermediate	Low	Very low	Very low
50-59	Intermediate	Intermediate	Low	Very low
60-69	High	Intermediate	Intermediate	Low
≥70	High	Intermediate	Intermediate	Low

Summary

The diagnosis of coronary disease involves a stepwise, incremental process that begins with a review of the medical history and findings from a physical examination. If the history and physical examination indicate the possibility of coronary disease, the patient should undergo a series of basic laboratory tests, including a 12-lead electrocardiogram, and evaluation of cardiac risk factors. If the patient's risk prediction is high or there is continued suspicion of the presence of CAD, a number of diagnostic procedures can be used to determine the likelihood of CAD. Selection of the appropriate diagnostic procedure from the vast number available can be difficult, and the clinician must consider the patient's safety and comfort, the diagnostic power of the test, and the cost-effectiveness of the procedure. Several organizations including AHA and the ACC (1, 2, 13) have developed algorithms to assist the clinician with this complex process. Furthermore, the AHA believes that development of cardiac imaging modalities must strike a balance between the development of their scientific potential and their premature clinical use (10).

CHAPTER 10

Pharmacologic Management

Nina B. Radford, MD

John S. Ho, MD

Larry W. Gibbons, MD

In the last 2 decades, research has provided a wealth of information about the value of certain drugs and drug combinations in preventing and treating clinical cardiovascular disease. Lifestyle modification is important and can be lifesaving. However, in the management of most cardiovascular diseases, the use of drugs or drug combinations has become the standard of care. Because this literature is vast and constantly changing as new studies emerge, treatment guidelines for various cardiovascular conditions have been created by expert panels to help health care providers establish optimal treatment plans tailored to the needs of their patients. However, patients with cardiovascular disease may have numerous clinical conditions, each with its own treatment guidelines. The patient with heart failure has hypertension and mitral regurgitation (MR). The patient with a coronary stent has elevated cholesterol and claudication. Treatment plans for these patients require that multiple standards of care be met, and often drugs that are useful for one condition also treat another. For example, angiotensin-converting enzyme (ACE) inhibitors can lower blood pressure in the hypertensive patient and prolong life in the normotensive patient with congestive heart failure. The use of antiplatelet agents can reduce the risk of myocardial infarction and stroke in the patient with coronary disease and transient ischemic attack, and there are many other examples.

The goal of this chapter is to bring the drug treatment components of the various guidelines together in a single resource so that when a patient with multiple cardiovascular conditions presents for cardiac rehabilitation, the clinician can quickly ascertain the rationale behind the patient's current drug treatment regimen and identify potential omissions. Why is the hypertensive patient with atrial fibrillation treated with β-blockers? A quick review of the guidelines for the drug treatment of hypertension and atrial fibrillation will provide the clues. When the patient with a 3-month-old paclitaxel-eluting coronary stent asks if she really needs to be on two blood thinners at once (aspirin and clopidogrel), the guidelines for secondary prevention of coronary disease will reveal the answer. An exhaustive review of all cardiovascular conditions

Address correspondence concerning this chapter to Dr. Nina Radford, Cooper Clinic, 12200 Preston Road, Dallas, Texas 75230. E-mail: nbradford@cooper-clinic.com is beyond the scope of this chapter; rather, we focus on the major cardiovascular conditions that are common in sufficiently stable patients referred for or enrolled in cardiac rehabilitation: primary prevention of cardiovascular disease and stroke, secondary prevention for patients with coronary and other atherosclerotic vascular disease, chronic atrial fibrillation, chronic heart failure, and valvular heart disease. While some mention of the mechanics of these drug treatments may be included in this chapter, a more detailed description of drugs used to treat cardiovascular disease (mechanisms of action, dosing, side effects, and cautions) as well as physiological effects of these drugs on exercise performance can be found in the appendixes in pages 347 and 354.

Primary Prevention of Cardiovascular Disease and Stroke

Primary prevention of cardiovascular disease has traditionally referred to the prevention of clinical or symptomatic cardiovascular disease such as myocardial infarction, angina pectoris, or transient ischemic attack. The treatment goals for primary prevention strategies intensify according to whether a patient is characterized as low, moderate, or high risk for the development of clinical cardiovascular disease using algorithms such as the Framingham Risk Score (FRS), which uses information about traditional cardiovascular risk factors. However, with the use of diagnostic imaging tests such as the ultrafast CT scan to measure coronary artery calcification or the use of ultrasound to measure carotid artery intimal–medial wall thickness, many patients are diagnosed with significant atherosclerotic vascular disease long before they develop symptoms. In these patients, the opportunity for true primary prevention of atherosclerosis is well passed; however, modification of cardiovascular risk factors can prevent clinically evident cardiovascular disease. Whether two asymptomatic patients with identical low or intermediate FRS categories ought to be treated similarly if one of them has a coronary artery calcification score of zero and the other a score of 400, or if one has an asymptomatic 50% carotid stenosis and the other does not, is the subject of much debate. As more data become available regarding the impact of aggressive cardiovascular risk factor modification on outcomes in asymptomatic patients who are diagnosed with significant atherosclerosis by various imaging modalities, the distinction between primary and secondary prevention strategies will continue to blur.

Targets for general risk factor interventions for primary prevention of cardiovascular disease and stroke include smoking, hypertension, dyslipidemia, diabetes, overweight and obesity, atherogenic diet, and physical inactivity (11, 14, 15, 18). Pharmacologic therapies that might be used to modify these risks are discussed subsequently. Two additional recommendations involve the use of adjunctive therapy to reduce thromboembolic risk: low-dose daily aspirin in persons at high risk for cardiovascular disease (unless contraindicated for other medical reasons) and anticoagulation with aspirin or warfarin, as clinically indicated, in patients with chronic atrial fibrillation.

The use of aspirin for primary prevention of cardiovascular disease has been studied and debated extensively. Although aspirin does not prevent atherosclerosis, it decreases the likelihood that an occlusive thrombus will form at an ulcerated plaque. The major side effects of aspirin use are hemorrhagic stroke and major gastrointestinal bleeding. The impact of aspirin on cardiovascular risk reduction may be different in men and women. For example, most primary prevention studies in men show approximately a 30% reduction in nonfatal MI but no clear benefit in nonfatal stroke and no overall mortality benefit. Conversely, the most recent large-scale study of aspirin in asymptomatic healthy women demonstrated a reduction in stroke, but not in first myocardial infarction, with benefit most evident in women ≥65 years of age (5). The use of aspirin for primary prevention of cardiovascular disease is recommended for individuals with an FRS greater than 10%, at which point the benefits of daily low-dose aspirin use are thought to outweigh the risks (2, 15, 18). Aspirin is usually withheld in patients with poorly controlled hypertension (systolic blood pressure ≥160 mmHg).

Although dietary modifications and physical activity are cornerstones of risk reduction for blood pressure lowering, lipid management, and diabetes treatment, many patients require drug therapy to achieve these goals. Table 10.1 lists pharmacologic therapies that might be used for primary prevention of cardiovascular disease (4, 8, 10, 13, 16, 17, 22). The names of drugs within a given class are listed along with a brief description of the mechanism of drug action for the class. With the ongoing development and approval of pharmacological therapies as well as postmarketing surveillance to identify serious drug side effects that may modify the application of certain drugs for the treatment of specific conditions, these kinds of lists in a medical textbook are often inherently incomplete by the time of publication. Furthermore, this list does not include drugs used to treat conditions that are off-label or outside the confines of FDA-approved uses.

TABLE 10.1   Pharmacological Therapies Used to Modify Cardiovascular Risk

Drug	Drug class/mechanism of action
SMOKING CESSATION	
Nicotine replacement therapy: patch, gum, inhaler, nasal spray, lozenge	Provides nicotine replacement so that the habit of smoking can be broken without the negative reinforcement of nicotine withdrawal symptoms
Varenicline	Partial agonist of α4β2 nicotinic acetylcholine receptor subtype where its binding produces agonist activity while simultaneously preventing nicotine binding
Bupropion	Weak neuronal uptake inhibitor of norepinephrine, dopamine and serotonin; chemically related to phenylethylamines; mechanism of action related to smoking cessation not well defined
BLOOD PRESSURE LOWERING	
Chlorothiazide, chlorthalidone, hydrochlorothiazide, indapamide, metolazone, polythiazide	Thiazide diuretics: Interfere with electrolyte transport in the distal convoluted tubule of the kidney
Bumetanide, furosemide, torsemide	Loop diuretics: Block electrolyte reabsorption in the ascending loop of Henle
Amiloride, triamterene	Potassium-sparing diuretics: Interfere with electrolyte transport in the collecting ducts of the kidney
Eplerenone, spironolactone	Aldosterone antagonists (receptor blockers)
Atenolol, betaxolol, bisoprolol, metoprolol, nadolol, propranolol, timolol, acebutolol, penbutolol, pindolol	β-blockers: Block β-adrenergic receptors
Carvedilol, labetolol	α- and β-receptor blockers: Nonselectively block β-adrenergic receptor and selectively block α1-adrenergic receptor causing vasodilatation without reflex tachycardia
Benazepril, captopril, enalapril, fosinopril, lisinopril, moexipril, perindopril, quinapril, ramipril, trandolapril	ACE inhibitors: Inhibit ACE conversion of angiotensin I to angiotensin II; there may also be an antiatherogenic effect
Candesartan, eprosartan, irbesartan, losartan, olmesartan, telmisartan, valsartan	Angiotensin receptor blockers: Block angiotensin II type I receptor that causes vasoconstriction and fluid retention
Diltiazem, verapamil	Nondihydropyridine calcium channel blockers: Block calcium channels that cause vascular smooth muscle vasoconstriction
Amlodipine, felodipine, isradipine, nicardipine sustained release, nifedipine long-acting, nisoldipine	Dihydropyridine calcium channel blockers: Block calcium channels that cause vascular smooth muscle vasoconstriction
Doxazosin, prazosin, terazosin	α1-receptor blockers: Block α1 receptor-associated vasoconstriction
Clonidine, guanfacine, methyldopa, reserpine	Centrally acting α2-receptor agonists: Decrease sympathetic outflow and blood pressure, thus lowering cardiac work
Hydralazine, minoxidil	Direct vasodilators: Relax vascular smooth muscle, preferentially dilating arterioles.

(continued)

Table 10.1 *(continued)*

Drug	Drug class/mechanism of action
LIPID MANAGEMENT	
Atorvastatin, fluvastatin, lovastatin, pravastatin, rosuvastatin, simvastatin	Statins: Inhibit hydroxymethylglutaryl coenzyme A reductase–mediated synthesis of cholesterol
Ezetimibe	Dietary cholesterol absorption inhibitor: Acts at the brush border of the small intestine to inhibit cholesterol absorption, reducing intestinal cholesterol transport to the liver, thus reducing of hepatic cholesterol stores and increasing clearance of cholesterol from the blood
Niacin, short-acting, long-acting forms	Nicotinic acid: Increases lipoprotein lipase activity, thereby reducing low-density lipoprotein and very low density lipoprotein synthesis
Fenofibrate, gemfibrozil	Fibrates: Activate the nuclear transcription factor peroxisomal proliferator-activated receptor-α
Cholestyramine, colestipol, colesevelam	Bile acid sequestrants: Increase stool elimination of bile acids and cholesterol by preventing enterohepatic recycling
WEIGHT MANAGEMENT	
Orlistat	Reversible gastric and pancreatic lipase inhibitor: Inhibits hydrolysis of triglycerides into free fatty acids and monoglycerides so they are excreted undigested
Sibutramine	Appetite suppressant approved for long-term use: Inhibits reuptake of norepinephrine, serotonin, and dopamine
Phentermine, phendimetrazine, diethylpropion	Appetite suppressants approved for short-term use: Affect centrally acting sympathomimetic amine stimulating release of dopamine, epinephrine, and norepinephrine
DIABETES CONTROL	
Acetohexamide, chlorpropamide, glimepiride, glipizide, glyburide, tolazamide, tolbutamide	Sulfonylureas: Stimulate the β-cells in the pancreas to release more insulin with slower onset and longer duration than rapid insulin releasers
Nateglinide, repaglinide	Nonsulfonylurea secretagogues (rapid insulin releasers): Stimulate β-cells to release more insulin over a short period of time only when glucose is high
Metformin	Biguanide: Reduces overproduction of glucose from the liver, increases insulin receptors on muscle and fat cells, reduces insulin requirements
Pioglitaxone, rosiglitazone	Thiazolidinediones: Improve receptivity of insulin receptors (reversing insulin resistance) in liver, muscle, and fat cells
Acarbose, miglitol	α-glucosidase inhibitors: Slow digestion of complex carbohydrates
Sitagliptin	Dipeptidyl peptidase-4 blocker: Slows the inactivation of incretin hormones (such as glucagon-like peptide-1) that are released by the intestine and results in increased insulin production and insulin release in a glucose-dependent manner
Insulin: rapid-acting, short-acting, intermediate-acting, long-acting, very long acting formulations	Facilitates entry of glucose into cells; stimulates liver to store glucose as glycogen and synthesize fatty acids

ACE = angiotensin-converting enzyme.

Adapted from Bonow et al. 2006; Fiore et al. 2000; Grundy et al. 2004; Krentz and Baily 2005; National Cholesterol Education Program (NCEP) Expert Panel on Detection, Evaluation, and Treatment of High Blood Cholesterol in Adults (Adult Treatment Panel III) 2002; Prescription Medications for the Treatment of Obesity 2004; treatobacco.net: Database and Education Resource for Treatment of Tobacco Dependence.

For any given risk factor modification goal, a specific class of drugs might be chosen because of its spectrum of effects, level of potency, side effect profile, or cost. Of the five classes of drugs used for lipid management, each has different effects on LDL-C, HDL-C, and triglycerides. These drug groups and their anticipated effects on various lipid parameters are shown in table 10.2 (10, 16). The choice of drug will be dictated by the specific lipid parameter targeted (LDL, HDL, or triglycerides) and the percentage change desired. For the patient with low HDL-C and elevated triglycerides but acceptable levels of LDL-C, niacin may be prescribed. For the patient with moderately high LDL-C requiring a 40% reduction to achieve treatment goals but acceptable levels of HDL-cholesterol and triglycerides, a statin would be preferred over a fibrate. The effect of lipid-lowering therapy will often give important clues regarding the primary underlying lipid abnormality (e.g., elevated LDL rather than low HDL).

Both systolic hypertension and diastolic hypertension are major risk factors for coronary disease. Numerous randomized trials show the benefit of blood pressure control in preventing cardiovascular disease. The practice of choosing a drug treatment based on its spectrum of actions is best illustrated by the drug treatment plans for hypertension. When a physician chooses an appropriate antihypertension agent, not only cardiovascular risk factors and the presence of clinical cardiovascular disease come into play but also the presence of other medical conditions that can serve as compelling indications or contraindications to the use of certain drug classes. For example, a β-blocker might be a compelling choice to treat hypertension in a patient with migraine headaches but not so in a patient with asthma. Table 10.3 lists potential compelling indications and contraindications for selecting drug classes to treat hypertension.

Secondary Prevention for Patients With Atherosclerotic Vascular Disease

There is no debate that secondary prevention treatment guidelines should be applied to patients who are at high risk for the development of cardiovascular disease such as diabetes; who have an FRS ≥20% (coronary heart disease risk equivalent) even in the absence of clinical cardiovascular disease; or who have established coronary heart disease (including myocardial infarction, angina pectoris, coronary artery bypass grafting, and percutaneous coronary interventions such as stent placement), clinically manifest peripheral vascular disease (including transient ischemic attack, stroke, and claudication), aortic aneurysm and asymptomatic peripheral vascular disease (including carotid and lower-extremity atherosclerosis in high-risk individuals such as those with multiple risk factors), poorly controlled risk factors (especially continued smoking), and metabolic syndrome. Many of the risk factors targeted for secondary prevention of cardiovascular disease are similar to those targeted for primary prevention: smoking, physical inactivity, atherogenic diet, diabetes,

TABLE 10.2 Treatment Effects for Drug Classes in Lipid Management

Drug class	LDL	HDL	Triglycerides
Statins	↓25-50	↑4-12	↓14-29
Ezetimibe	↓18	↑1	↓9
Bile acid sequestrants	↓10-18	↑3	Neutral or ↑
Nicotinic acid	↓10-20	↑14-35	↓30-70
Fibrates	↓4-21	↑11-13	↓30

Values are percentages. ↓ = decrease; ↑ = increase.

Grundy et al. 2004 and the National Cholesterol Education Program (NCEP) Expert Panel on Detection, Evaluation, and Treatment of High Blood Cholesterol in Adults (Adult Treatment Panel III) 2002.

TABLE 10.3 **Compelling Indications and Contraindications for Drug Therapy of Hypertension**

Drug class	Compelling indication	Contraindication
Nondihydropyridine and dihydropyridine calcium channel blockers	Atrial fibrillation rate control (nondihydropyridine) Angina pectoris Migraine Raynaud's syndrome (dihydropyridine)	Second- or third-degree heart block (nondihydropyridine) Status postmyocardial infarction (nondihydropyridine)
β-blockers	Systolic heart failure Postmyocardial infarction Atrial fibrillation rate control Essential tremor Hyperthyroidism Migraine Angina pectoris	Bronchospastic lung disease Depression Second- or third-degree heart block
Angiotensin-converting enzyme inhibitor	Systolic heart failure Postmyocardial infarction Proteinuric chronic renal failure Diabetes mellitus Lower extremity peripheral arterial disease	Angioedema Pregnancy Hyperkalemia Bilateral renal artery stenosis
Angiotensin receptor blocker	Systolic heart failure Proteinuric chronic renal failure Diabetes mellitus	Angioedema Pregnancy Hyperkalemia Bilateral renal artery stenosis
Diuretic	Systolic heart failure Diabetes mellitus Osteoporosis (thiazide)	Gout Hyponatremia
Aldosterone antagonist	Systolic heart failure Postmyocardial infarction Hypokalemia	Hyperkalemia
α-blocker	Benign prostatic hypertrophy	Depression

Adapted from Chobanian et al. 2003.

and hypertension. An important difference between primary and secondary prevention risk factor modification is that treatment goals are often more aggressive for secondary prevention. Thus, drug therapy is often necessary even if the patient has met goals for physical activity, dietary modifications, and weight control. Lipid-lowering goals that could be met with a single drug for primary prevention may require multiple drugs for secondary prevention. Thus, drug treatments listed in table 10.1 may be used more frequently in the patient with established atherosclerotic vascular disease. Several additional general recommendations for risk factor intervention are unique to secondary prevention:

- Evaluation for the presence of depression
- Influenza vaccination
- Initiation of low-dose aspirin
- Consideration of chronic β-blocker therapy in patients with coronary disease or other atherosclerotic vascular disease (unless contraindicated)

Beyond these general recommendations for secondary prevention in all patients with atherosclerotic vascular disease, there are additional recommendations for certain subgroups of patients, such as those status postmyocardial infarction or those status poststent placement. Table 10.4 lists drug treatment recommendations for secondary prevention of coronary and other atherosclerotic vascular disease in special subgroups (1, 4, 10, 11, 15, 16, 19, 20).

TABLE 10.4 **Secondary Prevention Drug Treatment Recommendations for Specific Populations of Patients With Coronary and Other Atherosclerotic Vascular Disease or With High-Risk Features**

Specialized populations	Treatment
s/p acute coronary syndrome	Clopidogrel: Start and continue 75 mg/day in combination with aspirin for up to 12 months. BBs: Start and continue indefinitely unless contraindicated.
s/p MI	BBs: Start and continue indefinitely unless contraindicated. Clopidogrel: 75 mg/day or warfarin may be used if aspirin is contraindicated. ACE inhibitors: In all patients indefinitely; start early in stable high-risk patients (anterior MI, previous MI, Killip class ≥II, LVEF 0.40). ARBs: In patients who are intolerant of ACE-I and have signs of heart failure or LVEF <0.40. Aldosterone blockade: In patients with potassium ≤5 mEq/L and creatinine ≤2.5 mg/dL in men or ≤2.0 mg/dL in women who are already receiving therapeutic doses of an ACE-I, have LVEF ≤0.40, and have either diabetes or heart failure.
s/p PCI with stent placement	Clopidogrel: Start and continue 75 mg/day in combination with higher dose aspirin (325 mg) for at least 1 month for bare metal stent, at least 3 months for sirolimus-eluting stent, and at least 6 months for paclitaxel-eluting stent, after which it should ideally be continued up to 12 months in patients who are not at high risk of bleeding. Aspirin: After duration of high-dose treatment with clopidogrel, lower dose (75-162 mg/day) should continue indefinitely unless contraindicated.
s/p CABG	Aspirin (100-325 mg/day) should be started within 48 hr of surgery and continued for up to 1 year, after which a lower dose (75-162 mg/day) should be continued indefinitely unless contraindicated.
s/p TIA or noncardioembolic stroke	Aspirin (50-325 mg/day): The combination of aspirin and extended-release dipyridamole, and clopidogrel are all acceptable options for initial therapy, with selection based on patient risk factor profiles, tolerance, and other clinical characteristics. Addition of aspirin to clopidogrel increases the risk of hemorrhage and is not routinely recommended for ischemic stroke or TIA patients. For patients allergic to aspirin, clopidogrel is reasonable.
Peripheral arterial disease	Cilostazol is indicated in patients with intermittent or limiting claudication (in the absence of HF). Pentoxifylline is second-line therapy in patients with intermittent claudication.
Left ventricular dysfunction (EF ≤40%)	See Chronic Heart Failure discussion and table 10.6.
Atrial fibrillation	See Chronic Atrial Fibrillation discussion and table 10.5.

s/p = status post; MI = myocardial infarction; PCI = percutaneous coronary intervention; CABG = coronary artery bypass graft; TIA = transient ischemic attack; EF = ejection fraction; BB = β-blocker; ACE = angiotensin-converting enzyme; LVEF = left ventricular ejection fraction; ARB = angiotensin receptor blocker; HF = heart failure.

Adapted from Antman et al. 2004; Chobanian et al. 2003; Fiore et al. 2000; National Cholesterol Education Program (NCEP) Expert Panel on Detection, Evaluation, and Treatment of High Blood Cholesterol in Adults (Adult Treatment Panel III) 2002; Sacco et al. 2006; Smith et al. 2006.

As indicated in table 10.4, there are some important differences between primary and secondary prevention recommendations regarding the use of antiplatelet therapy. Unless contraindications are present, the use of aspirin is universal for secondary prevention with doses in some settings higher than those recommended for primary prevention. The presence of enteric coating on aspirin does not appear to reduce the risk of serious side effects. Risks of aspirin use are higher in those already taking nonsteroidal anti-inflammatory drugs, making its use potentially more problematic in elderly patients with concomitant illnesses treated with these drugs. Whether aspirin resistance should be measured in high-risk individuals and how that measurement should affect the use of antiplatelet or anticoagulation therapy are the focus of ongoing research and are not addressed in any of the treatment guidelines. Clopidogrel is a second antiplatelet agent that comes into play for secondary prevention. Unlike aspirin, which irreversibly acetylates platelet cyclooxygenase, decreasing the formation of the procoagulant thromboxane A_2, clopidogrel inhibits adenosine diphosphate–induced platelet aggregation. Side effects of clopidogrel include bleeding, diarrhea, headache, dizziness, abdominal pain, nausea, and dyspepsia. Recent studies have shown that the combination of aspirin and clopidogrel is not superior to aspirin alone for primary or secondary prevention in patients at high risk for cardiovascular events.

Chronic Atrial Fibrillation

Atrial fibrillation is the most common sustained cardiac rhythm abnormality in adults; it is a supraventricular tachycardia manifested as an irregularly irregular rhythm caused by uncoordinated atrial activation. The ventricular response can be fast or slow, and atrial fibrillation can be sustained or paroxysmal. The three major treatment arms of atrial fibrillation treatment are rate control, rhythm control, and anticoagulation (9).

Some patients in atrial fibrillation with intrinsic conduction system disease will have adequate rate control in the absence of drug therapy. Rate control refers to the goal of controlling the ventricular response in patients with persistent atrial fibrillation in whom ventricular response is elevated. For patients with a rapid ventricular response and hemodynamic instability, urgent cardioversion will be required. However, for stable patients with a ventricular response that is higher than desired, drug therapy may be used to achieve rate control. Although there are no evidence-based criteria

for adequate rate control, common goals are ventricular rates between 60 and 80 beats/min at rest and between 90 and 115 beats/min during moderate exercise. Table 10.5 lists medications (and potential side effects) commonly used to control heart rate in stable patients in atrial fibrillation who might be encountered in a cardiac rehabilitation setting (9).

Restoration of normal sinus rhythm in patients in atrial fibrillation can occur spontaneously or can be achieved with electrical cardioversion, pharmacological cardioversion, or catheter ablation (for patients failing pharmacologic maintenance of normal sinus rhythm). Drug treatment is often required to prevent recurrent atrial fibrillation in patients in whom normal sinus rhythm has been restored. Table 10.5 also lists medications (and potential side effects) commonly used to maintain normal sinus rhythm in patients with a history of atrial fibrillation. The selection of therapy to maintain sinus rhythm is based on the presence of comorbid cardiovascular conditions. Flecanide, propafenone, and sotalol are most commonly used in the setting of no or minimal heart disease, whereas amiodarone is often used in the setting of substantial hypertensive heart disease or heart failure.

Chronic Heart Failure

The number of patients with chronic heart failure (HF) continues to climb in part because of the increasing number of patients who survive myocardial infarction with subsequent HF and the increasing life expectancy of HF patients attributable to improved therapies. Heart failure is a clinical syndrome that is characterized by symptoms of dyspnea, fatigue, and fluid retention (with peripheral edema or pulmonary congestion) and could result from any of a number of cardiovascular disorders that impair the ability of the ventricle to fill or eject, including myocardial infarction, hypertension, valvular heart disease, and genetic or metabolic cardiomyopathies. In the most recent treatment guidelines, four stages of HF were identified:

■ Stage A: high risk for HF but without structural heart disease or symptoms of HF

■ Stage B: structural heart disease without symptoms of HF

■ Stage C: structural heart disease with prior or current symptoms of HF

■ Stage D: refractory symptoms of HD requiring specialized treatment such as chronic inotrope administration or transplantation (12)

TABLE 10.5 Drugs Used to Treat Patients With Atrial Fibrillation

HEART RATE CONTROL

Drug	Potential side effects
Metoprolol, propranolol	Hypotension, heart block, bradycardia, worsening heart failure, depression, fatigue, worsening of lung disease
Diltiazem, verapamil	Hypotension, heart block, bradycardia, worsening heart failure, constipation, peripheral edema, digoxin drug interaction (verapamil)
Digoxin	Heart block, bradycardia, digoxin toxicity (anorexia, blurred vision)
Amiodarone	Hypotension, heart block, lung toxicity, skin discoloration, photosensitivity, thyroid dysfunction, corneal deposits, optic neuropathy, warfarin drug interaction, GI upset

RHYTHM CONTROL

Dofetilide	Torsades de pointes
Disopyramide	Torsades de pointes, heart failure, glaucoma, urinary retention, dry mouth
Flecainide	Ventricular tachycardia, worsening heart failure, conversion to atrial flutter with rapid conduction through the AV node
Propafenone	Ventricular tachycardia, worsening heart failure, conversion to atrial flutter with rapid conduction through the AV node, metallic taste, worsening of lung disease
Sotalol	Torsades de pointes, worsening heart failure, bradycardia, worsening of lung disease
Amiodarone	Hypotension, heart block, lung toxicity, skin discoloration, photosensitivity, thyroid dysfunction, corneal deposits, optic neuropathy, warfarin drug interaction, GI upset

ANTICOAGULATION

Aspirin	Bleeding, gastric ulceration, nausea, dyspepsia, heartburn
Warfarin	Bleeding, skin necrosis, alopecia, multiple drug interactions

GI = gastrointestinal; AV = atrioventricular.

Adapted from Fuster et al. 2006.

A number of drugs are recommended for routine use in patients with HF, with an increasing number of drug therapies used as the stage of HF worsens. Table 10.6 lists classes of drugs that are recommended for use in the clinical stages of HF based on published clinical outcomes data as outlined in the most current clinical guideline (12). As the results of additional clinical trials become available, this list will undoubtedly change.

The cornerstone of therapy at all stages of HF is the use of ACE inhibitors or, in ACE inhibitor–intolerant patients, angiotensin receptor blockers (ARBs). These agents prevent HF in high-risk patients (stage A) with a history of atherosclerotic vascular disease, diabetes, or hypertension with associated cardiovascular risk factors. The use of ACE inhibitors in asymptomatic patients with reduced left ventricular ejection fraction

(LVEF) (stage B) as a consequence of either ischemic or nonischemic cardiomyopathy delays the onset of HF symptoms and decreases the combined risk of death or hospitalization for HF; the use of ARBs is a reasonable alternative in these patients if they are intolerant to an ACE inhibitor. In symptomatic HF patients with reduced LVEF, ACE inhibitors have been shown to alleviate symptoms, improve quality of life, and prolong life. ARBs are used in stage C and stage D patients who are intolerant of ACE inhibitors or in combination with ACE inhibitors in patients who remain symptomatic on conventional therapy.

The use of β-blockers in the setting of HF was once thought contraindicated given their negative inotropic effects; however, these effects are significantly overshadowed by the ability of β-blockers to block the

TABLE 10.6   Classes of Drugs Used in the Four Stages of Heart Failure

Drug	Stage A	Stage B	Stage C	Stage D
CE-I: captopril, enalapril, fosinopril, lisinopril, perindopril, quinapril, ramipril, trandolapril	X	X	X	X
Angiotensin receptor blockers (if intolerant of angiotensin-converting enzyme inhibitor): candesartan, losartan, valsartan	X	X	X	X
β-blockers: bisoprolol, carvedilol, metoprolol succinate extended release		X	X	X
Oral diuretics: loop (bumetanide, furosemide, torsemide), thiazide (chlorothiazide, chlorthalidone, hydrochlorothiazide, indapamide, metolazone) potassium-sparing (amiloride, spironolactone, triamterene) sequential nephron blockade (metolazone, hydrochlorothiazide)			X	X
Aldosterone antagonists: spironolactone, eplerenone			X	X
Digitalis			X	X
Hydralazine/nitrates			X	X

Adapted from Hunt et al.

adverse effects of sympathetic nervous system activation in patients with HF. Unless contraindications are present such as symptomatic reactive airway disease or bradycardia, the use of β-blockers is recommended in asymptomatic patients with reduced LVEF and in stable patients with current or prior symptoms of HF and reduced LVEF. Treatment with β-blockers should begin with very low doses and should be titrated slowly as tolerated.

Additional medications used in stage C and stage D HF patients include diuretics, aldosterone antagonists, vasodilator combination of hydralazine and nitrates, and digitalis. The use of medication combinations mandates careful monitoring of blood pressure, heart rate, electrolytes, renal function, and volume status. Diuretics are used to treat fluid retention; thiazide diuretics may be preferred in the hypertensive HF patient with mild fluid retention because of their longer acting blood pressure–lowering effects. The addition of aldosterone antagonists to ACE inhibitor therapy in high-risk HF patients has been shown to reduce mortality, reduce the risk of hospitalization, and improve functional class. Close monitoring of potassium and renal function is required when treatment with aldosterone antagonists begins and if changes are made in the treatment plan that could affect electrolytes, volume status, or renal function (e.g., altering diuretic or ACE inhibitor

dose). The risk of hyperkalemia in patients treated with aldosterone antagonists increases in the setting of serum creatinine >1.6 mg/dL, use of high doses of ACE inhibitors, diarrhea or other causes of dehydration, and concomitant use of nonsteroidal anti-inflammatory drugs or cyclooxygenase-2 inhibitors. Aldosterone antagonists should not be used in conjunction with potassium supplements or if the baseline potassium is greater than 5.0 mEq/L. There are no data to recommend the use of digoxin in asymptomatic patients in sinus rhythm with reduced LVEF (stage B). The use of digitalis has been shown to reduce hospitalizations for HF in patients with current or prior symptoms of HF and reduced LVEF. However, because digoxin has a very narrow risk–benefit ratio even in this higher risk population and offers no mortality benefit, it is much less frequently added to multidrug regimens than are other therapies. The addition of hydralazine and nitrates in combination may be reasonable for patients with reduced LVEF and persistent HF symptoms who are already taking ACE inhibitors and β-blockers. A retrospective analysis and one prospective trial showed the addition of isosorbide dinitrate and hydralazine to an ACE inhibitor or a β-blocker to be beneficial. Compliance with this combination is reportedly poor because of the large number of tablets required and the high incidence of adverse reactions.

Valvular Heart Disease

Indications for pharmacologic treatment of chronic valvular heart disease in operable adult patients (3) are rare. The predominant features of valvular heart disease guidelines are recommendations regarding the appropriate frequency of follow-up imaging for specific clinical conditions and indications for valve repair or replacement. In some cases, limited medical therapies may be used cautiously in patients with severe valvular heart disease in whom severe comorbid conditions preclude appropriate surgical treatment. In other cases, critically ill patients may receive short-term medical treatment of acute valvular regurgitation in an effort to stabilize them prior to surgical intervention. These clinical scenarios are unlikely to be found in a cardiac rehabilitation setting. This discussion of pharmacologic treatment of valvular heart disease focuses for the most part on medications that might be used in patients with significant native aortic or mitral valve disease in whom indications for surgical treatment have not yet been developed and in whom cardiac rehabilitation might be recommended. The drug classes that might be used

by this patient population with four common valvular conditions (aortic stenosis, aortic regurgitation, mitral stenosis, and mitral regurgitation) are summarized in table 10.7 (3).

The most common reason to take medication (albeit intermittently) in the setting of valvular heart disease is endocarditis prophylaxis. Endocarditis in valvular heart disease patients is uncommon, but it can be catastrophic. It usually develops in individuals with underlying structural heart disease who develop bacteremia with certain organisms known to cause endocarditis. Transient bacteremia can occur during certain surgical, dental, or instrumentation procedures involving mucosal surfaces or contaminated tissue. Whether the administration of antibiotics prior to these procedures protects against development of endocarditis has not been established in prospective studies. Nonetheless, prophylaxis against infective endocarditis is recommended in valvular heart disease patients with prosthetic heart valves or valve repair, a history of infective endocarditis, congenital cardiac valve malformations (e.g., bicuspid aortic valve), acquired valvular dysfunction (e.g., rheumatic heart disease,

TABLE 10.7 **Drug Therapy That May Be Used in Patients With Chronic Valvular Heart Disease**

Condition	Drug classes
Aortic stenosis	Antibiotics for endocarditis prophylaxis in table 10.8
Aortic regurgitation	Antibiotics for endocarditis prophylaxis in table 10.8 Vasodilators (hydralazine, nifedipine, possibly angiotensin-converting enzyme inhibitors)
Mitral stenosis	Antibiotics for endocarditis prophylaxis in table 10.8 Negative chronotropic agents (β-blockers such as metoprolol, nondihydropyridine calcium channel blockers such as diltiazem or verapamil) Warfarin Drug treatment for atrial fibrillation including those listed for rate control, rhythm control, and anticoagulation in table 10.5
Mitral valve prolapse	Antibiotics for endocarditis prophylaxis in table 10.5 Aspirin or warfarin
Mitral regurgitation	Antibiotics for endocarditis prophylaxis in table 10.8 Drug treatment for atrial fibrillation including those listed for rate control, rhythm control, and anticoagulation in table 10.5 Drug treatment for stage B heart failure in table 10.6

Adapted from Bonow et al. 2006.

aortic sclerosis with restriction of leaflet motion and a peak velocity >2 m/s), and mitral valve prolapse (MVP) auscultatory evidence of valvular regurgitation or thickened leaflets on echocardiography (21). The standard oral prophylactic regimens for dental, oral, respiratory tract, and esophageal procedures in adults are listed in table 10.8.

Although cephalexin and cefadroxil (cephalosporins) are listed as alternatives to amoxicillin in patients who are penicillin allergic, cephalosporins should not be used in patients with immediate-type hypersensitivity reaction (urticaria, angioedema, or anaphylaxis) to penicillins. Because not all patients can recall the specific manifestations of their penicillin allergy, it may be prudent to avoid cephalosporins altogether in penicillin-allergic patients.

Aortic Stenosis

A discussion of the indications for surgical treatment of aortic stenosis (AS) can be found elsewhere. In the absence of a surgical indication, there are no other (medical) treatment indications for AS patients beyond antibiotic prophylaxis. Patients with mild or moderate AS commonly ask what they can do to prevent AS from worsening. Unfortunately, no medical therapies have been proven to prevent or slow the progression of AS. However, the association of AS with clinical risk factors for the development of atherosclerosis as well as the association of reduced AS progression with statin use in retrospective analyses has led to the hypothesis that lipid-lowering therapies may retard the development of AS. The single randomized trial of statin therapy published to date did not demonstrate a reduction in the progression of AS over 3 years in patients with moderate to severe AS at baseline (6). Additional randomized trials of statin use in patients with less severe AS at baseline with longer periods of follow-up may be warranted.

Chronic Aortic Regurgitation

Worsening aortic regurgitation (AR) is associated with left ventricular (LV) cavity dilatation and then worsening LV systolic function, at which time patients will often develop symptoms of dyspnea or exertional angina. In the setting of severe AR, surgery is the mainstay of therapy in symptomatic patients irrespective

TABLE 10.8   Prophylactic Regimens for Dental, Oral, Respiratory Tract, and Esophageal Procedures in Adults

Condition	Regimen
STANDARD GENERAL PROPHYLAXIS IN PATIENTS WHO ARE NOT ALLERGIC TO PENICILLIN	
Able to take oral medicines	Amoxicillin 2.0 g orally 1 hr before procedure
Unable to take oral medicines	Ampicillin 2.0 g IM or IV 30 min before procedure
STANDARD GENERAL PROPHYLAXIS IN PATIENTS WHO ARE ALLERGIC TO PENICILLIN	
Able to take oral medicines	Clindamycin 600 mg 1 hr before procedure
	■ Cephalexin* or cefadroxil* 2.0 g 1 hr before procedure
	Azithromycin or clarithromycin 500 mg 1 hr before procedure
Unable to take oral medicines	Clindamycin 600 mg IV 30 min before procedure
	■ Cefazolin* 1.0 g IM or IV 30 min before procedure

IM = intramuscularly; IV = intravenously.

*Cephalosporins should not be used in individuals with immediate-type hypersensitivity reaction (urticaria, angioedema, or anaphylaxis) to penicillins.

Adapted from Dajani 1997.

of LV function or in asymptomatic patients with LV systolic dysfunction or severe LV dilatation. However, medical treatment with vasodilator therapy may be used in three clinical settings, which are listed here in order of decreasing strength of recommendation:

- Vasodilator therapy *is indicated* in the treatment of patients with AR who have indications for surgery but are inoperable because of other cardiac or noncardiac conditions.
- Vasodilator therapy *is reasonable* in the short-term treatment of AR patients with severe LV dysfunction and severe HF symptoms to improve clinical status prior to proceeding with aortic valve surgery.
- Vasodilator therapy *may be considered* for long-term treatment of asymptomatic patients with severe AR and LV dilatation but normal systolic function.

Improved ejection fraction and reduced LV cavity size have been reported with hydralazine and nifedipine, but less consistent results have been reported with ACE inhibitors.

Mitral Stenosis

Because rheumatic fever is the primary cause of mitral stenosis (MS), prophylaxis against rheumatic fever is recommended, as is endocarditis prophylaxis. Unlike the patient with AS, the patient with MS should not automatically undergo mitral valve replacement. A patient with mild MS without symptoms at rest can develop symptoms in the setting of increased transmitral flow or decreased diastolic filling period (exercise, infection, pregnancy, or atrial fibrillation). Medications aimed at slowing heart rate (β-blockers, certain calcium channel blockers) may be prescribed for patients in normal sinus rhythm who develop exertional symptoms at high heart rates. More than one third of patients with symptomatic MS may develop atrial fibrillation, which can be associated with severe symptoms if a rapid ventricular response occurs in the setting of moderate or severe MS. In the hemodynamically stable patient, medical treatment of atrial fibrillation is indicated with therapies chosen for rate control or rhythm control as appropriate. Anticoagulation with warfarin is indicated in patients with MS and atrial fibrillation, a prior embolic event, and left atrial thrombus and may be considered in the setting of severe left atrial enlargement or left atrial enlargement and spontaneous echo contrast. The impact of MS on cardiac rehabilitation is discussed elsewhere.

Mitral Valve Prolapse

Antibiotic prophylaxis is recommended for patients with mitral valve prolapse (MVP) with thickened leaflets or mitral regurgitation. Aspirin therapy (75-325 mg/day) may be used in MVP patients in various clinical settings, which are listed here in order of decreasing strength of conviction:

- Aspirin therapy *is recommended* for MVP patients with transient ischemic attack and for MVP patients with atrial fibrillation who do not have a clinical indication for warfarin.
- Aspirin therapy *is reasonable* for MVP patients with a history of stroke in the absence of MR, atrial fibrillation, left atrial thrombus, leaflet thickening, or redundancy.
- Aspirin therapy *can be beneficial* in MVP patients with a history of stroke who cannot take warfarin.
- Aspirin therapy *may be considered* in MVP patients in sinus rhythm with echocardiographic evidence of high-risk MVP.

Anticoagulation with warfarin therapy (international normalized ratio 2.0-3.0) may be used in MVP patients in various clinical settings, which are listed here in order of decreasing strength of conviction:

- Warfarin therapy *is recommended* for MVP patients with atrial fibrillation who have one or more risk factores for stroke such as HF, hypertension, or diabetes and for MVP patients with a history of stroke in the presence of MR, atrial fibrillation, or left atrial thrombus.
- Warfarin therapy *is reasonable* for MVP patients with transient ischemic attacks despite aspirin therapy.

Chronic Mitral Regurgitation

There are a host of indications for MV surgery, which are discussed elsewhere. In asymptomatic patients with chronic MR and preserved LV function, there are no data from long-term studies to support the use of medical therapy such as vasodilators or ACE inhibitors. In patients with functional MR (resulting from dilated or ischemic cardiomyopathy) and LV dysfunction, medical treatment as outlined for stage B HF is indicated. If atrial fibrillation develops in the MR patient, medical treatment is indicated with drug therapy for rate control, rhythm control, and anticoagulation as appropriate.

Summary

Although the availability of a single medication to treat both blood pressure and heart failure simplifies the pharmacologic treatment, use of a single medication requires that the health care provider maintain a working knowledge of potential drug therapies for multiple cardiovascular conditions. Fortunately, expert panels have provided practice guidelines reflecting a consensus of expert opinion to assist health care providers in clinical decision making regarding management of specific diseases and conditions. These guidelines are invaluable tools for assessing medical treatment plans for patients with multiple cardiovascular risk factors and conditions.

CHAPTER 11

Surgical Management of Cardiovascular Disease

Sotiris C. Stamou, MD

Tomislav Mihaljevic, MD

Heart and vascular disease is the most common cause of death and disability in the Western world. Although cardiovascular diseases include a large number of clinical conditions, they can be broadly divided into ischemic heart disease and valvular heart disease. Ischemic heart disease, caused by atherosclerotic changes in the coronary arteries, affects millions of people worldwide. Valvular heart disease is less common and is mostly caused by degenerative processes that affect valvular tissue and structure.

Ischemic Heart Disease

Contemporary therapy of ischemic heart disease consists of medical management, percutaneous transcatheter balloon angioplasty (PTCA), and coronary artery bypass grafting (CABG). Although the choice of therapy needs to be individualized for each patient, medical therapy and percutaneous interventions are usually used for treatment of mild to moderate forms of coronary artery disease, whereas CABG is reserved for treatment of diffuse, severe coronary artery atherosclerosis. Treatment of coronary artery disease is one of

the most dynamic fields in clinical medicine, with rapid advances in diagnostic and therapeutic technologies and consequent improvement in outcomes of patients with ischemic heart disease. A review of treatment of ischemic heart disease is provided in this section.

Percutaneous Transcatheter Balloon Angioplasty

The objective of therapy for ischemic heart disease is to increase the supply of oxygen and nutrients in the ischemic myocardium. This goal can be accomplished by dilating or bypassing the coronary artery obstructions. Although medical therapy can be effective, in many cases the optimal treatment is interventional therapy with PTCA with or without stent placement, CABG surgery, or both. The term *angioplasty* comes from the Greek words *angio*, meaning "vessel," and *plasty*, meaning "to mold or shape." In PTCA, a catheter is

Address correspondence concerning this chapter to Tomislav Mihaljevic, Cleveland Clinic, 9500 Euclid Avenue, F24, Cleveland, OH 44195. E-mail: mihaljt@ccf.org inserted into one of the arteries of the leg or arm and is then advanced into the stenosed coronary artery, where the balloon is inflated for 1 to 2 min. As the balloon expands it compresses and redistributes the atherosclerotic plaque, thus dilating the artery.

PTCA Versus Medical Therapy

Several prospective randomized studies have compared the effectiveness of PTCA with that of the medical treatment of coronary artery disease. In the Angioplasty Compared to Medicine (ACME) trial, the efficacy of PTCA was compared with best medical management in 212 patients with one-vessel disease and stenosis greater than 70% (11, 18). In this study, patients undergoing PTCA demonstrated better relief from angina, reduced need for antianginal medications, a better quality of life, and improved exercise tolerance; there was no difference in mortality. Some PTCA patients (19%), however, required additional catheter-based interventions, and 7% underwent CABG surgery. In a follow-up study by the same investigators, 101 patients with stable angina and two-vessel disease were randomized to PTCA or medical therapy (7). At 6 months, both groups had freedom from angina, improved exercise duration, and improved overall quality of life. In the trial titled Coronary Angioplasty Versus Medical Therapy for Angina: The Second Randomised Intervention Treatment of Angina (RITA-2), PTCA provided better early symptomatic relief from angina compared with medical treatment. This, however, was not sustained over time, and at 2.9 years the PTCA group had a 3% greater risk of death or myocardial infarction (22). In the Atorvastatin vs. Revascularization Trial (AVERT), PTCA and medicine as initial strategy were compared among patients with hyperlipidemia (21). Among 341 patients with single- or double-vessel disease, ischemic events were less common in the medical than in the PTCA groups (13% vs. 21%, $p < .05$) (20).

Stents

Sometimes after PTCA, a stent is applied to the diseased artery. The stent is a metallic wire mesh tube that is used to form a scaffold in the stenosed coronary artery. A collapsed metal stent is positioned over a balloon catheter and transported to the stenosed coronary artery, where the stent is deployed with the inflation of the balloon. A limitation of PTCA is the risk of restenosis, which can be decreased with the application of stents. Randomized trials have shown that application of coronary stents in relatively large (>3.0 mm) native coronary vessels improves short- and long-term outcomes compared with conventional balloon PTCA. The Stent Restenosis Study (STRESS) and the Belgium Netherlands Stent (BENESTENT) trials showed that stent placement resulted in a 26% to 31% reduction in angiographic restenosis and a 27% to 31% lowering of 1-year clinical events compared with balloon PTCA (6). Self-expanding and balloon-expandable coiled and slotted tube stents have also been used to scaffold coronary dissections in patients with PTCA-induced complications.

Coronary Artery Bypass Graft Surgery

Coronary artery bypass grafting (CABG) is used to reroute the blood flow around the stenosed coronary artery using either arterial or venous conduits. Guidelines for surgical revascularization have been established by the American College of Cardiology and American Heart Association (table 11.1).

TABLE 11.1   Indications for Coronary Artery Bypass Graft Surgery Alone in Patients With Stable Angina, Unstable Angina, and Acute Myocardial Infarction

| Condition | CLASS* | | | |
	I	IIa	IIb	III
Asymptomatic or mild angina	▪ LMCA stenosis ≥60% ▪ LMCA equivalent: proximal LAD and LCA stenoses >70% ▪ 3VD (survival benefit greater with abnormal LV function: EF <0.50)	Proximal LAD stenosis with 1VD or 2VD†	1VD or 2VD not involving the proximal LAD‡	None

| Condition | CLASS* | | | |
	I	IIa	IIb	III
Chronic stable angina	■ LMCA stenosis ≥60% ■ LMCA equivalent: proximal LAD and LCA stenoses >70% ■ 3VD (survival benefit greater with abnormal LV function: EF <0.50) ■ 2VD with significant proximal LAD stenosis: either EF <0.50 or ischemia on noninvasive testing ■ 1VD or 2VD without significant proximal LAD stenosis but with myocardium and high-risk criteria on noninvasive testing ■ Disabling angina despite maximal medical therapy (acceptable-risk patient)	■ Proximal LAD stenosis with 1VD[†] ■ 1VD or 2VD without significant[§] proximal LAD stenosis, moderate area of viable myocardium, and demonstrable ischemia on noninvasive testing	None	■ 1VD or 2VD without significant proximal LAD stenosis, in patients who have mild symptoms that are unlikely attributable to myocardial ischemia or who have not received an adequate trial of medical therapy and have (a) only a small area of viable myocardium or (b) no demonstrable ischemia on noninvasive testing ■ Borderline stenoses (50-60%) other than in the LCMA, no demonstrable ischemia on noninvasive testing ■ <50% coronary stenosis
UA/ NSTEMI	■ LMCA stenosis ≥60% ■ LMCA equivalent: proximal LAD and LCA stenoses >70% ■ Ongoing ischemia unresponsive to maximal nonsurgical therapy	Proximal LAD stenosis with 1VD or 2VD[†]	1VD or 2VD not involving the proximal LAD[‡]	None
STEMI/AMI	None	Ongoing ischemia/ infarction unresponsive to maximal nonsurgical therapy	■ Progressive LV pump failure with coronary stenosis compromising viable myocardium outside the initial infarct area ■ Primary reperfusion in the early hours (≤6-12 hr) of an evolving STEMI	Primary reperfusion late (>12 hr) in evolving STEMI without ongoing ischemia

UA = unstable angina; NSTEMI = non-ST elevation myocardial infarction; STEMI = ST elevation myocardial infarction; AMI = acute myocardial infarction; LMCA = left main coronary artery; LAD = left anterior descending; LCA = left coronary artery; 1VD = one-vessel disease; 2VD = two-vessel disease; 3VD = three-vessel disease; LV = left ventricular; EF = ejection fraction.

*Class I: Conditions for which there is evidence or general agreement that a given procedure or treatment is useful and effective. Class IIa: Conditions for which weight of evidence and opinion is in favor of usefulness and efficacy. Class IIb: Usefulness and efficacy are less well established by evidence and opinion. Class III: Conditions for which there is evidence or general agreement that the procedure or treatment is not useful or effective and in some cases may be harmful.

†Becomes class I if extensive ischemia documented by noninvasive study or a left ventricular ejection fraction <0.50.

‡Becomes class I if there is a large area of viable myocardium and high-risk criteria on noninvasive testing.

§Becomes class I if arrhythmia is resuscitated or if there is sudden cardiac death or sustained ventricular tachycardia.

Adapted from Eagle 1999.

The choice of conduits for coronary CABG includes saphenous vein, internal thoracic arteries, radial arteries, inferior epigastric arteries, and gastroepiploic arteries.

The left internal thoracic artery (LITA) is used in most surgical revascularization procedures and is most commonly used for revascularization of the left anterior descending artery. The 10-year patency of the LITA exceeds 90%. The right internal thoracic artery is frequently used in younger patients for revascularization of the right coronary artery or circumflex artery. The right internal thoracic artery can be used as an in situ graft or as a free graft. The use of both internal thoracic arteries translates into long-term survival benefit when used in younger patients with coronary artery disease, at the expense of slightly higher incidence of sternal wound infection.

Saphenous vein grafts are commonly used to bypass other coronary arteries; however, their patency is inferior to that of internal thoracic arteries. The advantage of saphenous vein grafts is in the ease of harvesting and usually sufficient length of available conduit. Incidence of infections of the saphenous vein harvesting sites has been greatly reduced by the use of endoscopic harvesting techniques. These new techniques allow harvest of long segments of saphenous veins through a 1.5 to 2 in. long (3.8-5.1 cm) incision.

Radial arteries are an alternative arterial conduit for coronary revascularization. They can be safely harvested once the adequacy of the collateral circulation to the hand by ulnar artery is confirmed. Harvest of the radial artery is usually associated with very low morbidity, most commonly in the form of transient radial nerve palsy.

Inferior epigastric arteries are arterial conduits that are most commonly used in patients with limited conduit availability; these arteries can be used for revascularization of the right coronary artery. The conduit is usually harvested with a limited upper laparotomy and then advanced into the mediastinum through an incision in the diaphragm. Limited long-term patency and difficulty in harvesting the conduit in obese patients have limited the use of these arteries.

CABG Versus Medical Therapy

Several prospective, randomized clinical trials evaluated the survival benefit of CABG surgery in patients with chronic stable angina. These studies helped to identify categories of patients with angina who are most likely to benefit from CABG, namely patients with left main coronary artery disease; one-, two-, or three-vessel disease with proximal left anterior descending (LAD) involvement; and three-vessel disease with impaired left ventricular function (19, 27). In the Trial of Invasive Versus Medical Therapy in Elderly Patients With Chronic Symptomatic Coronary-Artery Disease (TIME), the incidence of major adverse events (death, nonfatal MI, or hospitalization) was lower and angina relief and quality of life were superior for those undergoing coronary angiography and surgical revascularization compared with those randomized to an initial trial of medical therapy without angiography (19% vs. 49%, $p < .0001$) (26). In the Asymptomatic Cardiac Ischemia Pilot (ACIP) trial, patients with anatomy amenable to CABG were randomized to angina-directed anti-ischemic therapy, drug therapy guided by noninvasive measures of ischemia, or revascularization by CABG or PTCA (3). At 2 years, mortality was 6.6% in the angina-guided group, 4.4% in the ischemia-guided group, and 1.1% in the revascularization group. The rates of death or MI were 12.1%, 8.8%, and 4.7%, respectively. The differences between revascularization and angina-guided therapy were statistically significant.

CABG Versus PTCA

Several prospective randomized studies comparing PTCA with CABG have been reported (23). The incidence of repeat revascularization has been higher among patients treated with angioplasty than those treated with surgery in all trials. The incidence of repeat revascularization in the PTCA-treated patients ranged from 36.5% in the Coronary Angioplasty versus Bypass Revascularisation Investigation (CABRI) trial at 1-year follow-up to 62% in the Emory Angioplasty versus Surgery Trial (EAST) at 3 years (12). In contrast to PTCA, CABG resulted in fewer repeat revascularization procedures in these same studies. The incidence of repeat revascularization procedures in multivessel patients randomized to CABG surgery was 3.5% in the CABRI trial and 13.5% in the EAST trial. Repeat revascularization procedures were required five to eight times more often in patients with multivessel disease initially treated with angioplasty compared with those randomized to initial CABG surgery. The use of stents has certainly reduced restenosis rates, and recent antimitotic drug-eluting stents appear to reduce the restenosis rates even further. The early results with rapamycin suggest that restenosis can be significantly decreased (17).

Coronary Artery Bypass Without Cardiopulmonary Bypass

The use of cardiopulmonary bypass is associated with a systemic inflammatory response, mediated in part by activation of complement, macrophages, and cytokines. This phenomenon has been related to the contact of blood components with the surface of the bypass circuit. It has been hypothesized that this inflammatory response contributes to postoperative bleeding, neurocognitive dysfunction, thromboembolism, fluid retention, and reversible organ dysfunction. In an attempt to minimize these complications, surgeons are increasingly using coronary artery bypass without cardiopulmonary bypass or off-pump surgery, and this procedure is considered an acceptable alternative method for myocardial revascularization. A number of studies and clinical trials have been performed to evaluate the efficacy and safety of this operation and define the subsets of patients who are most likely to benefit from this approach, and some trends have been observed. These trends include less blood loss and need for transfusion, less myocardial enzyme release up to 24 hr, less early neurocognitive dysfunction, and less renal insufficiency after off-pump CABG. Fewer grafts tend to be performed with off-pump CABG than with standard CABG (24). Length of hospital stay, mortality rate, and long-term neurological function and cardiac outcome appear to be similar in the two groups (24).

Valvular Heart Disease

Stenotic or regurgitant cardiac valves create hemodynamic compromise on one or both ventricles of the heart. Compensatory mechanisms of the ventricles allow the heart to compensate for these lesions for varying periods of time, before the need for surgical intervention. Significant valvular lesions, however, ultimately produce systolic or diastolic ventricular dysfunction, resulting in heart failure. Usually, surgery for stenotic valve lesions can be deferred until the patient becomes symptomatic. Regurgitant valve lesions, however, may produce significant ventricular dysfunction before the onset of symptoms, and thus surgery may be indicated in these patients. Among the heart's valves, the aortic and mitral valves are by far the most commonly affected and thus are the focus of this section.

Surgical Management of Aortic Valve Disease

Aortic stenosis, the most common valvular heart disease in developed countries, is most commonly caused by degeneration of the aortic valve tissue. Aortic stenosis is most prevalent in elderly people, although some congenital forms of aortic stenosis may affect younger patients as well. Aortic regurgitation is a less common form of aortic valve disease that is most commonly caused by a myxomatous degenerative process that causes prolapse of aortic valve cusps. Medical management is a mainstay of therapy for asymptomatic patients with preserved left ventricular size and function.

Aortic Stenosis

Aortic stenosis is a mechanical obstruction to flow from the left ventricle. Aortic valve replacement is the only effective treatment for severe aortic stenosis in the adult population. Percutaneous balloon aortic valvotomy has a role in the treatment of children with aortic stenosis and in the temporization of some symptomatic adults who are poor surgical candidates. Aortic valve replacement is usually recommended for patients who have any symptoms attributable to aortic stenosis in the absence of major comorbidities. The three principal symptoms of aortic stenosis are angina, syncope, and congestive heart failure. Angina and syncope warrant elective surgical therapy, whereas congestive heart failure mandates urgent intervention. The need for aortic valve replacement in patients with aortic stenosis who do not have symptoms is less clear. In patients with good ventricular function, aortic valve replacement is associated with an operative mortality rate of 2% to 8%. After aortic valve replacement, the projected 10-year age-matched survival rate is 80% to 85% (14). Bioprosthetic replacement aortic valves may be either porcine or bovine. Bioprostheses are less durable than mechanical prostheses but have the advantage of not needing lifelong anticoagulation to prevent blood clots from forming on the valve surfaces. The average life expectancy of an aortic valve bioprosthesis is 10 to 15 years. Bioprostheses rapidly calcify, degenerate, and narrow in young patients. Therefore, bioprostheses are primarily used in patients older than 75 years or patients who cannot take anticoagulants. Recently, aortic valves from human cadavers (aortic allografts) have been used in younger patients, particularly in the setting of endocarditis to avoid the need for anticoagulation medication. However, human aortic grafts are of limited quantity. The durability of allografts is limited. Structural valve failure (primary valve failure or deterioration) of allografts increases with time and approximates 19% to 38% at 10 years and 69% to 82% at 20 years (15). Mechanical prostheses have proven to be extremely durable and can be expected to last from 20 to 40 years. However, mechanical prostheses all require lifelong anticoagulation.

Aortic Regurgitation

Aortic regurgitation is the diastolic flow of blood from the aorta into the left ventricle. Regurgitation is caused by incompetence of the aortic valve or any disturbance of the valvular apparatus (e.g., leaflets, annulus of the aorta) resulting in diastolic flow of blood into the left ventricular chamber. Acute aortic regurgitation is treated by early valve replacement. With inadequate time for the left ventricle to compensate by myocardial hypertrophy, progressive congestive heart failure, tachycardia, and diminished cardiac output ensue rapidly. Patients with symptomatic chronic aortic insufficiency require surgical therapy because their prognosis when treated medically is only a few years. Determining the optimal timing of surgical intervention in patients with or without symptoms, however, may be very difficult. Aortic valve replacement is not recommended for patients who are asymptomatic and have normal ventricular function and good exercise tolerance (16). Surgical treatment is advisable for symptomatic patients with severe aortic regurgitation and for asymptomatic patients with an ejection fraction less than 0.50 and severe left ventricular dilation (end-diastolic diameter >75 mm or end-systolic diameter >55 mm) (1).

Aortic valve replacement is required for most patients with severe aortic regurgitation caused by primary valve disease (as opposed to aortic root disease) and for many patients with combined aortic stenosis and aortic regurgitation. In some patients with aortic root disease, the native valve can be spared when the aortic root is replaced or repaired. The mortality rate ranges from 3% to 8% in most medical centers. A late mortality of approximately 5% to 10% per year is observed in survivors who had marked cardiac enlargement or prolonged left ventricular dysfunction preoperatively (13).

Surgery of the Mitral Valve

Mitral stenosis is most commonly caused by rheumatic heart disease. At the beginning of 20th century, mitral stenosis occurred in epidemic proportions; however, modern antibiotic therapy has essentially eliminated this disease in developed countries.

Mitral valve stenosis—or mitral stenosis—is a condition in which the heart's mitral valve is narrowed. This narrowing prevents the valve from opening properly and obstructs blood flow between the left chambers of the heart. Mechanical relief of mitral stenosis should be considered when patients develop symptoms, when evidence of pulmonary hypertension appears, or when the mitral valve area is reduced to less than 1 cm². Other conditions that should prompt surgical consideration include systemic embolization, worsening pulmonary hypertension, and endocarditis. The options for mechanical relief of mitral stenosis include percutaneous balloon mitral valvuloplasty, closed mitral valvotomy, open surgical mitral valvuloplasty (commissurotomy), and mitral valve replacement.

Percutaneous Mitral Valvuloplasty

Percutaneous mitral valvuloplasty is a minimally invasive treatment that is used for a majority of patients with mitral stenosis. A specially designed balloon mounted on the catheter tip is used to dilate and widen the mitral orifice.

Percutaneous mitral valvuloplasty has provided good short-term and intermediate-term results in appropriately selected patients. Performed in the cardiac catheterization suite under fluoroscopic guidance, the technique includes advancement of one or two balloon catheters across the interatrial septum and inflation of the balloon within the stenotic mitral valve. Balloon inflation should increase the mitral valve area to about 2 cm². This is usually associated with a significant decline in left atrial pressure and transvalvular gradient and at least a 20% increase in cardiac output. The mortality rate associated with balloon mitral valvuloplasty is 0.5% to 2%. Other risks associated with percutaneous mitral valvuloplasty include systemic embolism, cardiac perforation, and creation of mitral regurgitation. Increased pulmonary vascular resistance has been shown to normalize after successful balloon valvuloplasty. Approximately 10% of patients have a residual interatrial septal defect. Three years after balloon valvuloplasty, at least 66% of patients are free of subsequent intervention. In appropriately selected patients, the results of balloon valvuloplasty compare favorably with those of surgical valvuloplasty (2).

Closed Mitral Valvotomy

Closed mitral valvotomy is used sporadically to treat patients with critical mitral stenosis who are not candidates for conventional mitral valve replacement. The operation is performed by blunt dilation of fused mitral leaflets.

Closed mitral valvotomy is performed without cardiopulmonary bypass but with the aid of a transventricular dilator. It is an effective operation, provided that mitral regurgitation, atrial thrombosis, or valvular calcification is not serious and that chordal fusion and shortening are not severe. Echocardiography may be used to select patients for the operation and exclude those with valvular calcification or dense fibrosis. When a satisfactory result cannot be achieved, the patient is placed on cardiopulmonary bypass and the valvotomy is carried out under direct vision, or the valve is replaced.

In a review of closed mitral valvotomy, English (5) reported that the hospital mortality rate after closed mitral valvotomy was 1.5%, and 0.3% of patients developed severe mitral regurgitation. Marked symptomatic improvement occurred in 86% of survivors. The actuarial survival rate was 89.5% after 18 years.

Open Mitral Commissurotomy

Open mitral commissurotomy is performed with the use of cardiopulmonary bypass. The stenotic orifice of the mitral valve is enlarged by partial division of leaflets at one or both commissures.

Surgical valvuloplasty (commissurotomy) allows the surgeon to directly see the mitral valve and the chordae tendineae and remove the left atrial thrombus. Cardiopulmonary bypass is established, and to obtain a dry, quiet heart, body temperature is usually lowered, the heart is arrested, and the aorta is occluded intermittently. The surgeon removes thrombi from the left atrium and left atrial appendage and often amputates the latter to remove a potential source of postoperative emboli. The commissures are incised, and, when necessary, fused chordae tendineae are separated, the underlying papillary muscle is split, and the valve leaflets are debrided of calcium. The surgeon may correct mild or even moderate mitral regurgitation. Furthermore, reconstruction of the valve may eliminate preexistent mitral regurgitation. In the presence of significant mitral regurgitation, however, the patient and physician should consider mitral valve replacement.

The mortality rate associated with open mitral valvuloplasty is less than 2%. When the procedure is performed in appropriately selected patients, the freedom from subsequent mitral valve intervention is about 75% at 5 years (2). Open valvotomy provides better hemodynamic results than does the closed procedure and lower risk of dislodging thrombi from the atrium or calcium from the mitral valve.

Mitral Regurgitation

Mitral regurgitation (MR) is the most common disease of the mitral valve in the developed world. It is caused by degenerative process of mitral valve leaflets and commonly affects middle-aged patients.

Mitral regurgitation, or mitral insufficiency, develops when the mitral valve does not close properly during systole, allowing the blood to flow backward from the left ventricle to the left atrium. The major causes of MR are mitral valve prolapse (MVP), rheumatic heart disease, infective endocarditis, annular calcification, cardiomyopathy, and ischemic heart disease. Less common causes of MR include collagen vascular diseases, trauma, the hypereosinophilic syndrome, carcinoid, and exposure to certain appetite-suppressant drugs. When considering operative treatment, the patient and physician must weigh the chronic and often slow but relentless progression of mitral regurgitation against the immediate risks and long-term uncertainties attendant on surgery, especially if valve replacement is required. The decision to replace or reconstruct the valve is very difficult: Replacement involves the operative risk as well as the risks of thromboembolism and anticoagulation in patients receiving mechanical prostheses, of late structural valve deterioration in patients receiving bioprostheses, and of late mortality, especially in patients with associated coronary artery disease who require coronary artery bypass grafting.

Mitral Valve Repair

Advantages of mitral valve repair over mitral valve replacement include improved long-term survival; better preservation of left ventricular function; and greater freedom from endocarditis, thromboembolism, and anticoagulant-related hemorrhage (10). With the introduction of standardized surgical techniques by Carpentier, Duran, and others, mitral valve repair has become reproducible and widely used (9). Symptomatic patients with degenerative mitral valve disease and 3+ or 4+ mitral regurgitation should be referred for surgery. Asymptomatic patients with 3+ or 4+ mitral regurgitation and a decrease in left ventricular function as demonstrated by resting or stress echocardiography, left ventricular dilatation, or new onset atrial fibrillation should also be referred for surgery (9).

Mitral valve repair restores the normal anatomy and function of the regurgitant mitral valve. The choice of specific repair technique is based on the primary cause of valve dysfunction.

- *Quadrangular resection.* Posterior leaflet prolapse is treated by quadrangular resection. The portion of the posterior leaflet with elongated or ruptured chordae is identified and resected. The resulting gap in the annulus is closed with one or two pledgeted sutures (figure 11.1). A ring annuloplasty completes the repair (9).
- *Sliding leaflet repair.* The sliding leaflet repair is used as an adjunct to quadrangular resection in patients with excess leaflet tissue and a posterior leaflet with a height of more than 1.5 cm. After quadrangular resection, the posterior leaflet is detached from the annulus for a distance of 1.5 to 2 cm on either side of the resection. Annuloplasty sutures are easily placed once the leaflet is detached. Then the leaflet is reattached to the annulus with a running 4-0 polypropylene suture (figure 11.2).
- *Anterior leaflet prolapse.* A variety of techniques have been used to treat anterior leaflet prolapse.

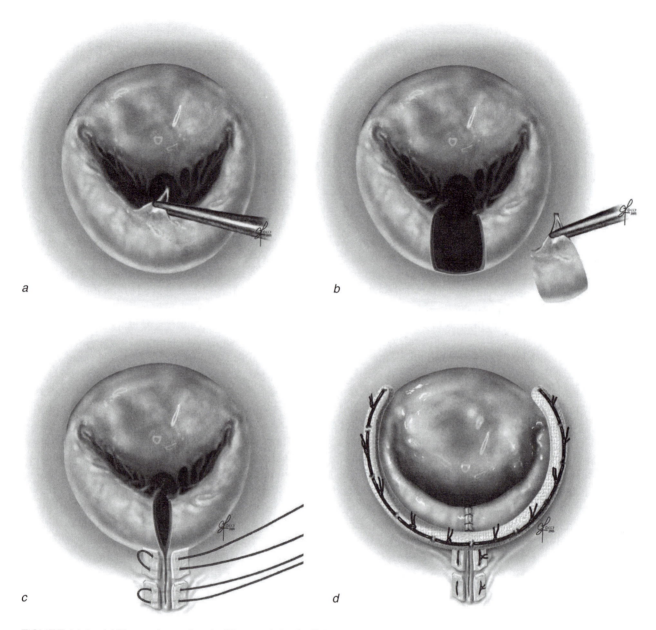

FIGURE 11.1 *(a)* The prolapsed part of the posterior leaflet is resected, and *(b)* edges of resected leaflet are approximated with *(c)* pledgeted sutures. *(d)* An annuloplasty ring is used to complete the repair.

Courtesy of Cleveland Clinic medical illustration department.

The most popular include chordal transfer, chordal replacement, and chordal shortening. Anterior leaflet resection is rarely indicated.

■ *Annuloplasty.* Annular enlargement is present in patients with degenerative disease. Annular dilatation usually occurs only along the posterior annulus because the anterior annulus is attached to the fibrous skeleton of the heart. Annuloplasty is a component of the repair in all patients with degenerative disease. Annuloplasty is performed to correct annular dilatation, increase leaflet coaptation, reinforce suture lines, and prevent further annular dilatation.

■ *Alfieri edge-to-edge repair.* Ottavio Alfieri described the edge-to-edge repair, a technique in which a suture affixes the free edge of a segment of normal posterior leaflet to the free edge of a prolapsing portion of the anterior leaflet.

Mitral Valve Replacement

Mitral valve replacement with prosthetic heart valves is an effective treatment of mitral regurgitation and mitral stenosis. Mechanical prostheses are made of specially processed carbon, with excellent durability and requirement for anticoagulation. Biological prostheses, most

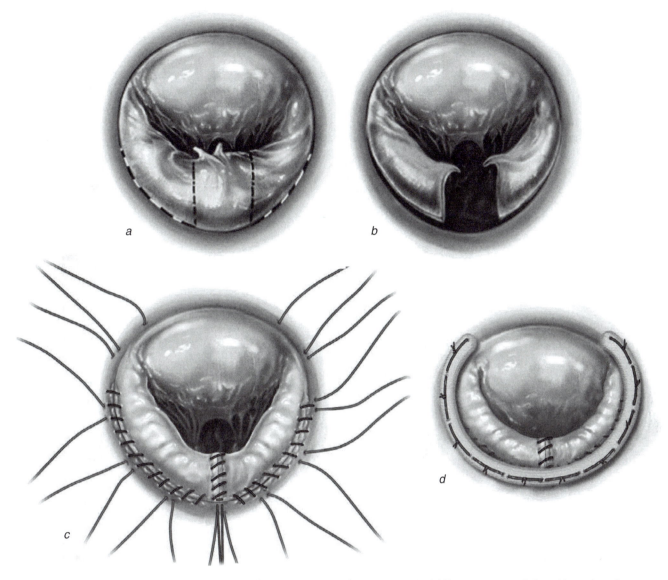

FIGURE 11.2 *(a)* Prolapsed midscallop of the posterior leaflet is resected. *(b)* Remaining medial and lateral scallops of the posterior leaflet are mobilized and *(c)* brought together using sliding repair technique. *(d)* The repair is completed by the insertion of the anuloplasty ring.

Courtesy of Cleveland Clinic medical illustration department.

commonly made from bovine or porcine tissue, are less durable but do not require anticoagulation.

Mitral valve replacement with a mechanical or bioprosthetic valve has been used successfully in treating MR for almost 4 decades. However, this operation carries some disadvantages. First, left ventricular function often deteriorates following this procedure, contributing to early and late mortality and late disability. This is not usually the case after mitral valve repair. Second, complications are associated with the prosthesis itself. These include thromboembolism or hemorrhage associated with mechanical prostheses, late mechanical dysfunction of bioprostheses, and the risk of infective endocarditis with both mechanical prostheses and bioprostheses. For these reasons, the current trend is to repair the mitral valve whenever possible, especially in patients with isolated or predominant mitral regurgitation. The Society of Thoracic Surgeons National Database Committee reported an operative mortality rate of less than 2% in 3,309 U.S. patients undergoing isolated mitral valve repair in 2002, comparing favorably to the 6% operative mortality for the 4,064 patients undergoing isolated mitral valve replacement (25).

Minimally invasive surgical techniques using a small, low sternotomy, although more demanding technically, are less traumatic and can be used for both valve repair and replacement. This approach has been reported to reduce cost, improve cosmetic results, and shorten the recovery time (8).

Summary

Cardiovascular disease is a major public health concern worldwide. Recent improvements in medical, interventional, and surgical treatment of ischemic heart disease have dramatically improved outcomes. An emphasis on disease prevention based on appropriate nutrition, exercise, and medical management could reduce the prevalence of this condition.

An increase in life expectancy leads to a greater number of elderly patients with valvular heart disease. Evolving treatment of valvular heart disease includes minimally invasive surgical approaches and percutaneous valve replacements.

CHAPTER 12

Cardiovascular Disease in Women

Nanette K. Wenger, MD

The landmark 2001 report of the Institute of Medicine, *Exploring the Biological Contributions to Human Health: Does Sex Matter?* (3), highlighted the importance of understanding the differences in human diseases between the sexes and translating these differences into clinical practice. In the area of cardiovascular disease, the escalating inclusion of women in registries, clinical trials, and case series has provided an increasingly robust evidence base for clinical practice. Public education about women and heart disease has burgeoned in the United States, including the Heart Truth Campaign of the National Heart, Lung, and Blood Institute and the Red Dress Campaign of the American Heart Association. The concordance of these efforts has the potential to improve the clinical outcomes of half of all patients seen in clinical practice—women.

Coronary Heart Disease

Cardiovascular disease is the leading cause of mortality for U.S. women, with coronary heart disease (CHD) responsible for approximately 250,000 deaths annually. Although CHD predominates in older age, it affects women across the life span. More than 9,000 women younger than age 45 incur myocardial infarction (MI) each year. Since 1984, more U.S. women than men have died annually from cardiovascular illness. Until 2000, cardiovascular mortality in the United States had decreased solely among men; favorably, since that time, there has been an annual continuing decrease in cardiovascular mortality for women. However, this improvement in women's survival is attributed to improved therapeutic approaches to established cardiovascular illness rather than to a decline in cardiovascular disease incidence. Therefore, an aggressive approach to coronary prevention is warranted for all women (18).

CHD is a major contributor to morbidity and disability for women. A third of women aged 55 to 64 years with documented CHD are disabled by their symptoms, with more than half of women older than age 75 disabled.

AHA Evidence-Based Guidelines for Coronary Prevention in Women: 2007 Update

The material in this section is based on recommendations from the American Heart Association (10). These guidelines emphasize a partnership between

Address correspondence concerning this chapter to Nanette K. Wenger, Emory University School of Medicine, 49 Jesse Hill Jr. Drive, Atlanta, GA 30303. E-mail: nwenger@emory.edu women and their physicians for coronary prevention, patterning the intensity of the intervention to the level of risk for the individual woman. Whereas the Framingham Risk Score (FRS) focuses on 10-year risk, the new guidelines focus on lifetime risk, because women develop the clinical manifestations of coronary disease 10 to 20 years later than do men. Women are categorized as high risk, at risk, or optimal risk. Women at high risk are those with documented coronary, cerebrovascular, or peripheral arterial disease; diabetes mellitus; chronic kidney disease; or a 10-year FRS global risk >20%. At-risk women are those with one or more major risk factors for cardiovascular disease, including cigarette smoking, poor diet, obesity (especially central adiposity), a family history of premature cardiovascular disease, hypertension, and dyslipidemia. As well, evidence for subclinical vascular disease such as coronary calcification, the metabolic syndrome, and poor exercise capacity on treadmill testing or abnormal cardiac rate recovery after stopping exercise defines the at-risk woman. A woman at optimal risk has an FRS global risk <10%, a healthy lifestyle, and no risk factors.

The first category of preventive approaches involves lifestyle interventions, all class I approaches. Women should be encouraged to not smoke and to avoid environmental tobacco smoke. A minimum of 30 min of moderate-intensity physical activity, such as brisk walking, is recommended on most and preferably all days of the week. When physical activity is used for weight loss or to sustain weight loss, 60 to 90 min of physical activity is recommended. For women with a recent acute coronary syndrome or coronary intervention, new-onset or chronic angina, a recent cerebrovascular event, peripheral arterial disease, or current or prior symptoms of heart failure and an LVEF <40%, a comprehensive cardiac rehabilitation regimen is advised. A heart-healthy diet includes a variety of fruits, vegetables, grains, low-fat or nonfat dairy products, fish, legumes, and protein sources low in saturated fat. Saturated fat intake should be less than 10% of calories and cholesterol intake less than 300 mg daily. Alcohol should be limited to no more than one drink a day and sodium intake to <2.3 g/day (approximately 1 teaspoon of salt). Consumption of trans fatty acid should be as low as possible, <1% of energy. Weight maintenance or reduction to achieve a body mass index between 18.5 and 24.9 kg/m^2 and waist circumference <35 in. (<89 cm) is recommended through a balance of physical activity, caloric intake, and formal behavioral programs. Evaluation for depression and referral and treatment as indicated are recommended for women with CHD (class IIa). Omega-3 fatty-acid supplementation maybe considered as an adjunct to diet for women with CHD

(class IIb), and higher doses may be used for high triglyceride levels.

The major risk factor interventions (class I) involve blood pressure, lipids and lipoproteins, and diabetes. An optimal blood pressure of <120/80 mmHg is recommended through lifestyle approaches, including weight control, increased physical activity, alcohol moderation, sodium restriction, and emphasis on consumption of fresh fruits, vegetables, and low-fat dairy products; pharmacotherapy is indicated for blood pressure ≥140/90 mmHg or at even lower levels (≥130/80 mmHg) in the presence of blood pressure–related target organ damage or diabetes. Thiazide diuretics should be part of the drug regimen for most patients unless they are contraindicated or unless there are compelling indications for other agents in specific vascular diseases. Initial treatment of high-risk women is with β-blockers, angiotensin-converting enzyme (ACE) inhibitors, or angiotensin receptor blockers (ARBs), with the addition of other drugs such as thiazides as needed to achieve goal blood pressure. Optimal levels of lipids and lipoproteins are a low-density lipoprotein cholesterol (LDL-C) <100 mg/dL, high-density lipoprotein cholesterol (HDL-C) >50 mg/dL, and triglycerides <150 mg/dL, with initial lifestyle intervention. For high-risk women, saturated fat intake should be <7% of calories and cholesterol should be <100 mg daily. In high-risk women, LDL-C-lowering therapy, preferably with a statin, should be initiated simultaneously with lifestyle changes to achieve an LDL-C <100 mg/dL. This is also applicable to women with other atherosclerotic CVD or diabetes or a 10-year absolute risk >20%. LDL-C reduction to <70 mg/dL is reasonable in very high risk women with CHD and may require LDL-lowering drug combinations (class IIa); statin therapy should be initiated in these women even with an LDL-C below 100 mg/dL in the absence of contraindications. With a low HDL-C or an elevated non–HDL-C in high-risk women, niacin or fibrate therapy should be initiated after the LDL-C goal is reached. For other at-risk women, the LDL-C level for initiation of pharmacotherapy is higher: LDL-C ≥130 mg/dL on lifestyle therapy with multiple risk factors and a 10-year absolute risk 10% to 20%, ≥160 mg/dL on lifestyle therapy with multiple risk factors even if the 10-year absolute risk is <10%, and LDL ≥190 mg/dL on lifestyle therapy regardless of the presence or absence of other risk factors or CVD. Niacin or fibrate is recommended after the LDL-C goal is reached. Both lifestyle and pharmacotherapy should be used to achieve a near-normal hemoglobin A$_{1c}$ (<7%) in women with diabetes if it can be accomplished without hypoglycemia.

Preventive drug interventions include routine aspirin use (75-325 mg daily) in high-risk women unless contraindicated. If the high-risk woman is intolerant to aspirin therapy, clopidogrel should be substituted. Aspirin therapy (81 mg daily or 100 mg every other day) should be considered in women ≥65 years old if blood pressure is controlled and the benefit for ischemic stroke and MI prevention is likely to outweigh the risk of gastrointestinal bleeding and hemorrhagic stroke (class IIa) and in women <65 years old when benefit for ischemic stroke prevention is likely to outweigh adverse effects of therapy (class IIb). β-blockers should be used indefinitely in all women following myocardial infarction, acute coronary syndrome, or left ventricular dysfunction with or without heart failure symptoms unless contraindicated. ACE inhibitors should be used (unless contraindicated) in women after myocardial infarction or in those with clinical evidence of heart failure or a left ventricular ejection fraction (LVEF) ≤40% or with diabetes; ARBs should be used if patients are intolerant to ACE inhibitors. Aldosterone blockade should be used in women after MI who do not have significant renal dysfunction or hyperkalemia who are already receiving therapeutic doses of an ACE inhibitor and β-blocker, have an LVEF ≤40%, and have diabetes or heart failure.

Class III interventions identify approaches to be avoided, given their lack of benefit and potential for harm. Hormone therapy and selective estrogen receptor modulators should not be used for the primary or secondary prevention of cardiovascular disease, nor should antioxidant vitamin supplements (e.g., vitamins C, E, and β-carotene). Folic acid, with or without vitamin B_6 and B_{12} supplementation, should not be used for the primary prevention of cardiovascular disease. Furthermore, in healthy women younger than 65 years of age, the routine use of aspirin is not recommended to prevent myocardial infarction.

Sex-Based Differences in Clinical Presentation

Angina is the predominant initial and subsequent CHD presentation in women (in contrast to MI and sudden death for men). Women with angina tend to be older than their male peers and more frequently have associated hypertension, diabetes, and heart failure. This presentation mandates prompt evaluation of chest pain in women, identifying the high-risk subset for whom intervention is warranted to prevent MI.

Although women with MI generally present with chest pain, women are more likely to have concomitant neck, back, shoulder, or abdominal discomfort and fatigue and dyspnea. Painless MI is more common in both sexes at old age. Atypical presentations contribute to a delay in recognition and therapy.

Diagnostic Testing in Women

A recent American Heart Association publication highlighted the importance of diagnostic testing for women with chest pain and emphasized its underutilization (9).

Although the exercise electrocardiogram (ECG) has lower sensitivity and specificity than imaging-based tests, it is appropriate for women who can exercise to adequate intensity and who have a normal resting ECG. When the resting ECG is abnormal, imaging-based testing with either echocardiographic or nuclear imaging procedures offers excellent diagnostic sensitivity and specificity for women. Pharmacologic stress testing is appropriate for women who cannot exercise to adequate intensity.

Emerging test modalities include coronary calcium scores, computed tomography imaging, and magnetic resonance imaging, but none are recommended for routine use.

MI: Differences in Management and Outcomes

About one third of all MIs occur in women, although women with an acute coronary syndrome are more likely to have unstable angina and less likely to have ECG- or biomarker-documented MI. Women are more likely to have non-ST-elevation MI than ST-elevation MI (18).

MI tends to be underrecognized in women or its recognition is delayed; women exhibit more delay in presenting to the emergency department after their onset of chest pain.

Recommendations for the management of acute coronary syndromes do not differ by gender, save for the consideration of an initial noninvasive strategy in low-risk women with unstable angina/non-ST-elevation MI (1). Nonetheless, recent surveillance of management of non-ST-elevation MI in the CRUSADE Registry showed that women were less likely to receive guideline-based therapies both at admission and at discharge. Bleeding with coronary thrombolysis for ST-elevation MI is greater in women, rendering acute percutaneous coronary intervention (PCI) the preferred management. The challenge is limited availability of primary PCI.

Women with MI, and in particular those younger than 50, have a doubled mortality compared with men during the acute hospitalization; during the initial 2 years following MI, women have an increased occurrence of both reinfarction and mortality. The contribution of suboptimal therapies to these adverse outcomes is not yet quantified.

Myocardial Revascularization: Differences in Management and Outcomes

PCI involves balloon angioplasty with and without stenting, although stenting with the use of bare metal or drug-eluting stents is the most common approach. Over time, PCI outcomes for women have improved dramatically. The acute procedural and clinical success rates are comparable for women and men, although women tend to be older and are more likely to have comorbidities including hypertension, diabetes, unstable angina, and peripheral vascular disease. Long-term outcomes are less favorable for women with increased mortality during hospitalization and less complete relief of angina than their male peers (18).

Coronary artery bypass graft (CABG) surgery is performed in about 180,000 women in the United States annually, without recent changes in the number of procedures. Women who undergo CABG have a doubled coronary mortality rate compared with men, and this difference is most prominent at younger ages. Women younger than age 50 who undergo CABG have a threefold increase in mortality compared with men of similar age. Much of the increased mortality seems related to comorbidities, rather than sex per se, with diabetes a major determinant of adverse outcome. Anemia may contribute to the adverse outcome. Early studies of off-pump CABG surgery suggest that this procedure, when applicable, may be advantageous for women.

With all revascularization procedures (including coronary thrombolysis for acute MI), women have an increased risk of bleeding compared with men. Contributors to this increased risk have not yet been ascertained.

Cardiac Rehabilitation: Sex-Based Differences and Recommendations

Women, and particularly older women, are less likely to be referred for cardiac rehabilitation and, when it is recommended, are less likely to attend and complete rehabilitation. Despite their lower baseline exercise capacity, older men and women of all ages experience an improvement in functional capacity comparable to that of younger men, even with 10 to 12 weeks of rehabilitation exercise training. Special effort is needed

to overcome obstacles to participation for women and to design programs for women with noncardiac morbidities such as arthritis and peripheral vascular disease. Resistance training can improve strength and enable increased performance of activities of daily living. Given the increased occurrence of depression following coronary events in women, a rehabilitation program may offer support, recognition, and therapy.

Hypertension: Sex-Based Differences

The Seventh Report of the Joint National Committee (7) defined a normal blood pressure as <120/80 mmHg. Prehypertension is 120 to 130 or 80 to 89 mmHg for systolic and diastolic blood pressures, respectively, whichever is higher. Stage I hypertension is 140 to 159 or 90 to 99 mmHg, and stage II hypertension is ≥160 or ≥100 mmHg for diastolic and systolic blood pressures, respectively, without sex-based differences. No antihypertensive drug therapy is indicated for prehypertension except in patients with chronic kidney disease or diabetes. Stage I hypertension may be controlled with one drug, but a two-drug combination is generally indicated for stage II hypertension.

Hypertension is the most common modifiable risk factor for women. Although it is less common in women than men at young and early middle-age, hypertension develops more prominently in women than men with aging such that it is more prevalent in women than men older than 60. The highest occurrence is in elderly black women, where hypertension is present in more than 75% of women older than 75 years. Women are more likely than men to be aware that they have hypertension and to have it treated, although less than half of all treated women have blood pressure controlled to goal levels. The major type of hypertension in elderly women is isolated systolic hypertension, defined as a systolic blood pressure >140 mmHg, with normal diastolic pressure.

A small but definite increase in blood pressure occurs in many women who use oral contraceptives; when contraceptive is discontinued, elevated blood pressure typically returns to normal, reinforcing the need to monitor blood pressure during contraceptive use. It remains uncertain whether menopause per se is associated with the occurrence of hypertension, whether hypertension is related to menopausal weight gain, or whether hypertension reflects increased prevalence of hypertension with aging.

All clinical trials of antihypertensive therapies showed significant reduction in stroke and major cardiovascular events in treated women, with treatment benefit comparable for women and men.

Recent data from the Women's Health Initiative (WHI) showed that one third of the women had hypertension; although two thirds were treated, only half had blood pressures controlled. Low levels of physical activity and the presence of obesity were associated with an increased frequency of hypertension. In WHI, most women were treated with a single drug, with the best control rates achieved with diuretic therapy. Current recommendations suggest that combination therapy may be warranted in many individuals. Lifestyle modification is important for all women with hypertension, with the most effective interventions being aerobic exercise and weight loss or weight control. Thiazide diuretics are of particular value for the older woman because they are associated with a decrease in bone loss and risk for hip fracture. Women are more likely than men to develop cough with ACE inhibitor therapy; diuretics may prove a problem in older women with urinary incontinence (16).

Hypertension in pregnancy occurs in about 5% of all pregnancies and includes women who had hypertension prior to pregnancy as well as those with pregnancy-induced hypertension with its adverse consequences of preeclampsia or eclampsia. Hypertension before the 20th week of pregnancy is assumed to be attributable to preexisting hypertension. As many as 25% of women have pregnancy-induced hypertension with the first pregnancy and 10% with a subsequent pregnancy (14). ACE inhibitor therapy is contraindicated during pregnancy because of its association with spontaneous abortion and fetal abnormalities.

Heart Failure: Sex-Based Differences

Although many cardiovascular diseases have decreased in prevalence, rates of heart failure in the United States have increased during the past 2 decades. The prevalence of heart failure also increases with aging; about 4% of women age 70 have heart failure in contrast to 15% at age 85. Women who develop heart failure, and particularly older women, are more likely to have preserved left ventricular systolic function. Heart failure with intact left ventricular systolic function, termed *diastolic heart failure*, reflects the limited ability of the heart to relax. Although hypertension remains a more prominent risk factor for development of heart failure in women than in men (who predominantly have heart failure attributable to MI), women who incur MI are almost twice as likely as men to subsequently develop heart failure (6, 11).

Peripartum cardiomyopathy is unexplained left ventricular systolic dysfunction that develops in the last month of pregnancy or within 5 months following delivery (14). Its occurrence varies greatly but averages about 1 in 3,000 to 4,000 pregnancies in developed countries. Its etiology is unknown, save for its excess occurrence with multiparity, older age, and hypertension or preeclampsia; the role of myocarditis remains uncertain. Peripartum cardiomyopathy includes marked fluid retention or overt cardiac failure; chest pain may be a confusing feature; and embolism and stroke may occur, as may supraventricular and ventricular arrhythmias—making it difficult to differentiate peripartum cardiomyopathy from other diseases. The physical findings are classic for acute ventricular systolic dysfunction—increased jugular venous pressure, pulmonary rales, a third heart sound, often a left sternal border systolic murmur, and edema. There is no classic electrocardiographic pattern, although sinus tachycardia is common. The chest X ray shows cardiomegaly and pulmonary venous congestion, and echocardiography demonstrates ventricular dilation and hypokinesis. Mitral and tricuspid valve regurgitation may be present, apical thrombi occur occasionally, and there often is a small pericardial effusion.

A woman with peripartum cardiomyopathy typically is managed with conventional treatment for left ventricular systolic dysfunction including diuretics, digitalis, and vasodilator therapy with hydralazine, nitrates, and spironolactone if needed. ACE inhibitor and ARB therapies are contraindicated until delivery has occurred, although anticoagulation is appropriate. The prognosis for peripartum cardiomyopathy is variable. In earlier years, one third of women recovered, one third remained stable, and one third progressed to more severe decompensated heart failure. Recent reports suggest a better prognosis, with about half of women returning to normal left ventricular function in about 6 months. A challenge with normalized left ventricular function is deciding whether a future pregnancy should be undertaken; cardiovascular reserve remains decreased even with grossly normal ventricular systolic function. Recurrent peripartum cardiomyopathy with subsequent pregnancies is described in up to 20% of women with apparent complete recovery of ventricular function and in almost half of women with persistent left ventricular systolic dysfunction (14).

Heart failure in general is diagnosed symptomatically by exercise intolerance, exertional dyspnea, and fatigue. The clinical findings include volume overload with pulmonary congestion and peripheral edema. The immediate evaluation should include an echocardiogram to differentiate diastolic and systolic heart failure and to determine possible remediable causes for heart failure such as coronary or valvular heart disease.

The majority of treatment trials for heart failure have involved left ventricular systolic dysfunction. The percentage of women enrolled in these trials was disappointingly small, generally about 20%, although there was no gross difference in the response of women to heart failure therapies. Treatment included diuretics, digitalis, ACE inhibitors, and β-blockers. Because of the underenrollment of women in clinical trials, there is only suggestive survival benefit for ACE inhibitors, although their use is recommended. β-blocker trials, when combined to reveal a significant number of events in women, have shown equal benefit for women as for men. ARB and aldosterone inhibitor trials have shown comparable benefit by sex. However, the Digitalis Investigation Group, examining the effects of digitalis therapy for long-standing heart failure, showed no benefit in the overall group but higher mortality for women; the latter may represent overdosing of digoxin in women (12).

Calcium channel blocking drugs have a role in the management of diastolic heart failure, but those with a negative impact on ventricular function are contraindicated in women with systolic heart failure.

Additional therapies include sodium restriction and, with systolic heart failure, substantial fluid restriction. Once symptoms are controlled, a low-intensity physical activity program is an important part of the regimen. In patients with diastolic heart failure, exercise may improve symptoms; hence, many women may be referred for cardiac rehabilitation.

For patients unresponsive to medical therapies, newer approaches include biventricular pacing (with early studies showing comparable improvement in women and men) and cardiac transplantation, the ultimate intervention. Women and men who undergo cardiac transplantation have comparable survival rates, and the vast majority attain good functional status. The safety of childbearing after transplantation has not been fully examined, although in general there are favorable outcomes for the mother and baby. Despite concerns about immunosuppressive therapy, no excess of birth defects or complications of pregnancy have been reported in transplanted women. The major concern is whether the woman with a transplanted heart will survive to raise her child to adulthood.

Implanted cardioverter defibrillators are recommended for women and men with severe left ventricu-

lar systolic dysfunction caused by both coronary and noncoronary heart disease (6, 11).

Valvular Heart Disease

In prior years rheumatic fever with resultant rheumatic heart disease (RHD) was the major cause of valvular heart disease in women. As rheumatic fever has declined in industrialized countries, most RHD in U.S. women occurs among those from developing countries (4, 5).

Rheumatic Heart Disease

Mitral stenosis is more frequent in women than men and predominates as a manifestation of RHD in women. Progressive narrowing of the mitral orifice, at times associated with recurrent episodes of rheumatic fever, limits cardiac output. The initial symptoms most commonly are associated with onset of atrial fibrillation or are related to the increased cardiac output of pregnancy. The diagnosis is made by physical examination and confirmed with Doppler echocardiography. Depending on the anatomic characteristics of the mitral valve, and in particular the degree of calcification, percutaneous mitral balloon valvotomy can be undertaken or surgical management chosen with mitral valve repair or replacement.

Mitral regurgitation often occurs in association with mitral stenosis in a woman with RHD. The increased workload on the left ventricle results in progressive ventricular dilatation, decreased exercise tolerance, and is often associated with atrial fibrillation. Diagnosis can be made by physical examination and confirmed by Doppler echocardiography. Surgical correction is warranted before the development of significant left ventricular dysfunction. Often mitral valve repair can be accomplished; alternatively, mitral valve replacement is undertaken.

Aortic stenosis commonly occurs in association with mitral valve disease in women with RHD. Progressive narrowing of the aortic valve orifice results in progressive symptoms of angina, heart failure, or syncope. The diagnosis can be made by physical examination and confirmed by Doppler echocardiography. Symptomatic aortic stenosis requires prompt surgical correction, typically with aortic valve replacement. In contrast to congenital aortic stenosis, calcification of the rheumatic aortic valve typically limits aortic balloon valvuloplasty.

Aortic regurgitation is also commonly associated with mitral valve disease in women with RHD.

Despite asymptomatic aortic regurgitation, surgical replacement of the aortic valve is indicated when left ventricular dilation occurs. Diagnosis is made by clinical examination and the severity assessed by Doppler echocardiography.

There is no medical treatment to reverse valve stenosis or regurgitation. Drug therapy can help maintain normal ventricular function or control the heart rate with atrial fibrillation. For the young woman contemplating pregnancy, however, *bioprosthetic or homograft valves* are preferable, despite their decreased durability compared with mechanical valves. Women with mechanical heart valves require anticoagulation, which is associated with considerable maternal and fetal complications of pregnancy.

Nonrheumatic Heart Disease

Nonrheumatic mitral stenosis is rare but occasionally occurs with congenital mitral stenosis or degenerative mitral valve disease with heavy calcification narrowing the mitral orifice.

Mitral regurgitation may be related to endocarditis, degenerative mitral valve disease, coronary heart disease, or mitral valve prolapse (discussed subsequently). Mitral regurgitation may be asymptomatic over a long period of time, but the woman subsequently develops dyspnea, orthopnea, and paroxysmal nocturnal dyspnea. Even in the absence of symptoms, surgical correction is warranted before there is progressive left ventricular systolic dysfunction. As is the case with RHD, diagnosis is made by clinical examination, and the severity of the regurgitation is confirmed by Doppler echocardiography. Surgical intervention involves either mitral valve repair or replacement, the choice of which depends on the anatomy of the mitral valve. Mitral repair, when feasible, is preferable because it improves left ventricular function and survival. Transcatheter repair is investigational.

Mitral valve prolapse, related to elongation of the mitral chordae, is more common in women than men and occurs in up to 3% of the U.S. population. Often mitral valve prolapse is asymptomatic, but many women describe chest pain, palpitations, fatigue, and anxiety. The diagnosis can be made by clinical examination and confirmed by echocardiography. Although women are more likely to have mitral valve prolapse than men, their long-term course is typically benign; predominantly men have progressive severity of mitral regurgitation and require mitral valve repair or replacement. Women with palpitations may have good response to β-blocking drugs.

Aortic stenosis is characterized by progressively increased valve narrowing and calcification. An atherosclerotic cause has been proposed, and studies are underway to determine whether statin therapy may decrease progression. Aortic stenosis is less common in women than in men, and among women it typically occurs at elderly age. The older age of occurrence in women may explain their less favorable outcomes with surgery. Symptoms of angina, heart failure, or syncope require urgent surgical valve replacement. Because women who experience aortic stenosis are typically elderly, coronary arteriography is required preoperatively to ascertain whether concurrent CABG surgery is required.

Bicuspid aortic valve, a congenital abnormality, is less common in women than in men, although it is another cause of late aortic stenosis. Diagnosis and management are as for aortic stenosis.

Aortic regurgitation occurs less frequently in women than in men. The chronic increased workload results in progressive ventricular dilation. Patients typically remain asymptomatic until late in the course of aortic regurgitation; physical activity increases the heart rate and thereby decreases the degree of regurgitation, limiting symptoms. Surgical correction is recommended with progressive ventricular dilation even for asymptomatic women. Diagnosis is by physical examination, and the severity of the aortic regurgitation can be determined by Doppler echocardiography. In some women, aortic regurgitation is associated with aortic root disease, such as in the Marfan syndrome.

Valvular Heart Disease Related to Appetite Suppressant (Anorectic) Drugs

With the progressive epidemic of obesity, prescription drugs have been increasingly used as anorectic agents, with the greatest prevalence of drug use in the 1990s. Concern subsequently developed with use of the combination appetite suppressant fenfluramine and phentermine (fen-phen). Although both drugs individually received U.S. Food and Drug Administration approval, combination therapy did not. Both agents were withdrawn from the U.S. market in 1997 because of their association with valvular heart disease and pulmonary hypertension. Earlier evidence of pulmonary hypertension with appetite suppressants had been available with other drugs in Europe. Women with pulmonary hypertension in Europe were more likely to have taken anorectic drugs, with increased duration of use associated with increased incidence of pulmonary hypertension.

The pulmonary hypertension rarely regresses, and management is with anticoagulant therapy, oxygen, diuretics, and vasodilator drugs. Early reports suggested abnormalities of cardiac valves with use of these drugs; an initial report suggested that a few women had severe valvular regurgitation requiring surgery. The true estimate of prevalence of valve disease is not known because most women had not had prior echocardiographic examination. The current estimate is that 4% to 9% of women using anorectic drugs will have aortic or mitral valve regurgitation, with the occurrence increasing with increased duration of use. Follow-up after diagnosis has shown that valvular disease either stabilizes or regresses with time. The American College of Cardiology recommends that these drugs be discontinued and patients be evaluated by echocardiogram (17).

Rehabilitation After Valve Repair or Replacement

Many women with symptomatic valvular heart disease restricted their physical activity prior to percutaneous and surgical repair in an attempt to avert symptoms. Hospitalization for surgery may also have induced deconditioning (4, 5). Cardiac rehabilitation exercise training can help restore physical work capacity.

Congenital Heart Disease

The diagnosis of congenital heart disease is suspected on clinical examination and confirmed with echocardiography. Although cardiac catheterization previously was recommended for complex congenital lesions, magnetic resonance imaging has obviated most of the need for cardiac catheterization, either for diagnosis or prior to surgery (2).

Because most hemodynamically significant congenital heart disease is corrected in childhood, most adult women have either nonhemodynamically significant congenital heart disease or surgically corrected disease. The major sex-based difference in management relates to pregnancy and its maternal and fetal risks and to the importance of women as caregivers. Congenital lesions differ little between the sexes, except that slightly more women have atrial septal defect, experience primary pulmonary hypertension, and develop the Eisenmenger physiology as a complication of shunt lesions.

Most women with mild to moderate congenital heart disease or corrected congenital heart disease can safely tolerate pregnancy. The major lesions warranting recommendations against pregnancy are those associated with pulmonary hypertension, hemodynamically significantly outflow obstruction, and the Marfan syndrome. Three to six percent of offspring may have congenital heart disease, although some studies cite an incidence as high as 10% to 15%. The Marfan syndrome may have a heritable risk as high as 50% for offspring.

Left-to-right shunt lesions include patent ductus arteriosus, atrial septal defect, and ventricular septal defect, with hemodynamically significant shunts typically corrected in childhood. There is a high rate of spontaneous closure of ventricular septal defect in the early years of life.

Stenotic lesions include coarctation of the aorta, which typically is corrected in childhood. There is a concomitant high occurrence of bicuspid aortic valve; its severity may worsen with the years. Aortic stenosis may result from a bicuspid aortic valve.

Pulmonic stenosis is typically corrected in childhood, currently with catheter-based valve dilation rather than with surgery as in earlier years.

Cyanotic congenital heart disease has a very high risk of maternal and fetal mortality during pregnancy attributable to a combination of hypoxemia and high hemoglobin levels.

Tetralogy of Fallot is the most common cyanotic congenital heart disease; complete correction in childhood rarely poses a problem in adult life. The Eisenmenger syndrome is pulmonary hypertension that results from a large-volume left-to-right shunt, with pulmonary hypertension subsequently producing shunt reversal with cyanosis. This poses a high risk with pregnancy, and physical activity exceeding usual daily activities is contraindicated.

The Marfan syndrome is a congenital multisystem abnormality whose major concern is aortic dilatation and rupture and aortic regurgitation. Even following valve replacement and aortic root dilation correction, pregnancy poses an increased risk.

Hypertrophic obstructive cardiomyopathy is characterized by abnormal thickening of the interventricular septum, often causing dynamic obstruction of the left ventricular outflow tract during systole and entrapment of the mitral leaflet toward the septum with resultant mitral regurgitation. Symptomatic women often have had therapy with surgery or catheter-based ablation. Pregnancy is well tolerated in the absence of hemodynamic obstruction, and exercise is not restricted. A substantial outflow gradient is a contraindication to competitive exercise. Patients have an unpredictable arrhythmia risk (8).

Rhythm Disturbances and Implications for Cardiac Rehabilitation

Ventricular premature beats are the most common rhythm disturbance and typically are described by patients as palpitations or skipped beats. The strong beat perceived by the patient is not the premature beat, which typically has a small stroke volume (because it occurs early in the cardiac cycle), but rather the beat following the premature one because of the larger filling volume. Ventricular premature beats commonly occur in the absence of underlying cardiovascular disease and typically require no treatment. For a patient who is highly symptomatic, low-dose β-blocking drugs may provide symptomatic relief. The prognosis of ventricular premature beats depends on the presence or absence of underlying cardiovascular disease. Per se, they constitute no contraindication to exercise training.

Supraventricular tachycardia (SVT) refers to rapid heart rate that originates in the atrium or the atrioventricular node. SVT attributable to an accessory pathway tends to be more common in women. Although in prior years pharmacotherapy was used to treat symptomatic supraventricular tachyarrhythmias, radio frequency ablation is highly successful and recommended for recurrent symptomatic supraventricular tachyarrhythmias. Radio frequency ablation has comparable success rates in women and men, although women tend to be more symptomatic and have a longer period of antiarrhythmic drug treatment before referral for ablation. Exercise is not contraindicated.

Atrial fibrillation is characterized by uncoordinated rapid atrial contraction that leads to stasis of the blood in atria and predisposition to thromboembolic complications. The occurrence and prevalence of atrial fibrillation increase with increasing age and with valvular heart disease, hypertension, coronary heart disease, and heart failure. Atrial fibrillation can be managed by pharmacologic rate or rhythm control. Current data suggest that both require anticoagulant therapy; therapy does not differ by sex. Atrial fibrillation with a controlled ventricular response rate is not a contraindication to exercise training.

Torsade de pointes, a polymorphic ventricular tachycardia, is the most serious ventricular arrhythmia, and its substrate is prolongation of the ECG QT interval. Drug-induced prolongation of the QT interval and resultant torsade de pointes are more common in women than men. Monitoring of the QT interval is recommended in women taking drugs known to prolong the QT interval, particularly the antihistamine terfenadine, the antipsychotic haloperidol, and the anti-infective erythromycin. Serious ventricular arrhythmias should be controlled before exercise training is undertaken.

Ventricular arrhythmias pose a high risk of sudden cardiac death for patients with severe left ventricular systolic dysfunction, typically an ejection fraction less than 35%. In clinical trials, antiarrhythmic therapy has been less successful than an implanted cardioverter defibrillator (ICD), currently the recommended therapy. Exercise testing is recommended for patients before undergoing exercise training to program the unit to appropriately perceive the exercise heart rate and not result in an unwarranted shock. ICD shocks cannot harm others exercising with the patient (13).

Cardiac pacemakers are implanted for serious atrioventricular conduction disturbances, sick sinus syndrome, and other arrhythmic etiologies. The most commonly implanted cardiac pacemaker today is a DDD (i.e., an atrioventricular pacemaker). Settings are programmed at implantation depending on the anticipated activity level of the patient, and many pacemakers are rate responsive. Less common is a VVI, a ventricular pacemaker, with settings also often programmed to reflect rate responsiveness. Exercise training can be performed in patients with implanted pacemakers; exercise testing can be used to determine the appropriate training heart rates.

Depression and Heart Disease

Because depression is highly prevalent in women, the role of depression in the occurrence and outcome of cardiovascular disease is particularly relevant to women (15). Women with CHD are more vulnerable to depression than are men, and depression likely more powerfully predicts cardiovascular disease for women. A recent study suggested that depression was particularly prominent among young women with CHD.

In a recent trial of cognitive behavioral therapy and interventions for social isolation in patients following MI, there was no evidence for benefit of this therapy. However, a subset analysis suggested potential benefit for antidepressant therapy, particularly selective serotonin reuptake inhibitors.

The AHA Prevention Guideline for Women recommends assessment for depression in women with CHD and referral for therapy (10).

Summary

This chapter highlights gender-specific data relevant to coronary heart disease, hypertension, valvular heart disease, congenital heart disease, cardiac rhythm distur- bances, and depression and heart disease. Expansion of the recruitment and enrollment of women in cardio- vascular clinical trials and emphasis on the reporting of gender-specific outcomes of such studies will increase the information available to the clinician and to women to guide the prevention, recognition, and diagnosis of cardiovascular disease.

Lifestyle Management of Cardiovascular Disease

Lifestyle management of cardiovascular disease is discussed in part III. Chapter 13 overviews the financial burden of this disease and the need for a clearly identifiable facility to manage specific clinical and financial issues. A review of the various strategies used to develop a comprehensive management plan for cardiovascular disease is presented in chapter 14. The remaining chapters (15, 16, and 17) discuss endurance, strength, and flexibility training specific to cardiovascular disease. Chapter 18 discusses nutrition and dietary factors that are associated with reducing likelihood or risk for developing disease.

Disease Management and Discharge Destinations

Linda Hall, PhD

In the United States, the disease burden in the first half of the 20th century was primarily caused by virus and bacteria that produced epidemics of typhoid, tuberculosis, and polio. As the industrial revolution and medical science progressed, those diseases were eliminated by development of vaccines. The industrial revolution brought forth a new way of living that led to sedentary lifestyles, increased consumption of fast foods, and other innovations that made life easier but also posed threats. These changes in the way many Americans lived led to the development of chronic diseases, especially obesity and type 2 diabetes, of almost epidemic proportions. This chapter develops a framework for creating a discharge destination in health care systems to manage chronic diseases and their causal risk factors. When patients are discharged from the hospital, often they are sent to as many as three or four outpatient offices and facilities to receive aftercare. By putting these services in one location, a discharge destination plan allows the patient to do one-stop health care shopping: easy parking, grouped appointments, and integrated delivery among and within diagnoses. For example, 80% of people with diabetes will die of heart disease. Why not group rehabilitation for heart disease and education for diabetes in the same facility?

Health Care Finance

Health care costs are a major concern for hospital chief financial officers, business and industry leaders, and human resource executives. A 12.6% increase in the U.S. national average for health care in 2004 served as a warning for these leaders; business and industry's contribution to employee health benefits will rise 54% and employee contributions may triple by 2010 (37). In 2001, health care spending in the United States was US$1.4 trillion, and according to the Centers for Medicare and Medicaid Services, health expenditures in the United States will reach US$2.6 trillion by 2010 and US$3.6 trillion by 2014 (4, 8). The United States spends twice the median level for health care of the 30 industrialized nations in the Organization for Economic Cooperation and Development, even though more than 15% of the U.S. population has no health insurance coverage. Astoundingly enough, U.S. citizens have worse outcomes than people whose nations spend much less (8).

Address correspondence concerning this chapter to Linda Hall, 9313 W. Hidden Valley Circle N., Sun City, AZ 85351. E-mail: LKHall317@aol.com

Hospitals today face huge strains in maintaining adequate bottom lines as reimbursement levels decrease, revenues decline, and costs increase (24). Tight labor markets (nursing shortage), lower payments from public insurers, and the growing cost of pharmaceuticals and technology decreased operating margins for America's hospitals from 3.7% in 2002 to 3.3% in 2003. Pending cuts in Medicare and Medicaid bring an additional cause for concern (16). Adding to the burden that hospitals face is the increasing amount of uncompensated care provided to the uninsured, who were estimated in 2004 to be 45 million Americans, although this number may have reached as high as 74 million over any 6-month snapshot in that year (30). Predictions are that as costs rise, more cost will be shifted to employers, who already bear a hefty portion of U.S. health care's financial burden. Ultimately, the employer will shift more cost to the employee or drop health care insurance coverage altogether, which then will increase the number of people without insurance (30).

Only 3% of the total budget for health care expenditures in the United States is dedicated to prevention of disease and injury (10). Although exercise, education, and lifestyle interventions are vitally important for people recovering from and managing chronic disease, insurance rarely pays for these interventions.

Insurance Reimbursement for Outpatient Education and Exercise

At the time of this writing, the Centers for Medicare and Medicaid Services (CMS) were remunerating US$31.03 for a session of cardiac rehabilitation (1). This amount is adjusted by the wage index for the region where the program is located. Pulmonary rehabilitation payments are determined by a local coverage determination that is regionally based, because there is no national coverage determination by CMS. Coverage is determined according to the personnel providing the service; for example, physical therapy is paid in 15 min increments, and a nurse or respiratory therapist or other health professional is paid by the session. For pulmonary rehabilitation, there is an additional remuneration for each 15 min of education appropriately documented in the patient's medical record (35). Diabetes self-management education is paid for by insurance, as are services for physical, occupational, and speech therapies. In all of these cases, the patient must be referred by a physician and have the appropriate diagnosis and accompanying code

per the International Classification of Diseases–Ninth Revision (20).

Cardiovascular exercise tests are covered under procedural terminology guidelines by the American Medical Association (AMA). These must be ordered by and supervised by a physician. There must be a clinically valid reason for ordering the test (e.g., suspected cardiovascular disease with accompanying risk factors such as hypertension, dyslipidemia, or diabetes), or otherwise insurance companies will not provide reimbursement (3). Insurance usually covers two stress tests per year unless physicians determine and document the need for more. As a result, 85% of patients entering cardiac rehabilitation programs are referred by their physicians without a preliminary stress test, a test that is recommended by ACSM and by many of the contributors to this book. Innovative program personnel have found ways to assess patients, such as using ECG to monitor heart rate and rhythm and using submaximal testing, such as a 6 min walk or bicycle tests, to monitor blood pressure (2). This submaximal procedure surveys for rhythm disturbances and provides information for exercise prescription and surveys. Otherwise, the physician will refer the patient and include a heart rate ceiling for safety.

Interventions to complete a disease management process (e.g., smoking cessation, weight management, exercise programming, behavior and risk factor modification) are not covered by any of the CMS-designated insurers and most commercial or business-affiliated self-insurance programs. Some managed care programs pay for interventions, and in all cases reimbursement should be sought with the insurance intermediary; however, these programs are usually only available as self-pay entities, and although they are recommended by physicians and advertised by hospitals, they are only used by patients and clients who have discretionary income.

Patient Satisfaction and Program Implementation

Health care is becoming extremely competitive, with hospitals competing against one another for occupied beds and physicians looking for increased income by performing screening tests and procedures in their offices rather than in hospitals. A health care system's market share is determined by its reputation as perceived by the public. The paying customer includes employers who determine health care contracts, health plans and provider groups that determine compensation formulas, and consumers who select their health plan based on whether it is a point of service or preferred provider plan (5). Patient satisfaction is a measure of patients' perceptions of their health and quality of life outcomes and their satisfaction with the quality of care and services they receive. Often these perceptions are as important as clinical measures such as reduced blood pressure or lipid profiles.

Press Ganey, the health care industry's leading patient satisfaction consultant, believes that services such as cardiac rehabilitation, pulmonary rehabilitation, physical therapy, occupational therapy, and speech therapy score high on the patient satisfaction grid of most health care organizations because these programs provide personal attention and care. These programs often are viewed as going the extra mile to ensure that everything is done to help the patient recover (33). Because these programs provide outpatient services, they may be viewed as the exit program from the hospital and will leave the patient with the perception of excellent service.

America's Health Problems

Approximately two thirds of all deaths in the United States are directly related to five chronic diseases— heart (cardiovascular) disease, chronic obstructive pulmonary disease, cancer, stroke, and diabetes. Chronic disease accounts for 75% of the nation's total health care costs. Because chronic disease, once diagnosed, is constant and prolonged, the resulting pain and suffering decrease the quality of life of millions of Americans (11). Chronic disease is costly because of increasing technology, improvements in environmental and social conditions, and the increase in life expectancy. Improvements in environment and social conditions have led to an increase in sedentary living, poor eating habits, and tobacco use as leisure time increases because of time-saving technology (12).

Three modifiable health-damaging behaviors are directly related to these five leading causes of death and suffering. These health-damaging behaviors—smoking, overweight and obesity, and a sedentary lifestyle—are preventable behaviors.

Smoking

Tobacco use is the single most preventable contributor to death and disease, responsible for more than 440,000 premature deaths in the United States annually. Tobacco use affects not only those who smoke but also those exposed to second-hand smoke, including infants, children, and adults. Each year, nonsmokers account for more than 3,000 deaths from lung cancer and 300,000 respiratory tract infections attributable to exposure to second-hand smoke. One half of all adolescents who try smoking will become addicted and will become lifelong smokers, and it is estimated that 6.4 million people who are currently under the age of 18 will die prematurely as a result of smoking (36). The direct and indirect costs of smoking exceed US$138 billion per year; a smoker currently pays approximately US$3.25 per pack of cigarettes and each pack smoked costs the United States US$7.18 in health care costs (36). Obviously, smoking cessation has the potential to affect health care expenditures in the United States and substantially reduce mortality and morbidity.

Obesity

Nearly two thirds of U.S. adults are overweight and more than 30% are obese (31). Classified as an epidemic because its prevalence has more than doubled in the last 20 years, obesity is seen as one of the top threats to the nation's health (28). Calling obesity and diabetes a health threat for our children that is growing into an international public health problem, former Surgeon General C. Everett Koop coined the term *diabesity* (31). Obesity is a function of an imbalance between calories consumed and calories expended through activity. Obesity stems from the increase in fast-food consumption, increases in consumption of soft drinks and supersized low-cost portions, and a concomitant decrease in the amount of physical activity in the U.S. population. The total cost for obesity is US$117 billion dollars per year, which is spent caring for the diseases associated with obesity listed in the section Chronic Diseases Caused by or Enhanced by Three Risk Factors. Obesity is costly to business and industry because 39.3 million work days are lost each year and 239.0 million more days involve restricted activity, losses that have a huge impact on productivity. This is a health risk that occupies the minds and efforts of many U.S. consumers, as evidenced by the expenditure of more than US$33 billion annually on weight loss products and services (31).

Sedentary Lifestyle

Booth and colleagues (6) described U.S. society as being at war with modern chronic disease, the roots of which lie primarily in one environmental factor that virtually did not exist before the 20th century. The antithesis of this environmental factor is able to prevent most chronic diseases, profoundly and positively affect all

Chronic Diseases Caused by or Enhanced by Three Risk Factors

Smoking

- Chronic lung disease
- Emphysema
- Asthma
- Heart disease
- Stroke
- Lung cancer
- Laryngeal cancer
- Esophageal cancer
- Oral cancer
- Bladder cancer
- Cervical cancer
- Pancreatic cancer
- Kidney cancer
- High blood pressure
- Peripheral vascular disease
- Sudden cardiac death
- Osteoporosis
- Peptic ulcer disease
- Impotence
- Dental disease

Obesity

- Heart disease
- Diabetes
- Congestive heart failure
- Angina
- Gout
- Stroke
- Hypertension
- Gallbladder disease
- Osteoarthritis
- Asthma
- Sleep apnea
- Uterine cancer
- Breast cancer
- Colorectal cancer

- Kidney cancer
- Gallbladder cancer
- Dyslipidemia
- Complications of pregnancy
- Menstrual irregularities
- Hirsutism
- Stress incontinence
- Psychological disorders
- Surgical risk

Sedentary Lifestyle

- Angina
- Heart attack
- Coronary artery disease
- Breast cancer
- Colon cancer
- Congestive heart failure
- Depression
- Gallstone disease
- High blood triglycerides
- High blood cholesterol
- Hypertension
- Poor cognitive function
- Low high-density lipoproteins
- Low quality of life
- Obesity
- Osteoporosis
- Pancreatic cancer
- Peripheral vascular disease
- Physical frailty
- Premature mortality
- Prostate cancer
- Sleep apnea
- Stiff joints
- Stroke
- Type 2 diabetes

Smoking data from U.S. Department of Health and Human Services 2005; obesity data from National Institute of Diabetes and Digestive and Kidney Diseases 2005; sedentary lifestyle data from Pate et al. 1995.

known chronic disease conditions, decrease morbidity and increase longevity, improve mental health, and decrease health care costs by billions of dollars (6). Called the *sedentary death syndrome* by Booth and colleagues (7), this environmental factor is inactivity or a sedentary lifestyle. According to Pate and colleagues (32), "Every American should accumulate 30 minutes or more of moderate intensity physical activity on most, preferably all, days of the week" (page 402). Twenty-eight percent of U.S. adults undertake no leisure-time activity, and 42% of U.S. adults do not meet the 30 min/day recommendation, which means that 70% of U.S. adults lead sedentary lives (7).

The direct and indirect costs of sedentary living as related to chronic disease exceeded US$150 billion in 2000 and account for approximately 15% of the total U.S. health care budget (7). The costs of cardiovascular disease and diabetes combined are US$396 billion a year. A 30% reduction in these two diseases would save US$119 billion a year. Is this feasible? Yes. Hu and colleagues (25-27) found that 2.5 hr of brisk walking per week reduced cardiovascular disease, stroke, and type 2 diabetes by 30%. All-cause mortality rates would be reduced by as much as 30% if every person expended an average of 1,000 kcal/week (approximately 2 miles/day, 5 days/week) (25). The list titled Chronic Diseases Caused by or Enhanced by Three Risk Factors on page 134 demonstrates the enormous effect that these three lifestyle choices or risk factors have on the development or exacerbation of chronic disease in the United States. The costs and the morbidity and mortality consequences of these account for more than 75% of health care expenditures and premature deaths annually.

Importance of Primary Prevention

The easiest way to reduce or eliminate the consequences of these three risk factors is primary prevention. At the time of this writing, Medicare was considering paying for two smoking cessation (13) opportunities per year, and many professional organizations were starting programs in which pedometers were used to encourage people to take 10,000 steps a day, which would affect both obesity and sedentary living (21). The information is available to educate Americans about the health risks from these three factors and how to change their behaviors. Newspapers and magazines publish articles on the topic. National television morning programs have started New Year's challenge programs each year, and even churches are starting health awareness programs (22). Business and industry support health education and awareness programs, often rewarding participants with financial or gift incentives. My own experience in running such programs at 4 health care organizations over the past 16 years is that only about 24% of employees in the organizations participated in these programs. Often they were the employees who would have participated in exercise and lifestyle programs on their own.

A cautionary note is worth mentioning here. Spending a lot of money on primary prevention, stopping disease before it starts, sounds like the answer; however, the cost savings for prevention measures applied in 2006 would not be realized until 2048 (9). Payors do not want to invest a large amount in a program that will provide no benefit within the current year, and they most assuredly want a benefit within 3 to 5 years. What are the chances that the person would still be enrolled in the original insurance program 30 years later? The implication is that a moderate approach to management of those with the disease and prevention for those at risk for it would over the long run provide the most cost-effective health care system. The majority of efforts to correct these major health risk factors occur as secondary prevention, after the patient has incurred the disease and is in the process of rehabilitating and managing the disease and its exigencies. Managing the disease will stem the exacerbations of these chronic diseases that would occur if the disease progressed unchecked and, as a result, will decrease the cost.

Disease Management

This book provides evidence-based exercise and medical interventions for many of the chronic diseases listed in Chronic Diseases Caused by or Enhanced by Three Risk Factors on page 134. In the last 15 years, a new process called *disease management* has developed, which is defined by the Disease Management Association of America as follows: "Disease management is a system of coordinated healthcare interventions and communications for populations with conditions in which patient self-care efforts are significant. Disease management:

- Supports the physician or practitioner/patient relationship and plan of care
- Emphasizes prevention of exacerbations and complications utilizing evidenced based guidelines and patient empowerment strategies, and
- Evaluates clinical, humanistic, and economic outcomes on an ongoing basis with the goal of improving overall health." (15)

CMS has initiated the Chronic Care Improvement Program, providing the opportunity for health care institutions to apply for grants to work with Medicare and Medicaid in helping beneficiaries to manage their health, adhere to physician plans of care, and obtain the medical care they need to reduce their health risks (34). The difficulty with all of these programs is that they have not been operational long enough to improve health outcomes and costs.

Janet Wright, MD, in testimony before the House Committee on Ways and Means, made the following observations:

> As an example of highly effective disease management, I call your attention to a mature and profoundly valuable program which has provided education in self-management and health preservation, linked patients and doctors through frequent progress reports, and not just satisfied, but indeed, life changed its participants. That program is one of the original disease management approaches known as Cardiac Rehabilitation. (14)

Thus, to intervene with all of the chronic diseases discussed in this book, we have a tried and true disease management program, the principles of intervention promoted by the example of cardiac rehabilitation.

Integrated Disease Management Facilities

We can learn much from the principles of managed care, which was the major focus of health care delivery in the 1990s as cost forced business and industry to look at new models of delivery. Managed care delivered health care services using five elements:

- Focus on prevention, early diagnosis, and monitoring of patients using specific clinical pathways.
- Provide comprehensive outpatient care in one centralized setting.
- Pay close attention to each patient's psychosocial needs.
- Identify and aggressively manage other chronic diseases and comorbidities.
- Look for creative cost-saving opportunities (23).

These focal points characterize the comprehensive outpatient cardiac programs that have been in operation since the late 1960s, which Dr. Wright described to the House Ways and Means Committee. It is appropriate to apply this model to other chronic diseases—diabetes, osteoporosis, cystic fibrosis, pulmonary disorders such as chronic obstructive pulmonary disease, arthritis, congestive heart failure, peripheral vascular disease, and many cancers, to name a few. The health outcomes of each of these diseases may be significantly affected by exercise, lifestyle, and nutrition intervention (see Chronic Diseases Caused by or Enhanced by Three Risk Factors on page 134).

Many health care institutions have answered the need for these services by creating centers throughout the medical complex. These poorly serve patients who have multiple comorbidities with their primary diagnosis, because these patients have to travel to different centers and undergo isolated programs. Creating a discharge disease management center, cross-training staff, and integrating certified licensed personnel present the following positives:

- Patients and customers do not get lost trying to find the office, program, or specialist.
- Parking and access are easier for patients.
- Providing all treatment in one facility rather than many separate entities reduces operational and bricks and mortar expenses.
- Leadership, management, clerical, billing, and housekeeping expenses are reduced because these services are supported by many cost centers in one facility rather than many small centers.
- An integrated program creates a patient's history in one facility, thus facilitating a continuum of care.
- Programs that are not well supported by insurance and are self-pay may be covered by programs that do well financially.
- Staff members increase their professional skills.
- Office, exercise, and monitoring equipment are shared in one center rather than being duplicated in many small centers (19).

Figure 13.1 depicts programming in the LiveWell Center, a comprehensive integrated disease management center developed by Forrest General Hospital. Because programs are connected, customers see what is happening as they participate in one program and ask to get involved in another. Tracking people throughout the center is facilitated by the interprogram and intraprogram involvement of staff.

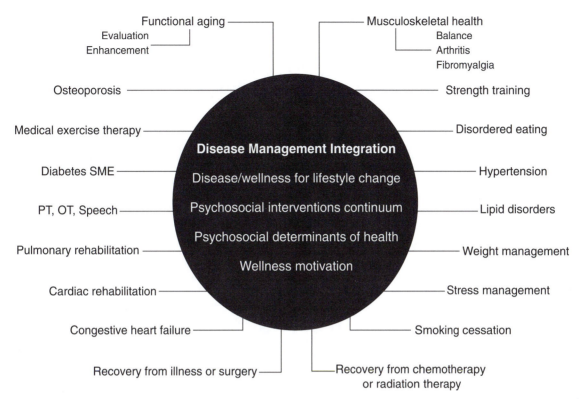

FIGURE 13.1 A model of disease management integration. PT = physical therapy; OT = occupational therapy; SME = self management education. Courtesy of LiveWell Center.

Summary

Creating a discharge destination is a win–win situation for the health care organization and the patient. Given the projected increase of chronic diseases developing as a result of lifestyle choices and behaviors, it makes sense for health care institutions to develop a one-stop facility for patients as they leave the physician's office or are discharged from the hospital or emergency room. A clearly identifiable facility that can produce positive clinical and financial outcomes has a marketing edge enviable in today's highly competitive market.

Intensive Comprehensive Lifestyle Modification

Beyond Conventional Cardiac Rehabilitation

Terri A. Merritt-Worden, MS

Health professionals accept without argument that modifying cardiac risk factors will affect the development and progression of coronary heart disease (CHD). Frustration with technology limitations that only bypass the problem rather than treat the underlying disease process has led physicians and scientists to consider intense risk factor modification as a treatment intervention. Some have hypothesized that if you aggressively and comprehensively treat modifiable risk factors, the progression of heart disease could be halted or even reversed. As discussed in other chapters in this book, there is significant evidence for the benefits of dietary intervention, therapeutic lipid lowering, and exercise, alone and in combination, in preventing and treating CHD. This chapter explores the effects of vigorously addressing *all* modifiable risk factors simultaneously, specifically targeting the behaviors that underlie lifestyle choices. Although there are other examples of intensive comprehensive cardiac rehabilitation, the model developed at the Preventive Medicine Research Institute is discussed here as a template for rigorous lifestyle modification that goes beyond conventional cardiac rehabilitation.

Research at the Preventive Medicine Research Institute

Since the late 1970s, Ornish and colleagues at the Preventive Medicine Research Institute (PMRI) have conducted a series of randomized controlled trials and demonstration projects that have shown that patients with CHD can be motivated to make and maintain intensive comprehensive changes in diet and lifestyle

The preparation of this chapter was supported in part by grants from the PepsiCo Foundation, Safeway Corporation, and the Department of Defense (#W81XWH-06-1-0565).

Address correspondence concerning this chapter to Terri A. Merritt-Worden, 150 Townsite Road, Nanaimo, BC V9S 1K4 Canada. E-mail: terri.merritt-worden@pmri.org that will slow, stop, or reverse the progression of CHD. After only 1 month, patients showed significant improvement in left ventricular function as measured by exercise radionuclide ventriculography (22). After 1 year, patients in the landmark Lifestyle Heart Trial (LHT) showed significant increases in exercise capacity, as measured by exercise treadmill testing, and regression in coronary atherosclerosis, as measured by quantitative coronary arteriography (20), and there was even more regression after 5 years than after 1 year (7). These arteriographic findings were corroborated by cardiac positron emission tomography (PET) scans demonstrating that blood flow to the heart improved significantly in experimental groups. The progression of CHD was stopped or reversed in 99% of perfusion abnormalities in the experimental group. In contrast, the control groups of each of these studies showed worsening of coronary heart disease by each of these measures even though they were following guidelines consistent with conventional cardiac rehabilitation (7).

The Multicenter Lifestyle Demonstration Project (MLDP) illustrated that it is possible to train physicians and other health professionals from hospitals in diverse regions of the United States to implement lifestyle modification programming (10, 18). Adherence to the program resulted in improvement in cardiovascular risk factors and clinical status of a greater magnitude than has been evidenced in any other community-based intervention (10, 18). Notably, results also indicated that the program was an effective alternative to revascularization. Most patients who were eligible for revascularization were able to safely avoid it by making comprehensive lifestyle changes. This decreased use resulted in an estimated US$29,529 per patient reduction in health care expenditures by Mutual of Omaha, the health plan that sponsored the demonstration (18).

In 1997, Highmark Blue Cross Blue Shield (HMBCBS) of Pittsburgh became the first health insurer in the United States to both provide and pay for a comprehensive lifestyle intervention. In 2001, HMBCBS partnered with Mountain State Blue Cross Blue Shield and the Public Employees Insurance Agency of West Virginia to initiate the first statewide outpatient program in West Virginia, which was soon followed by a similar initiative in Pennsylvania. The Multicenter Cardiac Lifestyle Modification Intervention Program (MCLIP) network continues to demonstrate the medical effectiveness (5, 13, 28, 29) and cost-effectiveness (23) of this treatment and prevention program.

Program Components

Most people recognize that diet and exercise are important to prevent and treat heart disease. Although the rigors of the Ornish program's dietary intervention are often focused on, less well known (and not systematically included in traditional cardiac rehabilitation programs) are the psychosocial aspects that comprise the other two cornerstones of the intensive comprehensive lifestyle change and cardiac rehabilitation program: group support and stress management (17, 19). See figure 14.1 for a summary of the four components of the Ornish program.

Low-Fat Plant-Based Dietary Plan

A plant-based diet is recognized by the American Dietetic Association (ADA) to be consistent with good nutritional status (25), and very low fat diets are also considered efficacious as long as patients are supervised and provided with support and long-term follow-up (11). Chapter 18 discusses the current dietary interventions and their effect on CHD risk factors, overall risk, and cardiac events. The dietary guidelines of the American Heart Association (AHA) are likely insufficient to stop the progression of coronary heart disease. Hunninghake and colleagues (9) demonstrated only a 5% improvement in low-density lipoprotein cholesterol (LDL-C) from an AHA step II diet compared with 27% improvement from lovastatin in the same patients. Also, in a number of randomized control trials studying coronary atherosclerosis regression, a majority of the patients who consumed an AHA step I or step II diet continued to show progression of disease. However, regression of coronary atherosclerosis may occur when dietary intakes of fat and cholesterol are much lower (7, 20). Dietary composition (i.e., percentage of calories from fat, carbohydrates, and protein) has been of great interest, both in the media and in scientific communities. Although some risk factors are positively affected by high-protein or high-fat diets, the AHA does not recognize them as healthful dietary plans for those with CHD (27). Also, most studies on diets with various macronutrients have been short term and only assessed risk factors (4), not clinical end points or measurements of disease regression. Additionally, the study intervention must include dietary changes large enough to sufficiently reduce risk or stop disease progression (8). In both of the aforementioned studies, adherence did not meet expectations, which may be a result of not including effective strategies to change the underlying behavior.

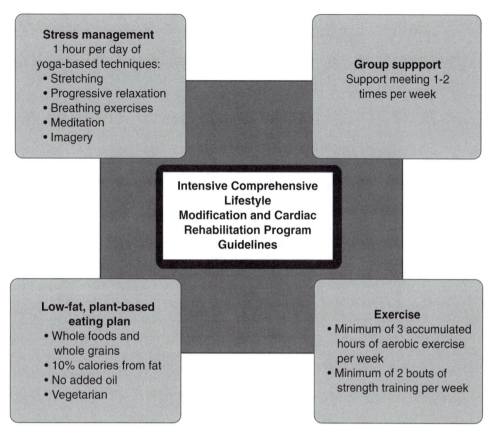

FIGURE 14.1 The four components of the intensive comprehensive lifestyle modification model developed at the Preventive Medicine Research Institute.

The Ornish program's dietary guidelines (see table 14.1) were designed to directly address the dietary factors known to promote CHD, such as increased risk factors associated with CHD and endothelial dysfunction (19). The rationale for stabilizing endothelial function, such as decreasing coronary spasm and platelet aggregation, has been previously described (16). The low-fat, whole-foods, plant-based diet is very low in both total fat and saturated fat and contains no added fats and oils as well as no trans fatty acids, a proven dietary cause of CHD. A diet low in oxidants may promote the oxidation of LDL-C and make LDL-C more atherogenic; therefore, a diet with abundant sources of antioxidants, such as bioflavonoids, carotenoids, phytochemicals, and other substances that are naturally prevalent in a plant-based diet and not prevalent in a meat-based diet, is recommended. The dietary guidelines from the Ornish program include six or more servings of whole grains and at least five servings of fruits and vegetables per day, resulting in more than 25 g of fiber per day. Generally accepted is the concept that soluble fiber-rich foods not only will improve diabetes but also may significantly reduce

other risk factors for heart disease, such as obesity and high total cholesterol, LDL-C, and triglycerides.

Adequate hydration is necessary to decrease the gastrointestinal side effects associated with a high-fiber diet. Although studies on the role of caffeine in the development and progression of CHD are not conclusive, caffeine is a stimulant and decreases the ability to successfully practice stress management, and thus it is not included in the dietary plan.

Group Support and Stress Management

The psychosocial status of the patient is of great importance when trying to modify CHD risk. A person's psychosocial status and the subsequent health-enhancing and health-damaging behaviors that result from it are certainly contributors to the pathogenesis of CHD. Specific to lifestyle modification, a person's psychosocial state may affect his or her ability to adhere to the desired behavior change. Treatment of disease may not be successful without first addressing adverse health risk behaviors and the underlying psychosocial causes. The four components of the Ornish program,

TABLE 14.1   Ornish Program's Dietary Guidelines

Dietary factors	Recommendation
Whole foods, complex carbohydrates	Whole grains ($\geq$6 servings per day) and fruits and vegetables ($\geq$5 servings per day), resulting in >25 g of fiber per day
Fat	10% fat of total calories from fat
Cholesterol	$\leq$10 mg/day
Animal products	None except nonfat milk products and egg whites
Calories	Unrestricted unless overweight and not losing weight
Sugar	In moderation
Caffeine	None allowed
Sodium	Moderate use unless medically indicated otherwise
Alcohol	Allowed in small amounts—1.5 oz (44.3 mL) of liquor, 8 oz (236.5 mL) of wine, or 12 oz (354.8 mL) of beer per day—but not encouraged
Soy	One serving per day of a full-fat soy product
Supplements	A low-dose multivitamin (without iron, unless childbearing age), plus a source of omega-3 fatty acids (fish oil for men and women; flaxseed for women only). Optional supplements may include antioxidants (vitamins E and C, selenium), folic acid, and possibly, on the advice of a physician, calcium supplements.

stress management and group support in particular, are designed to address various psychological states (e.g., depression, anxiety, anger, social isolation, and stress) that have been associated with CHD and its prognosis. Refer to chapter 24 for an in-depth discussion of the psychosocial risk factors and the mechanisms associated with increased risk for CHD.

The group support model in the Ornish program involves more than just sharing recipes and is not what most mental health professionals define as traditional group therapy. Group support sessions have the following objectives: to help patients overcome their sense of isolation, to teach communication techniques, to allow participants to become aware of their feelings, and to facilitate bonds that will help patients adhere to the other aspects of the program. Successful group support will greatly increase adherence to other parts of the program; reduce hostility, depression, and social isolation; and produce other effects that are not fully understood but may improve quality of life and clinical status (3).

Emotional stress that activates the sympathetic nervous system has long been suspected as a contributor to the pathogenesis of CHD and may lead to myocardial ischemia. Chronic stress can often result in depression,

anxiety, hostility, and inability to cope, thus decreasing a person's ability to make and maintain healthy lifestyle choices. Stress management elicits the relaxation response via the parasympathetic nervous system, which normalizes physiologic responses to stress.

The stress management techniques in the Ornish program, derived in part from hatha yoga, include stretching, progressive relaxation, breathing techniques, meditation, visualization, and imagery (20). Clinical trials show a variety of physical and psychological benefits of these techniques, which include lower resting oxygen consumption, reduced respiration rate, decreased muscular activity, increased peripheral blood flow, decreased stress hormones and catecholamines, decreased anxiety, decreased depression, and increased ability to concentrate.

Exercise

The role of exercise in primary prevention and cardiac rehabilitation is covered in detail in other chapters. Exercise also appears to play a role in helping to slow or stop the progression of CAD when combined with a low-fat diet (14) and pharmacologic lipid treatment (26). The latter study also showed that intensive lifestyle change combined with lipid active drugs reduced the severity of perfusion abnormalities in a dose–response fashion and that those changes independently predicted cardiac events. The exercise guidelines in the Ornish program are identical to the standard guidelines used in conventional cardiac rehabilitation. The on-site exercise programming, individualized exercise prescription, and home exercise programs follow the conventional American College of Sports Medicine guidelines and American Association of Cardiovascular and Pulmonary Rehabilitation guidelines.

Differences From Conventional Cardiac Rehabilitation

Although comprehensive lifestyle modification programs, like the Ornish program, are often seen as a variant of cardiac rehabilitation (in fact, intensive lifestyle modification programs were included in the Centers for Medicare and Medicare Services 2006 revised national coverage determination for cardiac rehabilitation), there are some significant differences.

Treatment Alternative

Because of the scientific evidence regarding the Ornish program's effectiveness in treating anginal symptoms, stopping the progression of heart disease, and, in some cases, reversing heart disease, this program is often used in addition to an intensive, comprehensive rehabilitation program. Many participants have chosen enrollment in the Ornish program over more costly and potentially dangerous revascularization procedures. In the MLDP, patients in the experimental group were able to avoid revascularization for at least 3 years by making comprehensive lifestyle changes at substantially lower cost without increasing cardiac morbidity and mortality. These patients reported reductions in angina comparable with what can be achieved with revascularization. Moreover, the angina symptom abatement occurs quickly for most patients. Within a few weeks after making comprehensive lifestyle changes, the LHT patients in the intervention group reported a 91% average reduction in the frequency of angina. Most of the patients became essentially pain-free, including those who had been unable to work or engage in daily activities because of severe chest pain (20, 21).

Outcomes

Traditional cardiac rehabilitation is effective in reducing cardiovascular risk and decreasing morbidity and mortality (30). Intensive risk reduction programming shows superior risk factor outcomes, in particular reduction of weight, depression, blood pressure, and lipids and control of glucose in diabetic patients. Minimal weight loss (<2%) at 12 weeks has been evidenced in traditional cardiac rehabilitation, whereas the Ornish program has reported a 6% decrease in men and women at 12 weeks (28) and >10% at 1 year (20). Significant decreases in levels of depression are reported for Ornish program participants compared with mixed results for cardiac rehabilitation enrollees (12). The program is particularly effective for those with diabetes, especially women (24). Results show improved blood pressure, improved LDL-C, no negative changes in high-density lipoprotein cholesterol (HDL-C) or triglycerides, improved glycemic control, and a >20% reduction in medication use (24, 29) compared with the minimal or null changes in those measures in conventional cardiac rehabilitation (2). With the onset of statin therapy and increased emphasis on achieving clinical practice guidelines for lipid therapy as part of conventional cardiac rehabilitation, fewer differences have been seen in some lipid results. Notably, the initial Ornish studies showed similar reductions in total and LDL-C without the use of medications (21). Table 14.2 reports outcomes on preliminary analysis for the first 1,951 subjects consecutively enrolled from 1997 to 2005 in the MCLIP.

In addition to the PMRI research, an independent replication of the intense lifestyle modification program compared patients undergoing the Ornish program, conventional cardiac rehabilitation, and no rehabilitative therapy. The Ornish program participants had significantly greater reductions in anginal frequency, body weight, body mass index, systolic blood pressure, total cholesterol, LDL-C, glucose, and dietary fat and increases in complex carbohydrates relative to the standard rehabilitation and no-rehabilitation groups. The study showed superior outcomes using the more intensive program for treating multiple CVD risk factors (1).

The excellent adherence to the program guidelines drives the clinical outcomes. Long-term adherence to the exercise surpasses the recidivism previously reported for conventional cardiac rehabilitation, where 6 months after participation, less than half of patients are still exercising at desired levels (15). Most people, both patients and health professionals, assume that the rigorous diet will be the biggest adherence challenge. Although making such large dietary changes is challenging, most participants find the dietary intervention to be one of the easiest changes to incorporate once

TABLE 14.2 **Multicenter Cardiac Lifestyle Intervention Program Data Preliminary Analysis (1998-2005)**

	Average at baseline	Average at 12 weeks	Average change	Percent change
Weight, lb (kg)	207.9 (94.3)	195.5 (88.6)	–12.4 (–5.7)	–6.0
Body mass index	32.7	30.7	–2.0	–6.1
Systolic blood pressure, mmHg	132.8	121.8	–11.0	–8.3
Diastolic blood pressure, mmHg	78.9	72.8	–6.1	–7.8
Functional capacity, METs	8.8	10.6	1.8	21.2
Total cholesterol, mg/dL	188.4	162.6	–25.8	–13.7
HDL-C, mg/dL	44.6	39.4	–5.2	–11.8
LDL-C, mg/dL	108.5	90.8	–17.7	–16.3
Triglycerides, mg/dL	183.8	167.8	–16.0	–8.7
HbA_{1c}, % (diabetics only n = 518)	7.5	6.7	–0.8	–10.7
General health, SF-36	52.5	68.2	15.7	29.8
Vitality, SF-36	47.5	68.4	20.9	44.2
Depression scale, CES-D	12.1	6.7	–5.4	–44.5
Hostility scale, Cook-Medley	8.0	6.6	–1.4	–18.3
Perceived stress scale	15.2	10.0	–5.2	–33.8
Dietary fat, % of total calories	27.5	9.4	–18.1	–65.9
Exercise, min/week	85.5	225.6	140.1	164
Stress management, min/week	23.0	373.9	350.9	1,529

MET = metabolic equivalent; HDL-C = high-density lipoprotein cholesterol; LDL-C = low-density lipoprotein cholesterol; HbA_{1c} = hemoglobin A_{1c}; SF-36 = Medical Outcomes Study 36-item Short Form Health Survey; CES-D = Center for Epidemiological Studies—Depression Scale. N = 1,951; attendance was 93.7% (unpublished data). Participants missing either baseline or 12-week data were not included in the analysis. Based on paired t test (two-sided). All baseline to 12-week changes are significant at $p < .001$.

the guidelines are understood and the palate begins to adapt to the low-fat foods. The most difficult aspect for most participants is the hourly stress management guideline, as many try to fit stress management into an already busy life. Despite the rigor, overall program adherence, both short term and long term, is excellent (5, 10, 20, 21). Refer to table 14.2 for data in progress.

One Ornish program outcome that has been interpreted by others as potentially problematic is the initial decrease in cardioprotective HDL-C levels. However, lowering HDL-C concentrations by dietary measures, in the context of a low-fat diet, does not present the same CHD risk as do low HDL-C concentrations in persons eating a high-fat diet, and the decline in HDL did not adversely affect the total cholesterol/HDL-C ratio (1, 5, 20, 21). HDL levels also have been shown to return to baseline after 1 year (10).

To illustrate the differences seen in traditional cardiac rehabilitation outcomes and intensive lifestyle modification program outcomes, see the case study on page 145.

Gender Differences

A higher percentage of women enroll in the Ornish program than in traditional cardiac rehabilitation. In comparison to enrollment rates as low as 5% in

■ Case Study

The following is an anecdotal case study that looks at the results of a large, exercise-based rehabilitation meta-analysis and the results from a large, metropolitan hospital located on the East Coast of the United States that delivers both a phase II cardiac rehabilitation program and the Ornish program essentially staffed by the same health professionals (where positions are the same). The meta-analysis includes the results from 48 exercise-based cardiac rehabilitation trials. (Note: Ornish data are included in the meta-analysis.)

In the phase II cardiac rehabilitation program (average annual enrollment = 310), participants attend an exercise class supervised by registered nurses and exercise physiologists and an education session three times per week for up to 12 weeks. A registered dietitian prescribes personalized dietary plans and provides follow-up counseling for each participant. A family nurse clinician and a psychologist provide group education and are available for individual or family counseling on coping with lifestyle changes. The Ornish program is delivered as described in this chapter.

The following are the metrics collected by both programs (the 12-week outcomes of participants consecutively enrolled in each program) and those reported in the meta-analysis.

	Exercise-based rehabilitation meta-analysis N = 8,940 (30)	Phase II cardiac rehabilitation program N = 104 (unpublished data)	Ornish program N = 106 (unpublished data)
Gender, % female/% male	20/80	24/76	39/61
Age, years	55	61	58
Weight, kg/lb (%)	NA	−0.4/−0.9 (0.4)	−6.4/−14.1 (6.5)
Total cholesterol, mmol/L (mg/dL)	−0.37 (−14.3)*	−0.49 (−19)*	−0.95 (−37)*
LDL-C, mmol/L (mg/dL)	−0.20 (−7.7)	−0.44 (−17)	−0.65 (−25.2)*
HDL-C , mmol/L (mg/dL)	−0.05 (−1.9)	0.05 (2)	−0.09 (−3.5)*
TG, mmol/L (mg/dL)	−0.23 (−20.4)*	−0.36 (−32)*	−0.52 (−46.4)*
SBP, mmHg	−3.2*	NA	−10.2*
DBP, mmHg	−1.2	NA	−6.9*

HDL-C = high-density lipoprotein cholesterol; LDL-C = low-density lipoprotein cholesterol; TG = triglycerides; SBP = systolic blood pressure; DBP = diastolic blood pressure.

*$p \leq .05$ for within-group baseline to follow-up differences.

The Ornish program evidenced the superior outcomes. Interestingly, the cardiac rehabilitation program staff, who were trained in intensive lifestyle modification, implemented a very comprehensive exercise-based program, which showed superior results compared with traditional cardiac rehabilitation in the meta-analysis.

cardiac rehabilitation, in the MLDP 21% of enrollees were women (10), and to date women make up 34% of those with diagnosed CHD in the MCLIP enrollment (5). One hypothesis is that this program places equal emphasis on all program components, whereas traditional cardiac rehabilitation is focused on exercise, a known barrier to women. In addition, women may be drawn to the psychosocial components of the Ornish program. Some health plans also provide coverage for the Ornish program for at-risk individuals. Interestingly, of those entering the program for prevention (three or more risk factors) 68% are women, suggesting that women are more likely to enroll prior to the development of disease, whereas men are more likely to enter after the disease has manifested (28).

Both genders evidence significant improvements in their program adherence and risk factors. Despite women's worse medical, psychosocial, and sociodemographic status at baseline, their improvement is similar to that of men's. Thus, this program may be particularly beneficial for women with CHD, who generally have higher mortality and morbidity than men after a heart attack, angioplasty, or bypass surgery (10, 28).

Program Delivery

The Ornish program is more intense than traditional programs with regard to the amount of hours participants engage in on-site activities, the program guidelines, and the degree of staff involvement. The program is usually delivered as a hospital-based outpatient program and is often delivered alongside a traditional cardiac rehabilitation program. Patients may be enrolled for up to 1 year and in the first 12 weeks attend approximately 100 hr of programming. Equal value and equal on-site session time are allocated for each of the four program components.

In the first 12 weeks, the twice-weekly sessions include 1 hr of each program component. In every program session, the participants engage in 1 hr of exercise and 1 hr of yoga-based stress management. A meal (either pot-luck or prepared by the hospital cafeteria) is served during an educational session, and the patients participate in a professionally facilitated support group session (6).

Although some didactic lectures are provided, the participants spend most of their time either participating in the actual activity (exercising, performing the stress management techniques, and participating in group support sessions) or engaging in a skill-building activities (e.g., cooking demonstration, grocery tours, interactive discussions). Within these experiences, two of the most important aspects of the program, the sense of community and imbedding of the health behaviors, are developed. For example, even the meal is an opportunity for community building as relationships develop while the participants dine together.

The time intensity of all program components and the staff's ability to create a healing environment may be the main factors in motivating participants to make and maintain lifestyle changes (to be discussed later) and largely account for the difference in clinical outcomes and program adherence between conventional cardiac rehabilitation and intensive comprehensive cardiac rehabilitation.

Required Staff Members

The team that delivers the Ornish program is more numerous and diverse than in most traditional cardiac rehabilitation programs. The staff includes a program director, a medical director, a chef–caterer–foodservice provider, an exercise physiologist, a group support facilitator (a licensed mental health professional or social worker), a nurse case manager, a registered dietitian, a stress management specialist (a certified yoga instructor), and an administrative assistant. Some program sites also employ a recruitment specialist, whose responsibility is to enroll eligible patients. The staff is central to program success and as such each staff member should have the following attributes:

- Personal *and* professional experience with lifestyle and behavior changes
- Belief in the philosophy and guidelines of the program
- Knowledge of the psychosocial, emotional, mental, physical, and spiritual dimensions of health and illness, especially heart disease
- Competence in her or his field of expertise and desire to build on this traditional foundation
- Willingness to become a part of a transdisciplinary team in an environment of transformational change
- Ability to communicate effectively with compassion and empathy

Expectations of Staff

As the primary role models for the participants, staff must understand the philosophical underpinnings of the program. Participants will observe how staff members adhere to the nutrition, stress management, and exercise guidelines and how they connect interpersonally.

After initial training, each staff member is asked to maintain the program lifestyle for a minimum of 3 months to gain the experience of living the program and understanding how patients feel when making major behavioral and lifestyle changes. The relationship that develops between staff member and participant is vital to the success of the program: a relationship built on trust, confidentiality, and shared experience.

The participants are not passive receivers of health care in this program. An important role of staff is to draw out and mobilize each participant to make multiple lifestyle changes and to influence the course of his or her disease. The program is built on the transformational process whereby the team educates and encourages the participants to activate their own healing process, both individually and as active members of the community.

Motivation of Participants

All participants are screened for motivation before they enter the program. It is assumed that the participant in this program is motivated to change her lifestyle. The staff's responsibility is to support the participant and provide the information and experience necessary to sustain or increase the motivation that the participant brought to the program.

In traditional models of health care, professionals expect shortcomings in their patients. A positive change in behavior, even short of the desired goal, is supported. In the Ornish model, making some progress is not enough. Participants diagnosed with this life-threatening disease must follow the minimum guidelines of the program, and the staff must be very clear about this. Although small changes are positively and compassionately acknowledged, the participant must be refocused on his ultimate goal and the need to progress more. The counseling provided must be explicit about expectation for the program.

Being the "holder of expectations" is one of the most important roles of a staff member. Everything about this program is an unreasonable expectation from the perspective of what is considered a normal life. The heart patient enrolls in the program because it provides hope for a normal life according to a new definition. Holding the expectation that the commitment required is reasonable may make it easier for patients to actively participate, ultimately for their lifetime. The program staff expects that the program can be followed by the average person. Program participants can succeed with the support of the program community, that is, the program team and staff and all participants. Fulfilling the role as the holder of expectations without creating pressure or tension for the participant and while maintaining the relationship with the participant can be difficult. The participant's right to choose whether to adhere to program guidelines is acknowledged. But program staff members should communicate clearly and without judgment or criticism that treatment benefits will be compromised if a participant does not adhere to minimum program guidelines. At times staff may need to say, "What you are doing is great, but it's not enough to achieve the result you enrolled in this program to obtain." Emphasizing that patients must meet the intensive guidelines is very important, because previous studies found that adherence to the Ornish intervention was strongly correlated with outcomes in a dose–response relationship: The more patients modified their lifestyles, the greater the improvement in coronary stenoses as measured by coronary angiography and cardiac PET scans (7, 20, 21).

Expectations of Participants

This intervention does not promote the conventional wisdom of slowly modifying risk factors. Participants are expected to begin following all the program guidelines as soon as they enroll in the program. Undertaking all of these large changes at the same time results in quick changes in angina, weight, and other symptoms, which motivate people to maintain the intensive lifestyle. Focusing on the "joy of living versus the fear of dying" is the strongest motivator for making and maintaining these intensive lifestyle changes (16).

A certain level of motivation is needed to initiate interest in enrollment, but surprisingly some of the most successful program participants are typical cardiac rehabilitation patients. More important than previous behavior is an antecedent event, whether that is a precipitating incident such as a myocardial infarction, worsening symptoms, or a new reason to live (e.g., child's upcoming wedding, new grandchild).

Intensive, comprehensive lifestyle modification is a program for life. Each component requires a lifelong commitment because, to the best of current knowledge, each aspect of the program is necessary to reverse CHD. Experience has shown that most people need substantial support to make and sustain the required lifestyle changes. Additionally, people who are part of a community that is living the same lifestyle are more successful at sustaining the lifestyle than an individual attempting to do the program on her own. In the LHT, the longer the participant was involved in the group-supported phase of the program, the more successful he was in maintaining lifestyle change, improving symptoms, and increasing physical activity and quality of life. For this reason, participants are encouraged to develop or join peer-led self-management communities after leaving hospital-based programs. Ornish program–based self-directed communities exist across the United States and Canada and help participants maintain the behaviors that resulted in the initial positive clinical outcomes. In fact, the surviving members of the LHT community continue to meet weekly after more than 20 years.

Comorbidities and Contraindications

Comorbidities and contraindications for the program modalities may affect program participation and must be considered on an individual basis for each participant. Because of the rapid changes experienced by some participants, hypertension, diabetes status, and medications must be monitored closely. Case management of each participant includes following specific guidelines for the following conditions: angina, arrhythmias, carotid atherosclerosis, claudication, colon irritability, diabetes, eye disease, gallstones, lipid abnormalities, hypertension, metabolic syndrome, obesity, and renal failure or kidney disease (6).

Summary

The landmark INTERHEART study of 29,972 people in 52 countries found that 9 risk factors related to lifestyle and nutrition accounted for more than 90% of the risk of a heart attack in men and women in almost every geographic region and in every racial and ethnic group worldwide (31). Often medical or surgical interventions are the first options given to CHD patients, because these options are perceived to be the quickest and easiest remedies. However, equal emphasis should be placed on intensive, comprehensive lifestyle modification and cardiac rehabilitation, because it is efficacious, is cost-effective, and has fewer side effects than medical or surgical interventions. It is hoped that as physicians and other health professionals receive more information and scientific evidence regarding lifestyle management, their perceptions that the average patient will not be motivated enough to follow the intensive guidelines will change. Health professionals need to become holders of the expectation that intensive comprehensive lifestyle modification is possible and can stop or even reverse heart disease progression and that lifestyle modification should be the first option for treatment when medically appropriate.

CHAPTER 15

Endurance Training

Carl Foster, PhD

John P. Porcari, PhD

Alejandro Lucia, MD, PhD

Milo was a farm boy in the Greek province of Crotonia who (in legend) lifted a newly foaled bullock every day until he became the strongest man in the world and one of the great champions of the classical Olympic Games. Beyond Milo's contribution to Olympic history, his story demonstrates the substantial adaptability of humans to repetitive exercise stress. Contemporary examples of this adaptability are common: for example, the 80-year-old who has trouble walking from the living room to the kitchen who, a year later, finishes a marathon. People's ability to adapt to exercise training despite the presence of cardiorespiratory disease is the conceptual underpinning of contemporary rehabilitation programs. This practice was anticipated more than 200 years ago by the Scottish physician Hebreden, who observed that one of his patients with exertional angina pectoris was "nearly cured" after a regime of sawing wood for half an hour per day for 6 months. We know that humans adapt to exercise, that the adaptation can quite substantially change exercise capacity, and that the adaptation can be profound enough to ameliorate many of the pathophysiologic sequelae of established disease.

However, we also know that exercise is not totally benign. Just as the legend of Milo suggests the possibility for adaptation to exercise, the legend of Phidippides (who supposedly died after running from Marathon to Athens to announce victory over the invading Persians) suggests the potential for risk posed by exercise. Although objective estimates of the cardiovascular risk of both exercise testing and exercise training are quite low (12), exercise carries much more than a theoretical risk, particularly in the beginning exerciser. Given that the first rule of medicine is valid even in the gymnasium, those charged with the exercise training of sedentary people and patients with cardiorespiratory disease must understand how to prescribe exercise to maximize the beneficial effects while minimizing the negative side effects.

This chapter provides a framework for designing endurance training programs for a variety of individuals, ranging from patients with cardiovascular disease to high-level performance athletes, but primarily for the beginning exerciser or patient with cardiovascular disease. The chapter draws extensively from controlled studies of exercise training in sedentary healthy individuals, many conducted by Pollock (cf. 2, 3, 27, 28, 32); from controlled studies in patients with cardiovascular disease (8, 29); and from recent studies with athletes (6,

Address correspondence concerning this chapter to Carl Foster, Department of Exercise and Sport Science, 133 Mitchell Hall, University of Wisconsin at LaCrosse, LaCrosse, WI 54601. E-mail: foster.carl@uwlax.edu

11, 13). Detailed rehabilitation protocols for patients with various manifestations of cardiovascular disease are presented separately (chapters 28-34).

Exercise Principles

Much of the exercise prescription literature is based on a series of well-controlled studies conducted largely by Pollock (cf. 2, 27, 28) in the early 1970s. The rationale for these studies was the acceptance of the maximal oxygen uptake ($\dot{V}O_{2max}$) as equivalent to endurance. Although such a simplistic criterion must be criticized today, this acceptance provided a common outcome measure that facilitated a generation of experimental studies. Interestingly, the $\dot{V}O_{2max}$ has reemerged in recent years as a powerful index of prognosis in patients with heart disease and retains a role in the most contemporary exercise training studies (3, 32). Thus, even though $\dot{V}O_{2max}$ may not necessarily equal endurance, it is a very important and powerful outcome measure.

Authors of these early studies recognized that exercise programs can be described in terms of the frequency, intensity, and time (or duration) of exercise training. Researchers also recognized that each of these variables probably had lower limits—in effect a lower threshold for the frequency, intensity, and time of training—likely to provoke training adaptations. Although we now know that the response to training is highly multifactorial (32), the overwhelming importance of frequency, intensity, and time of training to the adaptations provoked by training remains a principle of exercise programming.

Frequency

The relationship between the frequency of training on improvement in $\dot{V}O_{2max}$ and the incidence of side effects (primarily injuries) is presented in figure 15.1*a*. In previously sedentary individuals, training as little as 1 day per week can promote significant adaptations, particularly in individuals with a low pretraining exercise capacity (cf. 2, 27, 28). Beyond 3 days per week, the magnitude of the effect of training in beginning exercisers begins to saturate and the frequency of side effects begins to increase. In an alternative way of addressing the importance of frequency, intensity, and time of training, Hickson (16-18) systematically reduced these elements in already highly trained individuals (e.g., several weeks of training 6 days/week, 40 min/day, at intensities ≥90% $\dot{V}O_{2max}$). Hickson and colleagues demonstrated that when training was systematically decreased from 6 days/week of heavy training, reduced frequencies of training were not particularly harmful as long as the intensity and duration of training were maintained (16) (figure 15.1*b*). Interestingly, small reductions in training frequency were associated with improved performance, probably secondary to a reduction in the fatigue associated with heavy training (7).

Intensity

The relationship between the intensity of training and improvement in $\dot{V}O_{2max}$ and the incidence of side effects is presented in figure 15.1*c*. In previously sedentary people, the magnitude of increase in $\dot{V}O_{2max}$ increases rapidly with progressively more intense training (27, 28, 33), with comparatively little evidence of saturation. In studies in which training intensity was systematically decreased from very heavy training, despite preservation of frequency and time, $\dot{V}O_{2max}$ and performance capacity decreased rapidly (18) (figure 15.1*d*). Side effects related to intensity occasionally are catastrophic, particularly in previously sedentary people either with or at risk for cardiovascular disease (12). Even in younger or athletic people, higher intensity training is usually much less enjoyable and may require extrinsic motivation to be sustained.

The vast majority of the classical exercise training studies were based on interval exercise (e.g., walk–jog), and intensity was usually measured by palpation at the end of the difficult segments (e.g., jogging). Although palpation can be quite accurate if done correctly, it tends to bias toward underestimation because of the time required to find the pulse and start the count. Furthermore, these early studies did not account for the much lower heart rate (HR) during the recovery period. Therefore, the concept that the training response begins to saturate at intensities greater than ~85% of HR reserve (~90% HR_{max}) is probably not accurate, because the average HR during these studies was probably considerably lower than 85% of HR reserve (~90% HR_{max}) (33).

Time

The relationship between the time of training and changes in $\dot{V}O_{2max}$ and the incidence of side effects is presented in figure 15.1*e*. In previously sedentary people, the amount of enhancement in $\dot{V}O_{2max}$ increases rapidly with progressively longer exercise bouts, although there is evidence of saturation of the training response in sessions longer than 30 min. In studies in which training duration was systematically decreased in highly trained people, there were minimal decreases in $\dot{V}O_{2max}$ and performance, so long as training intensity

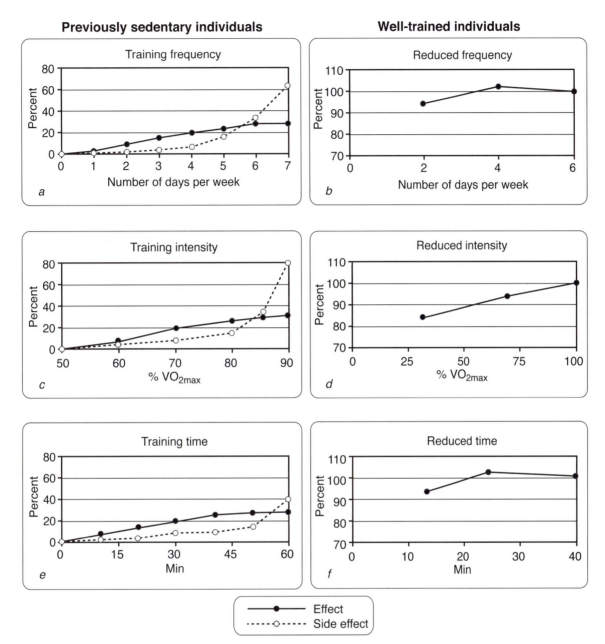

FIGURE 15.1 Schematic pattern of responses to the onset of training in previously sedentary people (left column) and to reductions in training in already well-trained people (right column). At the onset of training studies, there are generalized effects (positive adaptations) that follow a saturation curve and side effects that follow an accelerating curve. The percentage increase in $\dot{V}O_{2max}$ or endurance performance will average 20% to 30% in otherwise healthy sedentary people. The percentage of people with side effects will climb to more than 50% at higher training loads. The magnitude of saturation of the training effect usually will be less with progressively higher intensity training, although the percentage (and severity) of side effects may also be larger. In the reduced training studies, small reductions in training from very heavy levels (six times weekly for 40 min at >90% $\dot{V}O_{2max}$) may result in improved performance secondary to reductions in fatigue associated with heavy training. Despite maintenance of high frequency and duration of training, large reductions in training intensity are associated with rapid losses in endurance performance.

and frequency were maintained (17) (figure 15.1*f*). As is the case with training frequency, small reductions in training duration may have short-term benefits on performance, probably secondary to a reduction in

the fatigue associated with heavy daily training (26). Although decreases in frequency and time of exercise training have minimal impact in the short term, almost certainly such reductions would have a negative impact over a longer term, although specific evidence is lacking. In athletic people, the major way to increase the training load is probably in terms of training duration (31). Recent evidence shows that more prolonged training bouts that produce muscle glycogen depletion may be superior to an equivalent amount of training performed in a way that does not cause muscle glycogen depletion (15). At the same time, there is evidence that multiple short bouts of exercise designed to accumulate exercise time may be almost as beneficial as prolonged bouts in terms of improving $\dot{V}O_{2max}$ and endurance performance in sedentary people (5).

Mode

Any activity that involves large muscle groups is capable of producing adaptive responses in $\dot{V}O_{2max}$, although there is strong evidence that increases in $\dot{V}O_{2max}$ are dependent on changes in both peak cardiac output and in the ability of the muscles to extract oxygen from the blood. Although unproven, it is probable that exercise training intensity may exert relatively more influence on peak cardiac output and that training duration may exert relatively more influence on the ability of muscle tissue to extract oxygen from the blood. However, there is some evidence that relative muscle ischemia may be required to promote capillary growth (1), so higher intensity training that causes muscular oxygen desaturation (34) may be necessary to optimize peripheral delivery (e.g., capillary growth). Some evidence shows that activities that require a larger amount of muscle mass may lead to bigger adaptive responses. Some authors have reported strong evidence of mode specificity in terms of testing versus training mode (2, 27, 28). There is some evidence that mixed-mode training (cross-training) is about 50% as effective as single mode training in increasing endurance performance if it uses the same muscles as the criterion activity and about 25% as effective if it does not use the same muscles (10).

Threshold

The concept that the exercise intensity around the ventilatory or lactate threshold might be important relative to prescribing exercise training intensity is not new (21), and even the most recent discussions of the theoretical underpinnings of training theory suggest that a natural anchor point for training prescription is the intensity associated with a physiologic threshold (25). This intensity is usually in the middle range of the broad $\%\dot{V}O_{2max}$ or $\%HR_{max}$ windows recommended for endurance training and is an accurate marker of

the sustainable exercise capacity (25). Although direct measurement of either ventilatory or lactate threshold poses some technical challenges, the intensity of the threshold can be approximated by the intensity at which speech becomes difficult, the "talk test" (4, 30, 35). Most important, the exercise intensity at the ventilatory threshold often precedes electrocardiographic evidence of the ischemic threshold in patients with cardiovascular disease (23). Thus, it can be argued that in the absence of an exercise test to rule out exertional ischemia, advising exercisers to keep the intensity where speech is just comfortable may be a safety device to prevent exertion-related complications. Recent evidence from athletic populations suggests that despite the clear importance of a certain amount of high-intensity training to force the limits of adaptation, serious endurance athletes do remarkably little training at intensities above the ventilatory or lactate threshold (6, 31) and, indeed, seem to respond better to training when the relative amount of training above threshold is highly limited (6). This has led to discussions of a threshold-based training model (with a relatively high percentage of training above the ventilatory or lactate threshold) and a polarized training model (with most training at intensities either below the ventilatory or lactate threshold or above the respiratory compensation point) (31) (figure 15.2). Although a certain minimum of high-intensity activity seems to be required to improve performance in athletic groups, the evidence is

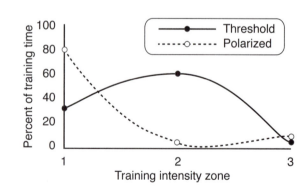

FIGURE 15.2 The percentage of training in the two primary models of endurance training performance. In the threshold-based training model, the majority of training is performed at intensities above the ventilatory or lactate threshold and below the respiratory compensation point (zone 2). There is limited evidence that this is the training model used by many recreational and fitness-level exercisers. In the polarized training model, the majority of training is performed below the intensity associated with the ventilatory or lactate threshold (zone 1) and, in more serious athletes, an appreciable percentage (~10%) of training may be performed at intensities above the respiratory compensation point (zone 3).

fairly clear that adaptations of endurance performance are more related to training volume at comparatively lower intensity than to increases in intensity (6, 31).

Training Impulse

Intensity, frequency, and duration, as components of the exercise prescription, interact to a large degree. Accordingly, to appreciate the combined effect of intensity, frequency, and duration, the concept of the training impulse as a combined marker of training intensity $\times$ training duration was developed some years ago (7, 26). Combining a marker of intensity (average heart rate, integrated time in various heart rate zones, or session rating of perceived exertion) (10, 11) with the duration of the exercise bout is an effective way of integrating intensity and time within a training session. If this is summed over a time period such as a week, it provides a convenient total training load that integrates the frequency, intensity, and time of exercise training. This integrated product is useful in predicting improved performance in healthy recreational exercisers and athletes (6, 10, 11, 31), describing the strain of exercise, and accounting for differences in prescribed and achieved exercise prescriptions (13). Some recent data demonstrate the effectiveness of the training impulse concept in terms of understanding the response to training in patients with cardiovascular disease (22).

The Art of Exercise Prescription

Cardiac rehabilitation specialists have used two approaches to exercise prescription, depending on the availability of graded exercise test results.

Top Down

Although prescriptive concepts related to markers of physiologic thresholds are more likely to be superior, the gold standard for prescribing exercise training intensity is based on accepted percentages of $\dot{V}O_{2max}$, $\dot{V}O_{2max}$ reserve, HR_{max}, or HR reserve (2). These reference values are based on maximal values observed during a graded exercise test to fatigue, hence the term *top down*. Strategies for translating exercise intensity into absolute workloads that yield desired HR or metabolic responses have been developed in our laboratory (9). Because standard exercise intensities ranging from 60% to 85% of $\dot{V}O_{2max}$ do not produce consistent responses during 30 to 60 min of exercise (21), exercise intensity prescription in the future will

likely be anchored to standard physiologic markers such as the ventilatory threshold (25).

Bottom Up

In many cases the results of a maximal exercise test are not available when a clinician wants to prescribe exercise. A common solution to this problem, pioneered by Pollock and colleagues at Sinai Samaritan Medical Center in Milwaukee (8, 27, 28) during the early days of highly structured phase II cardiac rehabilitation programs, is referred to as *bottom-up* exercise prescription. This practice recognizes that a rating of perceived exertion (RPE) of 13 to 15 (e.g., moderate to hard) on the classic scale, or 3 to 5 on the category ratio scale, gives exercise intensities that are generally well correlated with objectively measured exercise intensities. Using this logic, investigators have subjects perform an exercise bout that is similar to or only slightly more strenuous than normal ambulatory activity (hence the term *bottom up*). The RPE is monitored and HR noted. If the RPE is below 13 (classic scale) or 3 (category ratio scale) (e.g., moderate intensity), then the intensity for the next training session is increased. This is continued until the RPE is in the correct zone. At this point, values for training HR (which can be used for nonmonitored exercise) can be identified. Although the actual intensity in terms of $\%HR_{max}$ or $\%\dot{V}O_{2max}$ cannot be defined, this procedure has been associated with consistently appropriate responses to training (8, 27, 28). More recent data suggest that when the patient is just able to talk comfortably, then the exercise intensity is either at or just below both the ventilatory and ischemic thresholds and consistently within the window of accepted objective markers of exercise intensity (4, 30, 35).

Design of the Exercise Session

When designing an exercise session, one has to consider how to prepare for the session, which elements to include in the session, and how to recover from the session. These components are widely referred to as the warm-up, the training bout (aerobic phase or resistance phase), and the cool-down.

Warm-Up

Data demonstrate that warm-up activity performed prior to an exercise bout may be associated with improved performance (20), may reduce abnormalities of myocardial blood flow and ventricular function associated with the sudden onset of exercise (14), and may be associated with better overall responses to exercise. Recent evidence suggests that warm-up at low intensities may be as effective as that at higher intensities, although there is a persistent belief that less fit people, or those with atherosclerotic disease (with resulting endothelial functional abnormalities), may need more extensive warm-up (12, 14).

Aerobic Phase

The aerobic phase is, of course, the main part of the training session. In a hypothetical 30 min training bout for a beginning exerciser, approximately 20 min should be devoted to the aerobic phase. For safety reasons, in previously sedentary people, the intensity of training during the aerobic phase should be restricted during the first weeks of training (12). After the first weeks, the intensity of training may be increased for short periods of time (e.g., interval training), as in the classic studies (cf. 2, 27, 28). It is far easier for exercisers to perform very short intervals (20-30 s) with comparatively short recovery periods (60-80 s) than to perform longer intervals (3 min) even with very long recovery periods (6 min). Such a strategy has been shown to work well even in patients with advanced cardiovascular disease (24).

Resistance Phase

Resistance training is often a useful adjunct to endurance performance and can be thought of as an aid to endurance training. During the classical studies by Pollock, in which the sequence of aerobic training followed by resistance training was compared with the sequence of resistance training followed by aerobic training, the number of injuries occurring during aerobic training was markedly reduced when several weeks of resistance training were performed prior to the start of aerobic training (cf. 2, 27, 28). Furthermore, studies by Hickson and colleagues (19) suggested that a person's response to very heavy aerobic training was enhanced by the addition of resistance training.

Cool-Down

Very limited data address the value of a formal cool-down to the outcome of endurance training. Allowing time for the hemodynamic disturbances associated with exercise to slowly normalize makes sense. In people whose myocardial blood flow might be compromised, avoiding the acute hypotensive response associated with the end of exercise is highly reasonable. Thus, a good rule for exercise prescription is to include 5 min

of warm-up and 5 min of cool-down exercise on either side of the primary aerobic training bout. A case can be made for extending both the warm-up and cool-down in more debilitated people or in those with a higher likelihood of a compromise in myocardial blood flow associated with exercise.

Progression

The traditional concept of no more than a 10% increase in the overall training load during any week is well established (2). Furthermore, in previously sedentary people who either have or are at risk for cardiovascular disease, the concept of limiting the intensity of exercise during the early weeks of the exercise training program is well established (2, 12). Indeed, the concept pioneered by Pollock of progressing exercise duration from an initial 10 to 20 min up to 45 min before any progression in exercise intensity occurs is standard practice in many rehabilitation settings (8, 27, 28). This practice is probably one of the major factors in the excellent safety record of cardiopulmonary rehabilitation programs (12) and led to the general concept of progression of the total training load from about 300 kcal/week to about 1,000 to 2,000 kcal/week in patients with cardiovascular disease. Once a person is comfortable with a total energy expenditure of 1,000 to 2,000 kcal/week and can maintain this output, further progression of the training load is usually made on the basis of the client's needs or desires, because the primary adaptations to exercise are likely to have already taken place. Although there are limited data on more extensive training protocols in patients with cardiovascular disease, there is little reason to believe that they would not adapt much as do athletes (e.g., increased volume of relatively low-intensity training).

Limits of Adaptation to Training

The general expectation is that in healthy, previously untrained people, $\dot{V}O_{2max}$ will increase between 20% and 25% over the first 6 months of training. The total magnitude of response to training beyond this is generally remarkably small and most likely is attributable to increases in both the volume and intensity of training (6, 11, 31, 32). However, changes in endurance performance are often highly responsive to the volume of training, with high-intensity training having an upper limit of about 10% of the total training volume (6, 31). In less fit people and in patients with cardiorespiratory diseases, the increase in $\dot{V}O_{2max}$ and performance with training may be much larger than the nominal 20%

to 25% expectation (8, 27, 28), with changes of 50% being fairly routine and more than 100% occasionally observed, particularly if significant weight loss is associated with training. The magnitude of training seems to be strongly influenced by genetic factors (3, 32), with some people showing hardly any increase in $\dot{V}O_{2max}$ or performance with training and others showing a truly profound response to training. The causes of these highly individual responses to training are being investigated but almost certainly are regulated by multiple genes.

Summary

Humans are remarkably capable of responding to endurance training. Appropriate combinations of frequency, intensity, and time of training will produce on average 20% to 30% increases in $\dot{V}O_{2max}$ and endurance performance in otherwise healthy sedentary people. In more debilitated people and in patients with cardiovascular disease, the magnitude of improvement in endurance performance may be substantially larger, whereas in athletes the amount of improvement will be fairly small. In athletes, the main increase in training will be in the total volume of low-intensity training, and only about 10% of total training at higher intensities is well tolerated. The safety of exercise training in sedentary people and patients is probably optimized if the intensity of training is restricted during the first weeks of training. The response to training can be viewed as the interaction of the desired effects of training and the undesired side effects of training balanced against the needs and goals of the exerciser.

CHAPTER 16

Strength Training

Matt S. Feigenbaum, PhD

Kevin R. Vincent, MD, PhD

The role of strength training in disease prevention and rehabilitation is well established. Strength training is the most effective method for improving musculoskeletal function and is prescribed by the major health organizations to improve health and fitness levels and prevent disease (1-4, 17, 20, 21, 40). There is increasing evidence that strength training improves several risk factors associated with preventable chronic diseases (table 16.1). Strength training, particularly when incorporated into a comprehensive exercise program, has been shown to attenuate coronary artery disease (CAD) risk factors (5, 26, 33) and type 2 diabetes (11, 22, 42), prevent osteoporosis (35), improve body composition and reduce risk of metabolic syndrome (5, 44, 50), preserve functional capacity (25, 45, 46), and foster psychological well-being (6, 18, 45). These benefits can be safely obtained by most segments of the population when prescribed appropriate exercise programs, especially when program variables are manipulated to meet the needs of the participant.

Inadequate muscular strength and joint flexibility can lead to serious musculoskeletal disorders (e.g., low back problems) that result in considerable pain and discomfort, loss of income, increased disability, and premature retirement (10, 43). Although very few people die from a lack of muscular strength or flexibility, the overwhelming majority of elderly adults experience sarcopenia, and a substantial number suffer from chronic low back problems and disease- or disability-associated decreases in lean body mass. In addition to contributing to a muscle mass–related reduction in basal metabolic rate (BMR), inactivity, bed rest, and immobilization are accompanied by loss of bone mineral density and often result in osteoporosis-related fractures. Strength training can offset the age- and disease- or disability-associated declines in strength and musculoskeletal mass and improve functional capacity, which in turn can enhance a person's quality of life (10, 17). This benefit alone provides the rationale for incorporating strength training in exercise programs for healthy persons as well as for those with chronic diseases.

Primary Components of Strength Training Programs

Strength training improves musculoskeletal function through the progressive overload principle (i.e., by increasing more than normal the resistance to movement or frequency and duration of activity). Any magnitude of overload will result in strength development, but resistance loads performed to maximal or near-maximal effort will elicit a significantly greater training effect (20, 41). The intensity and volume of exercise can be manipulated by varying the weight load,

Address correspondence concerning this chapter to Matt S. Feigenbaum, Department of Health and Exercise Science, Furman University, Greenville, SC 29613. E-mail: Matt.Feigenbaum@Furman.edu

TABLE 16.1 Comparison of the Effects of Aerobic Endurance Training to Strength Training on Health and Fitness Variables

Variable	Aerobic exercise	Strength training
Bone mineral density	↑	↑↑
Body composition		
% fat	↓↓	↓
LBM	↔	↑↑
Strength	↔	↑↑↑
Glucose metabolism		
Insulin response to glucose challenge	↓↓	↓↓
Basal insulin levels	↓	↓
Insulin sensitivity	↑↑	↑↑
Serum lipids		
HDL-C	↑↑	↑↔
LDL-C	↓↓	↑↔
Resting heart rate	↓↓	↔
Stroke volume	↑↑	↔
Blood pressure at rest		
Systolic	↓↓	↔
Diastolic	↓↓	↓↔
$\dot{V}O_{2max}$	↑↑↑	↑
Endurance time	↑↑↑	↑↑
Physical function	↑↑	↑↑↑
Basal metabolism	↑	↑↑

% fat = percent body fat; LBM = lean body mass; HDL-C = high-density lipoprotein cholesterol; LDL-C = low-density lipoprotein cholesterol; $\dot{V}O_{2max}$ = maximum oxygen consumption; ↑ = slight increase; ↑↑ = increase; ↑↑↑ = large increase; ↓ = slight decrease; ↓↓ = decrease; ↔ = no change or no effect.

Reprinted with permission from M.L. Pollock and K.R. Vincent, *The President's Council on Physical Fitness and Sports Research Digest,* Series 2, No. 8, December 1996 (39).

the number of repetitions and sets completed, and the rest interval between sets and exercises.

When prescribing a strength training program, the clinician must determine an optimal balance of factors to maximize benefits. The person's health and fitness status, goals, time availability, and access to an appropriate training environment should be considered. For example, programs prescribed for competitive athletes often include exercises designed develop explosive power (e.g., Olympic lifts) and are not appropriate for elderly persons or patients with cardiovascular disease. During the 1990s, the major health organizations recognized the need to develop

strength training guidelines for specific segments of the population. Although these guidelines are the basis for prescribing individualized exercise programs, the primary components common to all strength training programs provide the framework for exercise prescription. The rationale for the recommendations for each component is described in the following sections.

Number of Repetitions

Muscular strength is best developed by using heavy weights (that require maximum or near-maximum tension development) with few repetitions, and muscular endurance is best developed by using lighter weights with a greater number of repetitions. To some extent, both muscular strength and endurance are developed under each condition, but each loading scheme favors a specific type of neuromuscular development (20, 41). The term *repetition maximum (RM)* refers to the maximal number of times a person can lift a load using appropriate technique before becoming fatigued. Thus, 8RM to 12RM per set is generally recommended to improve both muscular strength and endurance; however, a lower repetition range with a heavier weight (e.g., 6RM-8RM) may better optimize gains in strength and power (4, 20). Because orthopedic injury may occur in old or frail patients when performing efforts to volitional fatigue using a high-intensity, low- to moderate-RM training regimen, the completion of 10 to 15 repetitions or 10RM to 15RM is generally recommended for patients with cardiovascular disease (1, 21, 40).

Number of Sets

Three or more sets of 6 to 12 repetitions per exercise performed 3 days/week as part of a periodized training regimen are traditionally prescribed for many athletic programs. However, the minimal and optimal number of sets required to elicit significant gains in health parameters is substantially less for adult fitness participants and patients in comprehensive cardiac rehabilitation programs (19, 40). Over the past decade, several studies have examined the effects of single- versus multiple-set strength training programs (4, 19, 23). The rationale for using multiple sets is that the number of sets contributes to the total volume of work completed, which in turn is considered the most essential factor in eliciting physiological adaptations (20). Strength training guidelines recommended by the ACSM (2-4), AHA (21, 40), and AACVPR (1) reflect the empirical research conducted to determine the minimal and optimal levels of exercise needed to induce health- and fitness-related adaptations in the musculoskeletal systems. The amount of time required to complete a single-set program is less than half the time required to complete multiple-set protocols. This time efficiency often translates into improved program compliance, because exercise programs that last longer than 1 hr have higher dropout rates (29, 38). Because of the similarities in strength gains for single- and multiple-set programs, single-set programs are recommended for the adult fitness and clinical populations because these programs are less time-consuming, are more cost-effective, and produce health benefits that reduce disease risks.

Frequency of Training

The frequency of training is an important component of a strength training program (14, 20). The rest period must be sufficient to allow for tissue repair and development and to prevent overtraining; however, too much rest between sessions can result in detraining. A 48 hr rest period between concurrent training sessions is generally recommended (1, 4, 20), which corresponds with a 3 days/week frequency of training guideline for individual muscle groups. Although clinicians must consider the specific needs and goals of individual participants (i.e., time needed to recover from a training session), particularly for those who are frail or have orthopedic limitations, the conservative frequency of training guideline is a minimum of 2 days/week. Session frequencies of 2 days/week appear to produce 75% of the improvements made with frequencies of 3 days/week in cardiac patients (48) and 80% to 90% of the strength benefits of more frequent programs in the initially untrained person for the first few months (14). Participants who have time and want to achieve more benefits may choose to train 3 days/week. However, the guideline minimum of 2 days/week allows more time for recuperation, is less time-consuming, and thus may enhance adherence.

Modality of Exercise

Muscular strength and endurance can be developed by means of static (isometric) or dynamic (isotonic or isokinetic) exercises. Although each type of training has its advantages and limitations, dynamic resistance exercises are generally recommended because they best mimic activities associated with daily living. From a safety standpoint, resistance machines with weight stacks are recommended for several reasons:

1. The initial weight can be applied at a low level and increased in small increments (1 kg or less).
2. The equipment is usually designed to protect the low back and reduce the risk of injury.
3. Many machines are designed to avoid hand gripping, which reduces the risk of exercise-induced hypertension.
4. The machines are usually designed to allow the resistance to be applied evenly through the joint's normal range of motion.
5. Many types of machines can be double pinned to allow the subject to exercise through her pain-free range of motion.

6. Many resistance machines do not require the participant to balance or control the weight, as do dumbbells and barbells, which may reduce the risk of injury.

Using resistance machines requires less time than free weight exercises, allowing the participant more opportunity to pursue and obtain the benefits of aerobic endurance activities and flexibility exercises. The ability to complete a comprehensive exercise program within 45 to 60 min, 2 or 3 days/week, often improves program compliance.

Regardless of the training modality, strength training induces physiological adaptations (i.e., increased neuromuscular integration, muscle hypertrophy) that contribute to increases in muscular strength and function. The expected improvements from strength training are difficult to predict because increases in strength are affected by the participant's initial level of strength and his potential for improvement. Although the literature reflects a wide range of improvement in muscular strength with training programs (2-200%), the average improvement for previously sedentary persons during the first 6 months is 25% to 30% (19, 20).

Safety Considerations

Strength training is well established as an integral component of exercise rehabilitation for patients with CAD, orthopedic injuries, and neuromuscular and metabolic disorders, and it is increasingly being prescribed for many other clinical populations, such as patients with other stable cardiac conditions (e.g., stable congestive heart failure), patients with pulmonary diseases, and organ transplant recipients. Careful screening of potential participants is imperative prior to their enrollment in exercise rehabilitation programs (see Guidelines for Beginning Strength Training below). Patients with unstable angina, atrial fibrillation, uncontrolled hypertension, unstable congestive heart failure, or other unstable cardiac or cerebrovascular conditions are generally excluded from participation. In addition, patients with severe orthopedic disabilities or musculoskeletal disorders and patients with functional or cognitive impairments that preclude the safe performance of strength training should be excluded (1, 21, 40).

▪ Guidelines for Beginning Strength Training

Starting Point

- A minimum of 5 weeks after myocardial infarction, including 3 weeks of continuous participation in aerobic endurance exercise
- A minimum of 8 weeks after coronary artery bypass graft surgery, including 3 weeks of continuous participation in aerobic endurance exercise
- A minimum of 2 weeks after percutaneous transluminal coronary angioplasty, including 2 weeks of continuous participation in aerobic endurance exercise

Inclusion Criteria

The following criteria are similar to those for aerobic endurance exercise training:

- Aerobic capacity ≥5 METs
- Stable angina pectoris
- Resting systolic blood pressure ≤160 mmHg
- Resting diastolic blood pressure ≤100 mmHg
- Absence of uncontrolled dysrhythmias
- Absence of stenotic or regurgitant valvular disease
- Absence of hypertrophic cardiomyopathy
- Medically stable heart failure (AHA activity class B or C)

Adapted from AACVPR (American Association of Cardiovascular and Pulmonary Rehabilitation.2003, *Guidelines for cardiac rehabilitation and secondary prevention programs*, 4th ed. (Champaign, IL: Human Kinetics Publishers); G.F. Fletcher, et al.,1995, "Exercise standards: A statement for healthcare professionals from the American Heart Association," *Circulation* 91: 580-615; M.L. Pollock et al., 2000, "Resistance exercise in individuals with and without cardiovascular disease: Benefits, rationale, safety, and prescription," *Circulation* 101: 828-833.

The acute circulatory responses to strength training and safety concerns for patients with cardiovascular disease have been described previously (37). The primary concern for patients with cardiac conditions is a strength training–induced increase in pressure load on the heart. This pressure load is characterized by a moderate increase in cardiac output, a minimal change in peripheral vascular resistance, and a substantial increase in mean arterial pressure. It has been speculated that the resulting diastolic pressures cause unfavorable secondary remodeling of the ventricular wall. However, indicators of myocardial stress including rate-pressure product and estimated myocardial oxygen consumption are lower during strength training than aerobic endurance exercise at the same relative intensities. Furthermore, neither static nor dynamic strength training exercise has been demonstrated to elicit angina pectoris, ischemic ST-segment displacement, or ventricular arrhythmias in patients with stable cardiac conditions (37). The lower incidence of ischemic episodes and cardiac complications occurring during strength training is thought to be attributable to a lower peak heart rate response and higher diastolic pressure, which combine to enhance coronary artery filling and subsequently myocardial oxygen supply. The absence of cardiovascular complications in the studies reported to date infers that strength training is safe for cardiac patients, particularly those with good residual left ventricular function (1, 21, 37, 40).

To enhance safety and use time most efficiently, most strength training programs should incorporate a combination of resistance equipment and traditional calisthenics and flexibility exercises. Intensity should start low and progress slowly, allowing time for adaptation. Exercises should be rhythmic, performed at a moderate to slow controlled speed through a pain-free range of motion, with a normal breathing pattern during the lifting movements. Heavy resistance exercise can cause a dramatic acute increase in both systolic and diastolic blood pressure, especially when a Valsalva maneuver is used, and is generally not recommended for patients with cardiovascular disease (36, 37). If a 1RM test is administered to assess muscular strength at the beginning of a strength training program, then 30% to 40% of the 1RM for the upper body and 50% to 60% of the 1RM for the hips and legs should be used as the starting weight for the first exercise training session. When the patient can comfortably lift the weight for 12 to 15 repetitions using good form and perceives it to be light to somewhat hard (12-13 on the Borg RPE scale) (7), 5% can be added to the next training session. At this level of training, progression to a heavier weight should occur every 2 or 3 weeks. If the patient cannot lift the weight a minimum of 10 times, the weight should be reduced for the next training session.

Strength Training Guidelines

Recognizing that strength training can significantly improve a multitude of health factors, both the exercise science and medical communities recommend that people of all ages and both genders participate in comprehensive exercise programs. The major health authorities, including the Surgeon General (49), the American College of Sports Medicine (ACSM) (2-4), the American Heart Association (AHA) (21,40), and the American Association for Cardiovascular and Pulmonary Rehabilitation (AACVPR) (1), have developed strength training guidelines appropriate for the various segments of the population (table 16.2).

Guidelines for Healthy Adults

The recommendation for the initially untrained adult is one set of 8 to 12 repetitions to volitional fatigue of 8 to 10 exercises performed 2 or 3 times per week for persons younger than 50 years and the same regimen using 10 to 15 repetitions for persons older than 50 years (2-4). The research suggests that 80% to 90% of strength gains can be elicited using this regimen in the initial training period (i.e., up to the first 4 months) compared with high-volume program (multiple sets or greater intensity). The rationale for the recommendations regarding strength training program guidelines has been reviewed previously (2, 4, 19). For healthy untrained adults and most clinical populations, the research literature indicates that multiple-set programs may provide little, if any, additional stimulus for improving the rate of physiological adaptations in the initial training period compared with single-set programs. For the more serious lifter whose goal is to maximize muscle size and strength, there is compelling evidence for the multiple-set paradigm using periodization regimens (4). However, there is also increasing evidence that because the amount of time required to participate in formal exercise training is an important factor affecting program compliance, the majority of Americans who engage in strength training are more likely to adhere to the current ACSM recommendations in which strength training is but one component of the comprehensive exercise program model.

TABLE 16.2 Standards, Guidelines, and Position Statements Regarding Strength Training

	Sets; repetitions or RM; number of exercises	Frequency of training, days/week
HEALTHY SEDENTARY ADULTS		
1996 Surgeon General's report (49)	1-2 sets; 8-12RM; 8-10 exercises	2
1998 ACSM position stand (2)	1 set*; 8-12RM; 8-10 exercises†	2-3
1998 ACSM guidelines (3)	1 set; 8-12RM; 8-10 exercises	≥2
2002 ACSM position stand (4)	1 set*; 8-12RM; 8-10 exercises	2-3
ELDERLY OR FRAIL PERSONS		
1998 ACSM position stand (2)	1 set*; 10-15 repetitions; 8-10 exercises	2-3
PATIENTS WITH CHRONIC LOW BACK PAIN		
Carpenter and Nelson (10)	1 set; 8-15RM; isolated lumbar extension exercises	1
CARDIAC PATIENTS (AHA CLASS A & B)		
1995 AHA exercise standards (21)	1 set; 10-15RM; 8-10 exercises	2-3
2000 AHA position paper (40)	1 set; 10-15RM; 8-10 exercises	2-3
2003 AACVPR guidelines (1)	1 set; 12-15RM; 8-10 exercises	2-3
RECIPIENTS OF HEART TRANSPLANT		
Braith et al. (9)	1 set; 10-15 RM; 8-10 exercises	2
	1 set; 10-15RM; isolated lumbar extension exercises	1

ACSM = American College of Sports Medicine; AHA = American Heart Association; AACVPR = American Association of Cardiovascular and Pulmonary Rehabilitation; RM = repetition maximum.

*Multiple-set regimens may provide increased benefits.

†Minimum one exercise per major muscle group: e.g., chest press, pull-down (upper back), shoulder press, biceps curl, triceps extension, low back extension, abdominal crunch or curl-up, leg extension (quadriceps), leg curl (hamstrings), calf raise.

Guidelines for Elderly People

Aging is a complex process involving many variables (e.g., lifestyle factors, genetics) that interact with one another and greatly influence the quality of life during the life span. Strength training is a safe and effective modality for developing and maintaining the musculoskeletal system as well as improving physical function, endurance, psychological well-being, and health in older adults (>60 years) (17, 51). The ACSM exercise prescription guidelines (2-4) for young and middle-aged adults are also appropriate for elderly people, with slight but distinct differences in exercise prescription application. Because of the natural course of tissue degradation that encompasses loss of bone mineral density and sarcopenia, elderly adults may be more fragile and thus more susceptible to fatigue, orthopedic injuries, and cardiovascular and pulmonary complications. Clinicians must consider these factors when prescribing physical activity programs. Furthermore, many elderly adults are deconditioned, and it may be more beneficial over the long term to lower the intensity of the training regimen and progress more slowly than programs prescribed for younger adults. The mode of exercise is also an important consideration when designing strength training programs for the elderly. Resistance machines with weight stacks are usually recommended, for the safety-related reasons described previously. Exercise sessions should begin at a low intensity level (10-15 repetitions) and progress slowly (every 2-4 weeks). The initial resistance should allow the elderly participant to reach moderate fatigue (RPE 12 or 13) while completing the desired number of repetitions with good form. After an adaptation period of 3 to 4 weeks, the resistance can gradually be increased 5% with the goal of 13 to 15 on the RPE scale. Once this period of adaptation has been completed, healthy older adults without orthopedic or cardiovascular limitations may proceed to volitional fatigue (RPE 18-20) to obtain optimal benefits (17, 40).

Guidelines for Patients With Cardiovascular Disease

Similar to healthy adults, patients with advanced cardiovascular disease require a minimum level of muscular exertion to accomplish activities associated with daily living but often lack the physical strength, muscular endurance, or confidence to perform these tasks. Comprehensive rehabilitation programs for cardiac patients have traditionally emphasized dynamic aerobic exercise to maintain and improve cardiovascular fitness and gain other health benefits (53). The AHA (21, 40), ACSM (3), and AACVPR (1) recognize the importance of muscular fitness in preparing the cardiac patient to return to work and to participate in household and leisure activities. Many of these vocational and recreational activities place demands on the body that more closely resemble resistance exercise than aerobic endurance exercise. Therefore, it seems prudent to incorporate strength training into the patient's exercise program. Recent research indicates that complementary strength training has many favorable health and fitness benefits and can be safely

incorporated as early as phase II cardiac rehabilitation (see Guidelines for Beginning Strength Training on page 160) (1).

Updated strength training guidelines for traditional cardiac patients (i.e., post–myocardial infarction, with well-preserved left ventricular function) developed by the AHA (21, 40) and AACVPR (1) have been published (table 16.2 on page 162) and are similar to the guidelines established by ACSM for healthy adults (2-4). The primary differences involve reduced exercise intensity, slower progression of the training volume variables, and increased patient monitoring and program supervision. Strength training is widely prescribed for patients in phase III and IV cardiac rehabilitation, and standard recommendations include the use of weight machines or dumbbells in a circuit format for comprehensive conditioning (1, 21, 40). Circuits should include 8 to 10 exercises addressing each major muscle group—chest press, pull-down (upper back), shoulder press, biceps curl, triceps extension, low back extension, abdominal crunch or curl-up, leg extension (quadriceps), leg curl (hamstrings), calf raise—and patients should perform one set of each exercise using lighter weights that correspond to 30% to 50% of maximum and that can be performed for 10 to 15 (21) or 12 to 15 repetitions (1) consistently 2 or 3 days/week.

Although strength training has been shown to be safe in regard to precipitating a cardiovascular event (37), much variance exists among recommendations as to the level of fatigue (moderate to maximum) required in such programs (1, 3, 21). Thus, it appears that low-risk patients who have a MET capacity greater than 7 can be cleared for heavy strength training (10-15 or 12-15 repetitions to fatigue), whereas more high-risk patients should keep their fatigue to a moderate level (RPE ≤15). An additional point to consider when prescribing exercise programs for cardiac patients and other patient populations is that pharmacotherapy (e.g., β-blockers) may alter the normal hemodynamic responses to exercise. Because of this, the RPE scale (7) has gained increasing acceptance as an effective method for monitoring the cardiac patient's level of exertion during strength training (21).

Recently published studies indicate that strength training is safe and beneficial for patients with stable congestive heart failure (CHF) (13, 30) and for patients who have received heart transplants (8, 9). Heart failure is the leading hospital discharge diagnosis for patients older than 65, and approximately 500,000 new cases of CHF are diagnosed annually in the United States; with 70,000 of these newly diagnosed patients qualifying for heart transplantation. The incidence for CHF is increasing because of the growth in the elderly population and also because advances in thrombolytic and ischemia–reperfusion therapy prolong survival following acute cardiac insults. There is a growing clinical consensus that medically stable CHF patients (AHA activity class B or C) and heart transplant recipients respond favorably to strength training, and consequently an increasing number are enrolling in comprehensive rehabilitation and maintenance exercise programs (9, 21).

Guidelines for Patients With Metabolic Disorders

Strength training, particularly when combined with aerobic training, has been shown to attenuate coronary artery disease (CAD) risk factors. The following section discusses the effects of strength training for patients with metabolic disorders, including obesity, diabetes, hyperlipidemia, and hypertension.

Obesity

Identifying and addressing CAD risk factors (e.g., obesity, dyslipidemia, hypertension, inactivity) early in the progression of disease became the primary focus of preventive medicine in the past decade. According to the Centers for Disease Control and Prevention, the prevalence of overweight and obesity in the United States is greater than 60%, and these conditions carry an estimated annual economic burden exceeding US$110 billion (34). Obesity and overweight exacerbate many chronic conditions including CAD, hypertension, dyslipidemia, type 2 diabetes, osteoarthritis, and other musculoskeletal-related disabilities (15, 54). An excessive accumulation of visceral adipose tissue relative to gluteal or femoral adipose tissue is associated with several metabolic complications and increased risk for premature mortality. Although it is generally agreed that obesity occurs when energy intake exceeds energy expenditure, the issue of obesity is complex, and genetics, overeating, inactivity, and metabolic disorders are contributing factors (44).

A gradual weight management program including caloric restriction and a prescribed exercise regimen is recommended for overweight yet otherwise healthy people because it promotes numerous health benefits secondary to maintainable weight loss (38, 39). Aerobic endurance exercise has been widely prescribed as a nonpharmacological tool in the treatment of abdominal obesity and associated metabolic disorders, and studies of short-term aerobic endurance training indicate that it attenuates or prevents the reduction in BMR that can accompany calorie restriction (44). However, the effect of aerobic endurance exercise on lean body mass

and subsequently on long-term BMR remains controversial. Despite the increased reliance on lipolysis for energy use and subsequent reduction in adiposity, the loss of lean body mass often associated with a combined diet and aerobic endurance exercise program may decrease BMR and result in additional weight gain if exercise program compliance deteriorates (38). Strength training offsets the reduction in BMR associated with caloric deprivation, but the increased level of energy expenditure depends on the type, duration, and intensity of the exercise regimen. Recent studies have shown that strength training is an effective intervention for reducing abdominal adipose tissue and increasing metabolic rate (32).

Experts recommend incorporating strength training into a long-term weight management program. Although strength training is less likely than aerobic endurance exercise to acutely increase energy and lipid utilization, strength training may be more effective in maintaining or increasing lean body mass and BMR and thus can improve body composition, aid in weight reduction, and hence reduce the risk factors associated with atherosclerotic disease progression. The increases in lean body mass and BMR associated with strength training are, in part, related to the rate of protein synthesis, which is increased up to 24 hr after a workout (12). A meta-analysis conducted by Garrow and Summerbell (24) on the effect of exercise with or without dieting on the body composition of overweight subjects indicated that strength training had little direct effect on weight loss but consistently improved body composition and increased lean body mass by 2 kg in men and 1 kg in women.

Diabetes Mellitus

The relationships among obesity, non-insulin-dependent diabetes mellitus (type 2), and cardiovascular disease are well established, with the majority of people with type 2 diabetes classified as clinically obese (BMI >30 kg/m²) and at significant risk for a cardiovascular event. The pathogenesis of type 2 diabetes is complex, and multiple organ systems are involved; abnormalities of insulin secretion and hepatic and peripheral insulin resistance often contribute to endothelial dysfunction and atherosclerotic disease progression. In obese people with type 2 diabetes, strength training may improve insulin sensitivity and glucose metabolism and reduce the risks for developing hypertension, CAD, or peripheral vascular disease (52). Although the exact sequence of cellular mechanisms is not fully understood, strength training–induced muscle contractions elicit an insulin-like effect on glucose uptake and increase the levels of glucose-transport protein 4 in skeletal muscle (31, 47).

Hyperlipidemia

Hyperlipidemia is a modifiable risk factor associated with endothelial dysfunction and premature atherosclerotic plaque formation (16). Although aerobic endurance exercise has been well established as a means for improving serum lipid–lipoprotein concentrations, the results from cross-sectional and longitudinal strength training studies regarding specific changes in serum lipid profiles have been inconsistent (16). Considering the results of strength training studies, rehabilitation specialists encourage patients with elevated serum lipid–lipoprotein profiles to incorporate aerobic endurance exercise into their training regimen and consult their personal physicians for advice on dietary modifications and pharmacological treatment.

Hypertension

Hypertensive patients have been discouraged from participating in strength training for fear of placing an excessive demand on the myocardium, which may already display left ventricular dysfunction, or precipitating a cerebrovascular event. Such fears have arisen as a result of the marked pressor responses elicited during acute bouts of heavy strength training in bodybuilders (36). Contrary to what might be expected, however, studies investigating the impact of long-term participation in strength training programs have shown that strength training may improve resting blood pressure (27, 28). The benefits of strength training in lowering blood pressure appear to be most marked with circuit weight training and certainly can be enhanced when patients complete a comprehensive exercise program incorporating both aerobic endurance and strength training components. Although strength training is not recommended as the primary mode of exercise, the literature indicates that strength training is both safe and beneficial for hypertensive patients.

Summary of Current Strength Training Guidelines

The Surgeon General's Report *Physical Activity and Health* (49), the updated versions of the ACSM position stands for exercise training (2, 4), the *Guidelines for Exercise Testing and Prescription* developed by the ACSM (3), the AHA *Exercise Standards* (21), and the AACVPR *Guidelines for Cardiac Rehabilitation and Secondary Prevention Programs* (1) form the foundation for most recommendations regarding physical activity program design. These guidelines reflect the empirical research conducted to determine minimal and optimal levels of exercise to induce health- and fitness-related adaptations in the cardiovascular–respiratory and musculoskeletal systems. Although these recommendations may appear minimal, clinicians should incorporate strength training into a comprehensive exercise program that includes aerobic endurance training and flexibility exercises. The comprehensive exercise program should be designed so that it can be performed 2 or 3 days/week with each session not lasting more than 60 min. Although research indicates that greater frequencies of training or training volumes may elicit larger strength gains, the magnitude of difference within the first few months is usually small and is often associated with an increased incidence of injuries or a decrease in program adherence. The minimal guidelines are certainly appropriate for the patient enrolling in a comprehensive cardiac rehabilitation program. For safety and time considerations, most strength training programs should incorporate 8 to 10 exercises that condition the major muscle groups a minimum of 2 days/week. Intensity should progress slowly, allowing time for adaptation. To develop or maintain joint range of motion, calisthenic and flexibility exercises should be included. The goal is for healthy persons younger than 50 years to be able to complete one set of 8 to 12 repetitions to volitional fatigue (8-12RM). The AHA (21, 40) and AACVPR (1) guidelines for cardiac patients and the ACSM (2, 3) guidelines for persons older than 50 years recommend a lower-intensity program, incorporating one set of 10 to 15 or 12 to 15 repetitions. Depending on the patient's clinical status, this lower-intensity program should be performed to a level perceived as moderately hard or to volitional fatigue.

Summary

Participation in a strength training program has been shown to improve many health factors, such as lean body mass, basal metabolic rate, bone mineral density, walking gait, incidence of falls, pain caused by chronic low back problems, glucose tolerance and insulin sensitivity, and activity tolerance. There is also increasing evidence that strength training may favorably alter risk factors associated with a multitude of chronic diseases. Additional longitudinal studies are warranted to address these issues. However, the available evidence indicates that the current strength training guidelines for cardiac patient populations provide the minimal stimulus necessary to induce physiological adaptations that translate into improved health, function, and most importantly, quality of life. Recognizing that these benefits can be safely obtained by patients with many clinically diverse conditions, the major health organizations recommend incorporating strength training regimens into comprehensive rehabilitation programs.

CHAPTER 17

Flexibility Training

Ian Shrier, MD, PhD

Flexibility training is used to improve performance (24), prevent injury (23, 27), enhance rehabilitation following injury (15), and ease muscle aches and pains (5). Some of these effects have been well studied and some have not. Most of the research about stretching pertains to its effects in healthy young adults who are participating in vigorous sport. In patients who have significant cardiovascular disease or are undergoing cardiac rehabilitation, elite performance and rehabilitation following injury are less relevant. Therefore, this chapter focuses on potential benefits for older subjects who have not been active in the recent past and intend to increase their activity over the ensuing few months.

Physiology of Stretching

Stretching increases range of motion (ROM) through two different mechanisms: viscoelasticity and stretch tolerance.

Viscoelasticity

Human tissues exhibit viscoelastic behavior, which is a combination of elastic behavior (a change in length for a given force and the return to its original length immediately upon release, e.g., a rubber band) and viscous behavior (e.g., a substance that exhibits flow and movement that are dependent on time [7], such as molasses). Because of muscle's viscous behavior, if a constant force is applied to a muscle, the muscle length increases over time (termed *creep*, figure 17.1*a*). The corollary of creep is called *stress relaxation:* If the muscle is stretched to a constant length and held, force decreases over time (figure 17.1*b*). When the force is removed, the substance slowly returns to its original length. Another important concept is plastic deformation. If you damage the molecular structure of the tissue, the material remains permanently elongated even after the force is removed (similar to the way a plastic bag remains elongated after stretching) (7). Although stretching affects tendons and other connective tissue in addition to muscle, compliance of tissues in series is additive, and the compliance of the resting muscle is responsible for how easy it is to stretch a muscle–tendon–bone complex. For instance, if a rubber band is tied to the end of a stiff rope and the rope is tied to the end of the stick, the rubber band–rope–stick complex will still change length according to the compliance of the rubber band even though the rope is stiff (the compliance of the rope is low but not zero).

Stretch Tolerance

In the living person, ROM increases with stretching

Address correspondence concerning this chapter to Ian Shrier, Centre for Clinical Epidemiology and Community Studies, Lady Davis Institute for Medical Research, SMBD-Jewish General Hospital, 3755 Cote Sainte Catherine Road, Montreal, Quebec H3T 1E2 Canada. E-mail: ian.shrier@mcgill.ca

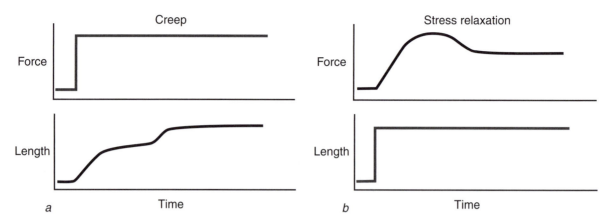

FIGURE 17.1 Viscoelastic substances exhibit both *(a)* creep and *(b)* stress relaxation. If a constant force is applied, the muscle will immediately stretch and then slowly increase in length *(a)*. If a muscle is stretched to a certain length and held, the force on the muscle gradually declines *(b)*.

through a mechanism termed *stretch tolerance*. When people stretch, they stop when they feel that the tension in the muscle is too high. If that sensation is masked (e.g., with ice), they can stretch further. In fact, an acute bout of stretching itself masks the sensation of tension and increases stretch tolerance (19). Therefore, both viscoelastic behavior and stretch tolerance are involved in the increase in ROM observed with an acute stretch (10, 19). The analgesia is at least partially attributable to the effects at the spinal cord or cerebral level, because during unilateral stretching using proprioceptive neuromuscular facilitation (PNF), the ROM in the nonstretched leg also increases (20).

The increased stretch tolerance that follows long-term stretching (i.e., over a period of weeks) may be attributable to an analgesic effect but could also be related to increased strength of the tissue. When a muscle is stretched 24 hr/day, some hypertrophy occurs even though the muscle has not been contracting (1, 30). This effect is known as stretch-induced hypertrophy. However, it is unknown whether stretching a muscle group for 30 to 60 s/day over months also results in hypertrophy.

Benefits of Stretching

Two principle health-related benefits are attributed to stretching: prevention of injury and alleviation of aches and pains.

Prevention of Injury

Stretching immediately before exercise has not been associated with a decrease in injury rate, even if the subject warms up before stretching (13, 23, 27). Of more importance to a cardiac rehabilitation program are the findings of three studies that examined injury rates in subjects who stretched regularly not immediately prior to exercise. In all three studies, the results suggested a clinically relevant benefit to stretching (risk ratio [95% confidence interval] = 0.82 [0.57, 1.14], 0.57 [0.37, 0.88], and 0.77 [0.54, 1.08]), but the results were only significant in one of the three studies (2, 11, 14). These results suggest that regular stretching should be part of a cardiac rehabilitation program.

Alleviation of Aches and Pains

As previously discussed, the increase in ROM with stretching is partly attributable to an analgesic effect (19). Therefore, stretching should theoretically decrease muscle aches of any cause. There is some evidence that stretching decreases the pain associated with unaccustomed exercise (8). Furthermore, several studies used stretching as a control intervention while examining the effects of other types of training in patients with fibromyalgia or unexplained physical symptoms (17, 22). In each study, subjects who stretched improved on at least one clinical scale of disability or pain, suggesting that stretching itself may be beneficial and should be studied against a nonactive control group to determine whether it is a real or placebo effect.

How to Stretch

Given the likely benefits of regular stretching in the cardiac rehabilitation population, clinicians must know how to prescribe stretching properly. Unfortunately, most studies examining different stretching techniques have been conducted on young, healthy subjects, and we must extrapolate these results to make inferences for the cardiac rehabilitation population. A full discussion of stretching techniques and positions is beyond the scope of this chapter. However, some common mistakes and adaptations are shown for the hamstrings in figure 17.2, the quadriceps in figure 17.3, the soleus in figure 17.4, and the pectoralis in figure 17.5.

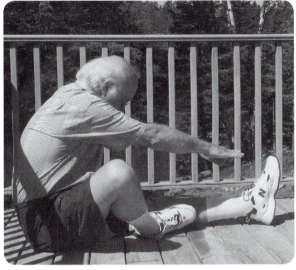

a

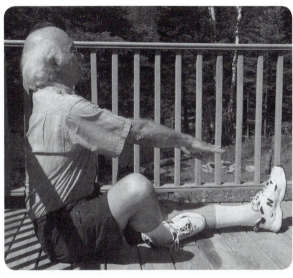

b

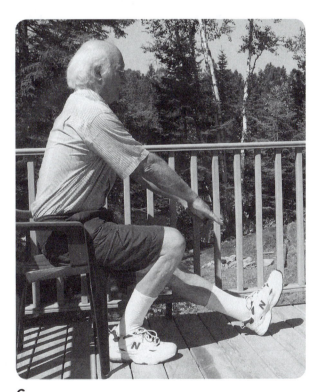

c

FIGURE 17.2 Stretching the hamstring. *(a)* The subject incorrectly rounds his low back. Although this allows him to reach further, it increases stress on the back and does not improve the effectiveness of the hamstring stretch. *(b)* The subject maintains a straight back in the correct posture. However, the hamstring muscles of this subject are not flexible enough to maintain the hip in 90° flexion, which is necessary to sit comfortably. *(c)* The subject performs the same hamstring stretch, but the chair allows a comfortable position with the hip flexed less than 90°.

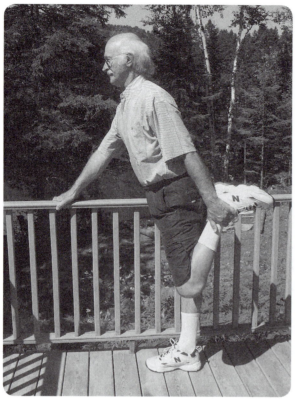

a

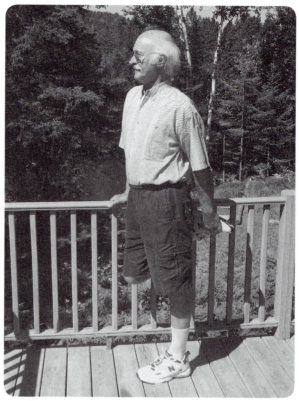

b

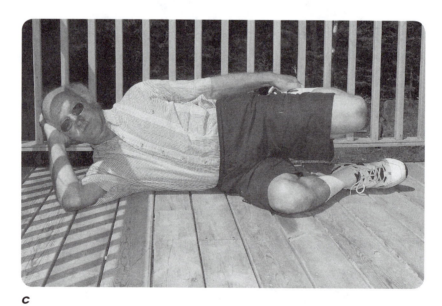

c

FIGURE 17.3 Stretching the quadriceps. *(a)* The subject incorrectly tries to bring his knee as far back as possible by bending at the waist, letting the thigh abduct, rotating the pelvis, and arching the back. *(b)* The subject maintains an appropriate posture for his back, keeps the thigh adducted (by holding the ankle with the contralateral hand), and contracts the appropriate muscles to prevent the pelvis from rotating and the back from arching. As a result, the quadriceps muscle is stretched even though the knee is anterior to the supporting leg. *(c)* The quadriceps stretch is shown while the subject lies on his side. This requires less balance capability, but it is not always possible to lie down.

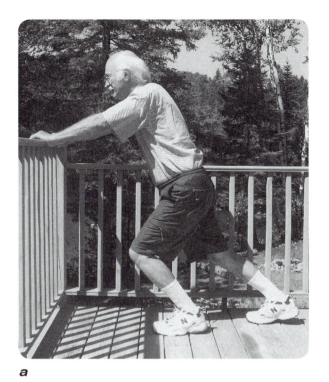
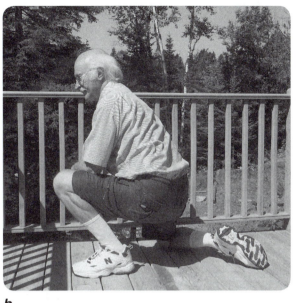

a

b

FIGURE 17.4 Stretching the soleus. (a) The subject uses the standard technique to stretch the left soleus; the ipsilateral gastrocnemius is relaxed by bending the knee and the subject leans forward over a dorsiflexed ankle. Because the leg must support the body weight, this position is sometimes difficult for people with sore knees. (b) An alternative position is shown where the subject bends his knee completely and rocks forward on the ipsilateral ankle. This position is not possible if the knee range of motion is limited, and it is sometimes difficult for the subject to find a comfortable position for the contralateral limb.

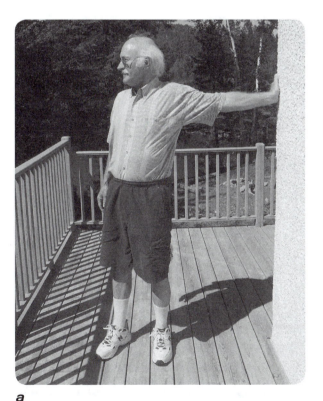
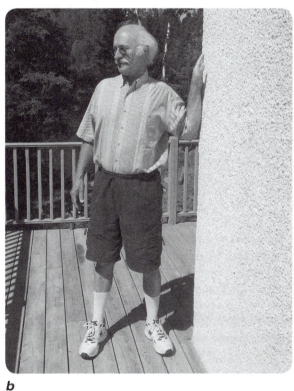

a

b

FIGURE 17.5 Stretching the pectoralis. (a) The subject has internally rotated his shoulder and "rolled" the shoulder anteriorly; the stretch is felt in the anterior shoulder instead of over the pectoralis muscle. (b) The subject bends his elbow, which makes it more difficult to internally rotate the shoulder; the subject is instructed to adjust the position until the stretch is felt over the anterior chest and not in the shoulder.

Duration

Many different stretching protocols are given to patients. This section describes some of the research supporting different approaches, with a focus on achieving long-term changes with regular stretching.

In humans, stretching the hamstring muscle using 30 and 60 s/stretches each day increased ROM much more than 15 s/stretches each day over the course of 6 weeks, but there was no difference between 30 s and 60 s (3). In a separate study, the same authors found that one hamstring stretch of 30 s/day gave the same results as three stretches of 30 s (4). However, the results of Borms and colleagues (6) appear to contradict these findings, because 10 s stretches were as effective as 20 s or 30 s stretches over the course of 10 weeks. The apparent contradiction may be resolved upon closer examination of the Borms study (6). In the groups who stretched for 20 s and 30 s, a plateau in ROM was reached after 7 weeks, but the group that stretched 10 s increased ROM gradually over the entire 10 weeks. Therefore, it is likely that 30 s stretches achieve the maximum benefit quicker (i.e., by 6-7 weeks) than 10 s stretches, but the two programs eventually achieve similar results by 10 weeks.

In the one study examining the effect of duration on hamstring ROM in elderly subjects (mean age 84.7 years), the authors found that 60 s stretches increased ROM faster than 30 s stretches (2.4°/week vs. 1.3°/week) (9). In addition, the gains achieved over 6 weeks of stretching were lost 4 weeks poststretching in subjects who stretched 30 s or less, but there remained a 5.4° increase in ROM in those who had stretched 60 s. These results suggest that individual subject characteristics such as age (perhaps via differences in baseline stiffness) may affect the most effective duration for stretching. Indeed, even among animal tissue studies, there is always variability between samples from different animals. Furthermore, Henricson and colleagues (12) found that different muscles differed in their response to heat plus stretching, perhaps attributable to differences in pennation, muscle length, or muscle fiber type. Finally, another possible explanation is that ROM in humans may be limited more by stretch tolerance than by viscoelastic behavior for certain muscles but not others. For instance, if viscoelastic effects limit the ROM of a particular muscle, stretching longer than 30 s would not be expected to increase the effectiveness. However, if stretch tolerance is the limiting factor, holding the stretch longer may indeed provide additional benefit. These results suggest that it is reasonable to assume interindividual (and intermuscle) variability, and therefore it may not be appropriate to give everyone the same stretching recipe. A more prudent approach may be to tailor the prescription according to the success of the intervention.

To produce an individualized program, the clinician should instruct the subject to hold an individual stretch as long as the subject feels tension (i.e., effects of stress relaxation or stretch tolerance continue to increase ROM). To obtain further benefit, once the tension stabilizes at a lower level, the subject may increase the stretch so that she feels the same tension as she did originally. The success of such a program is gauged by the increase in ROM over days and weeks. If a subject finds that tension stabilizes at a lower level within 15 s and that there are minimal increases in ROM, she should try holding the stretch for a longer period of time (although she should avoid forcing the stretch and causing muscle damage, i.e., overstretching).

Types of Stretches

PNF stretching usually results in greater increases in ROM compared with static or ballistic stretching, even though some studies did not achieve statistical significance (for references in this section, see reference 25).

When we compare the different types of PNF techniques, the agonist–contract–relax method (the hip flexors including quadriceps muscles actively stretch the hamstrings followed by a maximal quadriceps contraction and then passive holding) appears superior to the contract–relax method (a muscle contraction and then passive stretching of the muscle), which appears superior to the hold–relax technique (an isometric contraction with resistance gradually applied over 9 s). Although the original theory was that PNF techniques increase ROM through reciprocal inhibition of the muscle (i.e., decreased electromyographic activity), this was first disproved in 1979 and confirmed more recently. The mechanism of the increased ROM appears to be an increase in stretch tolerance.

Some people prefer static stretching (continuous stretching without any rest) for reasons of simplicity, and one study reported that static stretching is superior to cyclic stretching (applying a stretch, relaxing, and reapplying the stretch), whereas two studies suggested no difference. All of these studies examined the hamstring muscle, and there was no apparent methodological reason for the discrepancy. Although more research is needed before definitive conclusions can be made about the most effective way to stretch, cardiac rehabilitation patients should probably stick to the method that is easiest to teach and learn and to perform without a partner—static stretching.

Warming Up

If a warm-up is performed without stretching, there is no increase in the ROM (26). However, although heat does not improve ROM by itself, studies found that stretch plus heat was superior to stretch alone with respect to increases in hip flexion, abduction, and external rotation (12); shoulder ROM (18); and triceps surae ROM (28). With regard to activity-induced warm-up, most studies suggest that warming up before stretching increases the effectiveness of the stretch with respect to ROM (references 16 and 21, and specifically the ankle in reference 29), but there are some conflicting results (hamstring and quadriceps in reference 29). Finally, all of these studies examined the acute effect of a stretch, and there are no studies on the effect of warming up with respect to long-term changes in ROM. Given basic science observations, it is reasonable to recommend warming up prior to stretching, but if time is limited, stretching without warming up may be considered if the exercise session is limited to stretching. If the session includes other exercises in addition to stretching, pre-session warm-up may prevent injury, whereas pre-session stretching does not appear to prevent injury.

Summary

Current research suggests that stretching is likely to benefit the patient undergoing cardiac rehabilitation. Stretching should be done carefully and is likely to require longer periods of time for cardiac rehabilitation patients than for younger people. A reasonable approach is to use simple static stretches (preferably with a warm-up prior to stretching) for those not used to stretching and to individualize the duration of the stretch by showing the patient how to judge its short-term effectiveness. If long-term results are not achieved, the stretching technique and duration should be reviewed and modified.

CHAPTER 18

Effects of Dietary Patterns on CVD Risk Factors

Penny M. Kris-Etherton, PhD

Amy E. Griel, PhD

Diet is one of the cornerstones for the prevention and treatment of cardiovascular disease (CVD). Government agencies and scientific societies consistently advocate diet, weight control, and increased physical activity as the first steps to prevent and treat CVD (1, 6, 8, 13, 18, 25, 29). Dietary recommendations have been made that target important risk factors for coronary heart disease (CHD), including dyslipidemia, hypertension, overweight, and obesity. The recommendations are revised continuously based on new scientific discoveries about dietary factors, nutrients, and dietary patterns and how these modify CVD events and the associated risk factors. There has been an impressive expansion in the scope of dietary recommendations from the standpoint of nutrients and other dietary factors to modify, the resultant dietary patterns, and the risk factors they target.

The purpose of this chapter is to describe dietary recommendations for CVD prevention and treatment and discuss the expected effects on CHD risk factors and overall CVD risk. A second objective is to discuss the recent scientific literature that describes different dietary patterns that show remarkable effects on CVD risk factors and events. Last, we discuss how dietary recommendations can be implemented as dietary patterns that can have unprecedented effects on the prevention and treatment of CVD.

Dietary and Other Lifestyle Guidelines for CVD Prevention and Treatment

Major risk factors for CVD have been identified and form the basis of various treatment guidelines issued by government agencies and scientific societies. The major risk factors for CVD that are modifiable by diet and physical activity include elevated total cholesterol (TC) and low-density lipoprotein cholesterol (LDL-C), low high-density lipoprotein cholesterol (HDL-C), elevated triglycerides, hypertension, diabetes and insulin resistance, and obesity. In an analysis of three prospective studies (N = 20,995), at least one major CVD risk factor (e.g., elevated cholesterol level, high

Address correspondence concerning this chapter to Penny M. Kris-Etherton, Department of Nutritional Sciences, S-126 Henderson Building, The Pennsylvania State University, University Park, PA 16802. Email: pmk3@psu.edu blood pressure, diabetes, and cigarette smoking) was present in 87% to 100% of the population diagnosed with fatal CHD (12). In an analysis of 122,458 patients enrolled in 14 international randomized trials, Khot and colleagues (23) reported that at least one of four conventional CHD risk factors (i.e., cigarette smoking, diabetes, hyperlipidemia, and hypertension) was present in 85% of women and 81% of men with CHD. Collectively, the evidence demonstrates that controlling major CVD risk factors can significantly reduce CVD. The data from studies used for these analyses were instrumental in developing the treatment and prevention guidelines for CVD issued by government agencies and other scientific organizations.

The National Cholesterol Education Program's Adult Treatment Panel III (NCEP-ATP III) issued treatment guidelines for decreasing LDL-C. The initial therapeutic intervention recommended is diet along with lifestyle interventions that include weight loss and physical activity. The Therapeutic Lifestyle Changes (TLC) diet is recommended by NCEP-ATP III to lower TC and LDL-C levels. The TLC diet recommends appreciable reductions in saturated fat, trans fat, and dietary cholesterol (table 18.1). Therapeutic options to the TLC diet to achieve LDL-C goals include stanols and sterols (2 g/day) and viscous fiber (10-25 g/day). Weight loss and physical activity are also recommended as key components of the TLC diet. The effects of implementing the components of the TLC diet are shown in table 18.2. The cumulative estimate shows a marked reduction (20-30%) in LDL-C with implementation of all components of the TLC diet.

The Seventh Report of the Joint National Committee on Prevention, Detection, Evaluation and Treatment of High Blood Pressure recommended several lifestyle modifications. These include a weight loss of 10 lb (4.5 kg) in overweight persons; the Dietary Approaches to Stop Hypertension (DASH) eating plan (rich in fruits, vegetables, and low-fat dairy products, with reduced levels of dietary cholesterol, saturated fat, and total fat); a reduction in dietary sodium to <2,400 mg; 30 min of aerobic physical activity on most if not all days of the week; and moderate alcohol consumption (≤1 oz [2 drinks]/day of ethanol for men and ≤0.5 oz [1 drink]/day for women). The effects of these lifestyle modifications on systolic blood pressure (SBP) reduction are shown in table 18.3. Some individual interventions have effects as potent as pharmacotherapy. For example, weight loss, even a modest amount (i.e., 22 lb, or 10 kg), and the DASH eating plan (see page 181) lower SBP as much as 22 mmHg and 14 mmHg, respectively.

Overweight and obesity are major risk factors for CVD. The National Heart, Lung and Blood Institute (NHLBI) has issued Clinical Guidelines on the Identification, Evaluation and Treatment of Overweight and Obesity in Adults (30). The recommendations include caloric restriction (500-1,000 kcal deficit/day), physical activity (30-45 min of moderate levels of physical activity for 3-5 days/week initially), and behavior modification (self-monitoring, stress management, stimulus control, problem solving, contingency management, cognitive restructuring, and social support) for weight loss and maintenance of reduced body weight.

Diabetes is a major risk factor for CVD. In NCEP-ATP III, diabetes is considered a CHD risk equivalent (i.e., persons with diabetes are treated like persons with coronary disease). The American Diabetes Association issues yearly recommendations for nutritional practices and physical activity. These recommendations include achieving and maintaining a healthy body weight and good diabetes control with recommended lifestyle interventions (diet, physical activity) and prescribed therapeutic regimens for blood glucose control and management of plasma lipids and lipoproteins. Specific food-based recommendations for dietary carbohydrate for diabetes management include a dietary pattern that focuses on fruits, vegetables, whole-grain, legumes, low-fat milk, and a variety of fiber-containing foods. Dietary recommendations include a diet <10% kcal saturated fat (<7% kcal saturated fat for people at high risk), ~10% kcal polyunsaturated fat, 2 to 3 servings of fatty fish per week, minimal intake of trans fatty acids, 60% to 70% kcal carbohydrate (CHO) plus monounsaturated fat, 15-20% kcal protein, and <2,300 mg/day sodium.

The U.S. Dietary Guidelines 2005 were issued for Americans for health promotion and prevention of chronic disease. The dietary guidelines advocate achieving a nutritionally adequate diet that is high in nutrient-rich foods in all food groups and low in cholesterol-raising nutrients (saturated fat, trans fat, and cholesterol). Food groups to emphasize include fruits, vegetables, whole grains, low-fat and fat-free dairy products, and lean protein sources. Liquid oils are preferred to solid fats. Specific food-based dietary recommendations are listed in table 18.4 for 12 different levels of caloric intake.

Epidemiologic Studies of Dietary Patterns

Several studies have demonstrated the benefits of a healthy dietary pattern on CVD risk. In both women (11) and men (16), a prudent diet pattern (characterized

TABLE 18.1 Recommendations and Guidelines for Macronutrients*

	USDA dietary guidelines 2005 (8)	NAS DRIs (18)	NCEP-ATP III The TLC Diet (29)	AHA diet and lifestyle recommendations (25)	American Diabetes Association (1)
Total fat	Choose fats wisely for good health: 20-35%	20-35%	25-35%	25-35%	No recommendation
SFA	<10%	Low as possible	<7%	<7%	<7%
MUFA	Remaining fatty acids to achieve total fat	Remaining fatty acids to achieve total fat	Up to 20%	Unsaturated for SFA	—
PUFA	5-10%	5-10%	Up to 10%	Unsaturated for SFA	~10%
Linoleic acid (n-6 PUFA)	5-10%	5-10%	—	—-	—-
Linolenic acid EPA and DHA (n-3 PUFA)	0.6-1.2%	0.6-1.2%: up to 10% can be consumed as EPA + DHA	—	2 servings of fatty fish per week; 1 g/day EPA and DHA for coronary patients	2 or more servings of fish per week
Trans fat	Low as possible	Low as possible	Keep intake low	<1%	Minimize intake
Cholesterol, mg/day	<300	Low as possible	<200	<300	<200
Sodium, mg/day	<2,300	<2,300	<2,300	<2,300 Future goal: 1500	<2,300
Carbohydrate	Choose carbohydrates wisely for good health: 45-65%	45-65%	50-60%	≥6 servings, include 3 servings whole grains	60-70% from carbohydrates plus MUFA; one half of grain intake from whole grains
Protein	10-35% 2-3 servings	10-35%	15%	No recommendation	15-20%
Fiber	≥3 servings per day of whole grains	21-38 g/day	10-25 g/day soluble fiber	>25 g/day	14 g/1,000 kcal

NAS DRIs = National Academy of Science Dietary Reference Intakes; NCEP-ATP III = National Cholesterol Education Program—Adult Treatment Panel III; TLC = Therapeutic Lifestyle Changes; USDA = U.S. Department of Agriculture; AHA = American Heart Association; SFA = saturated fat; MUFA = monounsaturated fat; PUFA = polyunsaturated fat; EPA = eicosapentaenoic acid; DHA = docosahexaenoic acid, LDL-C = low-density lipoprotein cholesterol.

*Values are expressed as percentage of calories unless indicated otherwise.

by high intakes of vegetables, fruit, legumes, whole grains, fish, and poultry) was associated with lower relative risks of CHD (relative risk for women = 0.70 and 0.76 for men). In contrast, women and men consuming a Western diet pattern (characterized by high intake of red meat, processed meat, refined grains, sweets

and desserts, fried food, and high-fat dairy products) was associated with a higher CHD risk (relative risk for women = 1.46 and 1.64 for men). Another study conducted in women participating in the Framingham nutrition studies (28) reported that nutrient intake that was consistent with current dietary guidelines and smoking abstinence was associated with the lowest odds of carotid atherosclerosis. Dietary compliance was defined as meeting nutrient intakes defined by the American Heart Association (AHA) dietary guidelines, which are also consistent with the U.S. Department of Agriculture (USDA) Dietary Guidelines for Americans (≤30% kcal total fat, <10% kcal saturated fat, and <300 mg/day dietary cholesterol). Subjects who were considered to be noncompliant consumed diets that failed to meet one or more of these guidelines. Women with the highest dietary noncompliance (failed to meet one or more of the guidelines) in combination with cigarette smoking had an odds ratio of 3.49 compared with diet-compliant nonsmokers. Scientific information clearly indicates that a healthful dietary pattern and lifestyle practices can markedly reduce CHD risk in men and women.

TABLE 18.2   Components of the Optimal Diet for Low-Density Lipoprotein Cholesterol (LDL-C) Reduction

Dietary component	Reduction in LDL-C, %
Reduced saturated and trans fat (<7% of calories)	8-10
Reduced dietary cholesterol (<200 mg/day)	3-5
Viscous fiber (5-10 g/day)	3-5
Plant sterol and stanol esters (2 g/day)	6-15
Soy protein (25 g/day)	5
Weight reduction (loss of 10 lb, or 4.5 kg)	5-8
Cumulative estimate	30-48

Adapted from the National Cholesterol and Education Program 2001.

Controlled Clinical Studies of Dietary Patterns

Several secondary and primary prevention controlled clinical studies have demonstrated the power of a healthful dietary pattern to dramatically reduce risk

TABLE 18.3   Lifestyle Modifications to Manage Hypertension

Modification	Recommendations	Approximate systolic blood pressure reduction, mmHg
Reduce weight	Maintain normal body weight (body mass index 18.5-24.9)	5-20 for each 10 kg (22 lb) weight loss
Adapt DASH eating plan	Consume diet rich in fruits, vegetables, and low-fat dairy and low in saturated fat	8-14
Reduce dietary sodium	Reduce sodium to ≤2.4 g/day sodium or ≤6 g/day NaCl	2-8
Increase physical activity	Engage in regular aerobic activity such as walking (30 min/day on most days)	4-9
Moderate alcohol consumption	Limit alcohol to ≤2 drinks/day for men and ≤1 drink/day for women	2-4

From The Seventh Report of the Joint National Committee on Prevention, Detection, Evaluation, and Treatment of High Blood Pressure JNCVII. *JAMA.* 2003, 289: 2560-2572.

TABLE 18.4 Suggested Amounts of Food to Consume From the Basic Food Groups and Subgroups, as Well as Oils, to Meet Recommended Nutrient Intakes

TOTAL CALORIES PER DAY

	1,000	1,200	1,400	1,600	1,800	2,000	2,200	2,400	2,600	2,800	3,000	3,200
Fruit, cups (servings)/day	1 (2)	1 (2)	1.5 (3)	1.5 (3)	1.5 (3)	2 (4)	2 (4)	2 (4)	2 (4)	2.5 (5)	2.5 (5)	2.5 (5)
Total vegetables, cups (servings)/day	1 (2)	1.5 (3)	1.5 (3)	2 (4)	2.5 (5)	2.5 (5)	3 (6)	3 (6)	3.5 (7)	3.5 (7)	4 (8)	4 (8)
Dark green vegetables, cups/week	1	1.5	1.5	2	3	3	3	3	3	3	3	3
Orange vegetables, cups/week	0.5	1	1	1.5	2	2	2	2	2.5	2.5	2.5	2.5
Legumes, cups/week	0.5	1	1	2.5	3	3	3	3	3.5	3.5	3.5	3.5
Starchy vegetables, cups/week	1.5	2.5	2.5	2.5	3	3	6	6	7	7	9	9
Other vegetables, cups/week	3.5	4.5	4.5	5.5	6.5	6.5	7	7	8.5	8.5	10	10
Total grains, ounce equivalents/day	3	4	5	5	6	6	7	8	9	10	10	10
Whole grains, ounce equivalents/day	1.5	2	2.5	3	3	3	3.5	4	4.5	5	5	5
Other grains, ounce equivalents/day	1.5	2	2.5	2	3	3	3.5	4	4.5	5	5	5
Lean meat and beans, ounce equivalents/day	2	3	4	5	5	5	6	6.5	6.5	7	7	7
Milk, cups/day	2	2	2	3	3	3	3	3	3	3	3	3
Oils, g/day	15	17	17	22	24	27	29	31	34	36	44	51
Flexible calorie allowance, kcal/day	165	171	171	182	195	267	290	362	410	426	512	648

From Dietary Guidelines Advisory Committee 2005.

of CHD in men and women. Many of these landmark studies have served as the basis for current dietary guidelines and recommendations.

Secondary Prevention Trials

The purpose of secondary prevention trials is to evaluate the effects of an intervention in people who are already diagnosed with a particular disease. Beneficial results in secondary prevention trials thus indicate that the intervention has slowed the disease process, stopped it, or reversed it.

Diet and Reinfarction Trial (DART)

DART (5) evaluated the effect of three dietary factors: type and amount of fat, fish intake, and fiber consumption. Patients who had experienced myocardial infarction (N = 2,033) were randomly assigned to receive advice on one of these three dietary factors for 2 years. Those receiving fat advice were counseled both to reduce their total fat intake to 30% of total energy and to increase the polyunsaturated fatty acid (PUFA)/saturated fatty acid (SFA) ratio to 1.0. Those receiving advice regarding fish consumption were instructed to eat at least two portions (200-400 g) per week of fatty fish (mackerel, herring, kipper, pilchard, sardine, salmon, or trout). Participants receiving advice on fiber consumption were instructed to increase their intake of cereal fiber to 18 g/day. Although there were no significant changes in serum cholesterol levels in any of the three treatment groups, the group consuming the fatty fish did experience a significant decrease in both total mortality rate (29%) and coronary mortality rate (33%). A follow-up of the DART study indicated no substantial long-term survival benefits of the dietary advice were provided (31). Despite the results of the initial study, indicating a decrease in mortality for participants in the fish group, the mortality for this group was increased over the following 3 years. Throughout these 3 years of follow-up, however, there was no measure of dietary compliance or follow-up education.

Lyon Diet Heart Study

The Lyon Diet Heart Study (7), a randomized, single-blind secondary prevention trial (N = 423), tested the effects of a Western diet (AHA step I diet) versus a Mediterranean-type diet, which was rich in α-linolenic acid (ALA). This Mediterranean-type diet (30.5% kcal total fat, 8.3% kcal SFA, 12.9% kcal monounsaturated fatty acid [MUFA], 3.6% kcal PUFA, 0.81% kcal ALA) was rich in whole grains, root vegetables, green vegetables, fish, and fruits (at least once daily) and low in red meat (replaced with poultry). Margarine that had a fatty acid profile similar to that of olive oil (enriched with linoleic acid and ALA) was supplied by the study to replace butter and cream. Rapeseed and olive oils were used for salads and food preparation. Participants following the Mediterranean-type diet increased their consumption of fruits, vegetables, legumes, and fiber and decreased their consumption of meats, butter, and cream. Total fat intake was similar for both groups, approximately 31% of total energy. Following 2 years of treatment, levels of TC, LDL-C, HDL-C, triglycerides (TG), apolipoprotein B (ApoB), and apolipoprotein A-I were unchanged. Although both groups had similar lipids, lipoproteins, blood pressure, body mass index (BMI), and smoking status, subjects consuming the ALA-rich Mediterranean diet had significant reductions in all-cause death (–56%), cardiac mortality (–65%), nonfatal MI (–70%), and cancer (–61%). The Mediterranean diet plan improved many other aspects of the diet, including the fatty acid profile, antioxidant vitamins, and fiber, that have a beneficial impact on both recurrent CVD and cancer risk.

Lifestyle Heart Program

The Lifestyle Heart Trial was a secondary prevention trial in which subjects (N = 28) were randomized to either a usual-care group or an intensive lifestyle change group (34). Participants in the lifestyle change group received a very low fat vegetarian diet high in complex carbohydrates (15-20% kcal protein, 70-75% kcal CHO, 10% kcal total fat [PUFA/SFA ratio >1]), moderate aerobic exercise, stress management training, smoking cessation, and group psychosocial support. Following 1 year of the intervention, significant reductions occurred in TC, LDL-C, and ApoB levels by 28%, 40%, and 23%, respectively ($p < .005$). HDL-C levels decreased by 10%, whereas TG levels increased by 13% (not significant). When the same subjects were reassessed after 5 years of the intensive lifestyle change program, the experimental group experienced significant reductions in average percentage diameter stenosis (–3% vs. +12%, $p = .001$) and angina (–91% vs. +186%, $p < .001$) and experienced significantly fewer cardiac events than the control group (25 vs. 45, $p < .001$) (35). The results of this study came about through an intensive behavior modification program rather than diet alone.

Primary Prevention Trials

In primary prevention trials, an intervention is tested in a population that may be at risk for but not yet diagnosed with a particular disease or prevention. The results from primary prevention trials can be valuable in identifying appropriate dietary and lifestyle interventions for people based on their specific risk profiles.

Portfolio Diet

The Portfolio diet was designed to maximally lower LDL-C levels by using a variety of dietary interventions, each of which has specific hypocholesterolemic properties. The Portfolio diet is a vegetarian diet rich in soy protein (21.4 g/1,000 kcal), plant sterols (1.0 g/1,000 kcal), whole almonds (14 g/1,000 kcal), and viscous fibers (9.8 g/1,000 kcal) primarily from oats, barley, and psyllium (20). When the effects of the Portfolio diet (22% kcal protein [97% as vegetable protein], 51% kcal CHO, 27% kcal total fat, 4% kcal SFA, 12% kcal MUFA, 10% kcal PUFA, and 30.7 g fiber/1,000 kcal) were evaluated in hypercholesterolemic adults, TC levels decreased by 22% and LDL-C levels by 29% ($p < .001$), whereas HDL-C and TG levels decreased nonsignificantly (20, 21). Consistent with these changes, the TC/HDL-C ratio and ApoB decreased by 20% and 24%, respectively. Similar reductions in these risk factors were observed when the Portfolio diet was compared with an AHA step II diet (21).

The magnitude of cholesterol reduction observed following the Portfolio diet is similar to the reduction brought about by low-dose statin therapy (22). TC and LDL-C levels decreased by 22% and 29%, respectively ($p < .001$), on the Portfolio diet; by 23% and 31%, respectively ($p < .001$), on lovastatin treatment; but by only 6% and 8%, respectively ($p < .01$), on the vegetable-rich control diet when compared with baseline. Likewise, TC/HDL-C and ApoB decreased by 17% and 23%, respectively, following consumption of the Portfolio diet and by 22% and 27% following statin treatment ($p < .005$, compared with control diet). None of the diets affected HDL-C levels. In addition, a significant reduction in C-reactive protein (CRP) was observed for both the Portfolio diet group (33%) and the lovastatin group (28%). Thus, although traditional cholesterol-lowering dietary recommendations have focused on the reduction of saturated fat, current recommendations have been expanded to include foods high in viscous fiber, plant sterols, vegetable protein foods (soy), and nuts (almonds). The additive effect of these foods and their constituents appears to reduce LDL-C to levels similar to the levels that result from an initial therapeutic dose of a first-generation statin.

Dietary Approaches to Stop Hypertension (DASH) Diet Trials

The Dietary Approaches to Stop Hypertension (DASH) trial (3, 32, 37) was originally designed to compare the effects of three dietary patterns on blood pressure: (a) a control diet high in saturated fat and low in dietary fiber (15% kcal protein, 52% kcal CHO, 37% kcal total fat, 13% kcal SFA, 14% kcal MUFA, 7% kcal PUFA); (b) a fruit and vegetable diet with a similar macronutrient profile but high in dietary fiber (29.9 g/day); or (c) a DASH diet emphasizing fruits (4-5 servings/day), vegetables (4-5 servings/day), and low-fat dairy products (2-3 servings/day) (18% kcal protein, 58% kcal CHO, 27% kcal total fat, 7% kcal SFA, 10% kcal MUFA, 8% kcal PUFA, 29.7 g/day fiber). DASH decreased SBP and diastolic blood pressure (DBP) by 5.5 and 3.0 mmHg more, respectively, than the control diet ($p < .001$); the fruit and vegetable diet reduced SBP by 2.8 mmHg more ($p < .001$) and DBP by 1.1 mmHg more ($p = .07$) than the control diet. A secondary analysis of the DASH trial assessed the effect of the DASH diet on blood lipids. Following the DASH diet, TC, LDL-C, and HDL-C levels decreased significantly compared with the control diet (7%, 9%, and 8%, respectively, $p < .0001$), whereas nonsignificant reductions occurred in the fruit and vegetable group (2%, 2%, and <1%, respectively). TC/HDL-C and TG levels were unaffected in subjects on the DASH diet.

PREMIER Clinical Trial

The PREMIER clinical trial was designed to determine the effects of multicomponent lifestyle interventions on levels of blood pressure in people with above-optimal blood pressure and stage 1 hypertension (35). The study had a parallel-arm design with three treatment groups: (a) advice-only group (n = 273), which included one individual counseling session; (b) an established care (EC) group (n = 268), which had intensive behavioral intervention during the study; and (c) the DASH+EC group (n = 269), which had the same intensive behavioral intervention as the EC group plus counseling on the DASH diet (25% of calories from fat with ≤7% of calories from saturated fat, 9-12 servings/day of fruits and vegetables, and 2-3 servings/day of low-fat dairy) (2). Levels of blood pressure were reduced throughout the 6-month study period for all groups. Compared with baseline, mean (SD) SBP was reduced by 6.6 (9.2) mmHg in the advice-only group, 10.5 (10.1) mmHg in the EC group, and 11.1 (9.9) mmHg in the DASH+EC group following 6 months of treatment. The reductions in both SBP and DBP were significantly different in normotensive and hypertensive participants in the EC and DASH+EC groups compared with the advice-only group ($p < .01$) (2). Although the blood pressure reductions observed in the DASH+EC group were consistently greater than those seen in the EC group, these differences were not statistically different. Following 6 months of treatment, 34% of the DASH+EC group and 29% of the EC group had met the weight loss goal (>15 lb, or >6.8 kg), compared with 6% of the advice-only group. The DASH+EC participants also significantly increased their dietary intake of fruits and vegetables (an increase of 3.0 servings/day, for 7.8 servings/day total) and dairy products (an increase of 0.5 servings/day, for 2.3 servings/day total) compared with the advice-only group (4.9 servings/day total fruits and vegetables, 1.7 servings/day total dairy) ($p < .001$) (2). The results of this study demonstrate the potent beneficial effects of comprehensive behavioral interventions on levels of blood pressure in both normotensive and hypertensive people. In addition, the combination of the DASH eating plan and the comprehensive behavioral interventions did not have any additional benefits beyond those observed with the behavioral intervention alone. After 18 months, reductions in blood pressure were greater in the DASH + EC group and the EC group compared with the advice-only group (9). That the blood pressure reductions were similar in the two intervention groups after 18 months indicates that it is possible to make multiple lifestyle changes to decrease blood pressure, but that more research is needed to define the intervention that is required to achieve all of the behavior changes that are recommmended for the optimal reduction of blood pressure.

Diabetes Prevention Program (DPP) Trial

The DPP was the first large-scale intervention study designed to test the effectiveness of an intensive lifestyle intervention versus a medication in the prevention or delayed onset of diabetes (24). More than 3,000 people who were at risk for the development of type 2 diabetes (BMI ≥ 24 kg/m² and fasting plasma glucose 95-125 mg/dL or plasma glucose as measured by the oral glucose tolerance test 140-199 mg/dL) were randomly assigned to one of three intervention groups: (a) standard lifestyle recommendations plus metformin (850 mg twice daily), (b) standard lifestyle recommendations plus placebo (twice daily), and (c) an intensive program of lifestyle modification. The goal for the people in the intensive lifestyle modification group was to achieve and maintain a 7% weight loss. This weight loss was to be achieved by following a low-fat (<25% kcal total fat), hypocaloric (1,200-1,800 total kcal) diet and by engaging in at least 150 min/week of moderate intensity physical activity (e.g., brisk walking). The average length of follow-up for participants was 2.8 years.

The results of this study indicate that an intensive lifestyle intervention program is more effective at reducing the incidence of type 2 diabetes than is metformin in high-risk people. The incidence of type 2 diabetes was 58% lower in the lifestyle intervention group and 31% lower in the metformin group compared with the placebo group ($p < .001$). Furthermore, the incidence of type 2 diabetes in the lifestyle intervention group was 39% lower than in the metformin group ($p < .001$). In addition, the weight loss observed in the lifestyle intervention group (–5.6 kg) was significantly greater than the weight loss observed in the metformin (–2.1 kg) and placebo (0.1 kg) groups ($p < .001$).

In a follow-up study to the DPP trial, researchers evaluated the prevalence of the metabolic syndrome at baseline and the effect of the intensive lifestyle intervention and metformin therapy on the syndrome's incidence and resolution throughout the trial (33). At the beginning of the DPP trial, 53% of the participants fulfilled the criteria for the metabolic syndrome, as defined by the NCEP-ATP III guidelines. Following 3 years of the trial, 53% of the participants in the placebo group had acquired the metabolic syndrome, compared with 47% of the metformin group and 38% of the intensive lifestyle change group. The intensive lifestyle intervention reduced the incidence of the metabolic syndrome by 41% compared with placebo ($p < .001$) and 29% compared with metformin ($p < .001$). The results of the DPP trial thus indicate that an intensive lifestyle change program not only can reduce the incidence of type 2 diabetes but also can contribute greatly to reduction of the metabolic syndrome in a population of high-risk people.

Mediterranean-Style Diet

The dietary pattern characteristic of the Mediterranean region has been extensively studied to determine why inhabitants of this area have decreased rates of CHD. Diet composition varies in this region but tends to emphasize fruits, vegetables, breads, cereals, potatoes, beans, nuts, olive oil, and seeds. Other common characteristics of Mediterranean-style diets include dairy products (mainly cheese and yogurt), fish, poultry, wine consumed in low to moderate amounts, eggs consumed 0 to 4 times per week, and minimal consumption of red meat.

The results of a recent clinical trial indicate that a Mediterranean-style diet is also effective in reducing the prevalence of the metabolic syndrome and the associated CVD risk (10). In a randomized, single-blind trial, participants were randomly assigned to either an intervention group or a control group. Participants in the intervention group received dietary advice that was tailored to each person, based on a 3-day food record. The diet intervention consisted of 50% to 60% carbohydrates, 15% to 20% total fat (<10% saturated fat), and <300 mg/day sodium. In addition, participants were instructed to consume at least 250 to 300 g fruit, 125 to

150 g vegetables, 25 to 50 g walnuts, and 400 g whole grains (legumes, rice, maize, and wheat) per day and to increase their consumption of olive oil. Participants in the control group received oral and written information about healthful food choices and were encouraged to follow a diet similar to that of the intervention group (50-60% carbohydrates, 15-20% protein, <30% total fat). Following 2 years of the intervention, participants in the intervention group had significant decreases in body weight, BMI, waist circumference, homeostasis model assessment score, blood pressure, and levels of glucose, insulin, TC, and TG and had significant increases in HDL-C compared with the control group (p < .05). In addition, participants following the Mediterranean-style diet had significant reductions in serum markers of inflammation (interleukin-6, interleukin-7, interleukin-18, CRP) and improvements in endothelial function score compared with the control group (p = .01). As a result of the improvement in the numerous risk factors associated with the metabolic syndrome during the 2 years of follow-up, only 40 of 90 patients could still be classified as having the metabolic syndrome, compared with 78 of 90 patients in the control group who were still classified as having the syndrome (p < .001).

OmniHeart Trial

It is well established that dietary SFA raises TC and LDL-C levels (14, 15, 26, 27), and thereby increases the risk of CVD. Dietary strategies to reduce the risk of CVD therefore include a reduction in dietary SFA. Questions remain, however, about the type of macronutrient that should replace SFA to optimize the reduction in CVD risk. The Optimal Macronutrient Intake Trial to Prevent Heart Disease (OmniHeart Trial) was designed to compare the effects of three low-SFA diets, varying in the macronutrient profile, on serum lipids and blood pressure (4). Participants with prehypertension or stage 1 hypertension (N = 164) were randomized in this three-period, crossover, design-controlled feeding study. Each diet period lasted for 6 weeks, with a 2- to 4-week washout period between each of the diet periods. The three diets were (a) a rich diet in CHO (58% CHO, 15% protein, 27% total fat, 6% SFA, 13% MUFA, 8% PUFA); (b) a diet rich in protein (48% CHO, 25% protein, 27% total fat, 6% SFA, 13% MUFA, 8% PUFA); and (c) a diet rich in unsaturated fat (48% CHO, 15% protein, 37% total fat, 6% SFA, 21% MUFA, 10% PUFA).

When compared with baseline, levels of blood pressure and LDL-C and estimated CVD risk were lower on all three diets (4). Comparisons between the three test diets showed beneficial effects of the diets rich in protein and unsaturated fats, above those effects observed for the CHO-rich diet. When compared with the CHO-rich diet, the protein-rich diet decreased mean SBP by 1.4 mmHg (p < 01) in normotensive participants and by 3.5 mmHg (p < .01) in hypertensive participants. The protein-rich diet also elicited a greater decrease in LDL-C (3.3 mg/dL; p = .01), HDL-C (1.3 mg/dL; p < .05), and TG (15.7 mg/dL; p < .001) compared with the CHO-rich diet. The diet rich in unsaturated fatty acids had a similar blood pressure–lowering effect, decreasing mean SBP by 1.3 mmHg (p < .01) in normotensive participants and by 2.9 mmHg (p < .05) in hypertensive participants, beyond those effects observed following the CHO-rich diet. Compared with the CHO-rich diet, the diet rich in unsaturated fatty acids had no significant effect on levels of LDL-C but significantly increased HDL-C (1.1 mg/dL; p < .05) and lowered TG (9.6 mg/dL; p < .05). There were no differences between the effects on mean SBP and DBP following the protein-rich and unsaturated fatty acid–rich diets. The protein-rich diet did, however, significantly lower levels of TC (–5.0 mg/dL; p < .001), compared with the unsaturated fatty acid–rich diet, primarily attributable to the decrease in HDL-C observed on the protein-rich diet and the corresponding increase in HDL-C on the unsaturated fatty acid–rich diet. Levels of TG were also significantly reduced on the protein-rich diet (–7.1 mg/dL; p < .05), compared with the diet rich in unsaturated fatty acids. Overall, compared with a diet rich in CHO, diets rich in protein and unsaturated fatty acids similarly reduced the estimated 10-year CVD risk.

Food-Based Dietary Strategies for Achieving a Heart-Healthy Diet

Dietary recommendations for macronutrients, micronutrients, and other dietary constituents are consistent across different organizations and goverment agencies (table 18.1). These macronutrient recommendations provide the foundation for food-based recommendations that effectively allow for the translation of nutrition recommendations into practice. The focus of many of these food-based recommendations is on the type of dietary fat in the diet, the amount and type of fiber, and the amount of dietary sodium. Recommendations from all organizations and agencies include achieving and maintaining a healthy weight and participating in regular physical activity.

Major sources of SFA and trans fatty acids are listed in table 18.5. The major sources of SFA in the diet are meat, poultry, fish, eggs, and dairy, accounting for 60% of the SFA consumed in the American diet. Industrial or processed sources of trans fatty acids account for 80% of trans fat intake, whereas 21% comes from animal sources. The industrial sources of trans fatty acids are commonly found in commercially prepared baked products, including cakes, cookies, crackers, pies, and bread (40% of intake). Meat and dairy products con-

tain the naturally occurring trans fatty acids vaccenic acid and conjugated linoleic acid. Dietary strategies to reduce saturated and trans fatty acids in the diet should thus be aimed at reducing the consumption of these major contributors.

Dietary recommendations for the consumption of long-chain omega-3 fatty acids encourage the consumption of two fatty fish meals per week to achieve the recommended intake of 500 mg of eicosapentaenoic acid (EPA) and docosahexaenoic acid (DHA) per week. Different fish species contain varying amounts of EPA and DHA per gram, with herring, salmon, and mackerel the richest sources. Table 18.6 lists the nutrient profile of a variety of fish species, including the amount of fish needed to meet the recommended levels of EPA and DHA.

Dietary recommendations from major health organizations also include the reduction of dietary cholesterol to <200-300 mg/day and sodium to <2,300 mg/day for healthy people and and <1,500 mg/day for people at high risk for CVD. Major sources of dietary cholesterol are eggs, beef, and poultry, contributing 29.3%, 16.1%, and 12.2% of dietary cholesterol, respectively (table 18.7 on page 186). Dietary strategies that emphasis the inclusion of plant protein sources therefore decrease the amount of dietary cholesterol in the diet. The largest contributor of dietary sodium to the diet is the processing of food (77%). Emphasizing the consumption of fresh or frozen food products inherently reduces the consumption of dietary sodium. An additional 11% of dietary sodium is added during cooking (5%) and at the table (6%). The remaining contribution of sodium found in the diet is the 12% inherent in foods. Strategies to flavor foods with fresh herbs and spices would also decrease the amount of sodium consumed.

Consumption of dietary fiber, and whole grains in particular, is a major feature of any dietary recommendations. Recommended intakes range from 20 to 30 g/day of dietary fiber, with an emphasis on the incorporation of whole grains and sources of soluble fiber. Rich sources of total and soluble fiber are listed in table 18.8 on page 186; common examples of fiber-rich whole grains are listed in table 18.9 on page 187. Within the recommendations of NCEP-ATP III, the TLC diet recommends the consumption of 10 to 25 g/day of soluble fiber. This can be achieved with the consumption of 1 cup of oatmeal, one pear, 1/2 cup of cooked kidney beans, and 1/2 cup of cooked Brussels sprouts. An additional feature of the TLC diet is the inclusion of 2 g/day of plant sterol and stanol esters. Although plant sterol and stanol esters are found in a very low concentration in naturally occurring foods,

TABLE 18.5 Major Food Sources of Saturated and Trans Fatty Acids

Food source	Percentage of total dietary fatty acids
SATURATED FATTY ACIDS	
Meat, poultry, fish, eggs, dairy	60
Cheese (highest contributor)	13
Beef (second highest contributor)	12
Milk (third highest contributor)	8
Grains, vegetables, fruits, sweets, all other	30
Fats and oils	10
TRANS FATTY ACIDS	
Cakes, cookies, crackers, pies, and bread	40
Animal products (conjugated linoleic acid—natural trans fat)	21
Stick margarine	17
Fried potatoes, potato chips, corn chips, and popcorn	13
Shortening	4
Salad dressing	3
Breakfast cereal	2
Candy	2

TABLE 18.6 Nutrient Profile of Select Species of Fish (Per 85 g Cooked Fish Portion)

Fish type	EPA/DHA g	Total fat, g	SFA, g	Chol, mg	Na, mg	Grams fish needed to get 300 mg/day EPA/DHA	Grams fish needed to get 500 mg/day EPA/DHA
Herring							
Pacific	1.81	15.121	3.548	84.15	80.75	14.1	23.5
Atlantic	1.71	9.851	2.223	65.45	97.75	14.9	24.9
Orange roughy	0.002	0.765	0.02	22.1	68.85	12750.0	21250.0
Mahi mahi (dolphin)	0.118	0.765	0.205	79.9	96.05	216.1	360.2
Cod							
Pacific	0.24	0.689	0.088	39.95	77.35	106.3	177.1
Atlantic	0.13	0.731	1.43	47.75	66.3	196.2	326.9
Haddock	0.2	0.79	0.142	62.9	73.95	127.5	212.5
Tuna							
Light, canned in water, drained	0.26	0.697	0.199	25.5	287.3	98.1	163.5
White, canned in water, drained	0.73	2.525	0.673	35.7	320.45	34.9	58.2
Fresh	0.278	5.338	1.37	41.65	42.5	91.7	152.9
Salmon							
Sockeye	1.05	9.325	1.629	73.95	56.1	24.3	40.5
Chinook	1.48	11.373	2.732	72.25	51	17.2	28.7
Atlantic, farmed	1.83	10.498	2.128	53.55	51.85	13.9	23.2
Atlantic, wild	1.56	6.911	1.068	60.35	47.6	16.3	27.2
Mackerel							
Atlantic	1.022	15.138	3.55	63.75	70.55	25.0	41.6
Pacific	1.571	8.602	2.449	51	93.5	16.2	27.1
Trout, rainbow							
Farmed	0.98	4.947	1.376	57.8	35.7	26.0	43.4
Wild	0.84	6.12	1.789	58.65	47.6	30.4	50.6
Crab							
Alaska King	0.351	1.309	0.113	45.05	911.2	72.6	121.1
Blue	0.403	1.504	0.194	85	237.15	63.3	105.5
Shrimp (mixed species)	0.27	0.918	0.246	165.75	190.4	94.4	157.4
Scallop	0.17	0.646	0.067	28.05	136.85	150.0	250.0
White fish (mixed species)	1.37	6.384	0.988	65.45	55.25	18.6	31.0

EPA = eicosapentaenoic acid; DHA = docosahexaenoic acid; SFA = saturated fatty acid; Chol = cholesterol; Na = sodium. From US Department of Agriculture 2002.

TABLE 18.7   Food Sources of Dietary Cholesterol

Food	Ranking	% Total	% Cumulative
Eggs	1	29.3	29.3
Beef	2	16.1	45.4
Poultry	3	12.2	57.6
Cheese	4	5.8	63.4
Milk	5	5.0	68.4
Fish, shellfish	6	3.7	72.1
Cakes, cookies, doughnuts	7	3.3	75.4
Pork (fresh)	8	2.8	78.2
Ice cream, sherbet, frozen yogurt	9	2.5	80.7
Sausage	10	2.0	82.7

From US Dietary Guidelines Advisory Committee 2005.

TABLE 18.8   Total and Soluble Fiber Content of High-Fiber Foods

Food	Soluble fiber, g	Total fiber, g
Cereal grains (1/2 cup)		
Barley	1	4
Oatmeal	1	2
Oat bran	1	3
Seeds		
Psyllium (1 tbsp)	5	6
Fruit		
Apple (1 medium)	1	4
Banana (1 medium)	1	3
Blackberries (1/2 cup)	1	4
Pear (1 medium)	2	4
Prunes (1/4 cup)	1.5	3
Legumes (1/2 cup cooked)		
Black beans	2	5.5
Kidney beans	3	6
Lima beans	3.5	6.5
Lentils	1	8
Black-eyed peas	1	5.5
Vegetables (1/2 cup cooked)		
Broccoli	1	1.5
Brussels sprouts	3	4.5
Carrots	1	2.5

TABLE 18.9 Total Fiber Content of Whole-Grain Foods

Food	Amount of fiber (g) in a 100 g (3.5 oz) serving
Barley, pearled (minus its outer covering)	15.6
Wheat bran	15.0
Cornmeal, whole grain	11.0
Cornmeal, de-germed	5.2
Oat bran, raw	6.6
Rice, raw (wild)	5.2
Rice, raw (brown)	3.5
Rice, raw (white)	1.0-2.8

numerous supplemented food products are available to allow people to easily meet this recommendation. Examples of food sources that are supplemented with plant sterol and stanol esters include orange juice, margarine, yogurt, and granola bars.

Summary

Based on an extensive database as discussed herein, the optimal diet will provide a cornucopia of foods and nutrients to achieve dietary patterns that target multiple CVD risk factors (17, 19). A diet that is very low in saturated and trans fatty acids, cholesterol, and sodium; rich in vitamins and minerals; controlled in calories; high in dietary fiber; moderate in unsaturated fats, including n-3 fatty acids; and low in simple carbohydrates will most effectively improve the lipid and lipoprotein profile. As our knowledge base increases, scientists will continue to make science-based dietary recommendations that will target an increasing number of risk factors. Implementation of multiple dietary strategies will elicit unprecedented reductions in CVD risk by targeting an increasing number of lipid and lipoprotein risk factors for CVD. The consequence of this will be to accelerate the decline of CVD as an important cause of mortality and morbidity.

Common Comorbidities and Complications of Cardiovascular Disease

Part IV provides insight into some of the comorbidities and complications of cardiovascular disease. This section begins with a discussion of common comorbidities or risk factors including hypertension (chapter 19), diabetes (chapter 20), obesity (chapter 21), and dyslipidemia (chapter 22). Because arthritis is becoming more prominently associated with many disease states, chapter 23 provides insight into the complicating arthritic condition. Chapter 24 discusses psychosocial risk factors and the assessment and treatment in cardiac patients. The last three chapters in this part are concerned with complications attributable to stroke (chapter 25), neuropsychiatric disorders (chapter 26), and sleep disorders (chapter 27) as they pertain to the evaluation and treatment of cardiovascular diseases.

CHAPTER 19

Hypertension

Linda S. Pescatello, PhD

Sixty-five million (31.3%) Americans aged 18 years or older have hypertension, defined as systolic blood pressure (SBP) ≥140 or diastolic blood pressure (DBP) ≥90 mmHg, making hypertension a major public health problem in the United States (7). Hypertension prevalence rates continue to increase, yet awareness of the condition and control rates are poor (2, 7, 12). A person with normal blood pressure (BP) (SBP <120 mmHg and DBP <80 mmHg) at 55 years of age has a 90% lifetime risk of developing hypertension (2). Because of pervasiveness of this disorder, the term *prehypertension* (SBP 120-139 and DBP 80-89 mmHg) has been introduced, and nearly 30% of American adults have prehypertension (2, 22). Table 19.1 contains the Joint National Commission's Sixth Report (JNC VI) BP classification scheme (12) and the new JNC VII BP classification scheme, which includes the designation of prehypertension (2).

Because the majority of adults in the United Status have above-optimal BP and most will develop hypertension if they live long enough, all people are recommended to adopt healthy lifestyles to prevent hypertension (2). These healthy lifestyle recommendations include weight loss, reduced sodium intake, limited alcohol consumption, regular participation in physical activity, and consumption of a diet rich in fruits, vegetables, and low-fat dairy products. Table 19.2 displays the treatment guidelines for hypertension outlined in JNC VI (12) that are based on the BP staging scheme and the number of risk factors or presence of disease. As BP levels increase, the number of risk factors increase, or if disease is present, lifestyle interventions become adjuvant to drug therapy for the treatment and control of hypertension.

Overview of Clinical Pathophysiology

A variety of factors contribute to elevated BP and the vascular changes that characterize the condition. According to Ohm's law, mean arterial pressure (MAP) is the product of cardiac output (Q) and total peripheral resistance (TPR): MAP = Q × TPR. Consequently, the pathogenic mechanisms leading to hypertension must elevate Q, increase TPR, or do both. The factors contributing to these hemodynamic alterations include genetics, susceptibility to renal retention of excess sodium, sympathetic nervous system hyperactivity, renin–angiotensin system pressor and growth promoter actions, hyperinsulinemia or insulin resistance, and endothelial cell dysfunction, among others (20, 25).

Despite our knowledge of contributing factors, the cause of hypertension is not known in 95% of the people with hypertension; this is termed *essential hypertension*. Systemic hypertension with a known cause is referred to as *secondary hypertension* and primarily involves disorders and diseases of the renal (e.g., parenchymal disease and renovascular disease),

I thank my coauthors on the ACSM position stand on exercise and hypertension for providing the foundation of knowledge on which this chapter is based and my graduate students for the assistance, expertise, and time they provide to our investigations relating to exercise and hypertension. Funded in part by the American Heart Association Grant-in-Aid 0150507N.

Address correspondence concerning this chapter to Linda S. Pescatello, University of Connecticut, Department of Kinesiology, 2095 Hillside Road, U-1110, Storrs, CT 06269-1110. E-mail: Linda.Pescatello@uconn.edu

TABLE 19.1 Blood Pressure Classification for Adults Aged 18 and Older

JNC VI blood pressure category	JNC VII blood pressure category	Systolic blood pressure, mmHg		Diastolic blood pressure, mmHg
Optimal	Normal	<120	and	<80
Normal	Prehypertension	120-129	and	80-84
High normal	Prehypertension	130-139	or	85-89
Stage 1 hypertension	Stage 1 hypertension	140-159	or	90-99
Stage 2 hypertension	Stage 2 hypertension	160-179	or	100-109
Stage 3 hypertension	Stage 2 hypertension	≥180	or	≥110

JNC VI = sixth report of the Joint National Committee; JNC VII = seventh report of the Joint National Committee. Data are for patients not taking antihypertensive drugs and not acutely ill. When the systolic and diastolic blood pressure categories vary, the higher reading determines the blood pressure classification. For example, a reading of 152/82 mmHg should be classified as stage 1 hypertension and 170/116 mmHg should be classified as stage 3 hypertension.

In addition to classifying stages of hypertension on the basis of average blood pressure levels, clinicians should specify presence or absence of target organ disease and additional risk factors. This specificity is important for risk classification and treatment (see table 19.2). Optimal blood pressure with respect to cardiovascular risk is below 120/80 mmHg. However, unusually low readings should be evaluated for clinical significance. Data are based on the average of two or more readings at each of two or more visits after an initial screen.

Data from the Joint National Committee on Prevention, Detection, Evaluation, and Treatment of High Blood Pressure (1997) and Chobanian and colleagues 2003.

TABLE 19.2 Risk Stratification and Treatment

Blood pressure stages (mmHg)	Risk group A (no risk factors, no TOD/CCD)*	Risk group B (≥1 risk factor not including diabetes; no TOD/CCD)	Risk group C (TOD/CCD or diabetes, with or without other risk factors)
High normal (130-139/85-89)	Lifestyle modification	Lifestyle modification	Drug therapy†
Stage 1 (140-159/90-99)	Lifestyle modification (up to 12 months)	Lifestyle modification‡ (up to 6 months)	Drug therapy
Stages 2 and 3 (≥160/≥100)	Drug therapy	Drug therapy	Drug therapy

A patient with diabetes and a blood pressure of 142/94 mmHg plus left ventricular hypertrophy should be classified as having stage 1 hypertension with target organ disease (left ventricular hypertrophy) and with another major risk factor (diabetes). This patient would be categorized as stage 1, risk group C, and would be recommended for immediate initiation of pharmacologic treatment. Lifestyle modification would be adjunctive therapy for all patients recommended for pharmacologic therapy.

*TOD/CCD indicates target organ disease or clinical cardiovascular disease including heart disease (left ventricular hypertrophy, angina or prior myocardial infarction, prior coronary revascularization, and heart failure), stroke or transient ischemic attack, neuropathy, peripheral arterial disease, and retinopathy.

†For those with heart failure, renal insufficiency, or diabetes.

‡For patients with multiple risk factors, clinicians should consider drugs as initial therapy plus lifestyle modification. Major risk factors include smoking, dyslipidemia, diabetes mellitus, age >60 years, gender (men and postmenopausal women), and family history of cardiovascular disease (women <65 or men <55).

Data from Chobanian and colleagues 2003.

endocrine (e.g., acromegaly, Cushing's syndrome, or pheochromocytoma), and nervous (e.g., Guillain–Barré syndrome) systems. *Isolated systolic hypertension* (SBP ≥140 mmHg and DBP <90 mmHg) is rare before the age of 50 years but becomes the most common form of hypertension among older adults. *White-coat hypertension* is the transient and persistent elevation in BP when it is taken in the physician's office or other clinical settings. *Pulmonary hypertension* is a persistent elevation of pulmonary artery pressure characterized by dyspnea and fatigue that are likely to be accompanied by syncope and substernal chest pain. *Secondary pulmonary hypertension* often accompanies other forms of pulmonary and heart disease (16). The exercise guidelines put forth in this chapter do not pertain to people with pulmonary hypertension. The reader is referred to other sources for exercise recommendations relating to pulmonary hypertension (8, 16, 23).

The development of essential systemic hypertension is gradual, emphasizing the preventive importance of healthy lifestyle interventions. By the time hypertension is diagnosed, the causative factors may no longer be operative (i.e., elevated Q) because they have been normalized by compensatory mechanisms that attempt to maintain BP within normal ranges (20, 25). The developmental stage of hypertension is characterized by elevated Q, normal TPR, and enhanced endothelial dependent dilatation; however, as the condition progresses it is typically manifested in most people as normal Q, elevated TPR, and cardiovascular alterations that lead to endothelial dysfunction and left ventricular hypertrophy.

Hypertension is the most common primary diagnosis in America. Hypertension-related diseases include coronary artery disease, congestive heart failure, atrial fibrillation, cerebrovascular disease, end-stage renal disease, peripheral vascular disease, aortic aneurysm, and retinal disease. Hypertension has also been listed as a major contributing factor to the metabolic syndrome, a constellation of diseases and conditions that predispose people to cardiovascular disease (CVD) and diabetes mellitus (4). The current direct and indirect costs attributable to high BP in the United States are US$63.5 billion, underscoring the social and economic burden of the problem.

Preexercise Screening

This section contains the recommendations for evaluation prior to participation in exercise. The extent of the preexercise evaluation depends on the person's symptoms, signs, and overall CVD risk as well as the intensity of the exercise program, as detailed subsequently.

Medical Evaluation

The medical evaluation of a patient with hypertension includes a thorough individual and family history, physical examination, screening tests for secondary causes, and assessment of major risk factors, target organ damage, and CVD complications (2, 12, 18). The extent of the preexercise evaluation depends on the patient's symptoms, signs, and overall CVD risk (table

19.2) as well as the intensity of the exercise program (4, 18, 23). While formal evaluation and management are taking place, it is reasonable for most patients to begin a light- to moderate-intensity exercise training program (<60% maximal oxygen consumption, $\dot{V}O_{2max}$) such as walking. In patients with hypertension about to engage in more vigorous intensity exercise ($\geq$60% $\dot{V}O_{2max}$), a medically supervised peak or symptom-limited exercise test with electrocardiographic monitoring may be warranted (8, 18, 23). These patients include those with stage 3 hypertension (BP $\geq$180/110 mmHg), those in risk categories B and C (table 19.2), and those with documented CVD. Peak or symptom-limited exercise testing is also indicated in patients with symptoms suggestive of CVD such as exertional dyspnea, chest discomfort, or palpitations. Regular follow-up should be provided at intervals indicated by the American Heart Association (8) and the American College of Sports Medicine (ACSM) (23).

When pharmacologic therapy is indicated in physically active people with hypertension, it should reduce BP, decrease TPR, and not adversely affect exercise capacity. For these reasons, angiotensin-converting enzyme (ACE) inhibitors (or angiotensin II receptor blockers in case of ACE inhibitor intolerance) and calcium channel blockers are the recommended drugs for recreational exercisers and athletes (2, 4, 18, 23). If a third drug is needed, a low-dose thiazide-like diuretic, possibly in combination with a potassium-sparing agent, can be prescribed.

Abnormal Exercise BP Response and Exercise Contraindications

Factors that increase the risks associated with physical exertion are age, the presence of CVD, and exercise intensity, which is directly related to the pressor response and myocardial oxygen demand (4, 8, 20, 23). The normal BP response to endurance exercise is a progressive increase in SBP, typically 8 to 12 mmHg/MET, whereas DBP usually decreases slightly or remains unchanged. The expected peak BP on an exercise test is 180 to 210 mmHg SBP and 60 to 85 mmHg DBP. Patients with hypertension may experience an excessive increase in BP during exercise that exceeds these values and a delayed return to resting BP in recovery. The BP criterion for discontinuation of exercise testing is greater than 250/115 mmHg (4, 8, 23). However, hypertension-related cardiovascular complications are rare when BP increases above these levels. When resting BP is greater than 200/115 mmHg and for those with primary pulmonary hypertension, exercise is contraindicated. In patients in whom BP is uncontrolled, an exercise program should be undertaken only after medical evaluation and initiation of drug therapy. Finally, antihypertensive medications (e.g., β-blockers) may alter the hemodynamic response to exercise, so patients taking these medications should be tested for purposes of exercise prescription (4, 20, 23, 25). However, if the primary purpose of the exercise test is diagnostic, titrating the medication regimen of people with hypertension may be warranted.

Predictive Value of the Exercise BP Response

Resting BP, family history of hypertension, white-coat hypertension, overweight, physical inactivity, and poor physical fitness are predictors of hypertension (18, 20, 23, 25). Future hypertension is also predicted by an exaggerated BP response during or after exercise. Because evidence is limited, the use of exercise testing in the general population to predict future hypertension is not recommended. When exercise testing is performed for indicated reasons (8, 23), BP measurements may provide useful prognostic information. For example, a worse prognosis is associated with a hypotensive response during exercise in patients with CVD or heart failure, whereas prognostic information in patients with hypertension depends on their cardiac function (5).

Exercise and Blood Pressure Benefits

This section includes an evidence-based description of the influence of exercise on BP regarding the single session and training effects of endurance and resistance exercise.

Endurance Training

A thorough evidence-based review on exercise and hypertension was recently published by the ACSM (18). The reader is referred to table 19.3 for the evidence summary statements made in this position stand, including evidence categories A, the highest level consisting of a large number of randomized, controlled clinical trials; B, a smaller number of randomized, controlled clinical trials with inconsistent findings; C, observational and nonrandomized investigations; and D, expert opinion. Table 19.3 serves as a synopsis of the discussions in this chapter on exercise and hypertension and in particular associated BP benefits. One

such benefit is that higher levels of physical activity and greater physical fitness are associated with a reduced incidence of hypertension in white men. At this time, whether these BP benefits occur among women and in different ethnic groups is not known.

The effect of endurance training on resting BP has been examined extensively with meta-analytic techniques among people with normal and high BP (5, 6, 14, 18, 24). Most of the participants in these reviews were middle-aged white men. The training programs lasted about 16 weeks and consisted of 40 min sessions 3 times/week. The exercise modalities included walking, jogging, and running in about two thirds and cycling in about half of the studies. The exercise intensity ranged from moderate (40% to <60% $\dot{V}O_{2max}$) to vigorous (≥60% $\dot{V}O_{2max}$). Fagard (6) found that BP decreased an average of 7.4/5.8 mmHg among the groups with hypertension and 2.6/1.8 mmHg among the groups with normal BP. Similarly, Kelley and colleagues (14) concluded that BP reductions were greater in adults with hypertension (6/5 mmHg) than in those with normal BP (2/1 mmHg). Although evidence is limited, neither age, gender, nor ethnicity appeared to alter the response.

Even though all meta-analyses cited here concluded that overall BP was reduced in response to exercise training, the effect of training on BP among the individual studies was variable. Indeed, about 25% of the people with hypertension did not lower their BP after exercise training (18). Reasons for these discrepant findings are unclear but are thought to result from methodological inconsistencies, interactions among the factors that cause hypertension, and the mechanisms by which exercise lowers BP, which are poorly understood. Among randomized controlled trials using ambulatory BP, the reported decreases in SBP and DBP are less than those obtained in the laboratory or clinic with an average reduction of about 3 mmHg (18). An additional benefit of exercise training for those with hypertension is reduced BP at a fixed load during submaximal exercise.

Single Endurance Exercise Session Effects

Isolated aerobic exercise sessions produce immediate decreases in BP of similar magnitude to exercise training programs, and they persist for up to 22 hr after the exercise session (18, 19). The immediate BP reductions following an exercise session have been named *postexercise hypotension* (PEH, or short-term effect). Although evidence is limited, age, gender, and ethnicity

TABLE 19.3 **American College of Sports Medicine (ACSM) Exercise and Hypertension Position Stand Evidence Statements**

Section heading	Evidence statement	Evidence category*
Exercise BP and the prediction of hypertension and CVD morbidity and mortality	Exercise BP helps predict future hypertension in persons with normal BP.	C
	The prognostic value of exercise BP regarding CVD complications depends on the underlying clinical status and hemodynamic response and is therefore limited.	D
Exercise BP benefits	Higher levels of physical activity and greater fitness at baseline are associated with a reduced incidence of hypertension in white men; however, the current paucity of data precludes definitive conclusions regarding the role of gender and ethnicity.	C
	Dynamic aerobic training reduces resting BP in people with normal BP and in those with hypertension.	A
	The decrease in BP with aerobic training appears to be more pronounced in those with hypertension.	B
	Aerobic training reduces ambulatory BP and BP measured at a fixed submaximal workload.	B
	BP response differences among individual studies are incompletely explained by the characteristics of the training programs, that is, the weekly exercise frequency, time per session, exercise intensity, and type of exercise.	B
	Dynamic exercise acutely reduces BP among people with hypertension for a major portion of the daytime hours.	B
	Resistance training performed according to the ACSM guidelines reduces BP in normotensive and hypertensive adults.	B
	Limited evidence suggests that static exercise reduces BP in adults with elevated BP.	C
	Limited evidence suggests that resistance exercise has little effect on BP for up to 24 hr after the exercise session.	C
	No studies are available to provide a recommendation regarding the acute effects of static exercise on BP in adults.	None
	Regular endurance exercise reduces BP in older adults as it does in younger persons.	B
	Limited evidence suggests that PEH occurs in older adults.	C
	Endurance and resistance training do not reduce BP in children and adolescents.	B
	Endurance exercise training reduces BP similarly in men and women.	B
	Limited evidence suggests that acute endurance exercise reduces BP similarly in white men and women.	C
	No convincing evidence exists to support the notion of ethnic differences in the BP response to chronic exercise training.	B
	No convincing evidence exists to support the notion of ethnic differences in the BP response to acute exercise.	C
Exercise recommendations	For persons with high BP, an exercise program that is primarily aerobic-based is recommended.	A
	Resistance training should serve as an adjunct to an aerobic-based program.	B
	The evidence is limited regarding frequency, intensity, and duration recommendations; nonetheless, the antihypertensive effects of exercise appear to occur at a relatively low total volume or dosage.	C
	Limited evidence exists regarding special considerations for those with hypertension.	D
Mechanisms	Neural and vascular changes contribute to the decreases in BP that result from acute and chronic endurance exercise.	C
	Emerging data suggest possible genetic links to acute and chronic exercise BP reductions.	D

BP = blood pressure; CVD = cardiovascular disease; PEH = postexercise hypotension.

*See text for evidence category weighting description, A (highest) to D (lowest).

Reprinted, by permission, from L.S. Pescatello et al., 2004, "American College of Sports Medicine. Position Stand. Exercise and hypertension," *Medicine & Science in Sports & Exercise* 36: 533-553.

do not appear to alter PEH. It has been postulated that the single exercise session effect and chronic exercise training effect (long-term effect) of exercise on BP interact so that some of the BP benefit attributed to endurance exercise training programs may be related to recent exercise (18). However, in both endurance exercise training programs and a single endurance session, not all people with hypertension demonstrate PEH, for reasons that are not clear.

Single Exercise Session and Chronic Resistance Exercise Training Effects

Studies examining the effects of dynamic resistance training on BP are limited (3, 13, 18). When BP reductions are found to occur, the magnitude of the reductions resulting from resistance training are approximately 30% to 60% less than with endurance training, averaging approximately 3 mmHg (3, 4, 13, 23). Considering the excessive pressor response that occurs with isometric resistance training compared with endurance and dynamic resistance training, it is not surprising that there is a paucity of data regarding isometric exercise effects among people with hypertension. Nonetheless, limited evidence indicates that isometric resistance training lowers BP, and, interestingly, the effect seems to be of greater magnitude than with dynamic resistance training (20). The few investigations involving single resistance exercise sessions show equivocal effects on BP, and no studies were found that examined the single exercise session effects of isometric exercise on BP.

Exercise Prescription Recommendations

This section contains the exercise prescription recommendations for those with hypertension. These recommendations include the components of frequency, intensity, time, and type, or FITT.

Frequency: On Most, Preferably All, Days of the Week

Endurance training frequencies between 3 and 7 days/week lower BP (4, 6, 18, 23), but the number of weekly sessions needed to optimize the BP benefit is not known. A single exercise session results in immediate reductions in BP that last for the remainder of the day (i.e., PEH), and it contributes to the BP reductions

resulting from exercise training (23). In addition, many people with hypertension are overweight (5). The guidelines for weight loss and successful weight loss maintenance advocate considerable amounts of energy expenditure (a minimum of 1,000 kcal/week), which can only be achieved with daily or near-daily exercise (11). For these reasons, people with hypertension who are overweight should engage in physical activity on most, preferably all, days of the week to optimize BP benefit.

Intensity: Moderate Intensity Physical Activity

Fagard (6) reported the BP reductions from endurance exercise training to be similar between intensities of 40% and 70% $\dot{V}O_{2max}$. Findings from single-session endurance exercise studies agree with these endurance training reports that lower intensity exercise (40% $\dot{V}O_{2max}$) is a sufficient stimulus to reduce BP (19). When we consider the risk–benefit ratio, moderate-intensity (40 to <60% of $\dot{V}O_2$ reserve, $\dot{V}O_2R$) exercise training appears as effective as high-intensity training, if not more so, in lowering BP ($\geq$60% $\dot{V}O_2R$) exercise. Thus, the recommendation for those with hypertension is regular participation in moderate-intensity (40 to <60% $\dot{V}O_2R$) endurance exercise corresponding to approximately 12 to 13 on the Borg rating of perceived exertion (RPE) 6 to 20 scale (23).

Time: 30 to 60 Min Continuous or Intermittent Exercise Per Day

Exercise training programs prescribed either as long continuous bouts (30-60 min per session) or fractionated short bouts that accumulate throughout the day result in cardiovascular health benefits such as lower BP (4, 9, 11, 15, 18, 19). Evidence also suggests that exercise durations as short as 3 to 20 min reduce BP for several hours after a single exercise session.

Guidry and colleagues (9) compared the single exercise session effects of short- (15 min) and long- (30 min) duration endurance exercise performed at 40% $\dot{V}O_{2max}$ (n = 23) or 60% $\dot{V}O_{2max}$ (n = 22) on PEH among white, middle-aged overweight men with high normal to stage 1 hypertension. The investigators found that short- and long-duration exercise reduced SBP an average of 4 to 6 mmHg compared with control conditions for the remainder of the day, regardless of the intensity of the exercise session. Average DBP was not different between short- and long-duration exercise and control after 40% $\dot{V}O_{2max}$, but after 60% $\dot{V}O_{2max}$, DBP was reduced an average of 2.5 mmHg for up to 9 hr after long-duration exercise versus control. Guidry and colleagues (9) concluded that short- and long-duration, low- to moderate-intensity aerobic exercise immediately lowered BP for a major portion of the daytime hours. Nonetheless, Mach and colleagues (15) found the magnitude and duration of the BP reductions to be greater following longer than shorter bouts of moderate-intensity exercise. Thus, the recommendation is for 30 to 60 min of continuous or intermittent endurance exercise per day (minimum of 10 min intermittent bouts accumulated throughout the day to total 30-60 min of exercise) (18).

Type: Primarily Aerobic Activity Supplemented by Resistance Exercise

The majority of studies on exercise and hypertension (3, 6, 13, 14, 18) have used endurance exercises such as walking, jogging, running, and cycling as the treatment modality, and these studies convincingly show that endurance exercise lowers BP. The data on dynamic resistance training are limited (3, 13, 18). Although these data suggest that resistance training reduces resting BP, the magnitude of the effect is less than that for endurance exercise. Thus, the recommendation is for the exercise intervention to be primarily aerobic supplemented by dynamic resistance training (18).

Special Considerations

This section contains the special considerations in exercise prescription for those with hypertension.

■ Monitor BP before, during, and after exercise for purposes of management and as an incentive to increase motivation to exercise because of the immediate BP-lowering effects of exercise.

■ Extend the warm-up and cool-down periods to increase total energy expenditure and because antihypertensive agents such as α-blockers, calcium channel blockers, and vasodilators may provoke hypotension upon the cessation of activity.

■ Use the Borg RPE as an adjunct to heart rate to monitor exercise intensity when the hemodynamic response to exercise is altered by hypertension or is influenced by medications such as β-blockers.

■ Educate patients about fluid replacement and precautions when exercising in the heat, because their ability to dissipate heat may be compromised by antihypertensive medications such as β-blockers and diuretics.

■ Many people with hypertension are overweight and display features of the cardiometabolic dyslipidemic syndrome. These patients should be encouraged to follow the DASH diet (2), moderately restrict energy intake, and engage in moderate-intensity, prolonged aerobic exercise such as walking on a daily basis. They should also be made aware that some antihypertensive medications can aggravate dyslipidemia, particularly β-blockers and diuretics.

■ The majority of elderly persons will have hypertension. Additional exercise programming recommendations for the older adult can be found in a variety of resources on this topic (17).

■ Other precautions or modifications may be necessary for selected patients, particularly high-risk patients with comorbidities such as coronary artery disease, heart failure, or secondary pulmonary hypertension. The reader is referred to other resources, including part V: Rehabilitation of the Patient With Cardiovascular Disease in this textbook, regarding special populations (4, 8, 11, 16-18, 20, 21, 23, 25).

Mechanisms

As previously stated, MAP = Q × TPR. Consequently, reductions in BP following endurance exercise must be mediated by decreases in Q, TPR, or both. Because Q is typically maintained immediately following exercise attributable to elevations in heart rate, the primary mechanism by which BP is reduced following acute exercise is via decreases in TPR. As per Poiseuille's law, TPR is directly proportional to vessel length (L) and blood viscosity (n) and inversely proportional to the fourth power of the vessel radius (r^4), TPR = Ln/r^4. L and n do not change significantly with moderate-intensity endurance exercise, so that decreases in TPR are attributable to increases in r or a greater distensibility of the vasculature (4, 10, 18, 20, 25).

The reductions in TPR that result from endurance exercise are attributed to neurohumoral and structural changes, altered vascular responsiveness to vasoactive stimuli, or both. Neurohumoral adaptations include a diminished responsiveness to sympathetic nervous system stimulation, increased production of local vasodilators induced by muscle contraction, and increased muscle blood flow with exercise. The antihypertensive effects of endurance exercise may also be associated with genetic factors, notably those of the renin–angiotensin–aldosterone system, a proteolytic cascade with an important role in BP regulation and maintenance of fluid and electrolyte balance (1).

Because of multifactorial causes of hypertension and system redundancies in BP control at rest and during and after exercise, definitive conclusions regarding the mechanisms for the hypotensive effects of endurance exercise cannot be made at this time.

Summary

Hypertension is a major public health problem in the United States, with slightly more than 30% of Americans 18 years or older having prehypertension and 30% having hypertension (table 19.1). Because the majority of adults have above-optimal BP and most will acquire hypertension if they live long enough, all people are recommended to adopt healthy lifestyles to prevent hypertension, an essential component of which is habitual physical activity. Prior to undertaking an exercise program, people with hypertension should undergo a medical evaluation, the extent of which depends on the patient's symptoms, signs, and overall CVD risk (table 19.2) as well as the intensity of the exercise program. While formal evaluation is taking place, most patients may begin a light- to moderate-intensity exercise training program (<60% $\dot{V}O_2R$), such as walking.

Regular exercise participation results in numerous BP benefits for people with hypertension, as summarized in table 19.3. Higher levels of physical activity and greater physical fitness are associated with a reduced incidence of hypertension. Endurance exercise lowers BP approximately 5 to 7 mmHg after an isolated exercise session (i.e., PEH) or after exercise training. The magnitude of the effect is most pronounced in those with hypertension and appears not to be altered by age, gender, or ethnicity. The hypotensive influence of endurance exercise is a low-threshold event, meaning that BP benefits accrue at moderate exercise intensities and after short-duration exercise bouts. The mechanisms by which exercise lowers BP remain elusive because of redundancies in BP control at rest and during and after exercise.

The following exercise prescription is recommended for those with above-optimal BP:

- *Frequency:* on most, preferably all, days of the week
- *Intensity:* moderate intensity (40-<60% of $\dot{V}O_2R$)
- *Time:* ≥30 min of continuous or accumulated physical activity per day
- *Type:* primarily endurance physical activity supplemented by resistance exercise to achieve a caloric energy expenditure of a minimum of 1,000 kcal/week

CHAPTER 20

Diabetes

W. Guyton Hornsby, Jr., PhD
Irma H. Ullrich, MD

Patients with diabetes mellitus are frequently referred for cardiac rehabilitation. Effective and safe treatment of these patients requires attention not only to specific cardiac problems they may exhibit but also to management of their underlying metabolic disease. This chapter provides an overview of diabetes mellitus and discusses acute and chronic complications, cardiovascular disease risk, common acute emergencies, and pharmacologic and nutritional therapy in the context of exercise management of these patients during cardiac rehabilitation. Readers who are unfamiliar with the topic of diabetes may find the glossary on page 200 helpful.

Epidemiology

Diabetes mellitus is a chronic disease caused by insulin deficiency or resistance to insulin action, resulting in hyperglycemia. Close to 21 million people in the United States are believed to have diabetes, and the global estimate is more than 194 million cases (8, 15). The precise prevalence of diabetes is impossible to determine because there are more than 6.2 million undiagnosed cases in the United States, and approximately half of those with diabetes worldwide are unaware of their disease. Diabetes is increasing at an alarming rate. The increasing prevalence of diabetes is associated with a growing number of older people and a steady increase in obesity and physical inactivity.

There were 1.5 million new cases diagnosed in American adults in 2005, and it is projected that worldwide figures will increase to 366 million over the next 25 years (25).

Although the total prevalence of diabetes in the American population is 7%, there are distinct differences in prevalence by age and by race and ethnicity. In the United States, diabetes is found in approximately 176,500 people or less than 1% of those younger than age 20; however, 10.3 million or 21% of all Americans age 60 years or older have diabetes. The prevalence of diabetes is 9% of all non-Hispanic whites and 13% of all non-Hispanic African Americans age 20 years or older. Hispanic and Latino Americans aged 20 years or older are believed to be 1.7 times more likely to develop diabetes than non-Hispanic whites. American Indians and Alaska Natives are 2.2 times as likely to have diabetes as non-Hispanic whites. Prevalence of diabetes in this group ranges from 8% in Alaska Natives to 28% among American Indians in southern Arizona (21).

Diabetes results in serious morbidity and premature mortality. Long-term complications often affect the eyes, kidneys, and nerves, and there is an increased risk for heart disease, stroke, and peripheral vascular disease. Life expectancy of people with diabetes has

Address correspondence concerning this chapter to Guyton Hornsby, P.O. Box 9227, Division of Exercise Physiology, School of Medicine, West Virginia University, Morgantown, WV 26506-9227. E-mail: ghornsby@hsc.wvu.edu

■ Glossary

β-cell—Type of cell in the pancreas that produces the hormone insulin.

Charcot's joints—Also known as neuropathic arthropathy, occurs when a joint breaks down because of a problem with the nerves. In diabetes, this type of neuropathy most often occurs in the foot.

diabetic ketoacidosis—State of inadequate insulin levels resulting in hyperglycemia and accumulation of organic acids and ketones in the blood. Severe dehydration and significant alterations of blood chemistry are usually present.

hemoglobin A$_{1c}$—Also known as glycated hemoglobin, provides an indication of the average blood glucose concentration during the preceding 2 to 3 months.

hyperglycemic hyperosmolar state—Dangerous condition in which a person experiences very high blood glucose and dehydration without ketoacidosis. This condition is most often found in elderly people with type 2 diabetes and is usually triggered by an illness or infection.

hypoglycemia unawareness—Situation in which the usual adrenergic symptoms associated with a decrease in blood glucose are, for a variety of reasons, either not felt or not recognized.

metabolic syndrome—Combination of factors that place a person at high risk for heart disease. These factors are abdominal obesity, high triglyceride levels, high blood pressure, low high-density lipoprotein cholesterol, and high blood glucose levels.

nephropathy—Disease or abnormality of the kidney. Diabetic nephropathy is characterized by progressive decline in renal function and may result in end-stage renal disease.

neuropathy—Nerve pathology that may include focal, diffuse, sensory, motor, or autonomic damage.

polydipsia—Excessive thirst.

polyphagia—Excessive hunger.

polyuria—Passing of an excessive quantity of urine.

retinopathy—Damage to small blood vessels of the retina. Nonproliferative retinopathy includes development of microaneurysms, venous loops, retinal hemorrhages, and hard and soft exudates. Proliferative retinopathy is the development of new blood vessels.

been reported to be more than 12 years less than people without diabetes (20). Cardiovascular disease affecting the heart, brain, and peripheral vessels is 2 to 8 times higher in people with diabetes than in those without diabetes (17). Myocardial infarction, heart failure, cardiomyopathy, and silent ischemia occur earlier, occur more often, and are often more serious (13).

Twenty percent of all diabetes deaths are attributable to myocardial infarction. Patients with diabetes account for more than 33% of hospitalizations for heart failure, and heart failure in diabetes is often fatal. The poor prognosis in diabetes has been linked to hypertension, ischemic heart disease, and diabetic cardiomyopathy. Cardiomyopathy is a common finding in patients who have diabetes without heart failure. Studies using sensitive Doppler techniques to detect early and mild diastolic dysfunction have found diabetic cardiomyopathy to be present in more than 50% of patients with type 2 diabetes (7).

Sudden death occurs more frequently in diabetes and is attributable in part to underlying autonomic neuropathy. Patients with diabetes may have unrecognized symptoms of angina and may ignore shortness of breath, nausea, vomiting, sweating, sudden fatigue, or unexplained elevations in plasma glucose as symptoms of ischemia. It is estimated that 20% to 40% of myocardial infarction in those with diabetes is silent or undetected, and the delay in recognition is likely to contribute to poor outcomes.

Diagnosis and Classification

Diabetes is a group of metabolic diseases all having hyperglycemia in common. Diabetes is diagnosed when the patient demonstrates symptoms of diabetes with a random plasma glucose of 200 mg/dL (11.1 mmol/L) or higher, a fasting plasma glucose higher than 125 mg/dL (7 mmol/L) on more than one occasion, or a 2 hr plasma glucose of 200 mg/dL (11.1 mmol/L) or higher during an oral glucose tolerance test. The American Diabetes Association (2) has identified four major categories of overt diabetes mellitus:

- Type 1 diabetes
- Type 2 diabetes
- Other specific types of diabetes
- Gestational diabetes

Type 1 diabetes mellitus, which has formerly been known as juvenile-onset or insulin-dependent diabetes, accounts for only about 5% of total cases. This form of the disease usually has its onset in childhood or adolescence, but it also occurs in older adults. The most common cause of type 1 diabetes is the autoimmune destruction of pancreatic β-cells, which usually results in an absolute deficiency of endogenous insulin. Without insulin, glucose levels increase dramatically, causing the classic symptoms of polyuria, polydipsia, polyphagia, weight loss, and blurred vision. If hyperglycemia is not controlled, it can progress to ketoacidosis, coma, and even death. Treatment for type 1 diabetes involves providing exogenous insulin to normalize plasma glucose levels and attempting to prevent or delay long-term complications.

Type 2 diabetes mellitus, previously known as maturity-onset or non-insulin-dependent diabetes, accounts for almost 95% of total cases. Most patients with type 2 diabetes are obese. This disease used to be rare in those younger than 45 but is increasing at alarming rates in younger adults as well as in adolescents and children. This form of diabetes frequently goes undiagnosed for many years because its onset can be so gradual that classic symptoms do not appear or go unnoticed. The cause of type 2 diabetes is insulin resistance usually combined with an insulin secretory defect. There is a strong genetic predisposition for type 2 diabetes, and the risk of developing this disease increases with age, obesity, and inactivity. The goal of treatment for type 2 diabetes is to normalize plasma glucose and to prevent or delay chronic complications. Lifestyle changes such as weight reduction, exercise, and diet may be effective, but one or more drugs may also be necessary.

Other types of diabetes also exist, many which are accompanied by significant comorbidities. These types include genetic defects of β-cell function or defects in insulin action, diseases of the exocrine pancreas, endocrinopathies, drug- or chemical-induced diabetes, infections resulting in β-cell destruction, uncommon forms of immune-mediated diabetes, and other genetic syndromes sometimes associated with diabetes. The glycemic abnormalities associated with these specific types of diabetes may range from mild to moderate hyperglycemia to severe diabetes.

Gestational diabetes mellitus (GDM) is a transient form of diabetes that is diagnosed if glucose intolerance is first recognized during pregnancy. GDM is found in approximately 4% of all pregnancies in the United States. During pregnancy, treatment to normalize maternal blood glucose levels is important to avoid complications in the infant. Blood glucose in these women typically returns to normal on completion of the pregnancy, but 5% to 10% of women with gestational diabetes later develop type 2 diabetes. Women who have had gestational diabetes have a 20% to 50% chance of developing diabetes in the next 5 to 10 years.

Normal fasting plasma glucose levels should be no higher than 99 mg/dL (5.6 mmol/L) in the non-pregnant adult and the 2 hr postload value in an oral glucose tolerance test should be less than 140 mg/dL (7.8 mmol/L). Patients with a fasting plasma glucose or a 2 hr postload glucose higher than normal but less than the diagnostic criteria for overt diabetes are referred to as having *prediabetes*. An estimated 41 million people in the United States have prediabetes. Anyone with impaired fasting glucose or impaired glucose tolerance is at a relatively high risk for developing diabetes. Prediabetes is closely associated with the metabolic syndrome, a condition characterized by insulin resistance, abdominal obesity, dyslipidemia, and hypertension. Although diabetes may never appear in these patients, they still carry an excessive risk for cardiovascular disease

Complications

Complications may be generally divided into acute and chronic. Acute complications of diabetes are associated with extremes in plasma glucose levels. Hyperglycemia and other serious biochemical abnormalities leading to diabetic ketoacidosis (DKA) occur in type 1 diabetes and severe hyperglycemia, and a hyperosmolar state (HHS) may be seen in type 2 diabetes (4). Hypoglycemia is a common iatrogenic complication of both types of diabetes and can develop in anyone treated with insulin or oral hypoglycemic agents.

Chronic hyperglycemia is associated with microvascular, nerve, and macrovascular damage and can result in a number of serious long-term complications, including the following:

- Retinopathy with potential loss of vision
- Nephropathy, which can result in end-stage renal failure
- Peripheral neuropathy, which can result in foot ulcers, amputations, and Charcot's joints
- Autonomic neuropathy with gastrointestinal and genitourinary problems, sexual dysfunction, and inappropriate cardiovascular and sweating responses
- Atherosclerotic cardiovascular disease
- Peripheral arterial disease
- Cerebrovascular disease

Diabetes may increase susceptibility to many illnesses, and the prognosis for patients with diabetes who acquire illnesses such as pneumonia and influenza is often worse than in those who do not have diabetes. The emotional and social impact of diabetes and the demands of therapy may cause significant psychosocial dysfunction in patients and their families. Divorce, depression, and suicide are all increased in diabetes. Depressive disorders have been shown to increase patient care costs and lower quality of life in patients with diabetes (16), and the presence of major depression more than doubles the risk of cardiac death in patients with unstable angina or recent myocardial infarction.

Cardiovascular disease (CVD) is the major cause of mortality in both type 1 and type 2 diabetes. Diabetes has been recognized as an important independent risk factor for CVD. Patients with diabetes often have an assortment of major and contributing traditional CVD risk factors as well as several nontraditional factors unique to the diabetic state. A common finding is that diabetes, hypertension, abdominal obesity, dyslipidemia, and low cardiorespiratory fitness coexist and are often combined with cigarette smoking and detrimental psychosocial factors. Other nontraditional risk factors unique to the diabetic state include albuminuria, increased fibrinogen levels, hyperglycemia, and insulin resistance. Because of the excessive risk of CVD and subsequent cardiac events, the American Heart Association has designated diabetes as a "cardiovascular risk equivalent," meaning that those with diabetes belong in the same risk category as patients with already diagnosed CVD (17).

The pathogenesis of atherosclerosis in diabetic CVD has been linked to several factors:

- Metabolic factors—hyperglycemia, insulin deficiency or an insulin excess, insulin resistance, an excess flux of free fatty acids, and dyslipidemia underlie the diabetic state.

- Endothelial dysfunction—the altered metabolic state leads to a decrease in nitric oxide production combined with an increased production of endothelin 1 and angiotensin II, which disrupts normal blood vessel function and structure.

- Oxidation—hyperglycemia, in a milieu of oxidative stress, causes the nonenzymatic glycation and oxidation of cellular proteins, producing advanced glycation end products.

- Inflammation—advanced glycation end products set up harmful proinflammatory mechanisms in endothelial cells. Excess amounts of adipose tissue lead to the generation of cytokine growth factors that stimulate the proliferation and migration of smooth muscle cells, leading to atherosclerotic lesion formation and plaque instability.

- Prothrombotic state—hyperglycemia causes abnormal platelet cell activation and accumulation, augments blood coagulability, and decreases fibrinolytic activity, leading to detrimental formation and persistence of thrombi.

Management

Diabetes is a chronic illness requiring continuing medical care as well as extensive patient self-management. Effective medical management should involve a physician-coordinated team including physicians, diabetes educators, nurse practitioners, physician assistants, nurses, dietitians, exercise physiologists, pharmacists, and mental health professionals (3). Members of the cardiac rehabilitation staff have an important role in this team-oriented approach and should focus not only on the specific cardiac concerns of the patient but also on prevention and reduction of risk of acute and long-term complications of diabetes. Each aspect of the management plan should be understood by the medical team and agreed upon by the health care providers and the patient. Exercise sessions provide an excellent opportunity to provide education about diabetes and the effects of diet, exercise, and medications.

Control of blood glucose is a major goal of diabetes management. Improved glycemic control has been shown to decrease microvascular and neuropathic complications in prospective randomized clinical trials in both type 1 (11) and type 2 diabetes (22). The effects of improved control on cardiovascular disease risk are not as well documented, but at least one recent study demonstrated that intensive treatment of diabetes with improved glycemic control during a study period of approximately 6.5 years reduced the risk of a cardiovascular event by 42% and the occurrence of nonfatal myocardial infarction, stroke, or death from cardiovascular disease by 57% (12).

The American Diabetes Association recommends that glycemic control be monitored by hemoglobin A_{1c} (HbA_{1c}), that HbA_{1c} be less than 7% for patients in general, and that HbA_{1c} be as close to normal (<6%) as possible in individual patients as long as significant hypoglycemia can be avoided. Intense glycemic management with insulin has been shown to reduce morbidity in patients following myocardial infarction and in those with severe acute illness. The goal for HbA_{1c} may need to be increased for certain patients with a history of severe hypoglycemia, patients who are unaware of their hypoglycemic status, elderly adults, and patients with comorbid conditions.

Acute Glycemic Emergencies

The cardiac rehabilitation staff should be familiar with signs and symptoms of acute glycemic emergencies (see sidebar below) and should be prepared to take appropriate action (10). Supplies and equipment necessary for responding to acute emergencies must be available. These include blood glucose monitoring equipment and supplies; supplies to treat hypoglycemia including snacks or fluids, glucose tablets, and glucose gels; a glucagon injection kit; equipment and supplies for urine ketone testing; and phone numbers for anyone listed as an emergency contact. Syringes and lancets must be disposed of properly.

Hypoglycemia is common during exercise in patients taking insulin or any sulfonylurea medication. It may also occur with glucosidase inhibitors or short-acting insulin secretagogues if exercise is performed in the postprandial state. Exercise-induced hypoglycemia is even more likely during initiation of a training program. Blood glucose should be monitored before all exercise sessions or exercise testing, after exercise has concluded, and during exercise if any symptoms of hypoglycemia are noticed. Patients taking hypoglycemic medications should be advised to be more vigilant with self-monitoring of blood glucose after exercise as well because the hypoglycemic effects may continue for 24 hr or more as muscle glycogen is repleted.

If hypoglycemia does occur and the patient is conscious, it is advisable to give an initial oral glucose dose of 20 g. This should be repeated in 15 to 20 min if symptoms have not improved or if the monitored

▪ Signs and Symptoms of Acute Glycemic Emergencies

Hypoglycemia

- Blood glucose <70 mg/dL (3.9 mmol/L)
- Anxiety
- Behavioral changes (laughing, crying for no apparent reason)
- Poor coordination, stumbling
- Palpitations
- Tremors
- Sweating
- Hunger
- Numbness, tingling
- Cognitive dysfunction
- Seizures

Diabetic Ketoacidosis

- Blood glucose >250 mg/dL (13.9 mmol/L)
- Arterial pH <7.3
- Serum bicarbonate <15 mEq/L
- Nausea
- Vomiting
- Abdominal pain

- Rapid, deep respiration (Kussmaul breathing)
- Fruity breath odor
- Dry or flushed skin
- Dehydration
- Lethargy
- Extreme thirst

Hyperglycemic Hyperosmolar State

- Blood glucose >600 mg/dL (33.3 mmol/L)
- Serum total osmolality >330 mOsm/kg
- Absence of severe ketoacidosis
- Focal neurological signs (hemiparesis, hemianopsia)
- Seizures
- Drowsiness
- Confusion
- Fever >101 °F (38.3 °C)
- Dry skin, no sweating
- Extreme thirst

blood glucose remains low. However, the glycemic response to oral glucose is transient, typically less than 2 hr. Therefore, ingestion of a snack or meal shortly after the plasma glucose concentration is raised is generally advisable. If the patient is not conscious or is unable or unwilling (because of neuroglycopenia) to take glucose orally, parenteral therapy with glucagon may be necessary.

Medications and Nutrition

Effective management of diabetes involves appropriate selection of pharmacologic and nonpharmacologic measures combined with lifestyle intervention and self-care education. The goal is to achieve optimal glycemic control and to prevent or minimize acute and long-term complications. Therapy depends in part on the type of diabetes. Control of blood glucose in type 1 diabetes requires insulin replacement balanced with nutrient intake and physical activity, whereas in type 2 diabetes a number of options are available such as attempting to improve insulin action or increase insulin secretion or providing exogenous insulin.

All patients should receive instruction on nutrition therapy (14). Patients with type 1 diabetes usually are taught healthy eating behaviors and how nutrient intake should correspond with their specific insulin regimen. Patients with type 2 diabetes are typically counseled on healthy eating and weight loss. There is no single diet for patients with diabetes. The primary goal is to achieve optimal metabolic outcomes including blood glucose and HbA$_{1c}$ levels; low-density lipoprotein cholesterol, HDL-C, and triglyceride levels; blood pressure; and body weight. All patients with diabetes should receive individualized nutritional therapy provided by a registered dietitian familiar with all aspects of diabetes care.

Pharmacologic management of type 1 diabetes requires exogenous insulin replacement and may also include drugs to reduce CVD risk. Replacing insulin in a perfectly physiologic manner is not possible in conventional day-to-day living with available technologies for monitoring blood glucose and delivering insulin. Recent advances in analog formulations of insulin have dramatically changed treatment options, but the use of insulin still largely consists of adequately estimating the insulin required for prevailing glycemic needs based on sporadic glucose monitoring. Insulin delivered by subcutaneous injection results in a relative peripheral hyperinsulinemia and portal hypoinsulinemia compared with endogenous insulin, which is released directly into the portal vein.

The effect of injected insulin is highly dependent on the absorption kinetics from its subcutaneous depot. Most patients will inject insulin subcutaneously one to several times per day or will deliver insulin by continuous subcutaneous insulin infusion, called insulin pump therapy. A variety of insulin formulations are in use (see table 20.1). Different formulations may be combined to provide several peaks of insulin to coincide with meals, or patients can take multiple daily injections to provide basal and bolus dosing. Insulin pumps can be programmed to deliver varying basal rates and also deliver a patient-selected bolus dose at mealtimes or to correct unforeseen hyperglycemia.

Subcutaneous insulin absorption depends on the formulation being used, the volume injected, and the depth of injection as well as factors that may alter subcutaneous blood flow like temperature, massage, site of injection, and physical activity level. There is a strong likelihood that exercise will alter insulin absorption, leading to an inappropriate insulin level with hypoglycemia during or shortly after an exercise session. Anyone providing exercise therapy for those with diabetes should be familiar with symptoms of hypoglycemia and prepared to take appropriate action.

Pharmacologic management of type 2 diabetes should include medications to reduce CVD risk as well as agents to control glycemia, if lifestyle modifications are ineffective. A variety of options are available for control of blood glucose in type 2 diabetes. Increasing physical activity and decreasing nutritional intake can be effective, especially if there is a reduction in body weight. If lifestyle changes are unsuccessful, the pharmacologic choices include the use of insulin, oral agents, or combinations of these drugs. Insulin is an effective therapy for glycemic control in type 2 diabetes; however, some risks are associated with its use, including hypoglycemia and hyperinsulinemia.

Oral agents available for treatment of type 2 diabetes are listed in table 20.2. These medications may improve glycemic control by increasing insulin secretion or action or by decreasing glucose absorption. Sulfonylureas and meglitinides are insulin secretagogues. The main difference in the two classes of drugs is the rapidity and duration of stimulation of insulin secretion. The meglitinides are dosed at each meal and are intended to control postprandial hyperglycemia. There is risk of hypoglycemia with any insulin secretagogues, but this would be most likely to occur with the meglitinides when exercise is performed postprandially. Biguanides and thiazolidinediones are insulin sensitizers. There should be little or no risk of hypoglycemia with exercise when these agents are used alone. Acarbose and

TABLE 20.1 Insulin Preparations Commonly Used in the United States

Generic name	Trade name	Onset	Peak	Duration
RAPID-ACTING				
Insulin Lispro Insulin Aspart Insulin Glulisine	Humalog NovoLog Apidra	<15 min	30-90 min	1-3 hr
SHORT-ACTING				
Regular	Humulin R Novolin R	30-60 min	2-3 hr	3-6 hr
INTERMEDIATE-ACTING				
NPH Lente	Humulin N Novolin N Humulin L	2-4 hr	4-10 hr	10-16 hr
LONG-ACTING				
Insulin Glargine Ultralente	Lantus Humulin U	2-4 hr	Peakless	18-36 hr

miglitol inhibit glucose absorption. There is a slight risk of hypoglycemia with these agents when exercise is performed postprandially.

Other injectable medications can be used to treat diabetes including exenatide and pramlintide. Exenatide is an incretin mimetic sold under the trade name Byetta. This drug is used in treatment of type 2 diabetes and is found to increase postprandial insulin response, delay gastric emptying, suppress glucagon secretion, and reduce appetite. Pramlintide is a synthetic hormone similar to human amylin and is sold under the trade name Symlin. It can be used in combination with insulin therapy for treatment of either type 1 or type 2 diabetes. Pramlintide works by suppressing glucagon secretion and delaying gastric emptying. Both medications are typically used to reduce postprandial increases in blood glucose and may assist with weight loss. The most common side effect of these medications is nausea, but hypoglycemia may occur when these medications are combined with insulin or oral hypoglycemic medications. The timing of exanitide or pramlintide injections is an important consideration in exercise therapy because they may reduce absorption of oral medications and may interfere with absorption of dietary carbohydrate.

The choice of which pharmacologic agent to use for glycemic control will depend on cost and effectiveness, side effects that may occur, and additional goals of therapy such as CVD risk reduction (dyslipidemia, hypertension, and platelet abnormalities) and weight management. Other medications may be used to reduce CVD risk including statins and other lipid-lowering agents, angiotensin-converting enzyme inhibitors, angiotensin-receptor blockers, β-blockers, diuretics, calcium channel blockers, and aspirin. These drugs may be used alone or in combination. Special thought should be given to their cardiovascular and glycemic consequences, especially during exercise therapy.

Impact of Exercise and Exercise Training

Physical activity is one of the foundations of diabetes management. It is well known that exercise training can improve glycemic control, decrease insulin resistance, assist with weight management, and reduce CVD risk by improving hypertension, dyslipidemia, and cardiorespiratory endurance in those with type 2 diabetes. Exercise training has been recommended for treatment and prevention or delay of type 2 diabetes by both the American Diabetes Association (3) and the American College of Sports Medicine (1). Exercise training may also decrease insulin resistance, help with weight management, and reduce risk of CVD in type 1 diabetes.

TABLE 20.2 **Oral Agents Used to Treat Diabetes**

Generic name	Trade name	Concerns with exercise
BIGUANIDES		
Metformin Metformin (liquid)	Glucophage, Glucophage XR Riomet	
GLUCOSIDASE INHIBITORS		
Acarbose Miglitol	Precose Glyset	May produce hypoglycemia with postprandial exercise
MEGLITINIDES		
Nateglinide Repaglinide	Starlix Prandin	May produce hypoglycemia with postprandial exercise
SECRETAGOGUES		
Acetohexamide Chlorpromide Tolazimide Tolbutamide Glimepride Glipizide Glyburide	Generic only Diabinese Tolinase Orinase Amaryl Glucotrol, Glucotrol XL Diabeta, Glynase, PresTab, Micronase	Can produce hypoglycemia during or after exercise
THIAZOLADINEDIONES		
Pioglitazone Rosiglitazone	Actos Avandia	
DIPEPETIDYL PEPTIDASE-4 INHIBITORS		
Sitagliptin	Januvia	Produces no hypoglycemia unless given with another drug
COMBINATIONS		
Metformin + glyburide Metformin + rosiglitazone Metformin + glipizide Sitagliptin + metformin	Glucovance Avandamet Metaglip Janumet	See concerns for individual drugs

Although exercise training has considerable benefits for most patients with diabetes, there may also be risks of acute complications. Physical activity can cause hypoglycemia in any patient taking insulin or an insulin secretagogue. Appropriate precautions, such as medication dose or carbohydrate intake adjustments, are often needed to avoid hypoglycemia. Blood glucose in type 1 patients generally should be above 100 mg/dL (5.6 mmol/L) and below 250 mg/dL (13.9 mmol/L) at the start of exercise. Different preexercise glucose targets may be needed for some patients, and these should be provided by the primary care physician or diabetologist.

In patients susceptible to hypoglycemia, it is usually advisable that the patient consume a preexercise snack or drink containing carbohydrate if the preexercise glucose is less than 100 mg/dL (5.6 mmol/L). Blood glucose should be monitored in these patients before and after exercise and should be monitored during exercise if there are any symptoms of hypoglycemia. Fast-acting carbohydrates should be readily available in case hypoglycemia develops. These include glucose tablets, glucose gels, juices, sport drinks, or nondiet soft drinks. The usual starting dose for supplemental carbohydrate is 15 to 20 g, and treatment results should be noticeable within 15 min. Patients should never be allowed to leave an exercise facility until their blood glucose is above a safe level, especially if they are driving.

Patients with type 1 diabetes often need supplemental carbohydrate during or after exercise to keep glucose in a safe range. Patients with type 2 diabetes taking insulin or a medication that increases insulin production may need to take additional carbohydrate to treat hypoglycemia, but it is usually best to use glucose tablets or gels rather than food or drink, especially if weight management is a concern. If hypoglycemia does develop consistently in these patients, their managing physicians should be notified to determine whether medications should be adjusted. Many times exercise can lead to a significant reduction or discontinuation of hypoglycemic medications in type 2 diabetes.

Patients should avoid exercise during periods of very poor blood glucose control. Exercise can potentially worsen control, especially when hyperglycemia is found with ketosis in patients with type 1 diabetes or when a patient with type 2 diabetes is in an HHS. It is generally advisable to avoid exercise if signs or symptoms of DKA or HHS are present. If the patient with type 1 diabetes feels well and urine or blood ketones are negative, it is not necessary to postpone exercise based simply on blood glucose. Patients with type 2 diabetes may have blood glucose values greater than 300 mg/dL (16.7 mmol/L) in the postprandial state and still notice improvement in glucose with exercise. If the patient with type 2 diabetes feels well, has had no recent infections, and has no signs or symptoms of HHS, hyperglycemia by itself should not preclude physical activity. In a questionable case for proceeding with exercise, it is prudent to monitor blood glucose after 10 to 15 min of activity to see how the glucose is responding.

Before beginning any exercise program, patients with diabetes should be assessed for conditions that may predispose them to acute emergencies or injury such as hypoglycemia unawareness, severe autonomic neuropathy, or severe peripheral neuropathy as well as conditions that would require treatment prior to exercise training such as preproliferative or proliferative retinopathy or macular edema. These chronic complications may simply require exercise modifications, may require specific precautionary measures, may contraindicate certain forms of exercise, or may require therapeutic intervention to allow safe participation. For example, patients with severe peripheral neuropathy should have their feet examined for trauma-induced injury before and after weight-bearing exercise. They may also require special footwear.

Exercise training has been shown to reduce insulin resistance and improve glycemic control in type 2 diabetes and can decrease CVD risk in both type 1 and type 2 diabetes. Improvements in HbA_{1c} are consistent in studies using aerobic training programs of 50% to 80% $\dot{V}O_{2max}$ 3 to 4 times per week for 30 to 60 min per session (3). Improvements in HbA_{1c} appear to be greatest in patients with mild type 2 diabetes and in those who are most insulin resistant. Data are limited on the glycemic effects of resistance training in type 2 diabetes, but several recent studies suggest that resistance training may reduce HbA_{1c}, and the American Diabetes Association and American College of Sports Medicine have included resistance training in their exercise recommendations (1, 5).

Exercise training has not been shown to effectively improve HbA_{1c} in type 1 diabetes, although it can improve insulin sensitivity. Glycemic control in type 1 diabetes depends on the balance between insulin replacement, nutritional therapy, and physical activity. The challenge for those managing patients with type 1 diabetes in exercise programs is to adequately adjust insulin and nutritional therapy to allow safe participation. The benefits of exercise training for those with type 1 diabetes are primarily associated with reduction in CVD risk, and cardiovascular rehabilitation programs can contribute by providing exercise and nutritional educational programming in conjunction with behavioral modification to enhance overall reduction in CVD risk factors. Exercise training can be extremely effective in reducing the major CVD risk factors of hypertension, abdominal obesity, dyslipidemia, and low cardiorespiratory fitness in diabetes. Blood pressure has consistently been shown to be normalized or lowered with exercise training, and these effects appear to be more apparent in hyperinsulinemic patients. Exercise training has been shown to reduce abdominal obesity and to assist in moderate weight loss in type 2 diabetes. Weight loss of 10% to 15% can improve insulin resistance and aid in achieving metabolic goals. Patients with type 2 diabetes are usually very deconditioned and are often unable to expend enough energy with exercise to achieve even moderate weight loss. Therefore, in most patients, nutritional therapy should be combined with physical activity to reduce body weight.

Dyslipidemia can be improved with exercise training, most notably with reductions in levels of triglyceride-rich very low density lipoproteins. HDL-C may be increased, but this finding has not been found consistently in diabetes. This may be linked to the relatively modest training intensities that have been studied. Low cardiorespiratory fitness and physical inactivity are common characteristics of type 2 diabetes and have been recognized as independent predictors of all-cause mortality in this population (23). Moreover, there appears to be a steep inverse relation between fitness and mortality in diabetes, and this association is independent of differences in body weight (9). Low fitness has been shown to be a strong predictor of cardiac mortality in patients referred for cardiac rehabilitation (19), and these observations strengthen the importance of increasing fitness with physical activity in cardiac rehabilitation patients with diabetes.

Wexler and colleagues (24) reported that women with diabetes received less aggressive therapy for modifiable CVD risk factors than did men who had diabetes. Although coronary heart disease mortality has decreased over the past 30 years in the overall American population and in men with diabetes, coronary heart disease mortality in women with diabetes has increased over the same time period. Because women with diabetes have a relative risk of heart disease mortality that may be as high as 10-fold greater than women without diabetes, it is clear that CVD needs to be viewed as a serious, life-threatening complication for women with diabetes. Every effort should be taken to reduce the excessive CVD risk, including the use of exercise training.

Cardiovascular Rehabilitation for Patients With Diabetes

Patients with diabetes are frequently referred for cardiac rehabilitation, and the prevalence of diabetes is 20% to 40% in most programs. With the growing diabetes epidemic, the number of people with diabetes in cardiovascular rehabilitation will likely increase. Structured, professionally assisted exercise programs such as cardiac rehabilitation have even been recommended for general lifestyle and medical management for certain patients with diabetes (17). The cardiac rehabilitation staff should work as partners with the primary care physician or diabetologist and the diabetes management team.

Two studies reported outcome data after following patients with and without diabetes for a minimum of 7 weeks in cardiac rehabilitation. Patients with diabetes had greater CVD risk at entry, particularly for hyperglycemia, hypertension, abnormal triglyceride and HDL-C level, obesity, increased waist circumfer-

ence, and low cardiorespiratory fitness level. Hindman and colleagues (18) demonstrated similar proportional improvements with cardiac rehabilitation in all factors except those related to weight in patients with and without diabetes. Banzer and colleagues (6) improved cardiorespiratory fitness with cardiac rehabilitation in patients with diabetes, and these improvements were similar to improvements in those without diabetes, but the investigators were unable to improve other risk factors. The disappointing outcomes of Banzer and colleagues were likely attributable to the higher dropout rate in patients with diabetes.

High dropout rates in cardiac rehabilitation for patients with diabetes could be attributable to comorbid conditions, poor exercise tolerance, exacerbation of medical problems, or a greater incidence of intercurrent illnesses. The inability to achieve adequate weight loss in people with diabetes in cardiac rehabilitation may lead to dropouts and is most likely attributable to the low initial cardiorespiratory fitness levels and low energy expenditure with exercise sessions. Although improvement in fitness was proportionally similar for those with and without diabetes, posttraining cardiorespiratory fitness in those with diabetes was only increased to the pretraining values of those without diabetes. Although this is disappointing, it is clear that these improvements in cardiorespiratory fitness with cardiac rehabilitation should lower cardiac mortality risk in patients with diabetes.

Summary

Patients with diabetes present specific challenges to the cardiac rehabilitation staff. To effectively manage cardiac disease in people with diabetes, rehabilitation specialists should focus on achieving and maintaining glycemic control, avoiding acute complications, and reducing risk for long-term complications. Rehabilitation specialists must show patients how to prevent hypo- and hyperglycemia with exercise and avoid common exercise injuries that cause vascular and neural damage. Problems of compliance and adherence must be dealt with proactively to avoid exercise withdrawal, and risks of CVD must be modified aggressively. The cardiac rehabilitation staff should understand diabetes and its treatment so they can be part of a coordinated diabetes management team able to provide exercise therapy, lifestyle education, and secondary prevention to achieve the best possible short- and long-term results for cardiac patients with diabetes.

CHAPTER 21

Obesity

Wendy M. Miller, MD

Peter A. McCullough, MD

Obesity is a central risk factor for several conditions that promote cardiovascular disease, including hypertension, dyslipidemia, type 2 diabetes, and a proinflammatory state. This chapter reviews the epidemiology, evaluation, and management of the obese patient.

Epidemiology

Obesity has become a major public health concern for many developed countries. In the United States, obesity prevalence doubled in adults between 1980 and 2002 (5). By 2004, almost one third (32.2%) of adults in the United States were obese (20).

The human body can metabolize carbohydrate, protein, and fat to meet energy needs. When energy intake exceeds expenditure, excess energy can be stored. The revised World Health Organization equations for estimating energy expenditure are shown on page 210 (22). Fat is the major energy storage form, and unlike protein and carbohydrate, fat can be stored in very large amounts. When weight gain occurs as a result of excess calorie consumption, approximately 75% of the extra energy is stored as fat and the remaining 25% as lean tissue.

From a historical and evolutionary perspective, the ability of the body to store energy provided a survival advantage. Energy stores could be mobilized and used in times of famine and food deprivation. In developed modernized countries, however, where energy-dense foods are readily available with minimal physical activity, the prevalence of overweight and obesity attributable to positive energy balance is increasing (11).

In most people who are obese, their condition is the result of nonmedical causes such as sedentary lifestyle and increased calorie consumption. However, several factors can promote weight gain such as endocrine disorders, medications, or smoking cessation (see Conditions and Medications Contributing to Weight Gain on page 211). Treatable medical causes for obesity, such as Cushing's syndrome or newly discovered hypothyroidism, are uncommon.

Obesity and Cardiovascular Risk

Obesity is associated with an increased rate of death from cardiovascular disease as well as all causes (2). Excess fat deposition in the abdominal region,

Address correspondence concerning this chapter to Wendy M. Miller, William Beaumont Hospital, 4949 Coolidge Highway, Royal Oak, MI 48073. E-mail: wmiller@beaumont.edu

■ Revised World Health Organization Equations for Estimating Energy Expenditure

Step 1

Estimate basal metabolic rate:

- Men 18 to 30 years = (0.0630 × actual weight in kg + 2.8957) × 240 kcal/day
- Men 31 to 60 years = (0.0484 × actual weight in kg + 3.6534) × 240 kcal/day
- Women 18 to 30 years = (0.0621 × actual weight in kg + 2.0357) × 240 kcal/day
- Women 31 to 60 years = (0.0342 × actual weight in kg + 3.5377) × 240 kcal/day

Step 2

Determine activity factor:

- Low activity level (sedentary) = activity factor of 1.3
- Intermediate activity level (some regular exercise) = activity factor of 1.5
- High activity level (regular activity or demanding job) = activity factor of 1.7

Step 3

Estimate total energy expenditure:

- Total energy expenditure = basal metabolic rate × activity factor

---

commonly referred to as abdominal obesity or central obesity, is often associated with the *metabolic syndrome*, a term used to describe a constellation of risk factors that correlate with increased risk for cardiovascular disease as well as type 2 diabetes. Waist circumference is a fairly reliable surrogate for abdominal adipose mass and is a practical cardiovascular risk assessment tool. A waist circumference >100 cm (40 in.) in men and >88 cm (35 in.) in women is associated with increased morbidity and mortality (22).

The obesity comorbidities of hypertension, type 2 diabetes, dyslipidemia, and obstructive sleep apnea also increase cardiovascular risk. Unhealthy lifestyle habits found among many obese people, such as diets high in sugar, starch (simple carbohydrates), and saturated fat in combination with sedentary activity levels, promote cardiovascular disease through a variety of mechanisms.

Evaluation of the Obese Patient

Evaluation of the obese patient includes classification, clinical interview, physical exam, and diagnostic testing. Screening for potential etiologic factors and obesity comorbidities is an important component of the assessment.

Classification of Obesity

Classification of adult obesity is based on body mass index (BMI), which is calculated from weight and height measurements.

BMI = weight (kg) ÷ height (cm) ÷ height (cm) × 10,000

or

BMI = weight (lb) ÷ height (in.) ÷ height (in.) × 703

BMI nomograms enable clinicians to quickly assess degree of obesity (figure 21.1 on page 212). Disease risk can be further classified by waist circumference. Waist circumference should be measured with a flexible tape placed on a horizontal plane just above the iliac crest (19). The National Heart, Lung, and Blood Institute (NHLBI) obesity classification guidelines, shown in table 21.1 on page 213, demonstrate that a person's risk for hypertension, type 2 diabetes, and cardiovascular disease increases with a larger waist size (19). However, the utility of waist circumference in assessment of cardiovascular risk diminishes at a BMI of 30 kg/m^2. Beyond a BMI of 30 kg/m^2, the waist circumference is almost universally past the defined boundaries. In other words, among obese people, abdominal obesity

■ Conditions and Medications Contributing to Weight Gain

Lifestyle

- Excess calorie consumption
- Sedentary lifestyle
- Sleep deprivation

Endocrine

- Cushing's syndrome
- Polycystic ovarian syndrome
- Hypothalamic obesity
- Growth hormone deficiency
- Hypothyroid
- Pseudohypoparathyroidism
- Hypogonadism

Medications

- Narcoleptic/antipsychotic drugs (thioridazine, clozapine, quetiapine, risperidone)
- Antidepressants (amitriptyline, nortriptyline, imipramine, mitrazapine, paroxetine, olanzapine)
- Anticonvulsants (valproic acid, carbamazepine, gabapentin)
- Antidiabetic (insulin, sulfonylureas, nateglinide, thiazolidinediones)
- Antiserotonin (pizotifen)

- β-adrenergic blocker (propranolol)
- α-adrenergic blocker (terazosin)
- Steroid hormones (oral contraceptives, glucocorticoids, progestational steroids)
- Antihistamine (cyproheptadine)

Psychological

- Binge eating disorder
- Seasonal affective disorder
- Depression
- Anxiety

Genetic

- Laurence–Moon–Biedl syndrome
- Prader–Willi syndrome
- Turner syndrome
- Leptin deficiency

Other

- Low socioeconomic status (Hispanic men and women, African American women)
- Smoking cessation
- Sleep apnea
- Night-eating syndrome

---

is the rule with nonabdominal excess fat tissue present as the BMI increases.

Although BMI is the most widely accepted tool for defining overweight and obesity, it has limitations and should be interpreted carefully. One limitation is that BMI does not differentiate lean mass from fat mass. Therefore, a person with a large muscle mass may be classified as overweight or obese per BMI calculation but may actually have a low percent body fat. This is occasionally seen in professional athletes, although it is rare. Another limitation is in regard to ethnicity. Data reported on the associations among BMI, waist circumference, and disease risk have been collected predominantly from Caucasian subjects. There is evidence that different ethnic groups have significant differences in percent body fat for the same BMI. Asians, for example, tend to have a higher percent body fat than Caucasians at the same BMI, and African Americans tend to have a lower percent body fat compared with Caucasians at the same BMI. Thus, in some races, particularly Asians and Indians, a BMI of 22 to 25 kg/m^2 can be associated with abdominal adiposity and carry the same risk as a BMI >30 kg/m^2 in other races.

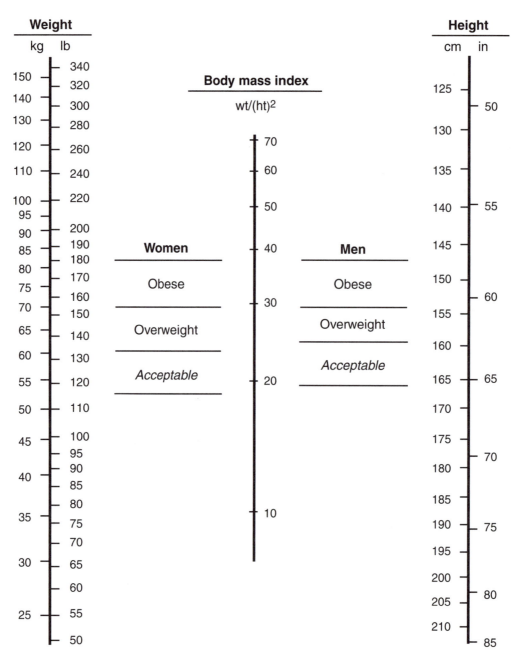

FIGURE 21.1 BMI nomogram. The nomogram is used by placing a ruler or straight edge between the body weight (on left) and the height (on right). The body mass index is read from the middle of the scale.

Clinical Interview, Physical Exam, and Diagnostic Testing

The clinical interview, physical exam, and diagnostic testing should include the following:

- Assessment of weight history, dietary habits, and physical activity
- Assessment of etiology and contributing factors of obesity (see Conditions and Medications Contributing to Weight Gain on page 211)
- Screening for obesity comorbidities and obesity-associated health risks (figure 21.2)
- Assessment for symptoms and diagnoses that may affect treatment
- Evaluation of family history of obesity and obesity comorbidities
- Assessment of current social support and psychosocial stressors
- Evaluation of motivation and readiness for change

TABLE 21.1 Classification of Overweight and Obesity by Body Mass Index (BMI), Waist Circumference, and Associated Disease Risk

	BMI, kg/m²	Obesity class	**DISEASE RISK* RELATIVE TO NORMAL WEIGHT AND WAIST CIRCUMFERENCE** Men <102 cm (<40 in.) Women <88 cm (<35 in.)	>102 cm (>40 in.) >88 cm (>35 in.)
Underweight	<18.5		—	—
Normal†	18.5-24.9		—	—
Overweight	25.0-29.9		Increased	High
Obesity	30.0-34.9	I	High	Very high
	35.0-39.9	II	Very high	Very high
	>40	III	Extremely high	Extremely high

*Disease risk for type 2 diabetes, hypertension, and CVD.

†Increased waist circumference can also be a marker for increased risk even in persons of normal weight.

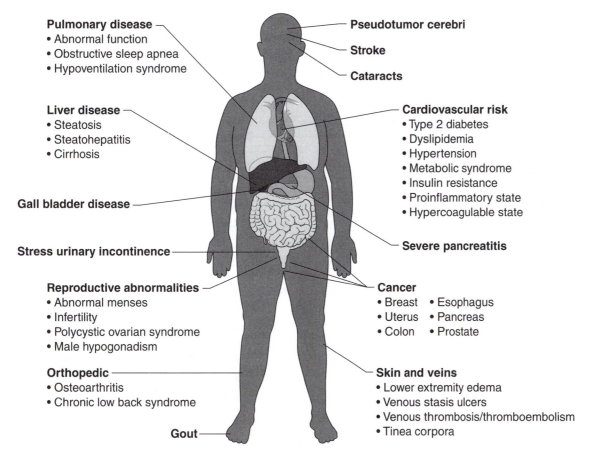

Pulmonary disease
• Abnormal function
• Obstructive sleep apnea
• Hypoventilation syndrome

Liver disease
• Steatosis
• Steatohepatitis
• Cirrhosis

Gall bladder disease

Stress urinary incontinence

Reproductive abnormalities
• Abnormal menses
• Infertility
• Polycystic ovarian syndrome
• Male hypogonadism

Orthopedic
• Osteoarthritis
• Chronic low back syndrome

Gout

Pseudotumor cerebri

Stroke

Cataracts

Cardiovascular risk
• Type 2 diabetes
• Dyslipidemia
• Hypertension
• Metabolic syndrome
• Insulin resistance
• Proinflammatory state
• Hypercoagulable state

Severe pancreatitis

Cancer
• Breast   • Esophagus
• Uterus   • Pancreas
• Colon   • Prostate

Skin and veins
• Lower extremity edema
• Venous stasis ulcers
• Venous thrombosis/thromboembolism
• Tinea corpora

FIGURE 21.2 Obesity comorbidities and health risks.

From NAASO, The Obesity Society

Many obesity comorbidities, including hypertension, hyperlipidemia, obstructive sleep apnea, and osteoarthritis pain, can dramatically improve or resolve with weight loss. Therefore, understanding the impact of the person's obesity on his health can help determine the magnitude of health improvement and cardiovascular risk reduction possible through weight loss. Education on potential quality of life improvement through weight loss can also be a motivational tool.

Screening for medical conditions and symptoms that may affect obesity treatment is an important component of developing a management plan. For example, severe osteoarthritis of the knees may prohibit or greatly limit weight-bearing exercises because of increased pain. Pool or water exercise may be a better option. Medical history can also affect dietary recommendations for weight loss. A patient with chronic kidney disease, for example, may need to follow certain dietary restrictions.

Laboratory studies to consider include thyroid stimulating hormone, fasting lipid profile, fasting glucose, fasting insulin level, liver enzymes, and high-sensitivity C-reactive protein. Blood pressure should be measured in all people and electrocardiogram should be considered, particularly in people with other cardiovascular risk factors or cardiovascular symptoms. Cardiac stress testing is indicated for people with symptoms suggestive of cardiac ischemia or for high-risk subjects, such as people with diabetes who plan to start a vigorous (>60% of maximal oxygen uptake) exercise program. Polysomnogram to screen for obstructive sleep apnea syndrome is indicated in all males with a BMI >45 kg/m^2, people who have snoring with observed cessation of breathing, and people with severe daytime somnolence.

Management of the Obese Patient

According to the NHLBI's evidence-based clinical guidelines on overweight and obesity in adults, treatment is recommended for patients with a BMI of 25.0 to 29.9 kg/m^2 or a high waist circumference and with two or more risk factors (19). Risk factors include established coronary heart disease or presence of other atherosclerotic disease, hyperlipidemia, hypertension, type 2 diabetes, impaired fasting glucose, family history of premature coronary heart disease ($\leq$55 years old in a first-degree male relative or $\leq$65 years old in a female first-degree relative), sleep apnea, and age (male $\geq$45

years or female $\geq$55 years or postmenopausal). Treatment is also recommended for patients with a BMI $\geq$30 kg/m^2 regardless of risk factors. The probability of restoring a normal body weight is inversely related to the BMI. Thus, it is important to catch the problem early in the course of excess body fat storage in order to reverse this process and restore body functions to the normal state.

Several prospective studies have demonstrated the health benefits of intentional weight loss, including a decrease in all-cause, cardiovascular, diabetes, and cancer mortality rates (6, 27). Resolution of obesity with subsequent improvement or resolution of obesity comorbidities is possible for patients who are motivated, ready to make positive lifestyle changes, and committed to practicing healthy long-term dietary and physical activity habits.

Realistic weight loss goals should be determined and discussed. A weight loss of 10% to 15% can often improve obesity-associated disorders such as dyslipidemia, hypertension, and diabetes mellitus (7). The patient should be educated that a loss of 15% or more of initial weight and maintenance of this loss signifies success, even if she does not reach a BMI <25 kg/m^2. Steady and progressive weight loss with normalization of body weight may take years and is the result of permanent diet and lifestyle changes.

Comprehensive obesity treatment includes a combination of three components:

■ Dietary treatment
■ Behavior modification
■ Physical activity and exercise

Additional components of treatment may include pharmacotherapy and surgical treatment.

Dietary Treatment

Reduction in caloric intake below energy expenditure results in a fairly predictable rate of weight loss. A reduction of 500 kcal/day (3,500 kcal/week), for example, usually results in a weight loss of 0.45 kg/week (~1 lb/week). Rate of weight loss can vary, however, depending on genetic factors, age, fidgeting, and amount of lean mass. Older people tend to lose weight more slowly than younger subjects because metabolic rate declines by approximately 2% per decade (16). A higher lean body mass is associated with a higher energy expenditure and therefore a quicker rate of weight loss.

The daily caloric intake necessary for a desired calorie deficit can be determined from the estimated total energy expenditure (see Equations for Estimating Energy Expenditure on page 210):

Daily caloric intake = total energy expenditure
– desired calorie deficit

Most overweight or obese adults will lose weight if they comply with a diet between 800 and 1,200 kcal/day. It is rare that a person would require a total caloric intake of <800 kcal/day for weight loss; therefore, very low calorie diets (400-800 kcal/day) should be reserved for people who require urgent weight loss, such as in preparation for a necessary surgery.

A registered dietitian experienced in weight management is a valuable resource in comprehensive weight management. A weight loss diet should provide adequate micronutrients (vitamins, minerals, trace elements) and macronutrients (protein, carbohydrate, and essential fatty acids). Therefore, energy-dense foods and beverages with minimal nutritional quality, such as sugar-containing beverages, starches, sweets, and alcohol, should be eliminated or extremely restricted during weight loss. Emphasis should be placed on appropriate portion sizes and adequate consumption of healthful foods such as high-quality protein and fruits and vegetables. This strategy provides all essential amino acids and fatty acids and sufficient calories for energy expenditure. In addition, significantly restricting or eliminating sugars, starches (foods made with refined flour, rice, and potatoes), and saturated fats (fried foods, high-fat spreads and condiments, and red meat) reduces calories considerably and provides a more favorable nutrient stream for glucose metabolism and insulin secretion, which in turn can improve appetite regulation and weight reduction.

Commercially packaged portion-controlled meal and snack replacement shakes, bars, soups, and entrees can be useful tools for weight loss, particularly when the BMI is greater than 30 kg/m^2 and the probability of success with food diets is greatly diminished. The meal replacement dietary approach has been shown to have beneficial short-term and long-term results for weight loss and cardiovascular risk factor reduction in obese people (4, 26). One prospective randomized 4-year trial found superior results with a meal replacement diet compared with a low-calorie all-food diet (figure 21.3) (4). Another recent randomized trial confirmed the superior weight loss achieved with meal replacements, and this correlated with improvement in biomarkers of longevity (10). Mean long-term weight loss following a

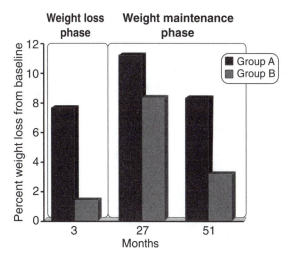

FIGURE 21.3 Mean percent weight loss and weight maintenance with a meal replacement diet and an all-food diet. Data from 100 patients, BMI >25 and ≤40 kg/m^2, randomized to a 12-week weight loss intervention of a 1,200 to 1,500 kcal/day diet: a diet consisting of two meal and snack replacements and one food meal (group A) or an all-food diet (group B). Dietary instruction and energy content for weight maintenance were the same for both groups and included use of one meal and one snack replacement per day. Over 4 years, average weight loss of group A was consistently greater than that of group B (p = .001).

Adapted, by permission, from M. Flechtner-Mors et al., 2000, "Metabolic and weight loss effects of long-term dietary intervention in obese patients: four-year results," *Obesity Research* 8(5): 399-402.

meal-replacement diet, although better than an all-food diet, is a modest ~8.4%. However, this degree of weight loss has been correlated with sustained improvement in fasting glucose level, insulin level, triglyceride level, and blood pressure.

Medical monitoring by an experienced physician should be considered when a client undertakes a diet consisting entirely or mostly of meal replacements. Certain medical risks such as gallstone formation, hypoglycemia, acute renal insufficiency, and electrolyte abnormalities can be minimized with appropriate medication adjustment, patient education, and monitoring by a physician experienced in meal replacement diets. Figure 21.4 summarizes a reasonable treatment approach based on body mass index.

Behavior Modification

Behavior modification is essential for short-term and long-term weight loss success. Techniques and tools for modifying behaviors and developing healthful lifestyle habits are usually taught by psychologists or other trained personnel. Behavioral strategies aimed

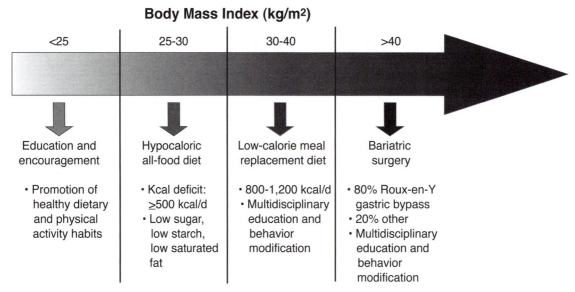

FIGURE 21.4   Reasonable treatment approaches based on body mass index.

at helping people develop healthful lifestyle habits, as listed in the NHLBI clinical guidelines on obesity (19), include the following:

- Self-monitoring—regular monitoring of dietary intake and physical activity

- Stress management—development and practice of strategies to cope with stress

- Stimulus control—identifying environments or situations that stimulate unhealthy eating; limiting exposure, implementing environmental control strategies, and practicing healthier responses

- Problem solving—brainstorming, developing, implementing, and evaluating strategies to overcome barriers to healthy lifestyle habits

- Contingency management—rewards, whether coming from the treatment team or the person

- Cognitive restructuring—positive self-talk, development of realistic goals, and restructuring of thoughts in regard to body image, diet, and physical activity

- Social support—support groups as well as family and friends working toward developing healthier habits

Physical Activity and Exercise

Exercise is a necessary component of obesity treatment for several reasons. Perhaps the most compelling reason is that regular physical activity appears to be the most reliable correlate of long-term weight control. Additionally, exercise is associated with improved preservation of lean mass during weight loss and overall improvement of cardiovascular risk factors. Glycemic control, insulin resistance, blood pressure, high-density lipoprotein cholesterol level, and triglyceride levels improve with regular exercise.

The amount and intensity of exercise necessary to control weight are not known definitively. However, a growing body of evidence shows that exercise ranging from 45 to 60 min/day on most days of the week is most effective for preventing weight regain in overweight and obese adults (figure 21.5) (3, 13, 14, 24). Accordingly, the American College of Sports Medicine recommends approximately 60 min/day on most days of the week (12) and the International Association for the Study of Obesity recommends 60 to 90 min/day on most days of the week (23) for weight control. Research on exercise intensity has demonstrated that moderate-intensity exercise (40-60% of maximal oxygen uptake) has a positive impact on health parameters (25) and is likely as effective for weight control as vigorous intensity exercise (13). Therefore, a reasonable recommendation for obese patients to work toward during weight loss, and continue long-term for weight maintenance, is a moderate-intensity exercise regimen for 60 min or more on most days of the week (or a total of 240 min/week or more).

Pharmacotherapy

Antiobesity medications may be useful for people who have failed to lose weight despite an adequate trial

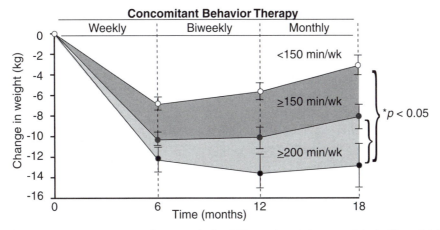

FIGURE 21.5 Moderate-intensity exercise for a total of ≥200 min/week is associated with weight maintenance in obese people.

of dietary calorie reduction, exercise, and behavior therapy. These agents should be used in conjunction with comprehensive obesity treatment. Approved indications by the U.S. Food and Drug Administration for use of antiobesity medications include a BMI ≥30 kg/m² or a BMI ≥27 kg/m² in the presence of other risk factors. Drugs that have received an approved indication for obesity treatment can be divided into two categories: appetite suppression and lipase inhibition. Disappointingly, a meta-analysis by Haddock and colleagues (8) found that in more than 100 clinical trials of weight loss medications, the placebo-subtracted weight loss was a modest ~4 kg and was not durable over time. Several other antiobesity drugs are under investigation, and two drug development approaches are being taken: (a) interfere with hunger and satiety signaling mechanisms or (b) direct adipocyte cytotoxicity resulting in apoptosis and reduction in fat mass (9).

Appetite Suppressants

Appetite suppressants include the sympathomimetic drugs phentermine, diethylpropion, benzphetamine, and phendimetrazine. Sympathomimetic drugs are central nervous system stimulants with pharmacologic activity similar to that of their prototype drugs, the amphetamines. Sibutramine is a nonsympathomimetic appetite suppressant that works via combined norepinephrine and serotonin reuptake inhibition. With the exception of sibutramine, all of the appetite suppressants are indicated for short-term use only. Overall, their effect on weight loss is modest. A meta-analysis of pharmacologic treatment for obesity found that relative to placebo, 12 months of sibutramine treatment resulted in a mean difference in weight loss of 4.45 kg, and 6 months of phentermine and diethylpropion treatment resulted in mean differences in weight loss of 3.6 kg and 3.0 kg, respectively (15).

Intestinal Lipase Inhibition

Orlistat, the only drug approved in the United States that alters fat digestion, inactivates gastric and pancreatic lipases, therefore prohibiting breakdown of dietary fat to absorbable free fatty acids and monoglycerides. This medication has been shown to inhibit dietary fat absorption by up to 30%. Effects on weight loss have been modest. In a meta-analysis of orlistat, the estimate of the mean weight loss for orlistat-treated patients was 2.89 kg at 12 months (15).

Experimental Drugs

Antiobesity medications in the experimental stage include rimonabant, leptin, peptide YY, and oxyntomodulin. Rimonabant is a cannabinoid receptor antagonist. The cannabinoid-1 receptor plays a role in regulation of appetite and body weight. In clinical trials, rimonabant has resulted in clinically meaningful weight loss as well as improvements in several metabolic risk factors. Leptin is a peptide produced primarily by adipose tissue, peptide YY is a gut hormone fragment peptide, and oxyntomodulin is a peptide produced in the L-cells of the gastrointestinal tract. All have been shown to reduce food intake.

Surgical Management

The term *bariatric surgery* is commonly used to describe the surgical management of obesity. The National Institutes of Health Consensus Development panel outlined the indications for bariatric surgery in 1991, and these guidelines continue to be widely used. Patients with a BMI >35 with obesity comorbidities or a BMI >40 regardless of comorbidities are potential candidates per the NIH guidelines (18). Additionally, candidates should have failed previous nonsurgical weight loss attempts, have acceptable medical risk for surgery, and be well informed and motivated. Contraindications to bariatric surgery include significant psychiatric illness that is not well controlled, current substance abuse, or inability to comply with lifelong nutritional requirements including daily vitamin replacement.

Bariatric surgery can induce weight loss by restrictive or malabsorptive mechanisms. Roux-en-Y gastric bypass (RYGB) surgery has both restrictive and malabsorptive mechanisms of action and is the most commonly performed procedure in the United States. The stomach is divided into a small (<30 mL) proximal gastric pouch, and a portion of the proximal small intestine is bypassed. RYGB has shown greater long-term weight reduction than purely restrictive procedures (17).

Laparoscopic adjustable gastric banding (LAGB), a purely restrictive procedure, is gaining in popularity since its approval in the United States in 2001. This is likely attributable to the reversibility and the lower complication rate compared with RYGB. LAGB involves placing a tight, adjustable prosthetic band around the entrance of the stomach.

Clinical trials on bariatric surgery have shown favorable results for significant weight loss, improvement or resolution of obesity comorbidities, and reduction in monthly medication expenses. A meta-analysis that included 136 studies in patients who had undergone a variety of bariatric procedures found a mean overall percentage of excess weight lost of 61% (95% confidence interval 58-64%). Seventy-seven percent of subjects experienced resolution of diabetes, 77% had improvement of hyperlipidemia, 62% had resolution of hypertension, and 86% had resolution of obstructive sleep apnea as a result of bariatric surgery (1).

Summary

The obesity pandemic will be the most important public health problem of this century. The projected rates of diabetes and related comorbidities will likely begin to decrease life expectancy of Western populations. Large public health obesity prevention interventions aimed at promoting and supporting healthy dietary and physical activity habits from infancy through adulthood are greatly needed. The retrievability of a normal body weight becomes less likely as the BMI moves beyond 30 kg/m². In obese people, a multidisciplinary behavior modification approach that includes meal replacement strategies is the most effective nonsurgical approach to obesity. In persons with diabetes who have a BMI ≥35 kg/m² and persons without diabetes who have a BMI ≥40 kg/m², bariatric surgery is the most effective obesity treatment. All forms of obesity treatment must be combined with professionally administered behavior modification and formal exercise training. These methods combined in an integrative manner form the nucleus of an effective weight control center. On the horizon, medical therapy for hunger control and perhaps direct cytotoxic therapy to adipocytes will be a welcome addition to the armamentarium for this difficult and important clinical problem.

CHAPTER 22

Dyslipidemia

J. Larry Durstine, PhD

J. Brent Peel, MS

Dyslipidemia is a primary risk factor in determining cardiovascular disease risk. Over the past 30 years, numerous epidemiological and clinical investigations have been conducted to better understand the relationship between dyslipidemia and atherosclerosis (2, 14, 22). The American Heart Association (AHA) estimates that approximately 107 million Americans have blood cholesterol levels exceeding 200 mg/dL (1). According to guidelines from the National Cholesterol Education Program (NCEP) Adult Treatment Panel (ATP) III, when blood cholesterol level exceeds 240 mg/dL, coronary heart disease (CHD) risk increases dramatically (7). Of the 107 million Americans with elevated blood cholesterol levels, about 38 million have blood cholesterol levels that exceed 240 mg/dL and therefore are considered to be at high risk for CHD events. The remaining 69 million people have blood cholesterol levels between 200 mg/dL and 240 mg/dL and are considered to have borderline–high CHD risk (7).

Investigations have identified key factors that link blood cholesterol, triglycerides, low-density lipoprotein cholesterol (LDL-C), and high-density lipoprotein cholesterol (HDL-C) with clinical manifestations of CHD. These lipid and lipoprotein factors were used by the NCEP to guide the development of medical and lifestyle interventions for the management of dyslipidemia and its related CHD risk. The initiation and progression of atherosclerotic CHD depend heavily on the presence of elevated LDL-C. Therefore, LDL-C is the primary lipoprotein target in the NCEP intervention algorithm (7) (table 22.1).

The evidence in support of elevated triglyceride as an independent risk factor for CHD is less clear. Hypertriglyceridemia appears to be more strongly associated with CHD risk in women than in men (2, 14). Nonetheless, large amounts of triglyceride are found in coronary atherosclerotic plaques, so elevated blood triglyceride levels should be determined when assessing a person's CHD risk (6, 9, 14). Recommendations for classifying levels of blood cholesterol, triglyceride, and LDL-C in regard to CHD risk are summarized in table 22.2.

LDL-C levels are broadly classified into three categories that match a person's CHD risk status with the type and intensity of medical and lifestyle intervention necessary for reducing CHD risk (table 22.1) (7). Because exercise and diet modifications work synergistically to enhance blood lipid and lipoprotein profiles, exercise and diet interventions are the cornerstone lifestyle changes incorporated into the NCEP-ATP III blood lipid management plan. If lifestyle changes do not achieve lipid goals, then pharmacological therapy is recommended. The intensity of drug therapy generally

Address correspondence concerning this chapter to J. Larry Durstine, University of South Carolina, Department of Exercise Science, 1300 Wheat Street, Columbia, SC 29208. E-mail: ldurstine@gwm.sc.edu

TABLE 22.1 Low-Density Lipoprotein Cholesterol (LDL-C) Goals and Cut Points for Therapeutic Lifestyle Changes (TLC) and Drug Therapy in Different Risk Categories

Risk category	LDL-C goal, mg/dL	LDL-C level at which to initiate TLC, mg/dL	LDL-C level at which to consider drug therapy
CHD or CHD risk equivalents (10-year risk >20%)	<100	≥100	≥130 mg/dL (100-129 mg/dL: drug optional)*
≥2 risk factors (10-year risk ≤20%)	<130	≥130	10-year risk 10-20%: ≥130 mgdL 10-year risk <10%: ≥160 mg/dL
≤1 risk factor†	<160	≥160	≥190 mg/dL (160-189 mg/dL: LDL-C-lowering drug optional)

*Some authorities recommend use of LDL-C-lowering drugs in this category if an LDL-C <100 mg/dL cannot be achieved by TLC. Others prefer use of drugs that primarily modify triglycerides and high-density lipoprotein, for example, nicotinic acid or fibric acid derivatives. Clinical judgment also may call for deferring drug therapy in this subcategory.

†Almost all people with ≤1 risk factor have a 10-year risk <10%; thus, 10-year risk assessment in people with ≤1 risk factor is not necessary.

Reprinted from Executive Summary of the Third Report of the National Cholesterol Education Program (NCEP), 2001, "Expert on Detection, Evaluation, and Treatment of High Blood Cholesterol in Adults (Adult Treatment Panel III)," *Journal of American Medical Association* 285: 2486-2497.

TABLE 22.2 Classification of Blood Triglyceride, Total Cholesterol, Low-Density Lipoprotein Cholesterol (LDL-C), and High-Density Lipoprotein Cholesterol (HDL-C) Levels

Range, mg/dL	Classification
TRIGLYCERIDES	
<150	Normal
150-199	Borderline high
200-499	High
≥500	Very high
TOTAL CHOLESTEROL	
<200	Desirable
200-239	Borderline high
≥240	High
LDL-C	
<100	Optimal
100-129	Near or above optimal
130-159	Borderline high
160-189	High
≥190	Very high
HDL-C	
<40	Low
≥60	High

Reprinted from Executive Summary of the Third Report of the National Cholesterol Education Program (NCEP), 2001, "Expert on Detection, Evaluation, and Treatment of High Blood Cholesterol in Adults (Adult Treatment Panel III)," *Journal of American Medical Association* 285: 2486-2497.

depends on whether primary or secondary CHD prevention is being targeted. The degree of lipid management achieved by lifestyle modification also influences the type and intensity of drug therapy.

Pathophysiology

Lipids are hydrophobic (not soluble in water) and do not mix well with body fluids. For lipids to move around the body they must combine with proteins (apolipoproteins) to form micelle particles or lipoproteins. Once formed, lipoproteins are spherical in shape and have a lipid core containing triglyceride, phospholipids, and free and esterified cholesterol surrounded by apolipoproteins. Lipoproteins are classified by density, and density is dictated by both the lipid content and the protein content. Lipoprotein separation is based on density characteristics (table 22.3) and is accomplished primarily through ultracentrifugation and precipitation techniques. Lipoproteins are divided into four major classes: chylomicrons, very low density lipoproteins (VLDL), LDLs, and HDLs. Chylomicrons are the largest particles, whereas HDLs are the smallest particle. Chylomicrons are derived from intestinal absorption of *exogenous dietary fat*

TABLE 22.3 Characteristics of Plasma Lipids and Lipoproteins

Lipid/ lipoprotein	Source	Protein, %	Total lipid, %	TG	Chol	Phosp	Free chol	Apolipoprotein
				COMPOSITION				
				PERCENTAGE OF TOTAL LIPID				
Chylomicron	Intestine	1-2	98-99	88	8	3	1	Major: A-IV, B-48, B-100, H Minor: A-I, A-II, C-I, C-II, C-III, E
VLDL	Major: liver Minor: intestine	7-10	90-93	56	20	15	8	Major: B-100, C-III, E, G Minor: A-I, A-II, B-48, C-II, D
IDL	Major: VLDL Minor: chylomicron	11	89	29	26	34	9	Major: B-100 Minor: B-48
LDL	Major: VLDL Minor: chylomicron	21	79	13	28	48	10	Major: B-100 Minor: C-I, C-II, (a)
HDL$_2$	Major: HDL$_3$	33	67	16	43	31	10	Major: A-1, A-II, D, E, F Minor: A-IV, C-I, C-II, C-III
HDL$_3$	Major: liver and intestine Minor: VLDL and chylomicron remnants	57	43	13	46	29	6	Major: A-1, A-II, D, E, F Minor: A-IV, C-I, C-II, C-III
Chol	Liver and diet		100			70-75	25-30	
TG	Diet and liver		100	100				

VLDL = very low density lipoprotein; IDL = intermediate-density lipoprotein; LDL = low-density lipoprotein; HDL = high-density lipoprotein; Chol = cholesterol; TG = triglyceride; Phosp = phospholipid.

(figure 22.1). Very low density lipoproteins are smaller and denser than chylomicrons and are synthesized primarily by the liver. Some VLDL particles are also derived from chylomicron breakdown (figure 22.1). Liver VLDLs are mostly responsible for movement of endogenous triglyceride. LDL particles represent the final stage of catabolism of VLDL and are the primary carrier of cholesterol. Intermediate-density lipoprotein (IDL) and lipoprotein(a) [Lp(a)] are intermediate steps in this pathway and are LDL subfractions. Other LDL subfractions include small and large particles (the smaller, denser particles are more atherogenic than the larger, less dense particles). HDL particles are involved in transporting cholesterol from all areas in the body back to the liver for degradation and disposal. This process, known as *reverse cholesterol transport*, is a major cardioprotective function of HDL because it counters the atherogenic effects of LDL within the arterial wall. HDL particles often are studied by their subfractions; the larger and less dense HDL$_2$ (cardioprotection is associated with HDL$_2$) and the smaller more dense HDL$_3$ particles.

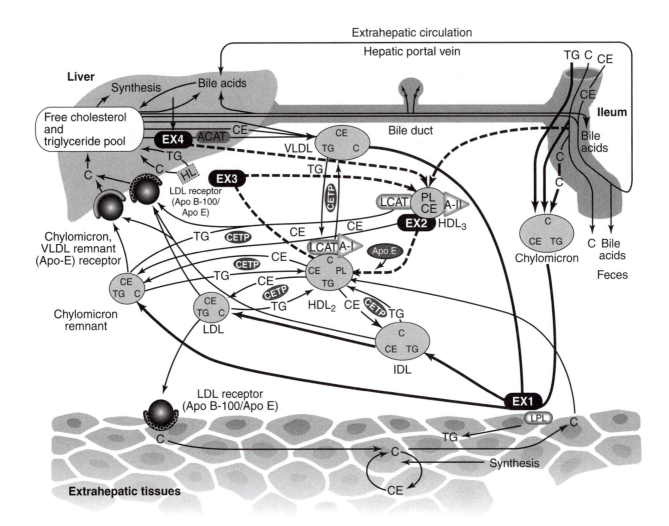

FIGURE 22.1   Transport of cholesterol and triglyceride between tissues in humans. PL = phospholipid; C = free cholesterol; CE = cholesteryl ester; TG = triglyceride; VLDL = very low density lipoprotein; IDL = intermediate-density lipoprotein; LDL = low-density lipoprotein; HDL = high-density lipoprotein; ACAT = acyl-CoA:cholesterol acyltransferase; LCAT = lecithin:cholesterol transfer protein; LPL = lipoprotein lipase; HL = hepatic lipase; CETP = cholesteryl ester transfer protein; A-I = apolipoprotein A-I; A-II = apolipoprotein A-II; Apo B-100 = apolipoprotein B-100; Apo E = apolipoprotein E. Heavy dark lines indicate major pathways, and lighter lines indicate minor pathways. EX1 to EX4 are points where exercise has a potential impact on lipoprotein metabolism: EX1 is the site for reduced synthesis of triglyceride, EX2 is the site for enhanced activity of LPL, EX3 is the site for enhanced LCAT activity, and EX4 represents enhanced reverse cholesterol transport.

Adapted, by permission, from J.L. Durstine and W.L. Haskell, 1994, "Effects of exercise training on plasma lipids and lipoproteins," *Exercise in Sport Science Review* 22: 447-521.

Several key enzymes regulate intravascular lipoprotein metabolism: lipoprotein lipase (LPL), hepatic lipase, lecithin-cholesterol acyltransferase (LCAT), and cholesterol ester transfer protein. Together with plasma lipoproteins, these enzymes foster the movement and exchange of triglyceride and cholesterol among lipoproteins, the intestine, the liver, and the extrahepatic tissue. Several lipoprotein metabolic pathways exist; however, the LDL receptor pathway and reverse cholesterol transport account for most of the cholesterol and triglyceride movement in the blood. When the function of these pathways is disturbed, either genetically or through adverse environmental influences, dyslipidemia results and CHD risk is increased.

Dyslipidemia is defined as the consequence of a variety of genetic, environmental, and pathologic factors resulting in elevated blood cholesterol and triglyceride levels. Factors associated with dyslipidemia include gender, age, body fat distribution, cigarette smoking, use of some medications, genetic inheritance, dietary habits, and physical inactivity.

Hypertriglyceridemia

Hypertriglyceridemia is defined as blood concentrations of triglyceride that exceed 150 mg/dL (7). Table 22.2 provides guidelines for characterizing the severity of hypertriglyceridemia. Although the primary causes for severe hypertriglyceridemia are related to genetic defects in triglyceride metabolism, secondary factors are physical inactivity, obesity, diabetes mellitus, smoking, high dietary fat intake, hyperthyroidism, and nephritic syndrome.

Postprandial Lipemia

Postprandial lipemia is the amount of time required for the removal of chylomicrons and their movement into extrahepatic tissue and chylomicron remnants by the liver. Exaggerated postprandial lipemia is believed to adversely affect endothelial function and therein contribute to atherosclerotic plaque formation. In apparently healthy persons, postprandial triglyceride levels return to baseline levels within 8 to 10 hr after consumption of dietary fat. Exaggerated or very prolonged postprandial hyperlipemia increases CHD risk (23).

Hypercholesterolemia

Hypercholesterolemia is a metabolic disorder leading to the presence of high blood cholesterol and LDL-C levels. Familial heterozygous hypercholesterolemia (affecting 1 in every 500 persons) is a genetic condition resulting in the inability of the LDL receptor to move cholesterol into body cells. This condition may be caused by a defective cell receptor that down-regulates LDL-C removal from the blood or it may occur because the blood LDL particles do not have the proper apolipoproteins to bind to LDL receptors in the cell membrane. Irrespective of the underlying cause, afflicted people have marked elevations in blood cholesterol and LDL-C and are at high risk for premature CHD.

High LDL-C

LDL-C is a product of the breakdown of chylomicrons and VLDLs by the action of the endothelial enzyme LPL. The resulting VLDL remnants and IDL particles are further hydrolyzed in a reaction catalyzed by LPL, eventually producing LDL particles (figure 22.1). LDL particles are normally removed from the blood through the interaction with LDL receptors found on all cells. Defects in this pathway can lead to elevated plasma LDL-C concentration. Diets high in saturated fat, trans fat, and cholesterol cause reductions in LDL liver receptors, prevent the catabolism of blood LDL, and result in increased blood LDL-C (see chapter 18 regarding dietary factors).

Lipoprotein(a) is a specific form of LDL that contains apolipoprotein A (ApoA) and is very similar in chemical makeup to blood protein plasminogen. Because of the structural similarities between Lp(a) and plasminogen, Lp(a) functionally competes with plasminogen for binding sites on fibrin and thereby inhibits fibrinolysis. Present information suggest that Lp(a) concentrations greater than 25 mg/dL are associated with an increased risk for premature CHD (13).

Low HDL-C

HDL-C levels are inversely associated with CHD risk independent of cholesterol and LDL-C levels. HDL, the smallest lipoprotein, is composed of primarily cholesteryl esters and some triglyceride. ApoA-I, a major component of all HDL particles, is synthesized by the liver and intestine. Primary causes of low HDL-C are genetic and include ApoA-I deficiencies and mutations, LCAT deficiency, Tangier disease, and familial hypoalphalipoproteinemia. In addition, low HDL-C is attributed to numerous secondary causes including central obesity, cigarette smoking, physical inactivity, and very low fat diets. Lipid disorders such as hypertriglyceridemia are associated with low HDL-C levels, as is the use of medication such as androgenic steroids, β-blocking agents, and progestins.

Diagnosis and Management

The first NCEP guidelines were developed in 1988, and subsequent versions of these guidelines have provided the scientific rationale for diagnosing dyslipidemia and for managing adults with high cholesterol and other dyslipidemias. These guidelines provide a strategy for primary and secondary CHD prevention primarily by targeting LDL-C assessment and treatment (7). Presently dyslipidemias are classified as hypercholesterolemia, hypertriglyceridemia, or combined hypercholesterolemia and hypertriglyceridemia. Whereas in the past, dyslipidemias were classified with elevated lipoprotein groups by the Frederick classification system, the recent NCEP guidelines give very specific clinical cut points indicative of relative CHD risk (table 22.1).

Screening for dyslipidemia begins with quantification of lipoprotein levels after an 8 to 12 hr fast. Cholesterol and HDL-C levels are usually measured every 5 years beginning at age 20 in patients who do not have CHD (7). LDL-C levels may be measured directly or may be estimated using the Friedwald formula (LDL-C = blood cholesterol – HDL-C – [triglyceride/5]) (10). This formula is not used when a person's triglyceride levels exceed 400 mg/dL. Depending on the results of initial measurement and the presence of other CHD risk factors, more frequent and more comprehensive lipoprotein assessments may be warranted.

The NCEP provides treatment guidelines for the management of plasma lipids and lipoproteins. Exercise, dietary modification, and weight loss are recommended as the initial therapy for at least 6 weeks. Pharmacologic therapy is based primarily on LDL-C levels (table 22.1). A core principle of the NCEP ATP III treatment guidelines is to match the initiation and intensity of therapy with a person's CHD risk status (e.g., 10-year probability of a CHD event), which is determined using a multiple risk factor prediction model such as the Framingham Risk Score (7).

Impact of a Single Exercise Session and Exercise Training

Regular exercise participation can benefit people with normal lipid and lipoprotein concentrations as well as most persons with dyslipidemia. This section discusses the benefits of a single exercise session and exercise training. A single exercise session is also referred to as a single exercise bout or period, whereas exercise training consists of a series of exercise sessions strung together over a period of months or years. The following discussion revolves around aerobic exercise.

Triglycerides and Exercise

The effects of a single exercise session on triglyceride concentrations are similar to those found for exercise training (3). Most well-conducted studies report reduced triglyceride concentrations after a single aerobic exercise session. These beneficial blood triglyceride reductions usually occur 24 hr after exercise and can last up to 72 hr postexercise.

Plasma triglyceride concentrations typically decrease after exercise training (table 22.4). Cross-sectional and longitudinal exercise training studies normally report decreases in plasma triglyceride concentrations, but not always (18). Exercise training–induced reductions in plasma triglycerides are related to baseline concentrations; previously inactive people with high baseline concentrations experience large reductions in plasma triglycerides (18), whereas people with lower initial baseline concentrations experience smaller reductions (21).

Postprandial Lipemia and Exercise

Investigators have reported that a single exercise session (both endurance and resistance) performed 12 to 24 hr before a meal decreased the magnitude of postprandial lipemia (4, 11). The magnitude of reduction of postprandial lipemia was primarily related to total energy expended during the previous exercise sessions, whether the exercise was performed in a single exercise session or in several intermittent sessions (23). Neither exercise intensity nor duration was a key factor in effecting the postprandial lipemia response; rather, the total energy expenditure (e.g., exercise volume) appeared to be the most important factor (23). Prior exercise training also affected the postprandial triglyceride response (23). Sedentary people may expect beneficial improvements in circulating lipids and lipoproteins from a single exercise session when 500 kcal is expended, whereas trained people may need to expend 800 kcal or more to elicit similar changes (11).

Blood Cholesterol and Exercise

Research evidence does not support changes in plasma blood cholesterol immediately after or in the days following a short-duration single exercise session (e.g., less than 30 min/day). However, some evidence does support changes in plasma blood cholesterol concentration immediately after and in the days following

TABLE 22.4 **Lipid and Lipoprotein Changes Associated With Exercise**

Lipid or lipoprotein	Single exercise session	Exercise training
Triglyceride	Decreases of 7-69% Approximate mean change 20%	Decrease of 4-37% Approximate mean change 24%
Cholesterol	No change*	No change†
LDL-C	No change	No change
Small, dense LDL-C particles	Literature unclear	Can increase LDL particle size, usually associated with triglyceride lowering
Lp(a)	No change	No change
HDL-C	Increase of 4-18% Approximate mean change 10%	Increase of 4-18% Approximate mean change 8%

LDL = low-density lipoprotein; HDL = high-density lipoprotein; Lp(a) = lipoprotein(a).

*No change unless the exercise session is prolonged.

†No change if body weight and diet do not change.

a very prolonged exercise session (e.g., marathon or triathlon), but only when a very large amount of energy is expended (18).

Neither cross-sectional nor longitudinal exercise training studies support an exercise-induced change in plasma blood cholesterol concentration (18, 21). When exercise training studies reported reductions in blood cholesterol concentration, these reductions were not related to either the baseline cholesterol concentration or the length of the exercise training program. Reduced body fat percentage was observed in some but not all studies that reported decreased cholesterol concentration. Blood cholesterol reductions occurring after an exercise training program were usually accompanied by reductions in body weight, percentage body fat, or dietary fat consumption.

LDL-C and Exercise

LDL-C levels are usually not affected after a single short-duration exercise session. However, after a prolonged exercise session, LDL-C levels may remain unchanged or may be lower (32). Studies reporting a decreased LDL-C level have typically used prolonged exercise in which a large amount of energy is expended. For example, Ferguson and colleagues (8) found that 1,300 kcal of energy expenditure after a single exercise session was associated with decreased LDL-C levels.

Plasma LDL-C is usually not changed after aerobic exercise training programs, but in some instances reductions have been noted (32). LDL particles are divided into several different subfractions, each having

different degrees of CHD risk. The smaller, more dense LDL particles correlate directly with CHD and are also associated with elevated triglyceride concentrations. Exercise training studies have reported differing effects on these smaller, dense LDL particles. Kraus and colleagues (19) recently reported that moderate-intensity exercise equivalent to the energy expenditure of running 17 to 18 miles/week decreased concentrations of small LDL and the number of LDL particles while increasing the size of the larger LDL particles. Overall plasma LDL-C remained unchanged. Williams and colleagues (30) found no change in small, dense LDL particles after 1 year of exercise training in overweight men, whereas Halle and colleagues (13) found lower triglyceride and small LDL particles in hypercholesterolemic men as physical activity levels increased.

Lp(a) and Exercise

Elevated Lp(a) concentrations greater than 25 mg/dL are associated with increased CHD risk. Lp(a) is an inherited trait and does not appear to change following a single exercise session or after regular physical activity participation (5, 15). Medications such as niacin can reduce Lp(a) levels (5).

HDL-C and Exercise

Data suggest that a single exercise session can change HDL-C and that the exercise volume necessary for HDL-C change is different for trained and sedentary people (4, 11). Exercise-trained people require an exercise energy expenditure of 1,100 kcal to significantly elevate HDL-C concentrations (5), whereas an energy expenditure of 500 kcal elicits significant elevations of HDL-C in sedentary people (11).

Exercise training programs lasting longer than 12 weeks usually increase HDL-C in a dose–response manner when exercise meets a certain threshold of energy expenditure, but not always (20, 21). Factors considered when evaluating HDL-C exercise training response include the exercise training volume as measured by the amount of calories expended during the exercise training program, body weight and body composition changes, and dietary changes (5). HDL-C exercise training–induced increases range from 4% to 22%, whereas the absolute HDL-C changes are more uniform and range from 2 to 8 mg/dL (table 22.4). Evidence suggests that an inverse correlation exists between initial HDL-C levels and the change in HDL-C after an exercise training program (17). Significant correlations have been established between distance run per week, time spent in exercise training, and the subsequent change in HDL-C concentrations. This relationship provides support for the strong positive relationship between exercise training volume and HDL-C change (17). Contrary to the popular notion that exercise-induced reductions in body weight or body fat are responsible for improvements in cholesterol levels, several studies reported that reductions in body weight or body fat are not prerequisites for significant changes in HDL-C. Thompson and colleagues (27, 29), whose subjects followed special diets with supplements to maintain body weight and body fat percentage during an exercise training program, found that exercise training resulted in HDL-C increases of 8 mg/dL and 3 mg/dL. Wood and colleagues (31) administered a weight loss program using caloric restriction alone or in combination with exercise training and found that body weight and percent body fat decreased in both groups whereas HDL-C increased only in the exercise-trained group. These studies support that exercise training with or without reductions in body weight or body fat can increase HDL-C, and this HDL-C increase may be augmented by reductions in percentage body fat and body weight.

ApoE Genotypes and Exercise

Studies suggest that the ApoE genotype has important implications in regard to exercise training adaptations. Taimela and colleagues (25) found no relationship between physical activity and ApoE phenotypes in women. Conversely, St-Amand and colleagues (24) reported significant interactions between physical activity, lipids and lipoproteins, and ApoE polymorphism among men. Hagberg and colleagues (12) found significantly decreased triglyceride concentrations in ApoE2 and ApoE3 subjects, whereas HDL-C increases were greater in only the ApoE2 subjects. Thompson and colleagues (28) reported that ApoE polymorphisms affect the lipid response after 6 months of exercise training. The LDL-C to HDL-C ratio in subjects with the ApoE3 homozygotes was decreased, but not for subjects with the ApoE4 allele. These studies provide support that exercise training is most effective at reducing blood triglycerides while increasing HDL-C and LPL activity in persons who have an impaired ability to clear triglyceride or subjects having an ApoE2 phenotype. Furthermore, these studies provide additional support that subjects who are homozygous for ApoE3 experience the most beneficial lipid changes as a result of exercise training.

Nutritional Management

Dietary intervention is important for altering blood lipid and lipoprotein levels (9). For a complete review of nutritional factors that affect LDL-C, refer to chapter 18. Because dietary cholesterol increases LDL-C levels, the primary strategy to reduce LDL-C is to replace cholesterol-raising foods (e.g., foods high in saturated and trans fatty acids) in the diet with complex carbohydrates or unsaturated fatty acids (9). An 8% to 10% reduction in LDL-C levels is expected with the adoption of diets low in saturated fat. An additional 3% to 5% decrease in LDL-C is found when dietary cholesterol is also reduced (7). The American Heart Association (9) issued the following dietary recommendations for achieving a desirable blood lipid profile:

- Limit food high in saturated fat.
- Replace saturated fat with lower-fat food.
- Increase food with unsaturated fat.
- Monitor intake of food high in cholesterol.
- Limit foods containing trans fatty acids.
- Increase food with viscous fiber.
- Increase foods containing plant stanols and sterols.

Increasing dietary consumption of soluble fiber and plant sterols is also recommended to enhance LDL-C lowering (7). Increases in soluble fiber of 5 to 10 g/day reduce LDL-C by 3% to 5%. The addition of 2 g/day of plant sterols reduces LDL-C by 6% to 15% (7).

HDL-C levels are improved by favorable dietary fatty acid composition and by interventions like exercise that reduce plasma triglyceride. Weight loss also improves HDL-C levels because increased weight and increased obesity both contribute to low HDL-C levels. Elevated triglyceride levels are a significant component of atherogenic dyslipidemia common among patients with diabetes, patients with metabolic syndrome, and people who are obese (7). The NCEP ATP III recommends reducing triglyceride levels to reduce CHD risk (7).

Excessive adiposity is a factor for atherogenic dyslipidemia, whereas dietary carbohydrates are a major determinant of elevated blood triglycerides. Hyperglycemia and hyperinsulemia contribute to dyslipidemia, and therefore replacing intake of simple sugars and rapidly hydrolyzed starches with complex carbohydrates and fiber may attenuate elevated triglyceride levels. A diet moderate in fat content (25-35% of total energy intake), high in complex carbohydrates, and high in fiber aids in lowering triglyceride levels, increasing both HDL-C levels and the larger, less dense, and less atherogenic LDL particles (9).

Pharmacologic Therapy

Pharmacological therapy is highly effective and generally well tolerated and is a core component for lowering blood lipids and lipoproteins. For a detailed review of pharmacology and cardiovascular disease, see chapter 10. In contrast, the effectiveness of hygienic therapies (therapies that have positive health benefits) including exercise, diet, and weight loss is greatly limited by patient compliance. Few patients achieve desired lipid levels by hygienic therapy alone; rather, most patients will require lipid-lowering medication to reduce blood lipids and lipoproteins. Because exercise profoundly decreases plasma triglycerides while improving glucose intolerance, which both contribute to reducing dyslipidemia, hygienic therapies are recommended for all patients under treatment for lipid disorders and are considered to be adjunctive to pharmacologic therapy in the management of blood lipid and lipoprotein.

HMG CoA Reductase Inhibitors (Statins)

Hydroxymethylglutaryl coenzyme A (HMG CoA) reductase inhibitors, or statins, are the first choice of medical therapy for patients with high LDL-C levels (7). Statins are the most effective and best tolerated drugs for reducing LDL-C. These drugs inhibit the liver enzyme HMG CoA, which regulates the rate of cholesterol synthesis. Inhibiting this enzyme lowers liver cholesterol synthesis and also increases liver cell surface LDL receptors, which also increase the liver's removal of blood LDL-C.

Six statins (atorvastatin, fluvastatin, lovastatin, pravastatin, rosuvastatin, simvastatin) are available in the United States. These medications when taken at their maximal dose reduce LDL-C by 20% to 60% and also reduce primary and secondary CHD events (7). Ezetimibe is a cholesterol absorption inhibitor and is also available in combination with the statin drug simvastatin. Ezetimibe acts at the brush border in the intestine to limit absorption of dietary cholesterol and primarily lowers LDL-C. It has little effect on triglycerides or HDL-C.

Various side effects are attributed to statin use including hepatotoxicity and myopathy. However, these side effects are rare. Other, less often reported side effects from statin use include muscle pain and discomfort. This muscle pain is associated with muscle protein and tissue breakdown and can lead to rhabdomyolysis, which is characterized by excessive muscle tissue breakdown and increased by-products found in the blood. Excessive amounts of these products in the blood can lead to acute renal failure and damage the kidney. Coenzyme Q-10 (ubiquinone) has been used to reduce statin-associated side effects (26). Because rhabdomyolysis may occur when statins are used in combination with other medications such as fibric acid derivatives, niacin, cyclosporine, and certain antibiotics, physicians rarely prescribe these medications in any combination.

The consumption of grapefruit or grapefruit juice should be minimized when taking statins. Grapefruit juice consumption reduces stain clearance from the blood and results in higher blood statin levels (16). Elevated blood statin levels can lead to induced liver myopathy and potential liver damage (26).

Bile Acid Sequestrants (Resins)

Bile acid sequestrants or resins are administered as a powdered resin dissolved in liquid or as a tablet. Three bile acid sequestrants are available: cholestyramine, colesevelam, and colestipol. If statins fail to achieve desired lipid level, bile acid sequestrants are administered. Resins inhibit the intestinal reabsorption of bile and its transport in the portal circulation to the liver. The loss of bile stimulates the up-regulation of hepatic LDL receptor activity, which in turn reduces plasma LDL-C concentration. The most common side effects of bile acid sequestrants are gastrointestinal related and include abdominal pain, constipation, bloating, and flatulence.

Fibric Acid Derivatives (Fibrates)

Fibrates are useful in reducing elevated triglyceride levels. Two fibrates are available in the United States: gemifibrozil and fenofibrate. Fibrates are normally well tolerated with few adverse side effects. In patients with hypertriglyceridemia, LDL-C levels can increase slightly because fibrates increase LPL activity, facilitating the breakdown of VLDL to LDL. Because fibrates when used in combination with statin therapy may produce rhabdomyolysis, this combination is often reserved for patients with high-risk CHD in whom the benefits exceed the risks. Fibrates also enhance the effects of other medications like the anticoagulant warfarin.

Niacin or Nicotinic Acid

Niacin is extremely useful in patients with low HDL-C levels with or without elevated triglycerides. Niacin has many potential areas of action, but its primary effect is inhibiting lipolysis. The most important niacin effect is an increased HDL-C, but decreased LDL-C also may be seen. Niacin supplementation is one of only a few ways to reduce Lp(a). A common adverse side effect associated with large doses of niacin is cutaneous flushing, which for many patients can dissuade its use. For some patients, the use of low daily doses either reduces or eliminates flushing. In other cases, flushing is reduced with the use of delayed-release niacin preparations. Also, because flushing is prostaglandin medi-ated, the effects are minimized by taking aspirin before the niacin dosage. Niacin also may produce reversible hepatitis, activate gout attributable to increased uric acid levels, produce peptic ulcers, and lead to or worsen glucose intolerance. As with several other drug therapies, patients undergoing niacin therapy must have liver function tests performed regularly to monitor the occurrence of adverse side effects.

Summary

Lipids and lipoproteins have prominent roles in the pathogenesis of CHD. Treatment guidelines for management of lipid and lipoprotein disorders are provided by the NCEP ATP III. Dietary modification, weight loss, and exercise interventions are recommended for the initial 6 weeks followed by pharmacological therapy of sufficient intensity to achieve desired lipid and lipoprotein goals. Scientific information provides strong evidence that regular exercise participation results in beneficial lipid and lipoprotein profile changes. Investigations are focusing on the molecular basis for lipid and lipoprotein changes in response to various interventions including exercise. These new studies should provide a better understanding of why some people respond to exercise whereas others do not. Clinicians should use this new information, coupled with the known effects of exercise on blood lipids and lipoproteins and the mechanisms responsible for these changes, to develop comprehensive individual medical management plans that will optimize pharmacological agents and adjunctive therapies.

CHAPTER 23

Arthritis

A. Lynn Millar, PhD

Exercise management in cardiovascular disease traditionally has emphasized screening and prescription for vascular indexes. However, failure to consider musculoskeletal limitations can undermine the potential benefits of a cardiac rehabilitation program. One of the most common factors that limit musculoskeletal function is the presence of arthritis. Arthritis is, more frequently than cardiac or pulmonary disease, the primary limitation on a person's ability to undertake physical activity. Approximately 43 million people in the United States have physician-diagnosed arthritis, and these numbers are expected to increase substantially within the next few decades (4). There are more than 100 types of arthritides, which can be subclassified as systemic or joint specific. More than 85% of those with arthritis have osteoarthritis (OA; joint specific), followed by rheumatoid arthritis (RA), fibromyalgia, and spondylopathies.

Arthritis interacts with cardiovascular disease both as a conditional risk factor and as a potential impediment to the exercise component of cardiac rehabilitation. Arthritis and cardiovascular disease share common risk factors that include excess body weight, age, and insufficient activity (5). Aerobic capacity is significantly lower in persons who have arthritis (both OA and RA) compared with similar-aged people without arthritis (15). In addition, recent studies have shown that people with rheumatoid arthritis have an increased risk of cardiovascular disease, diabetes, and hypertension (11). Although the cause of this increased risk has not been identified, the alteration in the immune system that is part of the systemic arthritides may provide an explanation, along with the other risk factors. People with ankylosing spondylitis (AS) have higher rates of aortic root and valve disease, which contribute to heart failure and stroke (18).

Pathophysiology

Joint pain and stiffness, usually with associated joint degeneration, are the primary symptoms of all of the arthritides. Over the long term, this results in loss of joint range of motion (ROM) and functional mobility. The pathophysiology that causes the joint degeneration is best addressed as joint specific or systemic. Joint-specific arthritis—osteoarthritis—is degeneration of the cartilage within one joint. The most common joints to be affected are the weight-bearing joints, thus the hips and knees. Often characterized as *wear-and-tear arthritis* associated with age, the risk of osteoarthritis is increased by several factors.

When a joint is injured or inflamed and painful because of arthritis, it is common to find muscle inhibition, or the inability of a muscle to contract. This inability is mediated by afferent nerves that inhibit central neural command (to prevent pain) or by reflex neural pathways that block efferent motor command to the muscle. The combination of muscle inhibition and decreased muscle strength is thought to alter the joint

Address correspondence concerning this chapter to A. Lynn Millar, Department of Physical Therapy, Andrews University, Berrien Springs, MI 49104. E-mail: lmillar@andrews.edu mechanics (21). Other risk factors specific to osteoarthritis include previous joint injury and malalignment of the joint (20). It is believed that these factors all result in abnormal load bearing of the cartilage and acceleration of the degeneration process.

The pathology of the systemic arthritides is variable but generally appears to include abnormalities in immune function. With rheumatoid arthritis, alterations in immune function affect the synovial fluid and tissues, leading to degeneration of the joint cartilage. Because of the systemic inflammation and immune response, pathologic changes are eventually evident in the cardiovascular system. Fibromyalgia does not have a pathophysiology that is as easily distinguished. Rather than affecting the joints, pain primarily affects the muscle tissues. Ankylosing spondylitis, the most common of the spondylopathies, is a systemic arthritis that targets the vertebral column. Loss of motion between the vertebrae occurs and eventually results in fusion of these joints, which can impair circulatory function, especially to the brain.

Diagnosis

The American College of Rheumatology (ACR) has identified diagnostic criteria for the various arthritides. During the early stages, osteoarthritis is often a self-diagnosis, based on the signs and symptoms of stiffness and pain with movement. Many people with osteoarthritis do not seek medical attention until they have significant pain that they are unable to control with over-the-counter medications or until they have a significant loss of function. The ACR guidelines for osteoarthritis vary slightly by joint; for example, in the knee, diagnosis is based on clinical and laboratory results (positive for 5 of 9 criteria), clinical and radiographic results (positive for 1 of 3 criteria), or clinical observation (positive for 3 of 6 criteria). Clinical criteria for osteoarthritis of the knee are as follows (1):

- Age greater than 50 years
- Stiffness lasting less than 30 min
- Crepitus (grating or crackling feeling within the joint)
- Bony tenderness
- Bony enlargement
- No palpable warmth of the joint

There are seven criteria for RA (2), four of which a patient must meet for a positive diagnosis. These criteria are as follows (2):

- Morning stiffness lasting ≥1 hr for ≥6 weeks
- Soft tissue swelling in three or more joints for ≥6 weeks
- Swelling in the proximal finger or wrist joints for ≥6 weeks
- Symmetric swelling for ≥6 weeks
- Rheumatoid nodules
- Positive rheumatoid factor
- X ray showing joint erosions or osteopenia in hand or wrist

In contrast to OA and RA, which have very specific diagnostic criteria, fibromyalgia is often a diagnosis of exclusion, with the criteria for a positive diagnosis including widespread pain in combination with tenderness at 11 or more of 18 specific sites (24). Ankylosing spondylitis is diagnosed using the patient's history, spinal X rays, and positive blood markers. Markers used in the diagnosis of several of the arthritides that also are associated with increased cardiovascular risk include blood levels of C-reactive protein and erythrocyte sedimentation rate. Human leukocyte antigen-B27 also is used in arthritis diagnosis.

Medications

Medications for arthritis focus on pain relief, inflammation control, disease modification, and biologic agents (i.e., some medications simulate biologic substances already in the body). Acetaminophen is often used for initial pain relief, but the most common medications for symptom relief with osteoarthritis are the nonsteroidal anti-inflammatories (NSAIDs). Over-the-counter medications within this category include aspirin, ibuprofen, and naproxen. For more severe pain, a second class of drugs, called cyclooxygenase-2 (COX-2) inhibitors, have proven effective; however, the side effects are potentially more serious and may include increased risk of cardiovascular events. Side effects of all the NSAIDs include gastrointestinal distress and the potential for gastrointestinal bleeding. Newer aspirins come with digestive buffers, and many physicians prescribe digestive buffers with other anti-inflammatory medications. The COX-2 inhibitors are less likely to cause gastrointestinal problems than are NSAIDs but have other side effects that include the potential for allergic reaction and liver damage. Some brands of COX-2 inhibitors were recently taken off of the market because of an increased risk of death from cardiovascular causes. Both NSAIDs and COX-2 inhibitors have been identified as potential causes of resistant hypertension, which increases the risk of cardiovascular disease. (17)

A third class of medications for osteoarthritis of the knee are synovial fluid supplements. These medications are a synthetic form of hyaluronic acid, which is the key component of joint synovial fluid. Hyaluronic acid has viscoelastic properties that enhance its lubricant and shock-absorbing functions. Synthetic synovial fluids injected directly into the joint space have been associated with diminished pain and a slower progression of joint destruction. The biological mechanisms of these compounds are not well understood.

Medications used by those with systemic arthritis include *disease-modifying antirheumatic drugs* (DMARDs) and several medications commonly called *biologics*, which mimic natural immune-modulating substances. Both of these types of drugs decrease the swelling and, more important, slow the progression of joint damage. Side effects are potentially serious and include an increased susceptibility to infections attributable to suppression of the natural immune response. The DMARDs can cause kidney or liver damage and carry a slightly increased risk of cancer. Some of the biologics are injected and can cause a reaction at the injection site.

Management

Arthritis may be an important consideration in both exercise testing and exercise training of cardiovascular patients. As previously noted, people with RA have a higher risk of heart disease, hypertension, and diabetes, and those with AS also have increased cardiovascular disease risk. Thus, thorough screening should take place prior to exercise testing and should include an assessment of signs and symptoms related to the previously mentioned cardiovascular conditions.

To ensure that an adequate stress is placed on the cardiovascular system during exercise testing, the selection of exercise test should address which joints are affected and the degree of joint involvement. Although OA is joint specific, with many older people both knees and hips may be involved. If the knee or hip motion is severely limited, a bicycle test or upper-body ergometry test may be indicated. For people with RA, the joints may also be swollen, thus limiting motion and causing significant pain. For those with severe joint disease, pharmacological stress testing offers a viable alternative to the exercise test.

Another consideration prior to exercise testing is lower-extremity strength and possibly muscle inhibition. People with arthritis often have decreased lower-extremity strength compared with people of a similar age who do not have arthritis. Decreased strength translates to poorer function, poorer balance, and increased pain (13). In addition, muscle inhibition could contribute to the sensation of "giving way," when the individual's knee temporarily fails to hold an extended position during weight bearing (10). Although knee extension strength is vital to normal gait, a rapid assessment of functional hip and ankle strength will give the clinician a better idea of a person's ability to perform a walking, bicycle, or upper-body exercise test.

Lower-extremity stability is often decreased concurrent with the changes in joint alignment and muscle strength. Stability and alignment of the joint should be assessed, because these directly affect a person's ability to safely participate in some activities. If a patient has lower-extremity instability, a bicycle test may be safer than a treadmill test. Malalignment of the joint is another issue related to progression of arthritis. Joint alignment and stability need to be protected so the individual can safely complete the exercise test or safely participate in the prescribed exercise.

Exercise Modifications

The exercise training component of a cardiac rehabilitation program may need to be modified for patients who also have arthritis. Potential areas for modification for each of the basic training areas (aerobic, resistance, and flexibility) are addressed in the following sections. In addition, some disease-related problems associated with exercise for this population are highlighted.

Aerobic Training

The primary concerns regarding exercise for those with arthritis have included potential exacerbation of symptoms and systemic inflammation and progression of joint degeneration. Many of the early studies addressed these concerns by using exercise doses well below ACSM guidelines (14, 15). Because these early studies reported positive effects of exercise, more recent studies included training regimens that were more intense. Munneke and colleagues (16) showed that people with rheumatoid arthritis were able to participate in a long-term, dynamic exercise program following ACSM guidelines, including a cardiovascular intensity that increased from 70% to 81% over 24 weeks (23). The investigators showed that progression of joint damage was independent of participation in the high-intensity program. There was an interaction between the baseline joint damage and activity;

participants with initially higher levels of joint damage had a faster rate of progressive joint damage. Follow-up analysis showed that the shoulder and subtalar joints also had additional damage. The authors concluded that most of those with RA could safely take part in high-intensity exercise, noting that bicycle exercise was the primary mode of cardiovascular training. Given these findings and others showing that malalignment of the joint can contribute to the progression of joint damage (20), bicycle training is the recommended mode for those with advanced lower-extremity arthritis or with significant lower-extremity malalignment.

Aquatic training has not shown significant changes in cardiovascular fitness; however, most of the studies have used the National Arthritis Foundation Program, which emphasizes joint movement. Melton-Rogers and colleagues (12) examined the effects of running in the water compared with bicycle riding on cardiovascular responses and exercise-related pain. Although the authors found similar cardiovascular benefits between the two activities, they did not find any difference in the pain levels reported during exercise. If alignment can be maintained and the participant has adequate ROM, walking and jogging are safe exercise modes. Intensity should be dictated by the participant's cardiovascular status and activity level. Frequency and duration should follow ACSM guidelines, with initial modifications based on the participant's activity and fitness level.

Resistance Training

As noted previously, lower-extremity weakness is related to decreased function, rapid progression of joint damage, and increased pain. Numerous studies have shown that patients with OA and RA experience significant improvements in function and pain with resistance training (3, 6-8). The types of resistance exercise and the intensity vary greatly. Even the more intense programs (70-80% of 1RM) have not reported detrimental effects. Studies that examined markers of disease activity reported decreases in disease activity following exercise training. Deyle and colleagues (6) noted that at the 1-year follow-up, the control group in their study had 15% more total knee replacements compared with those who received the exercise intervention. In their 5-year follow-up, Häkkinen and colleagues (7) found that subjects who had participated in the supervised exercise program maintained their strength improvements and that there was a significant difference in disease activity between exercisers and controls.

Modifications to resistance training include initial intensity, range of motion during the lift, body and joint position, and type of movement. If a participant has significant lower-extremity weakness and pain, decreasing the initial intensity to 40% of 1RM and using slightly more repetitions will help the participant adapt to the workload without exacerbating symptoms. Intensity can be progressively increased to 70% to 80% of 1RM, depending on the goals of the training program. For people with more severe joint damage, the joint range of motion is often limited. Motions that stress extreme range of motion, at either end of the movement, should be avoided. Such joint positions are usually painful and unstable. Even if the joint motion is kept to the middle ranges, some movements, such as a traditional squat, may put an increased torque through the joint. A simple modification of the squat position, such as sitting against a wall with the knees bent at a 90° angle and the feet away from the wall, can reduce the torque in the knee joint and strengthen the quadriceps without increasing joint pain. Open-chain resistance movements also may cause pain with high intensity levels.

Flexibility

The primary symptoms of arthritis are muscle stiffness and joint pain. Range of motion (ROM) for people with arthritis can be 20% to 60% of normal and is related to function. A relevant distinction is that of flexibility versus ROM. Flexibility refers to the way in which muscles affect motion, whereas ROM is the actual motion that is available at the joint. The available ROM is a composite function of the muscle's effect both on motion (i.e., the muscle's elasticity and ability to relax) and on mechanical limitations at the joint attributable to arthritis and other anatomical alterations. ACSM guidelines for activity focus on flexibility; however, both flexibility and ROM are vital to an exercise prescription for a person with arthritis. Both flexibility and ROM activities should be performed daily. Flexibility activities should emphasize gentle, sustained stretches. ROM activities should include full-range motions, repeated 10 to 15 times for the involved joints. People with more severe arthritis will benefit from doing ROM activities 2 to 3 times per day, because the repeated joint motion decreases pain and stiffness.

Additional Concerns

Several other factors need to be addressed when prescribing exercise for persons with arthritis. The appropriate footwear may help to control joint alignment and reduce impact to the lower-extremity joints. Older participants may need orthotic footwear if joints within the foot are involved with disease. People who have decreased hand function may need shoes with Velcro closure rather than ties.

As noted earlier, poor joint alignment will lead to greater degeneration in the joint, so alignment needs to be assessed by a specialist. Orthotics may help joint alignment for mild malalignment, whereas a splint or brace may be needed for more significant problems. If the alignment cannot be controlled, the activity must be modified.

Although exercise is very beneficial for people with arthritis, the disease activity must be considered. People with arthritis may fatigue more frequently, and regular rest should be scheduled into the daily activities. In addition, people with systemic arthritis often have flare-ups, episodes of increased joint inflammation and activity. During these episodes, participants should be counseled to continue with their program but to modify the program to avoid exacerbating the pain and inflammation. The primary activity that may need modification during a flare-up is the resistance component of the program. As inflammation and pain increase, the resistance should decrease, with a concomitant increase in repetitions.

A functional assessment may be helpful not only for the initial evaluation but also as a means to monitor progress. Several functional assessment tools have been validated, although many are specific to the type of arthritis. Hawley (9) presented an excellent review of the various instruments and their usefulness.

Summary

Arthritis is the most common condition that limits the ability to do physical activity, especially in middle-aged and older adults. In addition to maintaining strength, regular aerobic activity attenuates the progression of knee OA over 3 years (19). Contrary to common concerns, research has shown that appropriately prescribed exercise may decrease the pain and dysfunction that occur with arthritis. As noted in a recent Cochrane review on dynamic exercise for people with RA, no studies have shown negative effects of participating in exercise (22). Orthopedic limitations should be considered prior to cardiac testing as well as in the prescription phase. ACSM guidelines for exercise prescription are appropriate for adults with arthritis, although the flexibility component should receive added attention. Health care providers must be knowledgeable of arthritis, its pathology, its effects, and its management, because this will increase the patient's confidence and the likelihood of adherence to instructions.

CHAPTER 24

Psychosocial Risk Factors and Coronary Disease

Implications for the Assessment and Treatment of Cardiac Patients

Cara Frances O'Connell-Edwards, PhD

Emily York, PhD

James A. Blumenthal, PhD

Coronary heart disease (CHD) is the leading cause of death for American Indians and Alaska Natives, blacks, Hispanics, and whites. In 2002, 696,947 people died of heart disease (51% of them women), accounting for 29% of all U.S. deaths (20). In 2005, CHD was projected to cost US$393 billion, including health care services, medications, and lost productivity. We now know that the traditional risk factors—cigarette smoking, hyperlipidemia, diabetes, and hypertension—do not fully account for the timing and occurrence of CHD events, and it has been increasingly recognized that psychosocial factors play a significant role in the development and clinical manifestations of CHD (67, 68). This chapter provides an overview of the evidence that psychosocial risk factors are important considerations in cardiac rehabilitation and therefore require careful attention in the routine assessment and management of CHD patients involved in cardiac rehabilitation.

Empirical Evidence for Psychosocial Risk Factors in Cardiac Patients

Compelling evidence shows that in addition to lifestyle factors like smoking, diet, and exercise habits, personality factors and negative emotional states are associated with increased risk for adverse health outcomes. In the following sections, we review these key risk factors, which include depression, anxiety, and perceived stress as well as personality variables and social support, as

Address correspondence concerning this chapter to Cara Frances O'Connell-Edwards, The University of North Carolina at Chapel Hill School of Medicine, Department of Physical Medicine and Rehabilitation, Room 1181 Memorial Hospital, Campus Box 7200, Chapel Hill, NC 27599-7200. coconnel@email.unc.edu they relate to outcomes in both community samples and cardiac patients.

Depression

Of all the psychosocial risk factors that have been examined with regard to CHD, there is the most evidence for the link between depression and increased risk for adverse health outcomes among both healthy persons and cardiac patients. Evidence for the prognostic importance of depression in patients with CHD has been extensively reviewed (7, 30, 67-70). Prevalence rates of major depressive disorder (MDD) among patients with CHD have been estimated to be as high as 25%, with point prevalence rates estimated at up to 45% for patients with minor depression (mDD) or elevated depressive symptoms (25). A recent meta-analysis of 11 prospective cohort studies of initially healthy people indicated that depression conferred an increased relative risk between 1.64 and 2.69 for adverse cardiac events, including myocardial infarction (MI) and cardiac death, with the presence of MDD associated with the greatest risk (70) . Figure 24.1 shows that the presence of clinical depression is comparable to traditional risk factors, such as smoking and elevated blood lipids, as observed in the Framingham Heart Study.

Depression also is a significant risk factor for mortality in patients with established CHD. In an investigation of 222 patients who were assessed following MI, MDD was associated with more than a fivefold increase risk of cardiac mortality at 6-month follow up compared with no depression (30). Several recent meta-analyses documented the increased risk of morbidity and mortality in patients with CHD. Barth and colleagues (7) conducted a meta-analysis of 20 prospective studies of patients with various manifestations of CHD and demonstrated that depressive symptoms were associated with an odds ratio of 2.24 for mortality. The findings of the meta-analysis suggested that the presence of clinical depression or elevated depressive symptoms is associated with a significantly increased risk for the development of CHD among the general population and also is a risk factor for future cardiac events among patients with stable CHD, those who have experienced acute myocardial infarction (AMI), those who have undergone coronary artery bypass grafting (CABG), and patients with congestive heart failure (CHF).

Anxiety, Stress, and Distress

There is also evidence that anxiety, tension, and distress are risk factors for CHD morbidity and mortality

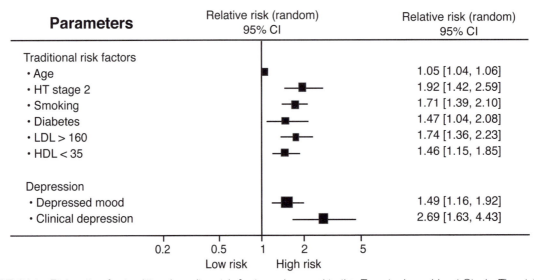

FIGURE 24.1   Risk ratios for traditional cardiac risk factors observed in the Framingham Heart Study. The risk ratios for depressive symptoms and depressed mood were derived from a recent meta-analysis by Rugulies (71). The risk conferred by depressive symptoms is comparable to traditional risk factors, and the presence of clinical depression appears to increase this risk. For traditional risk factors, risk ratios were calculated for cardiac death, myocardial infarction, coronary artery insufficiency, and angina. For depressive symptoms and clinical depression, the risk ratios were calculated for cardiac disease and myocardial infarction. CI = confidence interval; HT = hypertension; LDL = low-density lipoprotein; HDL = high-density lipoprotein.

Reprinted from *Journal of the American College of Cardiology*, Vol. 45(5) A. Rozanski, J.A. Blumenthal, K.W. Davidson, P.G. Saab, and L. Kubzansky, "The epidemiology, pathophysiology, and management of psychosocial risk factors in cardiac practice: The emerging field of behavioral cardiology." p. 15, Copyright 2005, with permission from Elsevier.

among both community samples and cardiac patients (42, 68). With regard to anxiety, the most consistent evidence has been found to support phobic anxiety and panic disorder. Elevated prevalence rates of anxiety disorders have been observed among cardiac patients, with estimated rates of panic disorder ranging from 10% to 50%; estimated rates for noncardiac patients who present with chest pain are as high as 56%. Patients with panic disorder experience recurrent panic attacks, demonstrate high levels of concern regarding future attacks, and often demonstrate behavioral changes (e.g., avoidance) in response to the panic attacks. Worry has also been recognized as a risk factor for cardiac events, and excessive worry that persists for at least 6 months is the hallmark symptom of generalized anxiety disorder (GAD).

Findings from three community-based, prospective investigations provide strong evidence for the relationship between phobic anxiety and sudden cardiac death (37, 46, 47). In a review of the literature, Januzzi and colleagues (42) found that the presence of phobic anxiety conferred a relative risk for cardiac mortality ranging from 3.8 to 6.1. There is also support for the association between worry and risk for MI, with one investigation reporting a 2.5-fold greater risk for MI among men who endorsed high levels of worry compared with men who reported low levels of worry (48).

Both chronic stress and acute stress have been linked to a range of cardiac end points (68). Job stress is among the most widely studied chronic stressor relative to CHD. It has been shown that the presence of high "job strain," that is, the combination of high demand (i.e., mental and physical effort) and low control (i.e., little decision latitude), confers increased risk for cardiac events (80).

Death of a loved one is a particular form of chronic stress, and evidence of substantially greater risks of mortality within a month of bereavement has been shown for both men and women (45). Furthermore, stressors may cluster with other psychosocial variables, promoting a synergistic effect on risk for CHD. For example, high levels of life stress and high levels of social isolation both individually increase the risk of subsequent cardiac events twofold, but when taken together these factors increase the risk fourfold (69).

Acute stressors also have been shown to trigger adverse pathophysiological processes, ranging from myocardial ischemia to sudden cardiac death. Retrospective reports of high levels of acute stress prior to MI have been noted, and increased rates of fatal and nonfatal MI are associated with a range of stressors ranging from earthquakes and war to sporting events

(for a review, see reference 78). Myocardial ischemia is induced by acute laboratory stressors such as public speaking and mental arithmetic, as well as by activities of daily living and negative emotions experienced during daily life. Indeed, a case-crossover design using daily diaries showed that feelings of tension and sadness were associated with a twofold greater risk for transient myocardial ischemia during 48 hr of Holter monitoring (80). All of these findings suggest that acute negative emotional states and chronic levels of distress are risk factors for cardiac events in CHD patients.

Personality Variables

More than 2 decades ago the type A behavior pattern (TABP) was established as a risk factor for CHD. TABP is characterized by competitiveness, excessive job involvement, speech stylistics (e.g., loud and rapid speech), impatience, and free-floating hostility. People who are more relaxed and easygoing are classified as type B. The landmark study in the field was the Western Collaborative Group Study (66), in which TABP was associated with twice the risk of new cardiac events and more than four times the risk of recurrent events compared with type B behavior in more than 3,154 middle-aged men in the San Francisco Bay area. A critical review of the literature in 1981 concluded that TABP was a significant risk factor for CHD and that the level of risk was comparable to cigarette smoking, hypertension, and elevated cholesterol (65). However, a series of subsequent investigations failed to support the role of TABP as a predictor of cardiac outcomes.

As a result of these negative studies, there have been efforts to identify the toxic elements of TABP. In the same way that some components of cholesterol (e.g., elevated LDL-C) are associated with greater risk whereas other cholesterol fractions (such as HDL-C) may be cardioprotective, certain components of TABP may be more damaging than others. A series of studies, including a reanalysis of the Western Collaborative Group Study study, revealed that high levels of anger and hostility may be especially pathogenic (56). High levels of hostility, as measured by the Cook–Medley Hostility (Ho) Scale, have been associated with increased atherosclerosis in cardiac patients and have been associated prospectively with increased rates of CHD in a variety of samples including middle-aged men and women (6), lawyers (5), and physicians (4). In a review of the literature, Smith (75) noted that in six of the eight prospective studies reviewed, hostility and anger were significant predictors of the development of CHD among healthy populations and were contributors to future cardiac events among people with CHD.

Notably, the effect sizes reported were comparable to those found with traditional cardiac risk factors.

Optimism is another personality trait that has received attention and may be relevant for cardiac patients. Positive expectancies have been linked to faster postsurgical recovery times and fewer postsurgical complications among patients undergoing CABG (73). A recent investigation found that optimism was associated with slower progression of carotid intima medial thickness and that women who were more optimistic demonstrated significantly less disease progression over a 3-year period compared with women who had lower levels of optimism (57).

Social Support

Both structural and functional aspects of social support are recognized for their impact on cardiac morbidity and mortality. Structural support is defined by a person's network of social contacts. Measures of the density of social support, frequency of interactions, number of close contacts versus peripheral acquaintances, marital status, group or church membership, and geographic proximity characterize this form of social support. Functional support includes both received support, which highlights the type and amount of resources provided by the social network, and perceived support, which focuses on the subjective satisfaction with available support or the perception that support would be available if needed. Received and perceived social support are often further delineated by type, including instrumental (e.g., help getting tangible tasks done), financial (economic support), informational (providing needed information), appraisal (help evaluating a situation), and emotional support (e.g., providing emotional support, feelings of being loved). Structural aspects of one's social support network, including marital status and frequent social contacts, are associated with lower rates of CHD. In contrast, social isolation is associated with increased cardiac mortality in healthy persons and among patients with established CHD (51). With regard to functional support, lower levels of perceived emotional support are found to predict MI in community-based samples and among patients with established CHD (52).

A number of psychosocial factors are associated with increased risk of CHD in both healthy populations and patients with established CHD. This evidence provides a strong rationale for including comprehensive psychosocial assessments as part of the routine evaluation of patients participating in cardiac rehabilitation programs. A list of potential instruments for assessing relevant psychosocial factors is presented in table 24.1.

Biobehavioral Mechanisms

A number of biobehavioral factors have been considered as potential mechanisms by which psychosocial risk factors may affect cardiac outcomes. These pathways may account for the influence of psychosocial variables on pathophysiologic processes, which in turn may affect the development and progression of cardiovascular disease. For example, lifestyle behaviors, including smoking, alcohol consumption, physical inactivity, and dietary practices, have long been recognized as contributors to the etiology and progression of cardiovascular disease. Health-compromising behaviors may, in fact, mediate the relationship between negative affective states and cardiovascular outcomes. For example, patients with depression demonstrate higher rates of smoking and sedentary behavior, which have been suggested to mediate the relationship between depressive symptoms and CHD (18). The relationship between depression and adherence to medication regimens has also been suggested as a behavioral mechanism linking depression to mortality among cardiac patients (83).

Pathophysiologic mechanisms have been proposed to link psychosocial variables to CHD, including (a) dysregulation of the hypothalamic–pituitary–adrenal (HPA) axis, (b) heightened activity of the sympathetic nervous system (SNS), (c) enhanced platelet reactivity, and (d) inflammatory responses associated with inflammatory cytokines. Dysregulation of the HPA axis has been linked to negative affective states (e.g., depression, anxiety) and environmental factors (e.g., social isolation, low SES) (for a review, see 50). HPA dysregulation may result in excess secretion of glucocorticoids, resulting in hypercortisolemia, which is associated with hypertension, insulin resistance, and truncal obesity. Anxiety and depression have been associated with heightened activity of the SNS, including higher resting heart rate and decreased heart rate variability (HRV) (35). Chronic activation of the SNS also may result in higher concentrations of circulating catecholamines (e.g., stress hormones), including norepinephrine, as well as decreased vagal tone, which has been linked to stress (61). Several blood markers are related to psychosocial factors and to CHD. For example, enhanced platelet reactivity is associated with atherogenesis and the development of CHD and has been observed in major depression and other negative affective states, including stress and hostility (59). Inflammatory cytokines, including interleukin-1 and interleukin-6, stimulate activity in the HPA axis and have been recognized for their role in the inflammatory processes associated with the stress response (55). Depressed patients also demonstrate increased levels of

TABLE 24.1 Suggested Measures for the Assessment of Psychosocial Risk Factors Among Cardiac Patients

Representative instrument	Format	Items	Scoring
RISK FACTOR OF DEPRESSION			
Beck Depression Inventory II (Beck, Steer, and Brown 1996)	Self-report	21	Multiple choice
Center for Epidemiological Studies Depression Scale (Radloff 1997)	Self-report	19	4-point Likert scale
Hamilton Rating Scale for Depression (Hamilton 1960)	Clinician-rated	17	Ratings based on the presence or absence of symptoms
Structured Clinical Interview for DSM-IV-TR (First et al. 1996)	Semistructured interview		Both structured, yes/no and open-ended items
RISK FACTOR OF STRESS			
General Health Questionnaire (Johnstone and Goldberg 1976)	Self-report	60	4-point Likert scale
Perceived Stress Scale (Cohen et al. 1983)	Self-report	10	5-point Likert scale
Spielberger State–Trait Anxiety Inventory (Spielberger 1983)	Self-report	40	4-point Likert scale
RISK FACTOR OF HOSTILITY			
Cook–Medley Hostility Scale (Cook and Medley 1954)	Self-report	50	True/false
Interpersonal Hostility Assessment Technique (Barefoot 1992; Haney et al. 1996)	Interview	4 categories of behavior	Summed frequency of behaviors
RISK FACTOR OF SOCIAL SUPPORT			
Perceived Social Support Scale (Blumenthal et al. 1987)	Self-report	12	7-point Likert scale
ENRICHD Social Support Inventory (Mitchell et al. 2003)			
Yale Social Support Index (Seeman and Berkman 1988)			
RISK FACTOR OF GENERALIZED OPTIMISM VS. PESSIMISM			
Life Orientation Test-Revised (Scheier and Carver 1985)	Self-report	6	5-point Likert scale

DSM-IV-TR = *Diagnostic and Statistical Manual of Mental Disorders*, 4th edition, text revision; ENRICHD = Enhancing Recovery in Coronary Heart Disease.

interleukin-6 and other inflammatory proteins associated with the development of CHD (2).

Psychosocial Interventions in Cardiac Patients

Recently, researchers have increased their efforts to establish criteria for evidence-based psychological interventions. Chambless and Ollendick (21) provide a summary of the American Psychological Association's task force report on category I, II, and III empirically supported treatments. Category I treatments are defined as treatments found to be superior to placebo or another plausible treatment in at least two studies. Category II treatments are supported by at least one study, and category III treatments are defined as having less rigorous support or emerging support. Table 24.2 summarizes the evidence-based psychological interventions for depression and anxiety. However, there are no empirically supported psychological interventions specifically targeting such factors as hostility and TABP, social support, or optimism.

TABLE 24.2   Evidence-Based Psychological Interventions for Two Psychosocial Risk Factors

Intervention	MDD		ANXIETY	
	Category I	**Category II**	**Category I**	**Category II**
BT	X	X		
BMT	X	X		
CBT	X	X	X	X
IPT	X	X		
BDT		X		
Self-control therapy		X		
Social problem-solving therapy		X		
Exposure			X	X
ERP			X	X
Stress inoculation + CBT + exposure			X	
Couples communication training + CBT + exposure				X
Partner-assisted CBT				X
Applied tension				X
Applied relaxation				X
Relaxation				X
Cognitive therapy				X
Family assisted ERP + relaxation				X
Systematic desensitization				X
EMDR				X

Criteria for efficacious treatment have not been met for social support, hostility, type A personality, optimism, or coping styles; BT = behavior therapy; BMT = behavioral marital therapy; BDT = brief dynamic therapy; category I treatments = superior to placebo or another plausible treatment in at least two studies; category II treatments = supported by at least one study; CBT = cognitive behavioral therapy; EMDR = eye movement desensitization and reprocessing; ERP = exposure with response prevention; IPT = interpersonal therapy; MDD = major depressive disorder.

Randomized Control Trials of Psychosocial Risk Factors

A limited number of randomized control trials (RCTs) have been conducted to examine the impact of treating psychosocial risk factors on clinical outcomes. Linden (53) reported that patients who received psychosocial interventions showed greater clinical improvement in psychological distress, blood pressure, heart rate, and cholesterol levels compared with a standard medical care and exercise training controls. Furthermore, patients who received psychosocial interventions were 40% less likely to die and were 65% less likely to have a recurrent coronary event than the control group over a 2-year follow-up period. A more recent meta-analysis conducted by the Cochrane Collaboration included 36 published psychological intervention trials among patients with CHD (n = 12,841) (64). Included in the meta-analysis were trials that offered stress management training (SMT) or other forms of psychological intervention and reported outcomes related to future cardiac events, such as death, all-cause mortality, and psychological functioning. The authors found that both SMT and psychological interventions improved symptoms of anxiety and depression. However, there was limited evidence that either SMT or psychological interventions reduced all-cause or cardiac mortality among patients with CHD. Patients who underwent SMT or other psychological intervention had fewer reinfarctions; however, the authors cautioned that these findings were not supported in the two largest RCTs included in the analysis. See table 24.3 for a summary.

TABLE 24.3 Randomized Controlled Trials of Interventions for Psychosocial Risk Ractors of Cardiac Outcome

Study	Participants	Intervention	End points	Medical outcome
Ibrahim et al. 1974	118 post-MI	Group therapy and control	Total mortality	1 year survival rate 10% higher in tx vs. control
Rahe et al. 1979	44 first MI	Group therapy; UC	Total mortality, nonfatal MI, CABG	Significantly lower coronary morbidity and mortality in group therapy vs. UC
Stern et al. 1983	106 post-MI (6 weeks to 1 year); Zung depression scale 40+; Taylor Manifest Anxiety Scale 19+	Includes SMT, ET, group counseling, UC	Total mortality; nonfatal MI, CABG	No significant effect on mortality; ET reported fewer cardiovascular sequelae
Vermeulen et al. 1983	98 acute MI	CCR, PI	Cardiac mortality, nonfatal MI	50% decrease in progressive CAD vs. control; higher rate of nonfatal MI in control; cardiac mortality significantly higher in control
IHD Life Stress Monitoring Program (Frasure-Smith & Prince 1985)	461 MI males	12 months UC and home-based PNI	Total mortality, cardiac mortality, nonfatal MI	Lower cardiac mortality in tx vs. UC; no difference in MI
Oldenburg et al. 1985	46 first acute MI	Includes SMT; CPI: individual counseling, RT, HE; RT + HE; UC	Total mortality, cardiac surgery, and heart attack inventory	No significant difference between UC, education, and counseling
RCPP (Friedman 1986)	1,013 MI	TABC + CC, CC, and control (nonrandom)	Recurrent MI, cardiac mortality	TABC + CC decreased MI recurrence rate more than CC and control; decreased cardiac deaths in experimental vs. control

(continued)

Table 24.3 (*continued*)

Study	Participants	Intervention	End points	Medical outcome
Fridlund et al. 1991	178 MI	PI + CR; UC	Total mortality, nonfatal MI, CABG/PTCA	Intervention had significantly fewer reinfarctions (1 year); total mortality significantly higher in control
PRECOR (Saint et al. (1991)	182 acute MI	RP; counseling; UC	Total mortality, nonfatal MI, CABG	NS
Burell 1995	261 CABG 3-12 months postsurgery	Includes SMT, CPI + CR, CR	Total and cardiac mortality, nonfatal MI, CABG (reoperation), PTCA	Total mortality significantly higher in control; nonfatal MI significantly higher in control
Jones and West 1996*	2,328 recent AMI	UC and psychotherapy + RT + SMT	Mortality, morbidity, use of medication	No significant decrease in risk for mortality or reinfarction at 12 months
Lidell and Fridlund 1996	116 acute MI	CCR + input from psychologist + ET + home-training program; UC	Total mortality, nonfatal MI, CABG/PTCA	NS difference between groups on cardiac events
Blumenthal et al. 1997*	107 CAD and ischemia	ET and SMT and UC (nonrandom)	Cardiac events: nonfatal MI, cardiac revascularization	SMT and ET decreased cardiac events vs. UC
MHART (Frasure-Smith 1997)	1376 post MI	12 months UC and home-based PNI	Total mortality, cardiac mortality, nonfatal MI, CABG	NS on 1-year survival; increased all-cause and cardiac mortality among women in tx group
Black et al., 1998	60; acute CHD events; identified level of psychopathology†	Includes SMT; CCR; SI (CCR+ ≥1 PI)	Total mortality, MI, CABG, PTCA combined, anxiety and depression	NS difference in rehospitalization rates in SI vs. control
Hofman-Bang et al. 1999	93 PTCA; 1-2 weeks postsurgery	Includes SMT, CPI + CR, UC	Total mortality, nonfatal MI, CABG, PTCA	NS; trend toward lower morbidity in intervention during 2nd-year follow-up
Van Dixhoorn and Duivenvoorden 1999	156 recent MI	ET and ET + RT	Cardiac events (cardiac death, reinfarction, heart surgery)	ET + RT decreased cardiac events and rehospitalizations after 5 years vs. ET only
Allison et al. 2000	441 unstable angina	Nurse-led counseling (exercise, diet, smoking cessation, drug management), UC	Clinical events (cardiac mortality, MI, CABG)	NS mortality; significantly lower recurrence rates and revascularizations in intervention vs. control
Cowan et al. 2001	133 survivors out-of-hospital VF or asystole	Includes SMT, psychosocial interventions (relaxation and BB; CBT; HE), UC	Total mortality, cardiac mortality, nonfatal MI	Risk of cardiovascular death reduced by 86% in psychosocial intervention; all-cause mortality reduced by 62%
Berkman 2003	2481 AMI with depression or LPSS	CBT + pharmacotherapy if needed and UC	Total mortality; nonfatal MI	29-month follow-up: no significant difference in tx vs. UC in event-free survival

Randomized controlled trials selected included medical outcomes; studies investigating only risk factors and biomarkers were not included. AMI = acute myocardial infarction; BB = biofeedback; CABG = coronary artery bypass grafting; CAD = coronary artery disease; CC = cardiac counseling; CCR = comprehensive cardiac rehabilitation; CPI = complex psychological intervention; CR = cardiac rehabilitation; ET = exercise training; HE = Health Education; IHD = ischemic heart disease; LPSS = low perceived social support; M-HART = Montreal Heart Attack Readjustment Trial; MI = myocardial infarction; NS = not significant; PI = psychological intervention; PNI = psychosocial nursing intervention; PTCA = percutaneous transluminal coronary angioplasty; RCPP = Recurrent Coronary Prevention Project; RP = rehabilitation program; RT = relaxation therapy; SI = special intervention; SMT = stress management training; tx = treatment; TABC = type A behavior counseling; UC = usual care.

*Partially randomized

†Global Severity Index T-score ≥63 (Symptom Checklist-90-Revised)

Depression

Published reports describe studies in which patients with depression were treated for depression with the goal of improving medical outcomes. The ENRICHD (Enhancing Recovery in Coronary Heart Disease Patients) trial investigated the effect of cognitive–behavioral therapy (CBT) on reducing risk for recurrent MI and mortality among post-MI patients who had major depression, minor depression, dysthymia, or low perceived social support (9). No significant differences were found in event-free survival between the psychosocial intervention and usual care group. Although sub-analyses revealed that some groups (i.e., white males) benefited from the intervention, overall the rates of mortality and nonfatal MIs were comparable between patients who received CBT and usual care.

Pharmacologic management of psychosocial risk factors is a relatively new area of interest. The SADHART (Sertraline Antidepressant Heart Attack Randomized Trial) study demonstrated that sertraline, a selective serotonin reuptake inhibitor, could be used safely to treat MDD in patients with unstable angina or acute myocardial infarction. Furthermore, depressed cardiac patients who received sertraline had better medical outcomes compared with patients who received placebo. However, no differences between groups in depression change scores were found (34). A secondary, post hoc analysis of the ENRICHD data noted that patients treated with antidepressants following MI demonstrated reduced risk of recurrent MI and all-cause mortality compared with patients not on antidepressant medication (79). Because this was not an RCT, however, the safety and effectiveness of antidepressant medication in reducing CHD events remain uncertain.

In the CREATE (Canadian Cardiac Randomized Evaluation of Antidepressant and Psychotherapy Efficacy) study, Frasure-Smith and colleagues (29) reported on the effects of an RCT of citalopram and interpersonal psychotherapy in a sample of 284 patients with CHD and major depressive disorder. Patients randomized to the treatment condition received 50 min interpersonal psychotherapy sessions and 20 min clinical management sessions for 12 weeks. The other half of the sample was assigned to a control condition, consisting of 12 weekly 20 min clinical management sessions. A second randomization was made for all patients, in which half were assigned to a 12-week citalopram condition and half to a matching placebo. Results revealed that citalopram was superior to placebo in reducing depressive symptoms; however, interpersonal psychotherapy was not more effective than clinical management in reducing symptoms of

depression in the sample. These findings provide further evidence for the safety and efficacy of selective serotonin reuptake inhibitors for the treatment of MDD in cardiac patients; however, the impact on cardiac events remains unknown.

Type A and Hostility

The first and most important RCT that examined the impact of TABP modification on medical outcomes was the Recurrent Coronary Prevention Project. This project examined the impact of type A behavior modification on mortality and reinfarction. Patients were randomized either to type A behavioral counseling plus cardiac counseling or to cardiac counseling alone, whereas a third, nonrandom comparison group consisting of patients who said they were too busy to participate formed an additional control group. The patients who underwent TABP modification exhibited reduced type A behaviors and lower cardiac recurrence rates (i.e., nonfatal MI and cardiac deaths) compared with patients receiving cardiac counseling alone and a nonrandomized control group. However, there was no difference in overall mortality rates between the type A modification group and controls (33).

Anxiety and Stress

Several RCTs have been conducted to examine the effects of psychosocial interventions designed to reduce stress, distress, and anxiety on cardiac risk factors and cardiac events. The Ischemic Heart Disease Study investigated the effects of a home-based psychosocial nursing intervention in post-MI males (31). Results revealed that the intervention resulted in lower stress ratings and reduced cardiac mortality after 1 year. However, in a subsequent effort to replicate this finding with a larger sample, including women, known as the M-HART trial, results revealed no group differences in rates of reinfarction or cardiac all-cause mortality, and there was a trend for worse outcomes in the treated women. The intervention did not reduce symptoms of anxiety or depression, which may have contributed to the negative results. A similar negative finding was reported by Jones and West (44), who examined the effects of a rehabilitation program consisting of psychological therapy, counseling, relaxation training, and stress management training in post-MI patients. Similar to M-HART, this study revealed no group differences in mortality rates, but there also were no differences in levels of anxiety and depression between the rehabilitation and the control conditions, indicating that the treatment failed to effectively reduce distress. Thus, it appears that interventions that do not successfully reduce distress also do not reduce risk of CHD.

Two RCTs from the Duke group provided more promising results. In an initial, semirandomized trial, 107 patients with stable CHD and evidence of exercise-induced myocardial ischemia were randomly assigned to stress management training (SMT) or exercise; patients who lived too far from Duke to participate in the interventions formed a usual care control group (15). As shown in figure 24.2, 22 (21%) of the 107 patients who participated in the trial experienced at least one event (median follow-up time = 44 months), defined as cardiac death, nonfatal MI, or revascularization procedure. Only 9% of the patients in the SMT group suffered an event, compared with 21% in exercise training and 30% in usual medical care. Compared with the usual care group, the SMT group had a relative risk of an event (after adjustment for baseline risk factors) of 0.26 (*p* = .04), and the exercise group had a relative risk of 0.68 (*p* = .41). In a longer term follow-up of this sample, SMT was associated with a significant reduction in subsequent cardiac events (MI, CABG, percutaneous transluminal coronary angioplasty, and death) compared with usual care, and these benefits persisted over a 5-year follow-up period (14). The SMT intervention was also associated with lower medical costs. Thus, the SMT intervention not only modified psychological outcomes but also significantly affected long-term clinical outcomes and medical expenditures.

In a subsequent, fully randomized RCT, Blumenthal and colleagues (16) examined the effects of an exercise training intervention and SMT in patients with stable CHD and exercise-induced myocardial ischemia. As in their previous study, both exercise and SMT interventions resulted in decreased depression and general distress relative to a usual care group. The active treatment groups also exhibited smaller reductions in LVEF during mental stress testing and improvement in flow-mediated dilation compared with the usual care group. Furthermore, patients receiving SMT showed improved baroreflex sensitivity and HRV compared with the usual care group.

Social Support

Although many social support interventions have proven to be effective, no established treatments exist for low social support and there is no evidence that treating low social support improves clinical outcomes. The ENRICHD trial increased perceived support among patients with low support, but there was no benefit in terms of medical outcomes (9).

Effects of Exercise on Psychosocial and CHD Outcomes

Exercise generally is considered safe for patients with stable CHD and is the cornerstone of most cardiac

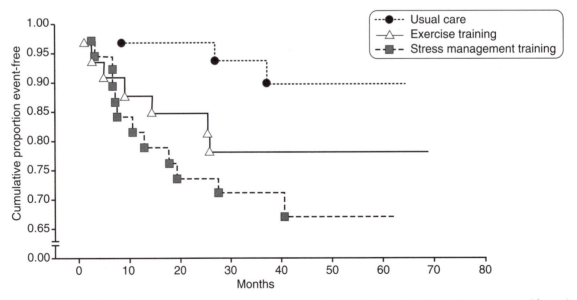

FIGURE 24.2 Cumulative time to event curves for exercise, stress management, and usual care groups. After adjustment for age, baseline left ventricular ejection fraction, and history of myocardial infarction, stress management was associated with a significantly lower risk (risk ratio [RR] = .26, *p* = .04) of an adverse cardiac event compared with usual care. Exercise was also associated with a lower relative risk compared with controls but was not statistically significant (RR = .68, *p* = .34).

rehabilitation programs. Exercise has well-documented cardiovascular benefits, as summarized elsewhere in this volume. Exercise training also is associated with several beneficial physiological changes including improvements in autonomic nervous system and hypothalamic–pituitary–adrenal axis functioning, endothelial function, hypertension, dyslipidemia, insulin resistance, and inflammation. Recent data from the ENRICHD trial suggest that exercise may reduce depression as well as risk for fatal and nonfatal cardiac events (11). After the investigators controlled for medical and demographic variables, patients who indicated that they exercised 6 months after their AMI had close to a 50% reduction in risk, even after adjustment for disease severity and other potential confounders.

In addition to improving medical outcomes, exercise is an effective treatment for psychosocial risk factors such as depression (49). In one of the larger studies on this topic (13), 156 depressed, adult patients with MDD were randomized to 4 months of treatment with supervised aerobic exercise, antidepressant medication (sertraline), or a combination of exercise and medication. Results revealed that exercise was as effective as antidepressant medication in treating depression by the end of the 16-week intervention. Moreover, 6-month follow-up of participants revealed that those patients who continued to exercise were half as likely to relapse. Recently, a placebo controlled trial showed that exercise produced comparable benefits to sertraline in patients with MDD and that both active treatments tended to be better than placebo (12).

Summary

There is now good evidence that psychosocial factors, particularly depression, stress, and low social support, place CHD patients at increased risk for untoward clinical events including recurrent MI and death. However, there is less compelling evidence that reducing psychosocial risk factors improves prognosis. For example, the only RCT to test a nonpharmacological treatment for depression in CHD patients with clinical depression is the ENRICHD trial. The results of the ENRICHD trial indicate that although CBT may reduce depression in patients with a recent MI, CBT did not reduce rates of mortality or cardiac events. Other behavioral treatments for psychosocial risk factors are emerging. Stress management training and aerobic exercise may be especially useful in this regard. However, because these interventions may not be accepted by everyone, strategies to increase motivation to engage in nonpharmacologic treatments and improve adherence may be especially useful. Ultimately, it may be possible to identify patients, based on individual difference characteristics (e.g., age, gender, level of stress), who are most likely to respond to particular treatments. Future research might also determine whether combination therapies (e.g., combining exercise with SMT) offer added benefit as part of a comprehensive program of cardiac rehabilitation.

CHAPTER 25

Stroke

Neil F. Gordon, MD, PhD

Stroke survivors are at a substantially heightened risk of another stroke. Recurrent stroke is a major source of increased mortality and morbidity. Fortunately, epidemiological studies have helped to identify the risk and determinants of recurrent stroke. Moreover, recent clinical trials have provided the data to generate evidence-based recommendations to reduce the risk of recurrent stroke. In this chapter, the epidemiology, pathophysiology, diagnosis, and medical management (especially exercise training) of stroke are briefly reviewed.

Epidemiology

Despite impressive technologic advances in cardiovascular medicine in recent decades, stroke remains a leading cause of morbidity and mortality in the United States. In the United States, there are an annual estimated 700,000 new or recurrent strokes. Approximately 500,000 of these are first strokes and 200,000 are recurrent strokes. On average, someone in the United States has a stroke about every 45 s. Stroke incidence rates are 1.25 times greater in men than in women. However, the difference in incidence rates between the genders is applicable mainly to young people and is nonexistent at older ages. Moreover, each year in the United States about 46,000 more women than men actually suffer a stroke. Black people have almost double the risk of first-ever stroke compared with white people. According to the American Heart Association's 2006 statistical update, the age-adjusted stroke incidence rates (per 100,000) for first-ever strokes are 323 for black males, 260 for black females, 167 for white males, and 138 for white females. Likewise, there is an increased incidence of stroke among Mexican Americans compared with non-Hispanic whites (2).

Stroke is an underlying or contributing cause of approximately 273,000 annual deaths in the United States and, when considered separately from other cardiovascular diseases, ranks third among all causes of death (behind heart disease and cancer). Stroke accounts for about 1 of every 15 deaths in the United States, and, on average, someone dies of a stroke about every 3 min. Because women live longer than men, women account for approximately 61% of stroke deaths in the United States each year. Stroke death rates are higher in blacks than in whites. Fortunately, from 1993 to 2003, the stroke death rate decreased in the United States by 18.5%, and the actual number of stroke deaths declined by 0.7% (2).

There are approximately 5.5 million stroke survivors in the United States. The estimated number of noninstitutionalized stroke survivors increased from 1.5 million to 2.4 million from the early 1970s to the early 1990s in this country. Unfortunately, stroke is a leading cause of serious long-term disability. Whereas 50% to 70% of stroke survivors regain functional independence, 15% to 30% are permanently disabled

Address correspondence concerning this chapter to Neil F. Gordon, Nationwide Better Health, 340 Eisenhower Drive, Building 1400, Suite 17, Savannah, Georgia 31406. E-mail: ngordon@interventusa.com and about 20% require institutional care at 3 months after stroke onset. More than 1 million American adults report difficulty with activities of daily living as a result of a stroke. It was estimated that annual direct and indirect costs for stroke care would total $57.9 billion in the United States in 2006 (2).

Pathophysiology

There are two major types of strokes: ischemic and hemorrhagic strokes. Ischemic strokes account for approximately 88% of all strokes. Risk factors for ischemic stroke can be classified into three groups: nonmodifiable risk factors (including age, race, gender, and family history); well-documented modifiable risk factors (including previous transient ischemic attack [TIA], carotid artery disease, atrial fibrillation, coronary artery disease, other types of cardiac disease, hypertension, cigarette smoking, hyperlipidemia, diabetes mellitus, and sickle cell disease); and less well-documented, potentially modifiable risk factors (including physical inactivity, obesity, alcohol abuse, hyperhomocysteinemia, drug abuse, hypercoagulability, hormone replacement therapy, oral contraceptive use, and inflammatory processes) (8). Because atherosclerosis is the most common underlying cause of ischemic stroke, it is not surprising that all of the major potentially modifiable risk factors for coronary artery disease are included in the preceding list.

Ischemic stroke can be subclassified into various categories according to the presumed mechanism of the focal brain injury and the type and localization of the vascular lesion. The classic categories have been defined as large-artery atherosclerotic infarction, which may be extracranial or intracranial; embolism from a cardiac source; small-vessel disease; other determined cause such as dissection, hypercoagulable states, or sickle cell disease; and infarcts of undetermined cause (4, 15). The certainty of the classification of the ischemic stroke mechanism is believed to be far from ideal, reflecting the inadequacy or timing of the diagnostic workup in some cases to visualize the occluded artery or to localize the precise source of embolism (4, 15).

Hemorrhagic strokes account for approximately 12% of all strokes. There are two major categories of hemorrhagic strokes: those that result from intracerebral hemorrhage and those that result from subarachnoid hemorrhage. Most intracerebral hemorrhages are related to hypertension. The most common cause of a subarachnoid hemorrhage is a ruptured aneurysm, which is also often precipitated by hypertension. Hemorrhagic strokes are less common

than ischemic strokes, but they are more likely to be fatal; 8% to 12% of ischemic strokes and 37% to 38% of hemorrhagic strokes result in death within 30 days. However, survivors of hemorrhagic strokes are less likely to be severely disabled compared with survivors of ischemic strokes (9).

Although approximately 14% of stroke survivors are estimated to achieve a full recovery in physical function, activity intolerance is extremely common among stroke survivors, especially elderly people. Ambulatory persons with a prior history of stroke may be able to perform at about 50% of peak oxygen consumption and 70% of the peak power output that can be achieved by age- and gender-matched people without a history of stroke. Such activity intolerance is likely to be multifactorial in etiology (10). Contributing factors are postulated to include bed rest–induced deconditioning, concomitant left ventricular dysfunction, the associated severity of neurological involvement, and the increased aerobic requirements of walking (10).

Energy expenditure during ambulation in hemiplegic patients varies with the degree of weakness, spasticity, training, and bracing, but in general, both the absolute (L/min) and the relative (ml $\cdot$ kg^{-1} $\cdot$ min^{-1}) oxygen costs of walking are elevated in hemiplegic patients compared with those of nondisabled subjects of comparable body weight. In some instances, the debilitating motor effects of a stroke can have a profoundly negative impact on mechanical efficiency, thereby increasing the energy cost of walking by up to twice that of nondisabled persons. Even everyday household tasks, such as making the bed and vacuuming, may be associated with markedly greater energy requirements among poststroke women than among their healthy counterparts (10).

Collectively, the previously mentioned factors can contribute to a vicious circle of further decreased activity and greater exercise intolerance in stroke survivors, leading to secondary complications such as reduced cardiorespiratory fitness, muscle atrophy, osteoporosis, and impaired circulation to the lower extremities. The latter may predispose to thrombus formation, decubitus ulcers, or both. Moreover, a diminished self-efficacy, greater dependence on others for activities of daily living, and reduced ability for normal societal interactions can have a profoundly deleterious psychological impact (10).

Diagnosis

In addition to the medical history and physical examination, computed tomography (CT) remains the most widely used neuroimaging technique for the evaluation of patients with suspected acute ischemic stroke (12). Advances in CT technology, including the development of CT angiography and perfusion studies, are likely to affect future recommendations about the use of CT in the evaluation of patients with suspected stroke. Magnetic resonance imaging techniques are also used widely in the assessment of patients with suspected stroke. Recent scientific statements of the American Heart Association have focused on perfusion imaging in the setting of acute ischemic stroke and provide information about the advantages and disadvantages of each imaging technique (3, 12).

The distinction between TIA and ischemic stroke has become less important in recent years because many of the preventive strategies are applicable to both groups (15). By conventional clinical definitions, if the neurological symptoms continued for >24 hr, a person was diagnosed with stroke, whereas a focal neurological deficit lasting <24 hr was defined as a TIA. With the more widespread use of modern brain imaging, however, many patients with symptoms lasting <24 hr are found to have a cerebral infarction. The most recent definition of stroke for clinical trials has required either symptoms lasting >24 hr or imaging of an acute, clinically relevant brain lesion in patients with rapidly vanishing symptoms. The proposed new definition of TIA is a "brief episode of neurological dysfunction caused by a focal disturbance of brain or retinal ischemia, with clinical symptoms typically lasting less than 1 hour, and without evidence of infarction" (15, p. 578). TIAs are important determinants of stroke, with 90-day risks of stroke reported to be as high as 10.5% and the greatest stroke risk apparent in the first week post-TIA (15).

In addition to the previously mentioned tests, appropriate tests are required to identify factors that may have precipitated the stroke as well as risk factors for recurrent stroke. Stroke typically does not occur in isolation, and stroke patients often have a high prevalence of associated comorbid conditions. In particular, cardiac disease has been reported to occur in up to 75% of stroke survivors (10).

Management

Stroke survivors should receive medical care from a physician-coordinated multidisciplinary team of health care professionals with expertise and special interest in stroke. Poststroke medical management is complex and typically requires that many issues be addressed in an integrated fashion. Exercise training is an important aspect of the medical management of stroke survivors. In this section, acute and chronic responses to exercise training are briefly reviewed and recommendations are provided for exercise prescription in stroke survivors.

Exercise Response

The World Health Organization's International Classification of Functioning, Disability, and Health organizes the effects of conditions such as stroke into problems in the "body structure and function dimension" and in the "activity and participation dimension" (10, p. 2032). Body structure and function effects (known as impairments), such as hemiplegia, spasticity, and aphasia, are the primary neurological disorders caused by stroke. Activity limitations (also referred to as disabilities) are manifested by reduced ability to perform activities of daily living. The magnitude of activity limitation is generally related to but not completely dependent on the degree of body impairment (i.e., severity of stroke). Other factors that influence the magnitude of activity limitation include intrinsic motivation and mood, adaptability and coping skill, cognition and learning ability, severity and type of medical comorbidity, medical stability, physical endurance levels, effects of acute treatments, and the amount and type of rehabilitation training (10).

The cardiovascular response to a single exercise session has been documented in several studies among stroke survivors. Oxygen uptake at a given submaximal workload in stroke patients is usually higher than in healthy subjects, possibly because of a reduced mechanical efficiency, the effects of spasticity, or both. In contrast, stroke patients have been shown to achieve a significantly lower peak oxygen uptake, workload, heart rate, and systolic blood pressure than control subjects during progressive exercise testing to volitional fatigue (10).

As is the case for the general population, the major potential risks of exercise for stroke survivors are musculoskeletal injury and sudden cardiac death. The foremost priority in formulating the exercise prescription for stroke survivors is to minimize the potential risks of exercise via appropriate screening, program design, monitoring, and patient education. Depending on the severity of disability and other coexisting medical conditions, certain patients may need to participate in a medically supervised exercise program (1, 7, 9, 10).

Before embarking on an exercise program, all stroke survivors should undergo a complete medical history (usually the most important part of the preexercise evaluation) and a physical examination to identify neurological complications and other medical conditions that require special consideration or that contraindicate exercise (10). Because up to 75% of stroke victims have coexisting cardiac disease and 20% to 40% of asymptomatic stroke patients may have abnormal tests for silent myocardial ischemia, it is recommended that stroke patients undergo graded exercise testing with electrocardiographic monitoring as part of a medical evaluation before beginning an exercise program (5, 10).

No studies have specifically evaluated how soon after a stroke graded exercise testing can be performed safely. Until such data become available, the American Heart Association recommends that good clinical judgment be used to decide the timing of graded exercise testing after stroke and whether to use a submaximal or symptom-limited maximal test protocol (10). In the absence of definitive evidence, the American Heart Association considers it prudent to follow exercise guidelines similar to those recommended for post–myocardial infarction patients and to use submaximal protocols (with a predetermined end point, often defined as a peak heart rate of 120 beats/min, or 70% of the age-predicted maximum heart rate, or a peak metabolic equivalent level of 5) if graded exercise testing is performed during the first 14 to 21 days after stroke (6, 10). The American Heart Association also considers it prudent to consider a systolic blood pressure >250 mmHg or a diastolic blood pressure >115 mmHg an absolute (rather than relative) indication to terminate a graded exercise test in a stroke patient (6, 10).

Graded exercise testing in stroke patients should be conducted in accordance with contemporary guidelines, as detailed elsewhere (1, 6, 7, 13). The exercise test modality or protocol for the stroke survivor is selected to optimally assess functional capacity and the cardiovascular response to exercise. The testing mode should be selected or adapted to the needs of the stroke survivor. Often, a standard treadmill walking protocol can be used (with the aid of handrails), and the Bruce protocol (or a modified version) is appropriate for many subjects. For some subjects, however, other modes may be needed. Special protocols are available for stroke survivors, especially those with hemiplegia or paresis. Such testing protocols may use arm cycle ergometry with the subject seated to optimize the load or arm–leg or leg cycle ergometry. If flexibility and adaptability are used in the selection of testing protocols, most stroke survivors who are deemed stable for physical activity can undergo exercise testing. For patients with disabilities that preclude exercise testing, pharmacological stress testing should be considered (10).

From a practical standpoint, it may not be feasible, for a variety of reasons, for many stroke survivors to perform an exercise test before starting an exercise program. For stroke patients for whom an exercise test is recommended but not performed, the American Heart Association recommends that lighter intensity exercise be prescribed and that the reduced exercise intensity be compensated for by increasing the training frequency, duration, or both (10).

Exercise Training Adaptations

Traditionally, the physical rehabilitation of stroke survivors ended within about 6 months after stroke because it was thought that most, if not all, recovery of motor function occurred during this interval. Recent research has shown that intensive rehabilitation beyond this time period, including exercise training, increases both aerobic capacity and sensorimotor function (10). Consequently, rehabilitation programs for stroke survivors increasingly have incorporated aerobic exercise training. This is usually complemented by specialized training to improve skill and efficiency in self-care, occupational, and leisure-time activities. In addition to improving quality of life, functional capacity, mobility, neurological impairment, and motor function, three major rehabilitation goals for the stroke patient are preventing complications of prolonged inactivity, decreasing recurrent stroke and cardiovascular events, and increasing aerobic fitness (10).

Recent evidence shows that the exercise trainability of stroke survivors may be comparable to that of their age-matched, healthy counterparts. The results of existing studies support the use of regular aerobic exercise to improve cardiovascular health and fitness after stroke, which is consistent with recent consensus statements on exercise for nondisabled people. Strength training also has been observed to have beneficial effects in stroke survivors. In particular, several studies have shown strong associations between paretic knee-extension torque and locomotion ability and between both hip flexor and ankle plantar flexor strength of the paretic limb and walking speed after stroke (10).

Recently, we provided guidelines on the recommended mode, intensity, frequency, and duration of exercise for stroke patients together with a brief summary of special considerations for exercise programming (table 25.1) (7). Our recommendations were adapted primarily from the American College of Sports Medicine's *Exercise Management for Persons With Chronic Diseases and Disabilities* (13). In recognition of the fact that the American College of Sports

TABLE 25.1 Summary of Exercise Prescription Guidelines for Stroke Patients

Mode of exercise	Major goals	Intensity, frequency, and duration
Aerobic ■ Large muscle activities ■ Arm and leg ergometry	■ Increase independence in ADLs ■ Increase walking speed and efficiency ■ Increase aerobic capacity ■ For patients with CHD, decrease BP and HR response to submaximal exercise, decrease submaximal myocardial oxygen demand, improve CHD risk factors, and induce other cardioprotective benefits	■ 40-70% $\dot{V}O_2$ reserve; 40-70% HR reserve; 55-80% HR_{max}; RPE 11-14 (6-20 scale) ■ ≥3 nonconsecutive days/week ■ 20-60 min/session ■ 5-10 min of warm-up and cool-down activities
Strength ■ Circuit training	■ Increase muscle strength and endurance ■ Increase ability to perform leisure and occupational activities and ADLs ■ For patients with CHD, decrease BP, HR, and myocardial oxygen demand at any given resistance (e.g., during lifting and carrying objects)	■ 40-50% maximal voluntary contraction ■ 2-3 days/week ■ 1-3 sets of 10-15 repetitions ■ 8-10 different exercises that work major muscle groups ■ Resistance gradually increased over time
Flexibility ■ Stretching (upper- and lower-body ROM activities)	■ Decrease risk of injury	■ Static stretches: hold for 10-30 s ■ 2-3 days/week

SPECIAL CONSIDERATIONS

■ Stroke patients often have CHD and hypertension; the combination of comorbidities, neurological deficits, and emotional barriers unique to each stroke survivor requires special consideration.

■ Subsets of stroke survivors (e.g., those with depression, fatigue syndrome, poor family support, or communication, cognitive, and motor deficits) require further evaluation and subsequent specialization of their rehabilitation program.

■ Treadmill walking is highly advantageous as an aerobic exercise mode.

■ Intermittent training protocols may be needed during the initial weeks because of the extremely deconditioned level of many convalescing stroke patients.

■ Adjunctive neuromuscular training is also recommended.

■ To enhance compliance, the issues of family support and social isolation need to be addressed and resolved.

Key revisions (to original table in Palmer-McLean et al. 2003)

■ Intensity guideline changed from 40-70% $\dot{V}O_2$ peak to 40-70% $\dot{V}O_2$ reserve or HR reserve; intensity guideline based on %HR_{max} included; target RPE changed from 13 to 11-14 (6-20 scale).

■ Frequency changed from 3-5 days/week to ≥3 nonconsecutive days/week.

■ Strength training guideline changed from 3 sets of 8-12 reps on 2 days/week to 1-3 sets of 10-15 reps of 8-10 different exercises on 2-3 days/week.

■ Flexibility training guidelines changed from 2 days/week to 2-3 days/week.

■ Additional strength and flexibility training guidelines included.

ADLs = activities of daily living; BP = blood pressure; CHD = coronary heart disease; HR = heart rate; RPE = Rating of Perceived Exertion; ROM = range of motion; $\dot{V}O_2$ = oxygen uptake.

Reprinted, by permission, from B.F. Franklin and N.F. Gordon, 2005, *Contemporary diagnosis and management in cardiovascular exercise* (Newtown, PA: Handbooks in Healthcare Co.).

Medicine's guidelines were provided by nationally renowned experts, the key revisions we made are noted in table 25.1 so that readers can revert to the original guidelines should they prefer to do so. Table 25.1 also briefly summarizes some of the key points from the American Heart Association's scientific statement "Physical Activity and Exercise Recommendations for Stroke Survivors" (10).

According to the American Heart Association, prescribing exercise for the stroke patient is comparable in many ways to prescribing medications; that is, one recommends an optimal dosage according to individual needs and limitations (10). Aerobic training modes may include leg, arm, or combined arm–leg ergometry at 40% to 70% of peak oxygen uptake reserve or heart rate reserve or 55% to 80% of peak heart rate, with perceived exertion (11-14, Borg 6-20 scale) used as an adjunctive intensity modulator. The recommended frequency of training is ≥3 days per week, with a duration of 20 to 60 min per session depending on the patient's level of fitness. Intermittent training protocols may be required during the initial weeks of rehabilitation due to the extremely deconditioned level of many convalescing stroke patients (7).

Treadmill training appears to offer several distinct advantages in the exercise training of stroke survivors. It requires the performance of a task required for everyday living, namely, walking, which helps enhance the generalizability of training effects. The use of handrail support and unweighting devices such as harnesses that lift patients, effectively decreasing their weight, allows patients who might otherwise be unable to exercise to walk on a treadmill. In patients with residual gait deviations, exercise intensity can be augmented by increasing the treadmill grade while maintaining a comfortable speed (10).

To maximize the generalizability of the training adaptations to daily activities, adjunctive upper-body and resistance training programs are also advocated for clinically stable stroke patients. Although there are no widely accepted guidelines for determining when and how to initiate resistance training after ischemic or hemorrhagic stroke, it may be prudent to prescribe 10 to 15 repetitions for each set of exercises rather than 8 to 12 repetitions (i.e., higher repetitions with reduced loads), similar to that recommended for post–myocardial infarction patients (9). Such regimens should be performed 2 to 3 days per week and include a minimum of 1 set of 8 to 10 different exercises that involve the major muscle groups (arms, shoulders, chest, abdomen, back, hips, and legs) (7, 9, 14). Adjunc-

tive flexibility and neuromuscular training to increase range of motion of the involved side, prevent contractures, increase activities of daily living, and reduce the risk of injury are also recommended (7, 10, 13).

Medications

The American Heart Association and American Stroke Association's guidelines for prevention of stroke in patients with ischemic stroke or TIA were updated in 2006 (15). The classes and levels of evidence used in these guidelines are defined in table 25.2. The key recommendations for the management of treatable vascular risk factors and modifiable behavioral risk factors are summarized in table 25.3.

As can be seen in table 25.3, stroke patients commonly take one or more cardioactive medications to optimize risk factor control. Moreover, stroke patients often receive treatment with oral anticoagulant and antiplatelet therapies to reduce their risk for recurrent events and other cardioactive medications (such as β-blockers, angiotensin-converting enzyme inhibitors, and angiotensin II receptor blockers) to manage comorbid conditions (15). Exercise professionals should be familiar with the effects of such prescribed medications on exercise tolerance and the hemodynamic responses to an acute bout of exercise and should modify the exercise prescription accordingly (1, 7). In particular, when exercise testing is performed for the purpose of exercise prescription in stroke patients, the test should be performed with the patient taking his or her usual cardioactive medications; ideally, the test should be performed at the same time of day when exercise training will typically be performed (1, 7).

Fortunately, cardioactive medications are unlikely to have a clinically relevant negative impact on the trainability of most stroke patients. Indeed, some cardioactive medications may allow certain stroke patients with cardiovascular disease (e.g., antianginal medications in stroke patients with myocardial ischemia) to exercise at higher intensities or for longer durations and, thereby, to derive greater benefit from exercise training. However, a given medication may have opposite effects on exercise tolerance when used in stroke patients with different types of cardiovascular disease. The best example of this paradox is β-blockers, which typically reduce exercise capacity in stroke patients with uncomplicated hypertension but may increase exercise capacity in stroke patients with angina or chronic heart failure (7, 13).

TABLE 25.2   Classes and Levels of Evidence Used in American Heart Association/American Stroke Association Guidelines for Prevention of Stroke in Patients With Ischemic Stroke or Transient Ischemic Attack

Class or level	Definition
Class I	Conditions for which there is evidence for or general agreement that the procedure or treatment is useful and effective
Class II	Conditions for which there is conflicting evidence or a divergence of opinion about the usefulness or efficacy of a procedure or treatment
Class IIa	Conditions for which the weight of evidence or opinion is in favor of the procedure or treatment
Class IIb	Conditions for which usefulness or efficacy is less well established by evidence or opinion
Class III	Conditions for which there is evidence or general agreement that the procedure or treatment is not useful or effective and in some cases may be harmful
Level of evidence A	Data derived from multiple randomized clinical trials
Level of evidence B	Data derived from a single randomized trial or nonrandomized studies
Level of evidence C	Expert opinion or case studies

Adapted from R.L. Sacco, 2006, "AHA/ASA guideline: Guidelines for prevention of stroke in patients with ischemic stroke or transient ischemic attack," *Stroke* 37: 577-617.

TABLE 25.3   American Heart Association/American Stroke Association Guidelines for Prevention of Stroke in Patients With Ischemic Stroke or Transient Ischemic Attack: Key Recommendations for Treatable Vascular and Modifiable Behavioral Risk Factors

Risk factor	Recommendations for treatable vascular risk factors	Class and level of evidence
Hypertension	Antihypertensive treatment is recommended to prevent recurrent stroke and other vascular events in persons who have had an ischemic stroke and are beyond the hyperacute period.	Class I, level A
	Because this benefit extends to persons with and without hypertension, this recommendation should be considered for all patients with ischemic stroke or TIA.	Class IIa, level B
	An absolute target BP level and reduction are uncertain and should be individualized, but benefit has been associated with an average reduction of ~10/5 mmHg, and normal BP levels have been defined as <120/80 mmHg.	Class IIa, level B
	Several lifestyle modifications have been associated with BP reductions and should be included as part of a comprehensive approach.	Class IIb, level C
	Optimal drug regimen remains uncertain; however, available data support the use of diuretics and the combination of diuretics and an ACE inhibitor. Choice of specific drugs and targets should be individualized on the basis of reviewed data and consideration as well as specific patient characteristics (e.g., extracranial cerebrovascular occlusive disease, renal impairment, cardiac disease, and diabetes).	Class I, level A

(continued)

Table 25.3 (continued)

Risk factor	Recommendations for treatable vascular risk factors	Class and level of evidence
Diabetes	More rigorous control of BP and lipids should be considered in patients with diabetes.	Class IIa, level B
	Although all major classes of antihypertensives are suitable for the control of BP, most patients will require >1 agent. ACE inhibitors and ARBs are most effective in reducing the progression of renal disease and are recommended as first-choice medications for patients with diabetes.	Class I, level A
	Glucose control is recommended to near-normoglycemic levels among diabetics with ischemic stroke or TIA to reduce microvascular complications.	Class I, level A
	The goal for HbA$_{1c}$ should be ≤7%.	Class IIa, level B
Cholesterol	Ischemic stroke or TIA patients with elevated cholesterol, comorbid coronary artery disease, or evidence of an atherosclerotic origin should be managed according to NCEP ATP III guidelines, which include lifestyle modification, dietary guidelines, and medication recommendations.	Class I, level A
	Statin agents are recommended, and the target goal for cholesterol lowering for those with coronary artery disease or symptomatic atherosclerotic disease is an LDL-C of <100 mg/dL and LDL-C <70 mg/dL for very high risk persons with multiple risk factors.	Class I, level A
	Patients with ischemic stroke or TIA presumed to be attributable to an atherosclerotic origin but with no preexisting indications for statins (e.g., normal cholesterol levels) can be considered for treatment with a statin to reduce the risk of vascular events.	Class IIa, level B
	Ischemic stroke or TIA patients with low HDL-C may be considered for treatment with niacin or gemfibrozil.	Class IIb, level B
Recommendations for modifiable behavioral risk factors		
Smoking	All ischemic stroke or TIA patients who have smoked in the past year should be strongly encouraged not to smoke.	Class I, level C
	Patients should avoid environmental smoke.	Class IIa, level C
	Counseling, nicotine products, and oral smoking cessation medications can be used for smoking cessation.	Class IIa, level B
Alcohol	Patients with prior ischemic stroke or TIA who are heavy drinkers should eliminate or reduce their consumption of alcohol.	Class I, level A
	Light to moderate levels, ≤2 drinks per day for men and 1 drink per day for nonpregnant women, may be considered.	Class IIb, level C
Obesity	Weight reduction should be considered for all overweight ischemic stroke or TIA patients to maintain body mass index of 18.5-24.9 kg/m^2 and a waist circumference of <35 in. (<88.9 cm) for women and <40 in. (<101.6 cm) for men.	Class IIb, level C
	Clinicians should encourage weight management through an appropriate balance of caloric intake, physical activity, and behavioral counseling.	Class IIb, level C
Physical activity	For those with ischemic stroke or TIA who are capable of engaging in physical activity, at least 30 min of moderate-intensity physical exercise most days should be considered to reduce risk factors and comorbid conditions that increase the likelihood of recurrence of stroke.	Class IIb, level C
	For those with disability after ischemic stroke, a supervised therapeutic exercise regimen is recommended.	Class IIb, level C

ACE = angiotensin-converting enzyme; ARB = angiotensin II receptor blocker; BP = blood pressure; HbA$_{1c}$ = hemoglobin A$_{1c}$; HDL-C = high-density lipoprotein cholesterol; LDL-C = low-density lipoprotein cholesterol; NCEP ATP = National Cholesterol Education Program Adult Treatment Panel; TIA = transient ischemic attack.

Adapted, by permission, from R.L. Sacco, 2006, "AHA/ASA guideline: Guidelines for prevention of stroke in patients with ischemic stroke or transient ischemic attack," *Stroke* 37: 577-617.

Summary

Stroke survivors should receive medical care from a physician-coordinated multidisciplinary team of health care professionals. Although additional research is warranted, current evidence provides a strong rationale for using exercise training as an integral component of the medical management of stroke survivors. Recent evidence shows that the exercise trainability of stroke survivors may be comparable to that of their age-matched, healthy counterparts. Aerobic training modes for stroke survivors may include leg, arm, or combined arm–leg ergometry at 40% to 70% of peak oxygen uptake reserve or heart rate reserve or 55% to 80% of peak heart rate, with perceived exertion (11-14, Borg 6-20 scale) used as an adjunctive intensity modulator. The recommended frequency of training is ≥ 3 days per week, with a duration of 20 to 60 min per session depending on the patient's level of fitness. Intermittent training protocols may be required during the initial weeks of rehabilitation because of the extremely deconditioned level of many convalescing stroke patients. Although there are no widely accepted guidelines for determining when and how to initiate resistance training after ischemic or hemorrhagic stroke, it may be prudent to prescribe 10 to 15 repetitions for each set of exercises rather than 8 to 12 repetitions (i.e., higher repetitions with reduced loads). Such regimens should be performed 2 to 3 days per week and include a minimum of 1 set of 8 to 10 different exercises that involve the major muscle groups (arms, shoulders, chest, abdomen, back, hips, and legs). Adjunctive flexibility and neuromuscular training to increase range of motion of the involved side, prevent contractures, increase activities of daily living, and reduce the risk of injury are also recommended.

CHAPTER 26

Neuropsychological Disorders

Mary Ann Kelly, PhD

Improvements in cognitive functioning are favorable by-products of the cardiovascular strengthening achieved through exercise. However, minimal attention has been given to the impairments of cognitive functioning that adversely influence exercise adherence. This is an especially critical concern for those suffering from—or at risk for—cardiovascular disease (CVD). The natural disease process and some corrective heart surgeries disrupt blood–oxygen transport and blood vessel integrity in ways that compromise brain function. A host of emotional, motivational, and cognitive processing problems can arise, even in minor forms of CVD. This chapter explores how these problems, collectively known as neuropsychological impairment, affect patients' abilities to learn about their illnesses and adhere to exercise prescriptions. The purpose of this chapter is twofold:

- Increase awareness about the risk for neuropsychological impairment (and more specifically, cognitive impairment) in individuals with CVD

- Help clinicians identify people at greatest risk for cognitive learning problems that may interfere with exercise adherence

Epidemiology and Pathophysiology

In a most basic sense, neuropsychological impairment in CVD is caused by cerebrovascular lesions and inadequate cerebral perfusion of oxygen-rich blood. Brain structure and function can be disrupted by these problems in focal and diffuse ways, but specific brain regions are more vulnerable, namely, frontal, subcortical, and medial–temporal structures and connections (9). This selective vulnerability creates an unfortunate supply and demand problem. These brain regions modulate various memory and executive functions, including attention and the initial encoding of information, factual recall, cognitive flexibility, strategic planning, and the capacity to self-monitor behavior. All of these cognitive processes are essential to learning new information and implementing behavioral change.

Address correspondence concerning this chapter to Mary Ann Kelly, Biomedical Science Tower, Room W1651, Translational Neuroscience Program, 3811 O'Hara Street, Pittsburgh, PA 15213-2593. E-mail: kellym3@upmc.edu

In essence, the cognitive skills in greatest demand for exercise adherence may be in shortest supply in those with CVD.

Stroke is the most likely problem that comes to mind when we think about disruptions of blood–oxygen transport and vessel integrity that negatively affect cognition. This is one of many causative factors, however. Two longitudinal studies demonstrated the more pervasive impact of other factors that can lead to progressive neuropsychological impairment in those with CVD. Using a large and relatively young, stroke-free population, the Whitehall II study showed that angina pectoris, myocardial infarction, coronary heart disease, and even peripheral vascular problems (i.e., intermittent claudication) were *all* predictive of cognitive impairment (21). Moreover, an increase in the number of CVD problems over a 6-year period was predictive of progressive cognitive decline in the Longitudinal Aging Study Amsterdam (4). Although the etiology of this impairment is undoubtedly multifactoral, silent cerebral ischemia and other vascular insufficiencies are likely contributors.

Population statistics compiled by the American Heart Association in 2005 indicate that approximately 13 million people in the United States have had silent cerebral infarcts (SCI) and that the risk for SCI increases with age and specific comorbidities (1). For example, Eguchi and colleagues (7) found a 58% incidence of SCI in individuals with hypertension, and this incidence rose to 82% when accompanied by diabetes. These SCIs most often involve ischemia in the small vasculature of the periventricular cerebral white matter that connects various brain regions. These widespread changes were once regarded as normal and age related, but this is no longer the case. It is now known that these changes predict a progressive course of cognitive decline (5). Therefore, although conventional wisdom may be that only major cerebrovascular events such as stroke produce significant cognitive impairment, it is clear that these problems are far more ubiquitous.

Common Neuropsychological Impairments

Several decades of research in clinical neuropsychology have characterized the most salient cognitive impairments associated with specific CVD processes and corrective cardiac surgeries. Beginning at the least severe end of the CVD spectrum, neuropsychological impairment can be present even before physical symptoms emerge. Using a group of young adults who were entirely asymptomatic but had parents with hypertension, Waldstein and colleagues (23) demonstrated that these people performed worse on specific visual–perceptual and spatial–constructional tasks than did controls without this heritable risk. More widespread problems are associated with symptomatic hypertension, especially in elderly people and those having the poorest blood pressure control (22). Like hypertension, congestive heart failure is a common problem that disrupts cognition, attributable in large part to heart pumping inefficiency (i.e., low ejection fraction). The combination of both low ejection fraction and hypertension is especially detrimental to cognitive function. Using a sample of cardiac rehabilitation participants, Moser and colleagues (13) showed that the combination of these two problems produced more significant cognitive impairment than all other CVD pathologies.

Acute coronary events such as myocardial infarction (MI) and cardiac arrest can cause impairment, although this typically varies in relation to the level of cerebral perfusion accompanying the event. MI is less likely to produce cognitive impairment than is cardiac arrest, which carries a specific risk for amnesia and explicit memory problems attributable to ischemic injury occurring in mesial–temporal brain structures. This does not mean that those who have had MI will be spared neuropsychological complications. As occurs in congestive heart failure, the inefficient function of the damaged heart after MI can negatively affect cognition along with the cumulative effects of underlying CVD factors. Post-MI depression is a common problem that is prognostic of poor medical outcomes as well as cognitive decline. Also, the cognitive profile of patients with post-MI depression may differ from what is seen in patients with non-cardiac-related depression and MI without depression (6).

The cumulative effects of multiple CVD factors contribute significantly to the level of neuropsychological impairment, although these cannot be reduced to simple additive effects. The expression and functional impact of CVD-related neuropsychological impairment are modulated by a variety of individual differences. A straightforward example is the increased risk for impairment in elderly people attributable to factors such as disease chronicity, normal age-related cognitive and physical decrements, and the risk for multiple comorbidities that carry additional neuropsychological risks. However, even in the face of advanced age and multiple CVD factors, the level of neuropsychological impairment will be less severe in those with greater cognitive, social, and physical reserve—that is, those with higher levels of education and higher quality of life, including cognitive, interpersonal, and physical engagement (8).

Cumulative effects and reserve factors are important to consider for patients whose CVD requires surgical intervention. Postsurgical cognitive impairments can be broadly classified into two risk categories: patient- and procedure-related factors (15). Age, education, and CVD severity are predominant patient-related risks, whereas risks associated with surgery are referred to as procedure-related risks. For example, percutaneous coronary intervention with stent implantation does not typically impair neuropsychological functioning as significantly as do more complex surgeries such as cardiac valve replacement and, especially, coronary artery bypass graft (CABG). Post-CABG neuropsychological impairment has received the most attention in the literature, with incidence rates ranging from 33% to 83% across studies (16). Moreover, this postsurgical impairment is predictive of further cognitive decline over time (17). Numerous procedure-related neuropsychological risks are associated with CABG, including the use of cardiopulmonary bypass, lengthy on-pump times, aortic cross-clamping, perfusion problems, higher levels of emboli in the circulating blood, hypotension during surgery, and rapid rewarming after surgery (3, 15).

Many comorbid medical problems can contribute to the neuropsychological impairment seen in the CVD population, although few problems have as deleterious an effect as diabetes mellitus. Diabetes is one of the most frequently occurring attendant diseases in the cardiovascular population, and apart from CVD-specific cognitive risks, diabetes alone can produce substantial neuropsychological impairment. Most studies have shown that both age and blood glucose levels moderate the nature and severity of neuropsychological impairment in people with diabetes. Elderly people with diabetes are at great risk for neuropsychological impairment, especially those with poor glucose regulation, those with hypertension, and those who have undergone CABG (11, 12, 20).

Although the neuropsychological impairments associated with CVD vary as a function of age, education, severity and type of CVD, surgeries, and comorbid disease processes, certain problems occur with regularity. Impairments of memory are a given, although the qualitative nature of memory problems can vary as a function of disease type and surgical factors. The most frequently occurring memory problems involve, but are not limited to, explicit (factual) memory and working memory. The distinction between these two types of memory is best understood through computer analogies. Working memory is akin to RAM, which holds information being worked on while it is being saved to the hard drive. Explicit memory is the file of information that has been stored and can be called up at a later time. Information processing (i.e., new learning) can be corrupted at either level—the initial processing or long-term storage of information—although the former may be of greater consequence in the context of new learning. The initial processing of information using working memory is one of the executive functions that mediate cognitive and metacognitive skills and thus enable learning and behavioral change. This primary problem with executive function may be the keystone of the cognitive supply–demand problem associated with CVD.

Identification Problems

In the context of routine clinical care, the presence of obvious neuropsychiatric symptoms such as paralysis, aphasia, or far-advanced dementia makes it more likely that cognitive impairment will be recognized. Less obvious problems will not be recognized, however. Kelly (10) showed that staff members were unable to accurately perceive cognitive impairments that predicted exercise adherence in cardiac rehabilitation participants, despite an intense level of contact (i.e., >100 hr of direct contact in 12 weeks). This underscores the need to identify patients who have learning-based adherence problems as early as possible in the treatment process, so the intervention program can be modified and enhanced to match the patient's learning needs.

Translational Neuropsychological Research

Combining neuropsychological assessment methods with information-processing theories of learning holds promise for both the identification and the accommodation of CVD-based cognitive impairments. This type of multidisciplinary approach attempts to translate the scientific evidence compiled through neuropsychological research into educationally relevant applications for CVD disease management. An example is to use neuropsychological assessment techniques to identify people at risk for poor adherence at the outset of treatment. If this can be done, this will drive further research examining the effectiveness of theoretically and empirically driven pedagogical accommodations designed to match the cognitive strengths and weaknesses of the learner. Extant research shows that neuropsychological measures, especially measures of working memory and other aspects of executive function, are useful for predicting activities of daily living (2, 14). These variables may be potent predictors of adherence to medical regimens, particularly if accompanied by other variables important to adherence such as demographic, disease, and specific psychosocial factors.

Kelly (10) conducted an initial study of this type with people participating in the rigorous Dr. Dean Ornish Program for Reversing Heart Disease. The primary goal of that study was to determine whether exercise adherence over the first 12 weeks of the program could be predicted using neuropsychological assessment data and other information routinely collected by the program. Exercise adherence was quantified through routine record keeping of both the participants and program staff. All participants received an exercise prescription requiring a minimum of 180 min of exercise per week, and a composite adherence percentage score was obtained for each subject by averaging his or her weekly percentage scores. Variables used to predict average exercise adherence were extracted from three sources: (a) subject variables relating to demography and disease, and scores on (b) psychosocial and (c) neuropsychological measures. Variables that correlated with the composite exercise adherence percentage score at $p < .10$ were considered eligible for inclusion in the predictive model, although additional selection rules were used to limit problems with statistical power and multicollinearity. Using hierarchical linear regression, Kelly found a highly significant predictive model that explained more than 50% of the variance in exercise adherence ($F_{4,40} = 10.322$, $p < .0005$). Although a diverse range of neuropsychological domains were represented in the test battery administered to all participants, the only neuropsychological variables that met inclusion criteria ($p < .10$) were two measures of executive function—conceptual flexibility for problem solving and working memory. Those who were less perseverative (i.e., better able to solve problems in situationally adaptive ways) and had fewer working memory problems had better exercise adherence. Together, these neuropsychological variables explained more than 20% of the variance in exercise adherence. An additional 31% of the variance in exercise adherence was explained by subjects' self-perception of physical vitality and busyness. The importance of these variables is not surprising. Adherence to an exercise prescription is strongly influenced by environmental demands (i.e., busyness) and the physical capacity for exercise (i.e., physical vitality). Figure 26.1 provides a visual representation of this preliminary predictive model for exercise adherence.

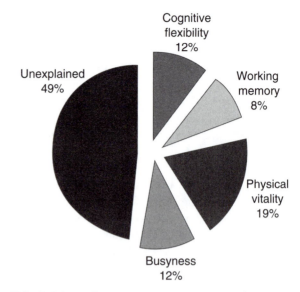

FIGURE 26.1 Preliminary predictive model for exercise adherence.

Practical Suggestions

Just as traditional psychological assessments (e.g., measures of depression, anxiety, quality of life, self-efficacy) have been incorporated into the screening of participants of cardiac rehabilitation programs, there is a need to routinely screen for neuropsychological impairment. Until this becomes common and accepted practice, existing research offers insight into specific CVD subpopulations at heightened risk for neuropsychological impairment. Table 26.1 provides a summary of CVD subpopulations at increased risk for learning-based adherence problems that may interfere with exercise adherence.

The pedagogical accommodation of CVD-based learning problems can be conceptualized as phenomenologically similar to learning disorders of childhood. For both problems, the clinician must select instructional methods and materials that match the cognitive profile and accommodate both the strengths and weaknesses of the learner. The qualitative nature of memory and executive function impairments associated with CVD contraindicates remedial instructional methods such as repetitive practice, simulated rehearsal, or other memory-enhancing exercises, and indeed several strategies are already known to be ineffectual for patients with CVD (18). These techniques are likely to increase (rather than decrease) the demand on key cognitive processes that are already in short supply. The most sensible approach is to teach people to use their residual cognitive supply along with "cognitive prostheses"—such as mnemonic (memory) aids and personal organizers—to help meet the cognitive demands of the exercise prescription (19). This shifts the focus from remediating the learner to adapting the environment to meet individual learning needs.

Table 26.2 attempts to illuminate the cognitive anatomy of a typical exercise prescription, highlighting how memory and executive control mediate learning and behavioral follow-through. Factual knowledge about both the disease process and the exercise prescription is foundational to adherence. Conceptualizing exercise as medicine is important, as is knowledge about the exercise prescription, personal parameters (i.e., heart rate and blood pressure values), and instructions for using exercise equipment. For all aspects of this learning, content-specific cues on instructional materials should be readily accessible to the learner to facilitate recall. Impairments of executive functions are expected to present even greater impediments

TABLE 26.1   Subpopulations With Heightened Risk for Neuropsychological Impairment

Problem (one or more)	Additional complications (one or more)		

Demography
    Advanced age
    Limited education
    Learning disability
    Intellectual limitations
	Multiple CVD risk factors
	CABG
	Diabetes mellitus
	Hypertension		

Disease factors
    Hypertension
    Diabetes
    Multiple CVD problems
	Poorly controlled blood pressure
	Advanced age		

Cardiac arrest or myocardial infarction	Extended period of cerebral ischemia		
CABG		Patient	Procedural
		Advanced age Diabetes Hypertension Advanced atherosclerosis	Rapid rewarming Multiple emboli Aortic cross clamping Greater on-pump time

CVD = cardiovascular disease; CABG = coronary artery bypass graft.

TABLE 26.2   Cognitive Anatomy of Exercise Prescriptions

	Factual learning: explicit and working memory	Behavioral implementation: executive functions
Disease knowledge	Exercise is medically necessary, not just a leisure activity. Physical vitality will improve through exercise. Memory and other cognitive skills will improve through exercise.	Specific current and future outcomes are associated with good and poor adherence.
Exercise prescription	Target heart rate: what it should be, when to check, how to cool down Components: recommended modalities and equipment Intensity and duration: each exercise component and total prescription Exercise equipment: specific instructions for use	Strategic planning to make time to exercise each week Flexibility to make last-minute changes if needed.

to exercise adherence because these modulate the dynamic enactment of learning and behavioral planning and initiation. Personal organizers that offer a weekly view—such as a calendar or day planner—may be especially useful cognitive prostheses. These may help accommodate the shortcomings in strategic planning that impede scheduling exercise into one's week and as well as shortcomings in cognitive flexibility needed to make as-needed, last-minute changes. Also, this offers a concrete way for clinical educators to help patients prospectively make time for exercise in their daily schedules.

Summary

Neuropsychological impairments have been identified in all forms of cardiovascular disease, but people participating in cardiac rehabilitation may be at heightened risk by virtue of both acute and cumulative effects of the disease process. Those referred for cardiac rehabilitation typically have recently had a cardiac event, have multiple risk factors or recent corrective surgeries, and are advanced in age. These primary disease and subject attributes—in the absence of any obvious or documented neurological problems such as stroke—heighten the risk for both cognitive and emotional problems that can impede program adherence and outcomes. Historically, greater attention has been given to the emotional rather than cognitive impediments of adherence. The goal of this chapter is to heighten awareness of the fundamental cognitive learning that underlies behavioral adherence.

Further research is needed to arrive at empirically based pedagogy for those participating in cardiac rehabilitation, but in the interim, a practical understanding of the problem of cognitive supply and demand is most important for clinical educators. Adherence to exercise prescriptions *demands* the ability to learn new facts and procedures and put these into action. Unfortunately, the cognitive processes needed for this learning may be in short supply in those participating in cardiac rehabilitation. A more individualized treatment plan that includes the use of mnemonic aids and personal organizers may help accommodate problems with memory, new learning, and the strategic execution of the exercise prescription. A great challenge lies ahead. Development and refinement of translational research in this area are needed to drive pedagogical adaptations and tip the cognitive supply–demand scale to a more favorable balance.

CHAPTER 27

Sleep

Shawn D. Youngstedt, PhD

Sunil Sharma, MD

Christopher E. Kline, MS

In healthy people, the nocturnal sleep period generally promotes rest and restoration of the heart via multiple mechanisms (15). Simply turning out the lights decreases blood pressure and heart rate. Lying down and refraining from movement increases parasympathetic tone, resulting in further lowering of heart rate and blood pressure. Conversely, increases in illumination and physical activity that accompany getting out of bed in the morning are associated with a surge in sympathetic nerve activity.

Sleep onset is associated with further increases in parasympathetic tone. Moreover, most of the sleep period (~75%) contains non–rapid eye movement (NREM) sleep, which is associated with relative parasympathetic dominance compared with wakefulness or rapid eye movement (REM) sleep (15). As sleep progresses to deeper stages of NREM sleep, heart rate, blood pressure, and the incidence of heart arrhythmias decline steadily, reaching their lowest levels during stages 3 and 4 sleep (slow-wave sleep). Sudden cardiac-related death also reaches a nadir at this time (20). Nocturnal changes in cardiovascular activity are influenced by circadian rhythms of sympathetic and parasympathetic nerve activity, which reach their nadir and peak, respectively, at night.

Ironically, for those with diseased hearts, who are most in need of heart recuperation, normal sleep processes can elicit unique autonomic, hemodynamic, and respiratory stresses. Indeed, approximately 20% of myocardial infarctions and 15% of sudden deaths occur between midnight and 6 a.m. (20). REM sleep, which comprises approximately 20% of the sleep period, is particularly associated with surges in sympathetic nerve activity, provoking tachycardia, hypertension, angina, arrhythmias, and irregular breathing. However, even NREM sleep poses cardiovascular challenges for people with diseased hearts. For example, myocardial ischemia can result from hypotension and increased coronary vasomotor tone during NREM sleep (20). Short bursts of sympathetic nerve activity are associated with K complexes and arousals from stage 2 sleep. Moreover, bursts of parasympathetic nerve activity, which often accompany transitions from NREM to REM sleep, have been associated with pauses in heart rhythm (15).

Numerous sleep abnormalities have been associated with deleterious effects on the cardiovascular and cerebrovascular systems. This chapter focuses on three of these abnormalities: sleep-disordered breathing, abnormal sleep duration, and shift work–related sleep disturbance. These conditions are reviewed with regard

Funded in part by National Institutes of Health grant HL71560 and a VA (VISN-7) Career Development Award.

Address correspondence concerning this chapter to Shawn D. Youngstedt, USC, 921 Assembly St, 3rd Floor, Columbia, SC 29208. E-mail: syoungstedt@sc.edu to epidemiology, putative pathophysiological mechanisms, treatment approaches, and potential efficacy of exercise as an alternative or adjuvant treatment.

Sleep-Disordered Breathing

There are several types of sleep-disordered breathing (SDB), including sleep apneas and sleep-related hypoventilation syndromes (1). Sleep apnea is the most common type of sleep-disordered breathing and is classified as central or obstructive sleep apnea. Obstructive sleep apnea is characterized by repetitive episodes of complete (apneic) or partial (hypopneic) upper-airway obstruction occurring during sleep. These events are often accompanied by oxygen desaturation and brief cortical arousals. Hypopneic and apneic episodes can occur hundreds of times per night. These episodes result in nonrestorative sleep, and many patients present with complaints of excessive daytime sleepiness.

Central sleep apnea is relatively rare and is associated with central nervous system disorders and failure of central respiratory drive mechanisms (1). Because obstructive sleep apnea (OSA) is the most common type of sleep apnea and its pathophysiology is perhaps best understood, this review emphasizes OSA.

Epidemiology of Obstructive Sleep Apnea

Most adults have at least some brief apneic episodes during sleep. Recently published guidelines by the American Academy of Sleep Medicine (1) include criteria for defining sleep apnea. The diagnostic criteria for adult OSA include either excessive daytime sleepiness or nighttime episodes of snoring and breath-holding plus an overnight polysomnography revealing five or more obstructed breathing events per hour of sleep (apnea–hypopnea index [AHI] >5) (1). Based on these criteria, the prevalence among adults has been estimated at 2% to 4% among middle-aged adults and 10% to 15% among adults older than 60 (23). The high proportion of patients with sleep apnea at sleep-disorder clinics and the serendipitous manner in which many of these patients have been referred to clinics have led to speculation that sleep apnea might be underdiagnosed. Furthermore, the increasing rates of obesity, hypertension, and diabetes in the developed world, which are all associated with sleep apnea, could forecast an increased prevalence of sleep-disordered breathing in the future.

The primary risk factors for OSA are body weight, gender, and age. A high body mass index (BMI) is clearly associated with a greater risk of sleep apnea.

Neck circumference of 17 in. (43.1 cm) or greater in males and 16 in. (40.6) or greater in females is also associated with higher risk of OSA. A relatively high prevalence of sleep apnea has been noted among football players, wrestlers, and weightlifters with low body fat percentages, suggesting that having a large neck is associated with OSA regardless of the fat or muscle composition of the neck. Indications are that these athletes suffer similar consequences (e.g., sleepiness) as others with OSA. Although SDB has been linked to obesity, it is clear that the risks associated with SDB (discussed subsequently) are independent of obesity (17).

Sleep apnea is approximately twice as common in men compared with women (24). However, this difference decreases substantially after women reach postmenopausal status, which is associated with OSA independent of age and BMI. Some evidence suggests that the gender difference in OSA is attributable to anatomical differences. Independent of body size, men tend to have longer pharyngeal airways and larger soft palate areas, both of which are associated with greater apnea risk. Hereditary or acquired bony or soft tissue abnormalities of the head and neck may predispose patients to OSA.

Aging is also clearly associated with a higher prevalence of sleep apnea (24). This pattern has been attributed to greater fat deposits around the pharynx with older age, even after controlling for BMI, and to a reduction of upper airway muscle tone. Enlarged tonsils and adenoids are considered the most important cause for OSA in children.

Racial differences in sleep apnea have been debated, but some evidence suggests higher rates of OSA among African Americans, Asians, Hispanics, and Pacific Islanders compared with age-matched Caucasians (16). Some evidence suggests that smoking is an independent risk factor for OSA (24). This could be attributed to pulmonary and respiratory effects of smoking and perhaps to nicotine withdrawal effects.

Because arousals associated with apneic events are typically brief, apneic patients are often unaware of them. Nonetheless, cardiovascular morbidity and mortality associated with sleep apnea are well documented. In a 10-year prospective study, untreated severe apnea was associated with a threefold increase in covariate-adjusted risk of fatal (relative risk = 2.7) and nonfatal (relative risk = 3.17) cardiovascular events compared with absence of severe apnea (9).

Sleep apnea is also associated with sudden myocardial infarction and death during sleep (17). Moreover, the incidence of stroke and all-cause death is correlated with the severity of apnea (22).

Multiple studies indicate that sleep apnea is an independent risk factor for hypertension and stroke (15). In data derived from the Wisconsin Sleep Cohort study, an AHI >15 was associated with a threefold-increased risk of developing new hypertension within a 4-year period (14). Approximately 65% of stroke patients have sleep apnea, which is associated with increased stroke mortality and greater morbidity (2).

Gami and colleagues (4) found a high prevalence of atrial fibrillation (approximately 50%) in subjects with OSA (adjusted odds ratio = 2.19), which was higher than that observed in high-risk patients with multiple other cardiovascular diseases. Preliminary evidence also links sleep apnea to diabetes, obesity, and the metabolic syndrome (21).

Sleep apnea clearly exacerbates other pathological conditions. For example, the presence of SDB is a major predictor of mortality after a person has a stroke (12). Moreover, mortality among patients with coronary artery disease is higher among those with apnea compared with those without apnea, even after investigators control for other covariates (10). Besides carrying cardiovascular consequences, sleep apnea also elicits profound daytime sleepiness, cognitive impairment, and decreased quality of life. It is also implicated in memory loss, impotence, and nocturia (16).

Pathophysiology of Obstructive Sleep Apnea

Patients with SDB tend to have a smaller upper airway. During the daytime, a reflex mechanism leads to increased activity of dilator muscles. However, with sleep onset these reflexes become absent, leading to collapse of the upper airways in people who are susceptible.

Each apneic event elicits a cascade of physiologic events that place a tremendous strain on the cardiovascular system (17). Of course, hypoxemia, which occurs with many apneic events, results in decreased oxygen delivery to the heart. Myocardial hypoxia can result in angina, myocardial infarction, arrhythmias, and impaired myocardial contractility (17). The number of cardiac arrhythmias has been correlated with the amount of oxygen desaturation. The resumption of breathing and reoxygenation following apneic episodes might also cause damage via massive production of free radicals.

Sympathetic nerve activity is activated by hypoxemia as well as by the resulting hypercapnia, changes in ventilation, and arousals from sleep. Increased sympathetic nerve activity during apneic events has been linked to endothelial cell dysfunction and pulmonary arteriolar vasoconstriction (17). Speculation is that chronic surges in sympathetic nerve activity contribute to insulin resistance and hypertension (17).

OSA also elicits release of inflammatory mediators (e.g., cytokines and C-reactive protein) and increased expression of cell adhesion molecules. Moreover, fluctuations in blood pressure associated with apnea and recovery can elicit stress in the walls of the myocardium and changes in coronary and cerebral blood flow, contributing to atherosclerosis.

Treatment of Sleep Apnea

The primary treatment of choice for OSA is continuous positive airway pressure therapy (CPAP). Positive airway pressure therapy is delivered with a system that generates airflow and delivers it via tubing to the patient. Acute use of CPAP has been shown to reduce the frequency of respiratory events, improve sleep and mood, and reduce blood pressure and sleepiness (17). Chronic use of CPAP has been associated with improved cognitive function, quality of life, and mood (7). CPAP use also has been shown to reduce the risk of fatal and nonfatal cardiac events in people with severe apnea (3).

Notwithstanding the benefits of CPAP, this therapy is judged to be too invasive by many patients. Complaints include discomfort in changing sleep position and wearing the mask, claustrophobia, disturbance of sleep of bed partners, and reduced intimacy with partners. Other side effects of CPAP include dry nasal passages and chafing of the face. Because treatment is typically indefinite, patients feel chronically burdened. For these reasons, compliance to CPAP is low. Nonadherence often begins with the first night of treatment, and 1-year compliance to CPAP treatment is only about 50%.

Considering the low compliance to CPAP, clinicians need to develop alternative or adjuvant treatments for sleep apnea. Some evidence suggests that exercise might help reduce the severity of OSA.

Exercise and Obstructive Sleep Apnea

It was previously surmised that exercise could be a helpful adjuvant to sleep apnea only to the extent to which it could help reduce body weight. However, recent epidemiologic and experimental evidence suggests that regular exercise might reduce sleep apnea and some of its negative consequences via other mechanisms such as improved muscle tone of upper-respiratory muscles.

A study of 1,104 men and women ages 30 to 60 years (13) found a significant inverse association between hours of reported planned exercise and AHI, after the investigators controlled for BMI and several other covariates. Adjusted mean AHI for those reporting >7 hr and 0 hr of exercise per week were 2.8 and 5.3, respectively. Sleepiness was also statistically controlled; thus, there was no obvious converse mechanism in which apnea produced sleepiness and, therefore, less ability or inclination to exercise.

To our knowledge, only two experimental investigations have focused on whether exercise training can decrease sleep apnea. Giebelhaus and colleagues (5) examined 11 patients with moderate or severe apnea (AHI >10) who had previously received CPAP treatment for 3 to 12 months. A 6-month exercise program involving one mild aerobic exercise session and one weight training session per week resulted in a 30% reduction in AHI, whereas there was no change in body weight. The data suggest that even modest exercise reduced sleep apnea beyond that noted after moderately long CPAP use. However, because there was no control treatment, the improvements might be attributable to the CPAP treatment or to spontaneous remission.

Norman and colleagues (11) conducted an uncontrolled, although intensive 6-month supervised aerobic exercise training program in a small group (n = 9) of obese people (BMI = 31.2 ± 4.6) with mild to moderate sleep apnea. Participants progressed to exercising 3 times weekly for 30 to 45 min, with ≥20 min of activity at 60% to 85% heart rate reserve. A significant improvement in AHI was noted (mean reduction of 47% from 21.7 to 11.8) as well as significant improvements in exercise capacity, sleep, blood pressure, mood, quality of life, and sleepiness. Although significant decreases in body weight, BMI, and neck girth were found, the changes (e.g., mean decrease in body weight of 6.2 kg) were not significantly correlated with changes in AHI. Additionally, literature suggests that the changes were insufficient to elicit the improvements in AHI that were found.

Regardless of its effect on apnea, exercise can help reduce the mortality and morbidity (e.g., fatigue) associated with sleep apnea. However, the cardiovascular consequences associated with chronic sleep apnea can make exercise both more risky and more difficult. For example, Tryfon and colleagues (19) found that blood pressure elevation during exercise was significantly greater among normotensive apneic patients compared with age-matched controls. Moreover, compared with control subjects, apnea patients have reduced aerobic and anaerobic capacity. Conversely, short-term (4-8 weeks) treatment of sleep apnea with CPAP has significantly improved anaerobic capacity, aerobic

exercise tolerance, and ratings of perceived exertion to a standardized workload (8).

Abnormal Sleep Duration and Cardiovascular Disease

Although the mechanisms are not clear, both short and long sleep have been associated with increased risk of cardiovascular disease.

Epidemiology

Epidemiologic studies have consistently found a U-shaped association of sleep duration with mortality and morbidity attributed to both cardiovascular and noncardiovascular causes. Both short sleep (i.e., ≤6 hr) and long sleep (>8 hr) have been associated with coronary heart disease, stroke, diabetes, hypertension, and hypercholesterolemia (25).

Pathophysiology

There are several potential mechanisms by which short sleep could elicit cardiovascular disease. Some evidence suggests that short-term sleep curtailment can increase sympathetic nervous system activity, increase blood pressure, and impair glucose tolerance.

In contrast with the risks of short sleep, the potential risks associated with long sleep have been scarcely addressed. One plausible mechanism by which long sleep could contribute to cardiovascular disease is via arousals from sleep. It has been shown that long sleepers have more fragmented sleep than average or short-duration sleepers (25). Both spontaneous and experimentally induced arousals from sleep are associated with surges in sympathetic nerve activity, cortisol, and blood pressure (25).

Treatment of Abnormal Sleep Duration

A host of treatment strategies are available to increase sleep duration. Simple sleep hygiene instructions, included in table 27.1, can be helpful (18). Sleeping pills are not recommended for chronic (>4 weeks) treatment because of associations of chronic use with mortality, tolerance, and rebound insomnia with discontinuance. Cognitive behavioral therapy is preferred for chronic management of poor sleep.

One of the most effective behavioral treatments for insomnia is sleep restriction treatment. Insomnia is often perpetuated or exacerbated by spending excessive time in bed in an effort to compensate for disturbed

TABLE 27.1 Sleep Hygiene Recommendations

Recommendation	Comment
Maintain a consistent bedtime and wake-time, even on weekends.	Keeping a consistent sleep period helps stabilize your circadian system.
Limit alcohol past dinnertime.	Although alcohol can help you fall asleep, it can also result in more awakenings.
Take a warm or hot bath about 2 hr before bedtime.	This aids in distal vasodilation, which promotes sleep onset.
Limit caffeine past lunchtime.	Stimulants will interfere with sleep if consumed too late in the day.
Use bed only for sleep (no watching TV, reading, or eating).	This helps build an association (conditioning) between your bed and sleeping.
Keep bedroom as dark and noise- and distraction-free as possible at night.	Excessive light can suppress production of melatonin, which has mild sleep-promoting effects.
If awake after 15 min of attempting sleep, leave bedroom and perform a monotonous task (e.g., reading) in dim light; when sleepy, attempt sleep again.	Avoid "trying" to fall asleep. Returning to bed when sleepy promotes an association of the bed with sleep.
Keep a consistent exercise schedule, exercising outdoors in bright light if possible.	Both exercise and bright light can promote sleep and synchronize your circadian system.
Allow 1 hr to unwind before bedtime.	Reducing anxiety (by relaxation, yoga, meditation) will improve subsequent sleep.
Keep naps to a minimum; no naps after midafternoon.	Napping too late in the day can disrupt subsequent nighttime sleep.

sleep. Having an insomniac spend less time in bed can result in consolidated and refreshing sleep. Clinicians have generally not addressed how to treat abnormally long sleep duration, which has not been regarded as harmful. Nonetheless, sleep restriction therapy would be an obvious treatment to consider (25).

Exercise for Short and Long Sleep

In epidemiologic studies, low levels of exercise have been one of the most robust correlates of both short and long sleep (25). A causal link between these variables could operate in either direction. Low levels of exercise could impair sleep or make one feel less energetic, resulting in long sleep. On the other hand, there is evidence suggesting that both short and long sleep may cause a person to become less active. Thus, epidemiologic studies of sleep duration and mortality and morbidity rates, which have typically controlled for exercise, might have underestimated the risks of long and short sleep. Short sleep could lead to fatigue, which is a significant predictor of low activity. Short-term sleep extension studies as well as anecdotal accounts

indicate that spending extra time in bed leads to feelings of lethargy, which could also make one less willing or able to engage in physical activity. Chronically, extra time in bed could also be hazardous because this would involve ≥1 hr of more of completely sedentary behavior and would allow less wakefulness time to engage in physical activity.

Exercise is a particularly attractive alternative or adjuvant sleep treatment for multiple reasons. First, epidemiologic studies have consistently shown that exercise is associated with better sleep. Second, exercise has been endorsed by most sleep experts as a means of improving sleep. Third, exercise would be far healthier than pharmacologic treatment and conceivably simpler and less expensive than traditional cognitive behavioral treatment.

Most of the literature on exercise and sleep has been restricted to normal sleepers and thus is probably limited by ceiling and floor effects (i.e., there is little room for improvement in sleep quality). Nonetheless, significant (albeit modest) improvement in sleep has been found in this population. Larger effects of exercise have been noted in people with insomnia, but this information has been limited primarily to self-report data.

Exercise could reduce sleep duration in long sleepers by increasing energy levels. Moreover, morning or evening exercise could facilitate sleep restriction therapy by helping the person maintain wakefulness.

Shift Work and Cardiovascular Disease

Shift work is a prevalent occupational practice despite its detrimental effects on worker health.

Epidemiology of Shift Work

Approximately 20% of U.S. workers are shift workers, who work during the evening or night or have constant shifting of their work schedules. Shift work is associated with an increased prevalence of cardiovascular morbidity and mortality as well as a host of other morbidities, including disturbed sleep, cancer, depressed mood, gastrointestinal problems, and accidents.

Pathophysiology of Shift Work

The associations of shift work with disease can be partly attributed to social and behavioral factors (e.g., stress). However, research suggests that although these factors contribute, the primary problem of shift work relates to chronic desynchronization between a person's circadian system and his or her environmental sleep–wake and work–rest schedule.

Circadian desynchronization has many potentially harmful consequences. Alteration in circadian rhythms of sympathetic nervous system activity relative to wakefulness could strain the cardiovascular system. Circadian desynchronization also alters postprandial glucose and lipid regulation, which has been implicated in the pathogenesis of cardiovascular diseases and other disease. Shift work might also be indirectly harmful via chronic sleep deprivation, one of the most common problems of shift work.

Current Treatment of Shift Work

The primary treatment for facilitating resynchronization of the body clock has been appropriately timed exposure to bright light, which works via a direct connection between the retina and the suprachiasmatic nuclei. However, the efficacy of light for shift-work adjustment has been less impressive than what might be theoretically predicted from short-term laboratory studies. Thus, alternative or adjuvant circadian treatments should be explored.

Exercise for Shift Work

Both animal and human research has suggested that exercise has significant phase-shifting effects. Available evidence suggests that exercise is helpful for shift workers. Cross-sectional and experimental studies indicate that exercise training reduces the complaints of shift workers (6). Moreover, short-term experimental studies have shown that nighttime exercise can facilitate circadian adjustment in shift workers.

Perhaps the most exciting findings in this area indicate that bright light and exercise might be combined to elicit synergistic circadian phase-shifting effects. This has been particularly well-documented in rodents but partly supported by human data as well. Conceivably, combining light and exercise could facilitate much more rapid adjustment to shift work and jet lag than previously realized.

Summary

Sleep is an essential behavior that normally contributes to health and optimal functioning. However, the nocturnal sleep period is a vulnerable time for those with cardiac disease. In addition, sleep abnormalities are commonly associated with cardiovascular disease. Obstructive sleep apnea, in which there are frequent airway obstructions during sleep, is an increasingly prevalent disorder, affecting up to 10% of adults worldwide. It exerts numerous health consequences, including increased blood pressure, increased risk of stroke, and increased systemic inflammation. Furthermore, both short sleep (≤6 hr) and long sleep (>8 hr) are associated with increased cardiovascular disease. Finally, shift work is associated with increased cardiovascular disease and all-cause mortality yet is a common occupational requirement. Exercise training has shown promise in attenuating the severity and consequences of these sleep abnormalities.

Rehabilitation of the Patient With Cardiovascular Disease

Part V presents insights into rehabilitation strategies for specific cardiovascular conditions. The specific conditions are coronary artery disease, myocardial infarction, and angina pectoris (chapter 28); coronary artery revascularization (chapter 29); cardiac arrhythmias and conduction disturbances (chapter 30); peripheral arterial disease (chapter 31); chronic heart failure (chapter 32); cardiac transplant (chapter 33); and thromboembolism and deep vein thrombosis (chapter 34).

CHAPTER 28

Coronary Artery Disease, Myocardial Infarction, and Angina Pectoris

Barry A. Franklin, PhD

Justin E. Trivax, MD

Thomas E. Vanhecke, MD

Coronary atherosclerosis involves a localized accumulation of lipid and fibrous tissue within the coronary artery, progressively narrowing the lumen of the vessel. Presumably, this degenerative process can result from the interaction of genetic, lifestyle, and environmental influences that are collectively known as coronary risk factors. Fatty streaks may progress over time to fibrous plaques and eventually to atheromata. Coronary blood flow is usually not significantly compromised until the obstruction exceeds 70% of the vessel's cross-sectional area. Such lesions can result in blood flow inadequate to meet myocardial oxygen demands, causing significant exercise-induced electrocardiographic (ECG) ST-segment depression, angina pectoris, or both. When ST-segment depression occurs in the absence of symptoms, it is referred to as asymptomatic or silent ischemia. Lesions that result in less lumen obstruction may still be complicated by hemorrhage, plaque rupture, or thrombosis, leading to angina pectoris, myocardial infarction, or sudden cardiac death.

Intensive risk factor modification may stabilize coronary plaques and lessen their vulnerability to rupture. In addition to stabilizing plaques, intensive risk factor modification can reduce clinical cardiovascular events by mitigating factors that may trigger plaque rupture (e.g., elevated blood pressure), exacerbate arterial inflammation (e.g., excess low-density lipoprotein [LDL] cholesterol), and adversely affect thrombogenic propensity (e.g., platelet stickiness). This chapter addresses the evaluation and treatment of patients with coronary artery disease (CAD), with specific reference to epidemiology, pathophysiology, diagnosis, medical management, exercise prescription, and rehabilitation outcomes.

Address correspondence concerning this chapter to Barry A. Franklin, Beaumont Health Center, Preventive Cardiology, 4949 Coolidge Highway, Royal Oak, MI 48073. E-mail: bfranklin@beaumont.edu

Epidemiology

Ischemic heart disease is the leading cause of death and disability in the Western world, encompassing several disease states (e.g., CAD and acute coronary syndrome [ACS]). An ACS may manifest as an acute myocardial infarction (AMI) with ST-segment elevation, unstable angina, or non–ST-segment elevation MI. Approximately 16 million people in the United States suffer from CAD (4). The American Heart Association predicts that >750,000 people will present to an emergency department with a new ACS in 2008 (4). Moreover, an additional 430,000 people will present with a recurrent coronary event (4).

Modifiable Risk Factors

The Framingham Heart Study identified several risk factors for the development of CAD that are largely modifiable via lifestyle changes or pharmacologic intervention: dyslipidemia, diabetes mellitus, hypertension, smoking, physical inactivity, and obesity. In contrast, nonmodifiable risk factors include age, gender, and family history of premature CAD.

Dyslipidemia

Cholesterol is a main constituent of coronary atherosclerotic lesions. Large epidemiologic studies have identified an increased risk of ACS in the presence of serum lipid abnormalities: mainly increased LDL cholesterol (LDL-C), elevated triglycerides, and decreased high-density lipoprotein (HDL) cholesterol or HDL-C. Furthermore, well-designed trials have shown that treatment of dyslipidemias reduces future coronary events and halts progression of CAD (41, 53). The National Cholesterol Education Program Expert Panel on Detection, Evaluation and Treatment of High Blood Cholesterol in Adults (NCEP ATP III) identifies LDL-C as the main target of cholesterol-lowering therapy (19). LDL-C may be reduced by lifestyle interventions (diet, fish oil supplementation, weight loss, and exercise), pharmacologic treatment (hydroxymethylglutaryl coenzyme A reductase inhibitors, bile acid sequestrants, nicotinic acid, fibric acid derivatives, cholesterol absorption inhibitors), or both. Despite multiple therapeutic approaches, fewer than one third of patients treated for hyperlipidemia achieve recommended LDL-C targets (19).

Diabetes

Approximately 20% to 25% of all patients who present with ACS are diabetic, and CAD accounts for 75% of all deaths in diabetes. People with diabetes exhibit a propensity for atherosclerosis with more extensive CAD, involvement of multiple vessels, unstable lesions, frequent comorbidities, and less favorable long-term outcomes with coronary revascularization (39, 54, 61). Accelerated progression and occlusion of atherosclerotic coronary lesions are also more common in diabetics. The International Diabetes Foundation and World Health Organization predict the prevalence of diabetes to increase from 7% of the U.S. population in 2005 to 9% of the population in 2025, which will undoubtedly lead to a significant increase of CAD over the next 2 decades (5).

Hypertension

Hypertension is the most common risk factor for CAD. According to the Joint National Committee on Prevention, Detection, Evaluation and Treatment of High Blood Pressure (JNC-VII), normal systolic and diastolic blood pressures are <120 and <80 mmHg, respectively (11). The risk of CAD increases with every increment in blood pressure over 110/75 mmHg. Therapy for hypertension should include lifestyle modification (weight reduction, exercise, dietary changes) and pharmacologic interventions, if necessary, to obtain goal blood pressures <140/90 mmHg (<130/80 mmHg with diabetes or chronic kidney disease).

Smoking

Major cohort studies conducted over the past 50 years have shown that the risk of dying from CAD is 70% greater among smokers than nonsmokers, and among smoking-related deaths, about 33% are from cardiovascular disease. Men and women who smoke at least 20 cigarettes per day are 6 and 3 times more likely to suffer an AMI, respectively, than age- and gender-matched nonsmokers (42). Smoking increases the risk for CAD and associated sequelae through many mechanisms, including direct promotion of atherosclerosis, platelet activation, increased thrombogenesis, decreased oxygen delivery, and increased sympathetic drive (augmented blood pressure and heart rate). According to the American Cancer Society, cigarette smoking in the United States declined from about 42% of the population in 1965 to approximately 21% in 2004 (9). Despite this favorable trend, an estimated 44.5 million adults continue to smoke.

Physical Inactivity

The American Heart Association and the JNC-VII classify obesity and physical inactivity as major modifiable risk factors for CAD (11, 17). Both physical inactivity and a reduced aerobic capacity are strongly associated with increased cardiovascular and all-cause mortality rates (63).

Obesity

The National Health and Nutrition Examination Survey data demonstrated that nearly two thirds of adults are overweight or obese and nearly one third are obese (20). Deaths attributable to obesity are projected to soon overtake tobacco as the number one cause of preventable death in developed countries. An increased body mass index is strongly associated with an elevated risk of cardiovascular disease, hypertension, and all-cause mortality.

Unmodifiable Risk Factors

Risk factors including age, gender, and family history of premature CAD are not modifiable. More than 71 million American adults have one or more types of cardiovascular disease, with >27 million estimated to be aged 65 or older (4). More than 80% of all AMI-related deaths occur in people who are 65 or older (25). In addition, heart disease is the leading cause of hospitalization among elderly adults, with one third dying during the acute phase. The risk for AMI increases after the age of 45 for men and 55 for women.

Gender

Gender differences have been observed in the epidemiology of the ACS. Excess risk has been documented in men compared with premenopausal women; however, after menopause the incidence of AMI in women increases to that of their age-matched male counterparts. Although this is presumably related to postmenopausal hormonal changes, the Women's Health Initiative demonstrated that hormone replacement therapy did not prevent or reduce CAD (51). Moreover, cardiovascular mortality is higher in women compared with men, which is likely attributable to associated comorbidities, including older age, dyslipidemia, and smoking history.

Family History

A family history of premature CAD, defined as heart disease in a male first-degree relative <55 years old or heart disease in a female first-degree relative <65 years old, is a major unmodifiable risk factor. Multiple studies have shown familial clustering of cardiovascular disease. This clustering is likely related to genetic mutations resulting in familial hypercholesterolemia (disorders of lipoprotein metabolism), diabetes, or collagen–vascular disorders. Environmental and acquired risk factors may also contribute to familial trends, including air pollution, smoking (personal or second-hand), and fetal environment.

Pathophysiology

Over the past 2 decades, major advances have been made in the understanding of AMI. Endothelial dysfunction and microvascular disease, inflammatory mediators, signals involved in coagulation and thrombosis, and defects in lipoprotein metabolism have become major areas of investigation. Although the classic theory of AMI, that is, a slow-growing plaque enlarging to near-complete obliteration of blood flow within the culprit coronary artery, has been largely discounted (3, 36), the paradigm of supply and demand remains the underlying mechanism of myocardial ischemia. Although the decreased oxygen supply during an AMI may result from hypotension, coronary spasm, coronary dissection, arrhythmia, or anemia, most patients presenting with an AMI have experienced coronary plaque destabilization or rupture resulting in formation of a superimposed occluding thrombus.

Atherosclerotic heart disease evolves silently over decades until it manifests with an acute plaque rupture or pain from chronic ischemia. Atherosclerosis begins with focal accumulation of lipoproteins within regions of the intima, which form fatty streaks before the second decade of life. In the Pathobiological Determinants of Atherosclerosis in Youth Study, 2,876 study subjects between 15 and 34 years of age underwent autopsy for noncardiac deaths. The majority of these subjects were found to have overt precursors of arterial atherosclerosis. In youths aged 15 to 19 years, intimal lesions appeared in all the aortas and more than half of the right coronary arteries (55).

Proliferation of the extracellular matrix is the first step seen histologically in the development of atherosclerosis. Thereafter, proteoglycans (mainly biglycan) on the luminal surface increase. As lipoproteins travel through the coronary arteries, proteoglycan interaction increases the time during which lipoproteins are at the luminal surface. This results in increased LDL oxidation by free radicals present along the endothelial surface. The LDL–proteoglycan interaction also appears to enhance intimal invasion. As LDL particles enter the intima, further separation from plasma antioxidants augments oxidation of the lipoproteins (34). The oxidized LDL entity increases leukocyte activity within the endothelium via increased expression of cellular adhesion molecules and cytokine production, and monocytes and T lymphocytes invade the subendothelial space (18). The mononuclear leukocytes engulf and phagocytize subendothelial oxidized LDL, becoming foam cells. As the foam cells accumulate, a fatty streak develops, which is the initial manifestation of atherosclerosis.

As the fatty streak matures, many inflammatory mediators are released and smooth muscle cells are attracted to the intima. The vessel wall accommodates the increasing cellular burden and inflammation by outward remodeling (figures 28.1 and 28.2) (35). This remodeling does not compromise blood flow in the vessel lumen until the plaque reaches its outward limit (>40% of the internal elastic lamina area), highlighting a major limitation of conventional coronary angiography in detecting the total atherosclerotic burden (23). At this point, the vessel lumen is gradually compromised by an expanding plaque that may be unstable (figure 28.1) or stable (figure 28.2). Multiple pathologic factors contribute to plaque instability and subsequent rupture, including plaque composition, fibrous cap vulnerability, and inflammatory mediators (1). If the

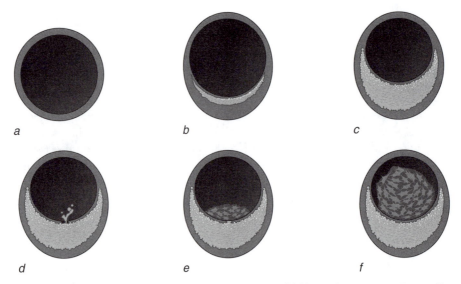

FIGURE 28.1 Unstable plaque in chronic coronary artery disease. *(a)* Normal coronary artery caliber without abnormalities. *(b)* Outward remodeling seen in the first steps of atherosclerosis and preservation of the luminal space. *(c)* Atherosclerotic lesion begins to obstruct luminal space (~30-40%), and the fibrous cap remains thin. *(d)* Plaque instability and rupture occur. *(e)* Platelets are attracted to ruptured plaque and begin to adhere to one another. *(f)* Plaque rupture acutely obstructs blood flow to the myocardium, with platelet interaction and subsequent blockage of coronary artery.

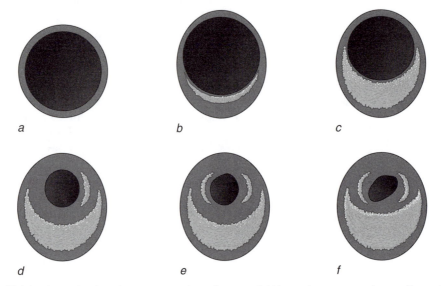

FIGURE 28.2 Stable plaque in chronic coronary artery disease. *(a)* Normal coronary artery caliber without abnormalities. *(b)* Outward remodeling seen in the first steps of atherosclerosis and the preservation of the luminal space. *(c)* Atherosclerotic lesion begins to obstruct luminal space (~30-40%) and the fibrous cap develops with large numbers of smooth muscle cells. *(d)* Further plaques form and the intima continues to grow with the recruitment of smooth muscle cells. *(e)* More plaques form, and the intima develops further. *(f)* Approximately 80-90% of the luminal space is obstructed.

plaque is stable, the patient is usually asymptomatic until luminal narrowing exceeds 70%. Thereafter, the patient may experience symptoms of stable angina or exertional angina that resolves with rest. Most patients experiencing an ST-segment elevation MI have not suffered from previous angina, because the culprit artery usually has <50% obstruction before the plaque becomes unstable (3).

Plaque composition in a vulnerable lesion consists of a macrophage-rich and lipid-rich core. Increased lipid composition leads to further LDL oxidation and subsequent inflammation. The increased population of macrophages further contributes to inflammation by releasing cytokines and inflammatory mediators. Subsequently, the fibrous cap becomes thin and collagen poor. With disruption of the frail fibrous cap, exposure of highly thrombogenic contents, including collagen fragments, crystalline surfaces, and tissue factor, further increases local thrombin generation. Platelet adhesion is the first step in the acute thrombosis of an unstable lesion occurring via platelet receptor glycoproteins and endothelial von Willebrand factor interaction. Platelets activate and adhere to one another, precipitating an ACS attributable to formation of an occluding thrombus within the coronary artery.

Diagnosis and Management of Acute CAD Events

A timely and accurate diagnosis of an unstable cardiac event (i.e., AMI or escalating anginal symptoms) is crucial. Although chest pain is the most common symptom in fatal AMI, it accounts for only 5.1% of all emergency department visits. Demographics, history, and risk factors can provide important clues to risk stratification. Stimuli that can trigger an AMI include unaccustomed vigorous physical exertion, cocaine use, exposure to cold temperatures, and severe emotional stress (64). During an acute cardiovascular event, minimizing time to treatment has the greatest potential to decrease morbidity and mortality (6).

The gold standard for the diagnosis of myocyte injury is an increase in serum cardiac enzymes. In 2007, the five major worldwide cardiovascular health groups set forth new definitions of AMI, subdividing it into five different types depending on mechanism of infarction (table 28.1) (2). These definitions emphasize using the serum level of troponin in making the diagnosis, along with adjunctive evidence of ECG ischemia or loss of viability through myocardial imaging (e.g., new wall motion abnormality). With its speed and

ease of attainment, the ECG is the single best test to immediately diagnose AMI. All patients with chest pain should undergo a 12-lead ECG as soon as possible, with specific reference to ST-segment displacement. Nevertheless, concomitant ECG changes may be absent during the initial presentation of an AMI. Many institutions have now embraced point-of-care cardiac marker analyzers to provide rapid quantitative results in ≤10 min rather than more time-consuming central laboratory testing. Given the time required to obtain serum markers, patients who present with a high index of suspicion should undergo reperfusion strategies. Patients with ST-elevation myocardial infarction should receive reperfusion therapy with percutaneous coronary intervention (PCI) with stenting within 90 min. If PCI is not available, a fibrinolytic should be administered within 30 min of symptom onset (6).

Recommendations presented here for the management of patients with an acute coronary event are from the American College of Cardiology and the American Heart Association consensus guidelines (6). Aspirin (160-325 mg) should be given immediately and continued indefinitely thereafter. Likewise, β-blockers should be administered promptly to patients without contraindications, because these attenuate myocardial infarction size, decrease cardiac oxygen consumption, and reduce mortality. Nitroglycerin should be used in patients with large infarctions, persistent myocardial ischemia, pulmonary congestion, hypertension, or combinations thereof. Nitroglycerin should not be used in patients with right ventricular infarction or those who are hypotensive or bradycardic. In the absence of hypotension or other contraindications, inhibitors of the renin–angiotensin–aldosterone system should be administered orally with the first 24 hr in patients with anterior infarction, pulmonary congestion, or an ejection fraction <40%. A landmark trial reaffirmed that clopidogrel should be given with aspirin in the setting of AMI, unless specific contraindications are present (i.e., hemorrhage or planned coronary artery bypass graft surgery) (10). If available, primary PCI should be performed in patients with AMI, especially within 24 hr. Heparin and glycoprotein IIb and IIIa inhibitors should be used as pharmacologic support during primary PCI, if appropriate (6).

In chronic stable CAD, hypertension, hyperlipidemia, family history of CAD, reduced aerobic fitness, sedentary lifestyle, diabetes, and cigarette smoking are the most common risk factors and should be used to assess a patient's risk. The most common clinical manifestation of CAD is angina pectoris (47). Atherosclerotic coronary artery obstruction creates an imbalance between myocardial oxygen supply and demand,

TABLE 28.1   Universal Definitions of the Five Types of Acute Myocardial Infarction by the American College of Cardiology, American Heart Association, European Society of Cardiology, World Health Organization, and World Health Federation

AMI type	Mechanism producing myocardial ischemia and infarction	Criteria to fulfill diagnosis
1	A primary coronary event, including plaque rupture or dissection	Troponin or creatine kinase-MB mass >99th percentile with additional evidence (ECG changes or wall-motion abnormality with imaging)
2	Decreased O_2 supply and demand (i.e., arrhythmia, coronary spasm, coronary embolism, anemia, or hypotension)	Troponin or creatine kinase-MB mass >99th percentile with additional evidence (ECG changes or wall-motion abnormality with imaging)
3	Sudden cardiac death, with signs and symptoms of ischemia, that occurred before blood samples could be obtained or before cardiac enzymes could be released	Symptoms, history, or limited data such as ECG changes
4	An event during a percutaneous coronary intervention	Serum markers to exceed 3 times the 99th percentile of normal
5	An event during a coronary artery bypass graft	Serum markers to exceed 5 times the 99th percentile of normal

AMI = acute myocardial infarction; ECG = electrocardiographic.

precipitating exertion-induced anginal pain, ischemic ST-segment depression, or both. An accurate history can often differentiate cardiac from other causes of chest pain. Typical anginal pain is best described as substernal squeezing, discomfort, or crushing pain, which may radiate to the jaw or arms, is worse with exertion, and is relieved by rest or nitroglycerin (47).

The physical examination of patients with CAD is variable and often unremarkable. Waist circumference, waist-to-hip ratio, and body mass index are useful indicators of a sedentary lifestyle, dietary indiscretion, or the metabolic phenotype. Atherosclerosis may manifest as peripheral vascular disease (i.e., carotid or renal artery bruits), and vascular insufficiencies may be assessed with simple tests such as the ankle–brachial systolic pressure index. Severe hyperlipidemia may be identified as lipid deposition in tendon xanthomata or retinal lipemia.

Protocol-driven exercise or pharmacologic stress tests are useful, noninvasive studies for diagnosing CAD. The sensitivity and specificity of these tests increase when combined with thallium (or sestamibi) imaging, to evaluate myocardial perfusion defects, or with echocardiography, to identify wall motion abnormalities. Indications for coronary angiography, the gold standard of assessing the severity of CAD, are listed in table 28.2. Many new diagnostic technolo-

gies are available, although their roles have not been completely defined. Multidetector computed tomography (MDCT) provides a two-dimensional array of detector elements that noninvasively acquire images of multiple slices or sections of an artery instantaneously, facilitating remarkable visualization of coronary atherosclerosis. For example, with a 64-slice MDCT, each rotation captures 64 images simultaneously. Although MDCT is used in an acute setting, studies are lacking that justify routine clinical application of this diagnostic modality (28).

Electron beam computed tomography (EBCT) may be useful for evaluation of patients with suspected CAD. Like MDCT, EBCT lacks consensus guidelines for its use. The presence of any calcification is indicative of CAD. Whereas stress testing is usually abnormal in the setting of more advanced disease (e.g., with a >50% stenosis), CT detection of coronary disease may be able to identify disease at earlier stages. With EBCT, a calcium score is generated. The higher the calcium score, the greater the potential for extensive calcification with a high probability for significant stenosis and an abnormal stress test result. A negative EBCT finding makes the presence of atherosclerotic plaque, including unstable plaque, very unlikely; however, a positive or equivocal test suggests the need for additional diagnostic testing.

Medical Management

Treatment of the coronary patient begins with addressing modifiable risk factors. Increasing physical activity, reducing body weight and fat stores, quitting smoking, controlling diabetes, and managing lipids and hypertension are essential. Varied cardioprotective medications are available for the treatment of CAD, and the potential therapeutic effects of three main classes of drugs have been reported (figure 28.3). Addressing depression and social isolation is also important, because these psychosocial factors, if left untreated, may form significant barriers to achieving lifestyle changes. For more on psychosocial factors, see chapter 24.

TABLE 28.2 Indications for Coronary Angiography

Absolutely appropriate	May be appropriate	Not appropriate
Patients undergoing AMI reperfusion and PCI	Patients with contraindications to or high risk for stress testing with high suspicion	Asymptomatic patients who are being screened for CAD
Patients with suspected abrupt closure or subacute stent thrombosis after PCI	Patients who are symptomatic with serial deterioration on noninvasive testing	Patients with stable angina who respond to medical therapy
Patients who are severely symptomatic (CCS class III or IV)	Low-risk patients with angina that accelerates or intensifies despite adequate medical therapy	Patients who refuse or are not candidates for future revascularization
High-risk patients undergoing noninvasive tests (stress ECG, echo, or perfusion studies with symptoms)	Patients who are asymptomatic without known CAD with >2 major clinical risk factors and who are found to be abnormal (intermediate) but not high risk on noninvasive testing	
Patients who have failed fibrinolysis (as a rescue strategy)	Patients with upcoming major surgery (for risk stratification)	

PCI = percutaneous coronary intervention; AMI = acute myocardial infarction; CAD = coronary artery disease; CCS = Canadian Cardiovascular Society.

Beta blockers	Statins	ACEIs/ARBs
↓ Blood pressure	Improved lipid profile (i.e., ↓ LDL, ↓ trig, etc.)	↓ Blood pressure
↓ Heart rate	↓ Inflammation	↓ Fibrinolysis
↓ Contractility	↑ Endothelial function	↑ Plaque stability
↓ Myocardial O_2 demand	↑ Plaque stability	↑ Arterial compliance
↑ Coronary flow	↓ Macrophages	↓ Oxidative stress
↓ Cardiac remodeling	↓ Reactive O_2 species	↓ Inflammation
Antiarrhythmic	↑ NO bioactivity	↓ Collagen matrix
↓ Adrenergic activity	↓ VSMC proliferation	↓ VSMC proliferation
	↑ EPCs and CACs	

FIGURE 28.3 Proposed physiologic and clinical effects of three widely prescribed cardioprotective drugs. LDL = low-density lipoprotein cholesterol; trig = serum triglycerides; NO = nitric oxide; VSMC = vascular smooth muscle cell; EPC = endothelial progenitor cell; CAC = cultured angiogenic cell; ACEI = angiotensin converting enzyme inhibitor; ARB = angiotensin receptor blocker; ↑ = increased; ↓ = decreased.

Smoking cessation is mandatory, and cessation rates can be increased as much as 30% with as little as 3 min of physician counseling (60). The importance of smoking cessation was recently reiterated from a 50-year follow-up study on male British physicians (15). This study demonstrated that cessation at age 60, 50, 40, or 30 years gained, respectively, about 3, 6, 9, or 10 years of life expectancy. Approved by the Food and Drug Administration in 2006, varenicline (Chantix) is a highly effective medication to aid in smoking cessation (24). Likewise, bupropion, nicotine replacement products, and counseling may help, especially when used in combination.

β-blockers reduce mortality rates in chronic CAD patients and should be given unless absolutely contraindicated. These medications should be titrated to maintain resting heart rate at 50 to 60 beats/min and systolic blood pressure >95 mmHg. In asymptomatic men at risk for coronary disease and patients with chronic stable angina or documented CAD, aspirin (81-325 mg) can reduce the incidence of initial or recurrent AMI.

The statins (hydroxymethylglutaryl coenzyme A reductase inhibitors) have a firmly established role in reducing mortality and future cardiovascular events in patients with CAD, postmyocardial infarction, hyperlipidemia, diabetes, or other coronary risk equivalents (8). Intensive lipid lowering decreases the progression of CAD more effectively than standard treatment, and there is a linear reduction in cardiovascular disease mortality and LDL-C. An LDL goal of <70 mg/dL is desirable in patients with CAD or chronic angina or those who have experienced a myocardial infarction (41). Statins may need to be combined with bile acid sequestrants, niacin, or ezetimibe to achieve this goal. On the horizon are medications that potentially can halt or reverse atherosclerosis. Infusion of recombinant phospholipid complexes of the apolipoprotein A1 Milano human genetic variant of the HDL protein in human subjects has shown promising results (40).

The goals of treatment in chronic angina are to decrease the frequency of angina, increase longevity, and improve quality of life. Increasing exercise tolerance through rehabilitation is a highly effective and beneficial intervention. Medical therapies for anginal symptoms include β-blockers, calcium channel-blockers, and nitrates. Nitroglycerin (0.3-0.6 mg) given sublingually is effective when symptoms arise. Most anginal patients do not respond to monotherapy, and a combination of long-acting β-blockers, nitrates, and calcium channel blockers often is required. Ranolazine is FDA approved for chronic angina; however, it prolongs the QT interval and should be reserved for patients who have not achieved an adequate response with other antianginal drugs. Ranolazine can be used in combination with amlodipine, β-blockers, or nitrates.

Exercise Management

Regular physical activity and structured exercise programs are widely recognized as important interventions in the rehabilitation of patients with AMI and exertion-induced signs or symptoms of myocardial ischemia as well as in those who have undergone coronary artery bypass graft surgery, percutaneous transluminal coronary angioplasty, or both. This section briefly reviews contemporary issues in exercise prescription, including inpatient and outpatient therapy after an acute coronary event, upper-body and resistance training, lifestyle activity, and modulators of exertion-related cardiovascular events. Enhanced external counterpulsation therapy to improve angina and functional capacity in patients with symptomatic CAD is also addressed.

Early Convalescence After Acute Myocardial Infarction

Prolonged bed rest has been shown to result in physiologic deconditioning (e.g., muscle atrophy, weakness) and a significant decrease in aerobic capacity. Although a traditional explanation for these sequelae has been the absence of daily physical activity, it appears that the deterioration in cardiorespiratory fitness may simply reflect the lack of exposure to chronic orthostatic stress. Accordingly, research suggests that the impairment in exercise tolerance with bed rest may be lessened by regular exposure to orthostatic stress, such as intermittent sitting or standing during the hospital confinement period and early convalescence (13). Formalized in-hospital exercise programs after AMI appear to offer little additional physiologic or behavioral (self-efficacy) benefits over routine medical care (52).

Outpatient Exercise Prescription

In addition to requiring sustained compliance, the safety and effectiveness of an exercise program depend on an appropriate exercise prescription. The typical aerobic exercise session has three phases: warm-up, endurance phase, and cool-down. Recreational games and activities can also be used after the endurance phase and before the cool-down. A brief review of the physiologic basis and rationale for each phase is provided next.

Warm-Up

The warm-up (~ 5-15 min) serves as a period of adaptation by increasing blood flow and enhancing the efficiency of working muscle. Moreover, a preliminary warm-up may decrease the likelihood of musculoskeletal injury and the occurrence of ECG signs that are suggestive of myocardial ischemia or ventricular irritability—abnormalities that may be provoked by sudden strenuous exertion (7). Thus, the warm-up has cardioprotective value and enhances performance capacity.

Endurance Phase

The endurance phase (≥30 min) is either continuous (a 30 min daily bout) or intermittent (e.g., three 10 min daily bouts or two 15 min bouts), and its purpose is to directly stimulate the oxygen transport system and maximize caloric expenditure. The most effective exercises for the endurance phase use large muscle groups, are maintained continuously, and are rhythmic and aerobic. Brisk walking has several advantages over other forms of exercise for improving cardiorespiratory fitness (e.g., it is an easily tolerable activity that requires no special equipment). Moreover, walking provides an activity intense enough to achieve an aerobic training stimulus in ≥90% of men and women with documented CAD (50).

The concept of oxygen uptake reserve (i.e., a percentage of the difference between maximum and resting oxygen consumption) has been introduced for prescribing exercise intensity (56). For most deconditioned patients with CAD, the threshold intensity for improving cardiorespiratory fitness corresponds to ~45% of the oxygen uptake reserve (56), which approximates 69% of highest heart rate achieved during peak or symptom-limited exercise testing. However, the most consistent benefit appears to occur with exercise training at least three times a week for ≥12 weeks duration, 20 to 40 min per session, at an intensity approximating 70% of 85% of maximum heart rate (62). Although vigorous-intensity exercise may provide greater improvements than moderate-intensity exercise in some coronary risk factors (57), such as increased aerobic fitness, vigorous-intensity exercise is also associated with a heightened risk for musculoskeletal and cardiovascular complications (21). Because symptomatic or silent myocardial ischemia may be arrhythmogenic (27), the potential for exercise-related cardiovascular events can be reduced by establishing the target heart rate safely below (≥10 beats/min) the ischemic ECG or anginal threshold. Patients who have angina or have experienced myocardial infarction who have not undergone a preliminary exercise test may initiate exercise training at 2 to 3 metabolic equivalents (METs; 1 MET = 3.5 ml·kg^{-1}·min^{-1}) and, in the absence of abnormal signs and symptoms, can safely progress while monitoring heart rate (ideally through continuous ECG surveillance) and perceived exertion (38).

Cool-Down

The cool-down (5-10 min) provides a gradual recovery from the intensity of the endurance phase. Continued low-level movement (e.g., slow walking or pedaling) permits appropriate circulatory readjustments and return of the heart rate and blood pressure to near-resting values; enhances venous return, thereby reducing the potential for postexercise lightheadedness; facilitates the dissipation of body heat; promotes more rapid removal of lactic acid than stationary recovery; and combats the potential deleterious effects of the postexercise increase in plasma catecholamines (14). Thereafter, muscle-stretching or muscle-lengthening exercises are encouraged.

Upper-Body and Resistance Training

The limited degree of crossover of training benefits from the legs to the arms, and vice versa, appears to discredit the general practice of restricting exercise to the legs alone (e.g., walking, jogging, stationary cycle ergometry). Consequently, patients with CAD who rely on their upper extremities for occupational and leisure-time activities should train their arms as well as their legs to develop muscle-specific cardiorespiratory and hemodynamic adaptations to both forms of effort. Guidelines for dynamic arm training are shown in table 28.3 (22).

Resistance training can safely and effectively increase muscular strength and endurance, improve cardiovascular function, favorably modify coronary risk factors,

---

TABLE 28.3 Guidelines for Arm Exercise Prescription

Variable	Comment
Target heart rate	~10-15 beats/min lower than for leg training
Work rate	~50% of the power output (kg · m · min^{-1}) used for leg training
Equipment	Arm ergometer, combined arm–leg ergometer, rowing machine, wall pulleys, simulated cross-country skiing devices

and enhance psychosocial and physical well-being in clinically stable coronary patients (48). It has also been shown to attenuate the rate–pressure product when a given load is lifted (37), which may reduce cardiac demands during daily activities that involve the upper extremities (e.g., carrying packages, lifting objects). Single-set resistance training exercises to volitional fatigue, especially among novice exercises, are as effective as multiple-set programs in improving muscular strength and endurance and are less time consuming. Such regimens should be performed a minimum of 2 times a week and include 8 to 10 different exercises at a load that permits 10 to 15 repetitions per set for cardiac patients (48).

Lifestyle Activity

A recent consensus statement (53) on preventing recurrent cardiovascular events in patients with coronary and other atherosclerotic vascular diseases extolled the importance of 30 to 60 min of moderate-intensity aerobic activity, such as brisk walking, on most and preferably all days of the week, supplemented by an increase in daily lifestyle activities (e.g., walking breaks at work, gardening, household work). Over the last decade, confirmatory data regarding the independent and additive cardioprotective benefits of increased lifestyle activity have been reported. Randomized clinical trials have shown that a lifestyle approach to physical activity among previously sedentary adults has similar effects on cardiorespiratory fitness, body composition, and coronary risk factors as a traditional structured exercise program (49). The Activity Pyramid (figure 28.4) has been suggested as a model to facilitate public and patient education to combat our increasingly hypokinetic environment (33). Pedometers can also be helpful in this regard to enhance awareness of physical activity by progressively increasing daily step totals.

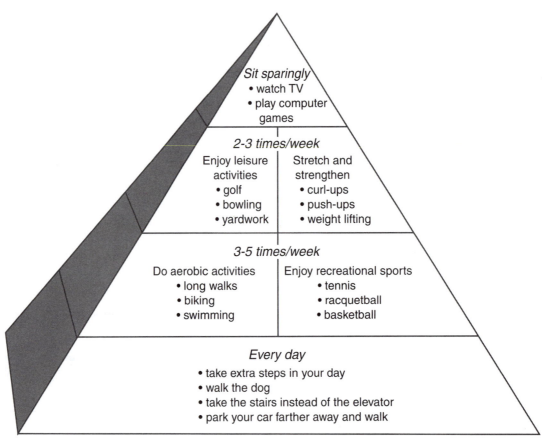

FIGURE 28.4 The Activity Pyramid presents a tiered set of weekly goals to improve cardiorespiratory fitness and health, emphasizing the importance of accumulating ≥30 minutes of moderate-intensity activity on most, and preferably all, days of the week. The second and third tiers include structured aerobic activities and recreational sports (3-5 times/week) and leisure-time sports (e.g., golf) and stretching and strengthening activities (e.g., resistance training) (2-3 times/week). Collectively, these activities should reduce the amount of time spent at the top of the pyramid, that is, in sedentary pursuits.

Adapted from *The Activity Pyramid* ©Park Nicollet Health Source® Minneapolis, U.S.A. Used with permission.

Modulators of Exertion-Related Cardiovascular Events: High-Risk Activities

The relative risk of AMI and sudden cardiac death appears to increase transiently during strenuous physical exertion compared with the risk at other times. This seems to be particularly true among habitually sedentary people who have underlying structural cardiovascular abnormalities (e.g., hypertrophic cardiomyopathy) or CAD who perform unaccustomed vigorous physical activity (21). Ways that clinicians can reduce their patients' risk of exertion-related cardiovascular events have been published (21): Encourage coronary patients to engage in regular, moderate intensity activity to move them out of the least fit, least active, high-risk cohort; counsel inactive people to avoid unaccustomed, vigorous physical activity and recreational and domestic activities that impose combined physical, emotional, and environmental stresses (e.g., snow removal, deer hunting) (12, 26); advocate appropriate warm-up and cool-down procedures (7, 14); emphasize strict adherence to prescribed training heart rates; and educate patients about forewarning signs and symptoms (e.g., chest pain or pressure, lightheadedness, threatening ventricular arrhythmias).

Enhanced External Counterpulsation: An Alternative Therapy for Patients With Vascular Disease and Chronic Angina

Enhanced external counterpulsation (EECP) is a noninvasive treatment that can reduce anginal symptoms and improve functional capacity in symptomatic patients with CAD who are no longer responsive to drug therapy or repeated revascularizations (45). An EECP device consists of a series of modified blood pressure cuffs wrapped around the calves, thighs, and buttocks of the patient, who is lying on a comfortably padded bed. The cuffs are connected by hoses to an inflation–deflation valve assembly and air compressor, which are synchronized to the cardiac cycle via the R wave obtained by continuous ECG telemetry monitoring. Cuff pressure is increased in small increments to a peak pressure, usually 260 to 300 mmHg. The program consists of 35 one-hour treatments, 5 days a week over the course of about 7 weeks.

Although the exact physiologic mechanisms by which EECP provides clinical benefits to patients remain unclear, there is evidence that the benefits are multifactorial and involve augmented blood flow to ischemic myocardium, enhanced vasomotor function, improvements in left ventricular diastolic perfor-

mance, or combinations thereof (45). One study (44) demonstrated that EECP acutely increases oxygen consumption at rest, in small amounts but in a sustained fashion, during a single therapy session in unfit coronary patients with refractory angina and in healthy sedentary adults. Thus, EECP therapy may simulate a very low level of exercise and serve as a sufficient aerobic training stimulus in selected patients.

Rehabilitation Outcomes

Increased functional capacity, symptomatic relief of angina pectoris, favorable risk factor reduction, enhanced psychologic status, decreased cardiovascular mortality, and improved quality of life appear to be sufficient end points to recommend an exercise-based cardiac rehabilitation program. The physiologic basis and rationale for selected outcomes are detailed next, with specific reference to proposed mechanisms of action.

Cardiorespiratory Function

Regular aerobic exercise decreases heart rate and blood pressure at rest and at any given oxygen uptake or submaximal work rate. Consequently, cardiac demands are reduced and anginal symptoms may be alleviated. Such changes may be manifested as decreased ST-segment depression, attenuated myocardial perfusion abnormalities, or both, at matched–rate pressure products after exercise training. On the other hand, exercise training does little to improve left ventricular ejection fraction, regional wall motion abnormalities, resting hemodynamics, and coronary collateral circulation, regardless of the intensity, frequency, or duration (62).

Endurance exercise also improves muscle function and increases the coronary patient's ability to consume and use oxygen, commonly referred to as the maximal oxygen consumption or aerobic capacity. Because a given task requires a relatively constant supply of oxygen, expressed as milliliters of oxygen per kilogram of body weight per minute ($ml \cdot kg^{-1} \cdot min^{-1}$) or as metabolic equivalents (METs; 1 MET = 3.5 $ml \cdot kg^{-1} \cdot min^{-1}$), the unfit coronary patient may have to work at the high end of his aerobic capacity to accomplish a brisk walk (figure 28.5). However, an augmented aerobic capacity following an exercise-based rehabilitation program would allow this same patient to accomplish the walk at a lower percentage of his aerobic capacity, with less fatigue. This benefit is especially important for the patient who is working below, rather than above, his anaerobic or ventilatory threshold.

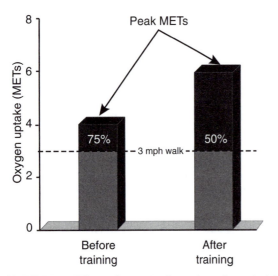

FIGURE 28.5 Effect of exercise-based cardiac rehabilitation on peak oxygen uptake (metabolic equivalents, or METs) and relative oxygen cost (activity METs/peak METs) of walking at 3 mph on a level grade (~ 3 METs). Following a physical conditioning program, peak oxygen uptake increased from 4 to 6 METs, decreasing the relative oxygen cost of a 3 mph walk from 75% to 50%.

Fitness and Mortality

Studies in persons without known CAD have identified a low level of cardiorespiratory fitness as an independent risk factor for all-cause and cardiovascular mortality. Recently, researchers extended these data to men and women with established CAD who were referred for exercise-based cardiac rehabilitation and followed for an average of 7.9 and 6.1 years, respectively (29, 30). For each 1 ml·kg^{-1}·min^{-1} increase in aerobic capacity, as directly measured during cycle ergometer testing, there was a 10% reduction of cardiac mortality in women and a 9% decrease in men. Another provocative report, using the well-described Primary Angioplasty in AMI (PAMI-2) database, found that exercise capacity more accurately predicted 2- and 5-year mortality than did left ventricular ejection fraction in patients with ST-elevation AMI treated with PCI (16). There are multiple mechanisms by which moderate to vigorous physical activity and improved cardiorespiratory fitness may decrease recurrent cardiovascular events, including antiatherosclerotic, anti-ischemic, anti-arrhythmic, antithrombotic, and psychosocial effects of endurance exercise (figure 28.6). Adaptations in autonomic control may favorably influence several of these mechanisms, especially with more vigorous exercise intensities (57).

Coronary Risk Factors

Aerobic exercise can result in modest decreases in body weight, fat stores, and blood pressure. A recent meta-analysis (31) found that chronic aerobic exercise increases HDL-C and decreases triglycerides in adults with cardiovascular disease, especially men. Although there is little evidence of beneficial outcome in smoking cessation resulting from chronic exercise as a sole intervention, well-designed education, counseling, and behavioral strategies (relapse prevention) have been shown to reduce cigarette smoking (62). Approximately 20% ± 5% of patients can be expected to stop smoking as a result of such interventions, a rate that occurs in addition to the spontaneously high smoking cessation rates in most populations soon after AMI. In summary, cardiac rehabilitation regimens reporting the most favorable impact on coronary risk factors are multifactorial (i.e., providing exercise training, dietary education, and counseling, and in some studies pharmacologic therapy, psychological support, and behavior training).

Psychological Functioning

A review of the scientific literature concluded that exercise training enhances some measures of psychological and social functioning, particularly as a component of multifactorial cardiac rehabilitation (62). On the other hand, exercise training did not consistently improve measures of anxiety and depression. Group therapy or stress management may be more effective interventions in this regard.

Morbidity and Mortality

Three meta-analyses (32, 43, 46) of controlled clinical trials conducted in the 1970s and early 1980s showed that exercise-based cardiac rehabilitation provides a 20% to 24% reduction in total and cardiovascular-related mortality (vs. 15% in exercise-only trials) (62) after AMI (figure 28.7), with no difference in the rate of nonfatal recurrent cardiac events. However, these results cannot necessarily be extrapolated to patients following coronary artery bypass surgery or PCI. In addition, the influence of reperfusion therapy and emergent and elective coronary revascularization procedures, as well as improved adjunctive pharmacologic

Antiatherosclerotic	Psychologic	Antithrombotic	Anti-ischemic	Antiarrhythmic
Improved lipids	↓ Depression	↓ Platelet adhesiveness	↓ Myocardial O_2 demand	↑ Vagal tone
Lower BPs	↓ Stress	↑ Fibrinolysis	↑ Coronary flow	↓ Adrenergic activity
Reduced adiposity	↑ Social support	↓ Fibrinogen	↓ Endothelial dysfunction	↑ HR variability
↑ Insulin sensitivity		↓ Blood viscosity	↑ EPCs and CACs	
↓ Inflammation			↑ Nitric oxide	

FIGURE 28.6 A structured endurance exercise program sufficient to maintain and enhance cardiorespiratory fitness may provide multiple mechanisms to reduce nonfatal and fatal cardiovascular events. BP = blood pressure; HR = heart rate; ↑ = increased; ↓ = decreased; O_2 = oxygen; EPCs = endothelial progenitor cells; CACs = cultured angiogenic cells.

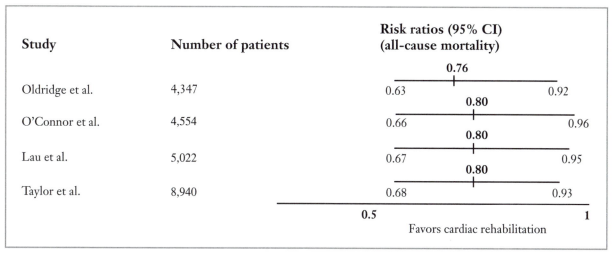

FIGURE 28.7 Reduced all-cause mortality in coronary patients who participated in exercise-based rehabilitation programs in four meta-analyses (32, 43, 46, 58). CI = confidence interval.

agents, which markedly decrease early postinfarction mortality, may diminish the impact of adjunctive exercise-based cardiac rehabilitation programs on survival.

Recently, researchers used a meta-analysis of 48 randomized trials of cardiac rehabilitation including 8,940 patients to address the effect of cardiac rehabilitation on mortality rates (58). Compared with usual care, cardiac rehabilitation reduced all-cause mortality by 20% (figure 28.7) and cardiac mortality by 26%, independent of whether the trial was published before or after 1995. Approximately half of the decrease in cardiac mortality achieved with exercise-based cardiac rehabilitation may be attributed to reductions in major risk factors, notably cigarette smoking, cholesterol, and systolic blood pressure (59). Collectively, these data suggest that the mortality benefits of cardiac rehabilitation persist in modern cardiology.

Summary

The growing worldwide burden of CAD and its sequelae mandates the development and implementation of effective population-based interventions for secondary prevention. A major limitation of one approach, coronary revascularization, is that it embraces a common response of many in the medical community, that is, the use of coronary artery bypass graft surgery or percutaneous coronary intervention as a first-line strategy to stabilize overt cardiovascular disease. These costly procedures, which are not without risk (e.g., AMI, stroke, fatal arrhythmias, and cognitive difficulties), have been largely unsuccessful in halting and reversing the epidemic. Contemporary studies suggest that multifactorial risk factor modification—

especially diabetes, cigarette smoking, hyperlipidemia, and hypertension—may slow, halt, and even reverse the progression of atherosclerotic CAD. Exercise tolerance or, more specifically, aerobic capacity also provides one of the strongest and most consistent prognostic markers in persons with and without CAD.

The benefits of aggressive risk factor modification include a reduction in anginal symptoms, decreases in exercise-induced ischemic ST-segment depression, fewer recurrent cardiac events, and a diminished need for coronary revascularization. The challenge (as a clinician) is yours!

CHAPTER 29

Coronary Artery Revascularization

Peter H. Brubaker, PhD

Henry S. Miller, Jr., MD

During the past 25 years, the frequency and variety of coronary artery revascularization procedures, such as coronary artery bypass grafting (CABG) or percutaneous transluminal coronary angioplasty (PTCA), with or without intravascular stenting, have substantially increased in the United States and around the world. These procedures are being conducted more frequently in elderly and high-risk patients than ever before (5). Moreover, emerging interventions including transmyocardial laser revascularization and infusion of vascular growth factors to stimulate angiogenesis are progressing from experimental procedures to clinical use. Consequently, clinicians working in secondary prevention and cardiac rehabilitation programs must understand the surgical and interventional procedures available, their risks, and the appropriate pre- and postprocedure medical management for patients undergoing these procedures. Finally, clinicians must be well aware of the modifications required to develop safe and effective preventive and rehabilitative exercise programs for these patients.

Epidemiology

According to the American Heart Association (5), the total number of cardiovascular operations increased 470% from 1979 to 2002 in the United States. This rapid increase in cardiovascular procedures can be attributed to the development and improvement of interventional procedures and the continued increase in the incidence of coronary artery disease (CAD). More than 1.46 million cardiac catheterizations and 657,000 PTCA procedures were performed on Americans in 2002. Moreover, the rate of coronary stenting increased 147% from 1996 to 2000, and it is estimated that 515,000 CABG procedures were performed in the US in 2002. Consequently, data from the latest Healthcare Cost and Utilization Project (5) indicate that the mean charges for diagnostic cardiac catheterizations, PTCA, and CABG procedures are US$17,763, US$28,558, and US$60,853, respectively. Consequently, the collective cost of these procedures contributes significantly to the more than US$393 billion spent in 2005 to treat all cardiovascular diseases.

In 2002, males were significantly more likely than females to have a diagnostic catheterization (884,000 vs. 579,000), PTCA (434,000 vs. 223,000), stent (363,000 vs. 174,000), or CABG (373,000 vs. 142,000) (3).

Address correspondence concerning this chapter to Peter H. Brubaker, Departments of Medicine and Health and Exercise Science, Box 7628, Wake Forest University, Winston-Salem, NC 27109. E-mail: brubaker@wfu.edu

Furthermore, the majority of these procedures were performed in the patients older than 65. In 2002 there were essentially twice as many cardiac procedures done for CAD in the south region of United States versus the northeast, the Midwest, or the west regions of the country (119,800 vs. 59,000, 77,900, 59,300, respectively) (5). These trends indicate that men, elderly people, and people who live in parts of the country where unhealthy lifestyle habits (i.e., physical inactivity, poor dietary habits, overweight and obesity) are more likely to be practiced have an increased risk (or at least treatment) of CAD.

Pathophysiology

Coronary revascularization with CABG, percutaneous coronary intervention (PCI), or emerging revascularization procedures (transmyocardial laser, infusion of growth factors) is necessary in cases of myocardial ischemia, a condition in which inadequate oxygen is available to the myocardial cells. Diagnostic tests used to identify the presence of myocardial ischemia are described in chapter 9 (Contemporary Approaches to Cardiovascular Disease Diagnosis). Myocardial ischemia is of concern because it transiently increases the risk for arrhythmias and alters cardiac muscle (myocyte) contractile function, which subsequently affects systolic and diastolic function of the ventricle (8). Moreover, severe or sustained myocardial ischemia increases the risk for myocardial infarction and related complications. Ischemia occurs when there is an imbalance between myocardial blood supply and demand (figure 29.1), which, for the majority of people, will result in the symptom of angina pectoris.

However, approximately 20% of patients with CAD will have "silent" or nontraditional anginal symptoms (20). Angina is often described as discomfort in the chest, back, or neck region that may radiate to the jaw or arms. Myocardial ischemia and the accompanying symptom of angina are generally precipitated by physical exertion, emotional stress, environmental changes (temperature, altitude), or large meals (postprandial ischemia). However, less specific symptoms of ischemia and angina include dyspnea, fatigue, and generalized discomfort.

As seen in figure 29.1, a variety of conditions that increase wall tension (e.g., hypertension, left ventricular hypertrophy, or dilated cardiomyopathy), elevate heart rate (e.g., metabolic conditions or tachycardia), or increase myocardial contractility may disproportionately increase myocardial oxygen demand (MVO_2) relative to the normal oxygen supply and result in myocardial ischemia. Patients with demand-induced myocardial ischemia are generally not candidates for revascularization because coronary artery occlusion is not responsible for the ischemia. Appropriate pharmacologic therapy and alternative surgical interventions to reduce myocardial demand are subsequently considered for these patients (8).

Although other factors, such as anemia (decreased oxygen-carrying capacity), coronary vasospasm (extrinsic compression of coronary artery), and decreased diastolic perfusion pressure (figure 29.1) may reduce myocardial blood supply, the primary cause of myocardial ischemia in most people is the presence of atherosclerotic lesions in the coronary arteries. The pathogenesis of atherosclerosis is described in chapter 6. Cardiac myocytes, in contrast to many other muscle cells in the body, are very effective at extracting oxygen

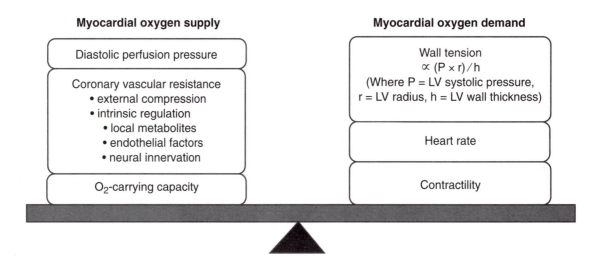

FIGURE 29.1 Major determinants of myocardial supply and demand.

from the blood and thus have a near-maximal arteriovenous oxygen content difference at rest. Without a significant oxygen extraction reserve, the coronary arteries must vasodilate to increase flow and compensate for the increase in myocardial demand. Nondiseased segments of the coronary arteries will normally dilate in response to increased myocardial demand; however, arterial segments with atherosclerotic disease appear to lose their vasodilatory reserve (8). Although small atherosclerotic lesions may permit adequate myocardial perfusion at rest, narrowing of the coronary artery lumen by 70% or greater will likely result in ischemia as myocardial demand increases from physical exertion or stress (11). As the obstruction becomes larger than 70% of the coronary artery, ischemia symptoms are likely to occur at lower levels of exertion and even at rest. Recent studies suggest that small endocardial coronary arteries as well as larger epicardial coronary arteries with minimally obstructive lesions can demonstrate abnormal endothelial function and therefore are unable to appropriately vasodilate in the face of an increased myocardial demand (11). Impaired endothelial function and subsequent inability to vasodilate may explain, at least in part, the presence of angina symptoms in people with normal coronary angiograms (e.g., nonobstructive atherosclerosis), a condition often referred to as cardiac syndrome X (15).

Medical Management

The medical management of patients who have undergone PCI, CABG, and alternative procedures is discussed in the following sections.

Post-PCI Patient

Patients treated by PTCA with or without stent (PCI) clearly require medications to prevent thrombosis during and after the procedure. Recent recommendations from AHA/ACC on secondary prevention of CAD suggest that after PCI with stent placement, the initial aspirin dose should be 325 mg/day for 1 month in bare-metal stent recipients, 3 months in sirolimus-eluting stent recipients, and 6 months in paclitaxel-eluting stent recipients (18). In the higher risk patients (angina at mild to moderate exertion or complex coronary lesions), clopidogrel (Plavix) should be given at a loading dose of 300 mg before the procedure and 75 mg daily for 3 to 6 months after stenting and 6 to 12 months after drug-eluting stent placement (7).

Patients with unstable angina or non-ST-elevation myocardial infarction should be prescribed GP2B/3A

inhibitors. These drugs can also be prescribed for patients who have taken clopidogrel (Plavix) before PCI. In patients undergoing PCI who have had a myocardial infarction with ST-segment elevation (commonly called STEMI) with or without stent placement, a GP2B/3A drug should be administered. Low molecular weight heparin or bivalirem can be used in patients with and without STEMI and can be combined with GP2B/3A inhibitors in the low-risk patients in this category. Early experience (in the mid-1980s) with PTCA alone resulted in 6-month restenosis rates of 30% to 40%, but the development of intracoronary stents and platelet inhibiting drugs has contributed significantly to a decreased risk of restenosis after PCI. Furthermore, drug-coated versus bare-metal stents have been associated with lower rates of restenosis in randomized controlled trials (17).

Post-CABG Patient

The management of CABG patients depends on the comorbidities present and the operative procedure performed. These operations are done with and without extracorporeal circulation (bypass pump machine) as well as with or without a median sternotomy (separation of sternum) using the minimal access approach through the anterior chest wall (9). Obviously, the postoperative management of these patients depends on the procedure performed. Anticoagulant therapies, including aspirin, are discontinued before CABG but are restarted postoperatively and generally continued indefinitely. The AHA/ACC guidelines on secondary prevention of CAD suggest that for CABG patients, aspirin dosing regimens ranging from 100 mg/day to 325 mg/day appear to be efficacious (18). The use of other, more potent thrombolytic agents is dependent on the risk of thrombi and the presence of arrhythmias (e.g., atrial fibrillation). Routine postoperative care, including early ambulation, usually results in discharge within 4 to 7 days postoperatively. Until the last decade, vein grafts were the predominant conduit vessel of choice for CABG, but high graft failure associated with vein grafts has led to the use of arterial grafts. Ten years after CABG, the patency rate for arterial and vein grafts are 93% versus 60%, respectively. Figure 29.2 describes the vein and artery graft options for CABG (9).

In all patients with coronary artery disease who have undergone PTCI or CABG, the control of risk factors is essential to prevent progressive atherosclerosis. Comprehensive rehabilitation programs that emphasize appropriate lifestyle modification and risk reduction have been shown to be highly beneficial (7). In addition to using antithrombotic therapy, patients often are

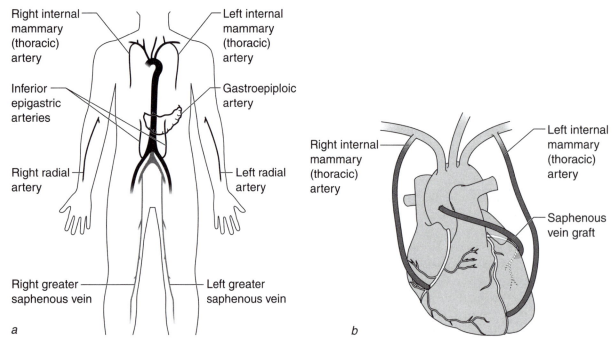

FIGURE 29.2 *(a)* Arterial and venous grafts used for myocardial revascularization procedures. *(b)* Coronary artery bypass graft surgery. Three-vessel (often called triple) bypass using right internal mammary artery (RIMA), left internal mammary artery (LIMA), and a saphenous vein graft to bypass occlusions in the right coronary artery, the left anterior descending coronary artery, and the circumflex coronary artery, respectively.

Reprinted, by permission, from P. Brubaker, L. Kaminsky, and M. Whaley, 2002, *Coronary artery disease: essentials of prevention and rehabilitation programs* (Champaign, IL: Human Kinetics), 101.

prescribed β-blockers, angiotensin-converting enzyme inhibitors, or angiotensin receptor blockers depending on degree of myocardial dysfunction (i.e., reduced ejection fraction). Hydroxymethylglutaryl coenzyme A reductase inhibitors (statins) are widely used after revascularization because of their lipid-lowering and anti-inflammatory (pleiotropic) effects as well as their ability to prevent and potentially reverse atherosclerotic lesions (16). Antiarrhythmic drugs, pacemakers, and implanted cardiodefibrillator devices are considered individually in the revascularization patient depending on the type of arrhythmia and degree of myocardial dysfunction.

Alternative Revascularization Interventions for Refractory Patients

Because of an unacceptably high operative mortality rate, a significant number of patients with severe CAD are not appropriate candidates for the surgical and interventional procedures previously described. Consequently, several alternative therapies to improve myocardial blood flow and reduce anginal symptoms in patients with severe CAD have been investigated. One such approach involves the injection of growth factors,

particularly recombinant human vascular endothelial growth factor (rhVEGF), to stimulate the growth and proliferation of new blood vessels, a treatment termed *therapeutic angiogenesis*. Initial studies in animal models and in peripheral vascular beds have demonstrated that several growth factors could safely and effectively stimulate angiogenesis. Henry and colleagues (14) evaluated the effects of infusing rhVEGF on treadmill exercise time as well as on angina frequency in 178 patients unsuitable for standard revascularization. Although high-dose rhVEGF showed no benefit over placebo or low-dose rhVEGF infusion at 60 days of follow-up, at 120 days of follow-up high-dose rhVEGF infusion resulted in a significantly higher treadmill exercise times and less frequent angina compared with the other two groups. Furthermore, infusion of rhVEGF was well tolerated and demonstrated excellent short-term safety in this small, short-term study. These findings warrant larger and longer studies of safety and efficacy for patients considered nonoptimal for standard revascularization.

Another approach for reducing myocardial ischemia involves creating small channels in the myocardium with a laser. The technique, called transmyocardial revascularization, involves applying a carbon dioxide or holmium laser directly to the beating heart to make 10 to 50 1 mm channels. These channels presumably allow oxygen-rich blood from the left ventricle to perfuse the myocardial cell, reducing the ischemia caused by occluded coronary arteries. Five prospective trials of ischemic patients not amenable to conventional revascularization (CABG or PCI) demonstrated that after 1 year, transmyocardial revascularization provided superior angina relief, decreased hospitalization, improved quality of life, and greater rates of event-free survival compared with usual care medical therapy (4). Furthermore, patients randomized to transmyocardial revascularization treatment have demonstrated improved survival at 5 years compared with patients receiving usual care medical management (3).

Although revascularization procedures with transmyocardial laser and endothelial growth factor are promising, there are inadequate data to provide specific evidence-based recommendations regarding exercise testing and training guidelines for patients revascularized with these techniques.

Exercise Management

Although exercise testing, endurance training, and resistance training are valuable for managing patients who have undergone revascularization, exercise must be performed properly to avoid injury. Details on exercise testing and different modalities of exercise training for revascularization patients are described next.

Exercise Testing

Exercise stress testing is often used after revascularization procedures to determine functional status, evaluate vocational readiness, and develop an individually based exercise prescription. For patients who have undergone successful and uncomplicated CABG, routine exercise testing appears to provide little clinical benefit and can impose an unnecessary financial burden (10). For patients with incomplete revascularization (i.e., coronary vessels cannot be bypassed or opened via PCI), an exercise test to evaluate the presence and severity of ischemia is warranted before initiating an exercise program. The most appropriate time to perform an exercise test in CABG patients is generally 3 to 4 weeks after surgery, when most of the complications (sternal stability, incisional pain, rib soreness, hypovolemia, anemia, muscle weakness) have resolved and the patient is able to give a near-maximal physiologic effort during the test.

Although some debate exists regarding the need for and potential risks of exercise testing after PCI, many clinicians support the use of early postprocedural exercise testing (1-2 days) to evaluate the functional status of the PCI patient (1). More routinely, exercise testing is conducted at 2 to 5 weeks and again at 6 months postprocedure. Testing at these intervals can enable the clinician to detect potential restenosis, assess functional capacity, provide advice concerning physical activity restrictions, and develop an exercise prescription (1).

Endurance Exercise Training

Historically, patients who had undergone CABG did not enter formal cardiac rehabilitation programs until 4 to 6 weeks after surgery, usually initiated only after approval by the surgeon. It has become more acceptable for patients with uncomplicated CABG to begin cardiac rehabilitation as soon as possible after discharge (often within 1 week of surgery) as the benefits of light upper-extremity range of motion exercises and low-level ambulation have become more apparent (1). After the patient has undergone appropriate screening for contraindications (2), endurance exercise training can begin, with exertion limited to resting heart rate + 30 beats/min or Rating of Perceived Exertion 11 to 13 until more objective data from a symptom-limited exercise test are generated. When using these arbitrary and subjective approaches to exercise prescription, the clinician must recognize that significant intersubjective variability exists (2). As the CABG patient progresses through outpatient cardiac rehabilitation, a more traditional exercise prescription that specifies type, intensity, frequency, and duration can be used (2). Some CABG patients may initially need lower intensity or other exercise modifications because of musculoskeletal discomfort (chest and back) or healing at the incision sites (sternum and legs).

For patients who have undergone PCI, endurance exercise can begin almost immediately as long as the catheter access site, generally in the groin, has healed properly. The exercise prescription for the PCI patient is generally similar to that for other cardiac patients, although PCI patients may be able to progress more rapidly, particularly if there was no myocardial damage, and they are less likely to have had extended periods of physical inactivity pre- and postprocedure. As described in an earlier section, stenting and aggressive pharmacotherapy have considerably reduced the risk for restenosis after PCI, compared with early experiences with PTCA alone. However, the PCI patient should still be observed closely in the exercise program for potential recurrence of ischemic signs and symptoms indicative of restenosis (1).

Resistance Exercise Training

Even just a few days of bed rest can result in a significant loss of lean body mass and cardiovascular function. To counteract the deleterious effects of bed rest and other complications associated with CABG, patients should begin range-of-motion activities and exercises with very light (i.e., 1-3 lb, or 0.45-1.36 kg) hand weights, as well as mobilization, while in the hospital or soon after leaving the hospital. Stretching and flexibility activities can begin as early as 24 hr after CABG. As outlined in Patient Criteria for a Resistance Exercise Program, CABG patients should avoid traditional resistance training exercises (with moderate to heavy weights) until the sternum has healed sufficiently, which generally takes 3 months (1). Surgery patients who experience sternal movement or wound complications should perform lower-extremity exercises only. Nevertheless, significant soft tissue and bone damage of the chest wall can occur during surgery. If this area does not receive range-of-motion exercise, adhesions may develop and the musculature can become weaker and shorter, accentuating postural problems and hindering strength gains.

PCI patients can begin light resistance training with elastic bands and small hand weights almost immediately for the upper-body muscles; training can begin for the lower body when the catheter access site has healed properly (assuming the catheter access site was the leg). More aggressive resistance training for the PCI patient can be safely initiated 3 weeks (including 2 weeks of endurance activity) postintervention.

General resistance training guidelines for cardiac patients (shown on page 291) are generally thought to be appropriate for stable PCI and CABG patients (1).

▪ **Patient Criteria for a Resistance Exercise Program**

A resistance exercise program is defined as one in which patients lift weights 50% or greater of 1RM. The use of elastic bands, 1 to 3 lb (0.45-1.36 kg) hand weights, and light free weights may be initiated in a progressive fashion at phase II program entry, provided no other contraindications exist. Criteria for participation include the following:

- Minimum of 5 weeks after date of MI or cardiac surgery, *including* 4 weeks of consistent participation in a supervised cardiac rehabilitation endurance training program (entry should be a staff decision with approval of the medical director and surgeon as appropriate)

- Minimum of 3 weeks following transcatheter procedure (PTCA, other), *including* 2 weeks of consistent participation in a supervised cardiac rehabilitation endurance training program (entry should be a staff decision with approval of the medical director and surgeon as appropriate)

- No evidence of the following conditions:
  - Congestive heart failure
  - Uncontrolled dysrhythmias
  - Severe valvular disease
  - Uncontrolled hypertension. Patients with moderate hypertension (systolic blood pressure >160 mmHg or diastolic blood pressure >100) should be referred for appropriate management, although these values are not absolute contraindications for participation in a resistance training program.

- Unstable conditions

■ Resistance Training Guidelines

To prevent soreness and minimize the risk of injury, the initial load should allow 12 to 15 repetitions comfortably. If a 1RM pretest is used, this load would be approximately 30% to 40% 1RM for the upper body and 50% to 60% for the hips and legs. Low-risk stratified, well-trained patients may progress to higher relative loads depending on program goals.

Perform 1 set of 8 to 10 exercises (major muscle groups) 2 to 3 days/week. An additional set may be added, but additional gains are not proportionate.

Some specific considerations are as follows:

- Exercise large muscle groups before small muscle groups.
- Increase loads by 5% when able to comfortably lift 12 to 15 repetitions.

- Raise weights with slow, controlled movements; extend the limbs completely when lifting.
- Avoid straining.
- Exhale (blow out) during the exertion phase of the lift (e.g., exhale when pushing a weight stack overhead and inhale when lowering it).
- Avoid sustained, tight gripping, which may evoke an excessive blood pressure response to lifting.
- Use an RPE of 11 to 13 as a subjective guide to effort.
- Stop exercise if warning signs or symptoms occur, especially dizziness, dysrhythmias, unusual shortness of breath, or anginal discomfort.

Reprinted, by permission, from AACVPR, 2004, *Guidelines for Cardiac Rehabilitation and Secondary Prevention* (Champaign, IL: Human Kinetics), 119.

Rehabilitation Outcomes

Given the differences in patient selection and procedures performed, appropriate outcomes may differ for CABG and PCI patients. Further discussion on specific outcomes for each intervention is provided next.

Post-CABG Patient

At entrance to cardiac rehabilitation, patients who have undergone CABG have a significantly reduced exercise capacity compared with patients entering cardiac rehabilitation after other cardiac conditions or procedures (e.g., myocardial infarction, PCI), even after adjustment for age. Consequently, a primary role for cardiac rehabilitation after CABG is to return these patients to a reasonable level of functional independence.

In a controlled trial of cardiac rehabilitation after CABG with 10-year follow-up, patients who participated in cardiac rehabilitation had a decrease in total cardiovascular events and a reduction in hospital admissions (13). Additionally, in a mixed population of 147 post-CABG patients, improvements in peak exercise capacity after cardiac rehabilitation correlated with a decrease in long-term mortality rates. That is, the greater the increase in peak exercise capacity obtained through participation in cardiac rehabilitation, the greater the reduction in cardiovascular mortality.

Post-PCI Patient

Participation in cardiac rehabilitation for post-PCI patients can markedly improve functional capacity, lipid profile, and exercise tolerance; decrease morbidity rate (clinical events) and hospital readmission rate; improve sympathovagal balance; improve quality of life; and decrease inflammatory biomarkers (e.g., C-reactive protein). Furthermore, endurance exercise training has been shown to increase treadmill time, improve myocardial perfusion, and reduce risk of restenosis (12) in PCI patients. Endurance exercise training in the PCI patient has also been shown to improve a variety of psychosocial outcomes (1).

In a randomized trial of patients who underwent PCI, those who participated in cardiac rehabilitation not only improved their lifestyle habits more significantly than the non–cardiac rehabilitation group but also were more likely to retain this healthier lifestyle over a 5-year follow-up. Furthermore, patients who have undergone PCI in the presence of myocardial infarction have been shown to have improved endothelial function as a result of 6 months of exercise training. A randomized trial by Belardinelli and colleagues (6) demonstrated that PCI patients who participate in cardiac rehabilitation tended to experience a significant increase in maximal oxygen consumption and quality of life compared with a control group, which experienced no change in those variables. Furthermore, after participation, the cardiac rehabilitation group had significantly less residual coronary artery stenosis and significantly improved myocardial perfusion (based on thallium scores). In addition, clinical events were significantly reduced in the cardiac rehabilitation group versus the control group (18.6 vs. 46%, respectively).

Endothelial dysfunction and inflammation are known to play an important role in the development and progression of CAD and restenosis following PCI. Exercise training prevents endothelial dysfunction and restores endothelial function in a variety of cardiac patients, including those who are post-PCI. A recent study demonstrated that cardiac progenitor cells are able to differentiate into various mature cell types, including endothelial cells, and play a role in repairing damaged endothelium (19). Exercise training, as part of cardiac rehabilitation, results in increased integration of these cells into the endothelium of patients with CAD. Furthermore, exercise training reduces fibrinogen and plasminogen activation and modulates platelet activation following acute exercise. Exercise appears to moderate inflammation, as indicated by reduced levels of cardiac rehabilitation in post-PCI patients who participated in cardiac rehabilitation. Thus, exercise training results in a variety of physiological adaptations that appear to reduce the occurrence of restenosis after PCI.

Summary

Until recently, there was a relative paucity of information regarding exercise therapy and other lifestyle interventions designed specifically for patients who have undergone revascularization. However, contemporary research has demonstrated that exercise therapy has a variety of benefits, some of which are particularly important and unique to the revascularization patient. Consequently, patients who have undergone PCI and CABG should participate in a comprehensive secondary prevention and rehabilitation program that includes aggressive risk factor interventions as well as endurance and resistance exercise training components to maximize quality and quantity of life.

CHAPTER 30

Cardiac Arrhythmias and Conduction Disturbances

Frank G. Yanowitz, MD

Michael J. LaMonte, PhD

Cardiac arrhythmias and conduction disturbances are among the many issues that confront health care professionals working with athletes, healthy sedentary and active people, and patients with cardiovascular and other diseases. Advances in the recognition, evaluation, and management of cardiac electrical abnormalities have paralleled recent progress in diagnostic and treatment modalities. An ongoing challenge for health care and exercise professionals is to provide patients with a sound understanding of the seriousness of these conditions and to deliver safe and effective recommendations for physical activity programs in the context of primary and secondary disease prevention. To meet this challenge, health care practitioners need to be familiar with the electrocardiographic characteristics of these abnormalities and the appropriate evaluations and treatments. This chapter considers the anatomic and electrophysiologic basis of common cardiac arrhythmias and conduction abnormalities and discusses various diagnostic and management approaches to several common electrical problems. For a more detailed discussion of electrocardiogram (ECG) interpretation, readers are referred to several excellent textbooks (7, 10, 34) and an extensive tutorial that is available on the Internet (36).

Anatomy of the Heart's Electrical System

A four-chamber diagram of the heart's electrical system including pacemaker sites and conduction pathways is illustrated in figure 30.1. The electrical impulse normally originates in pacemaker cells located in the *sinoatrial (SA) node* high in the right atrium. Internodal tracks preferentially conduct the impulse from the SA node to the *atrioventricular (AV) node*, while simultaneously the atria are activated primarily by direct cell-to-cell electrical transmission that spreads outward from the SA node like ripples in a pond through the right and left atria and into the AV junction. Another conduction tract, *Bachmann's bundle*, preferentially transmits activation through the interatrial septum into the left atrium. Activation of atrial muscle cells produces the P wave of the electrocardiogram. In normal hearts, the AV node and *bundle of His* provide the only electrical connection between the atria and

Address correspondence concerning this chapter to Frank G. Yanowitz, 1575 E. Stablewood Circle, Salt Lake City, Utah 84117. E-mail: fyanow@mac.com ventricles. The AV node is made up of slow-conducting calcium-channel cells that delay conduction to allow the contribution of atrial contraction to ventricular filling. The bundle of His immediately divides into *right* and *left bundle branches*; the left bundle branch further divides into *anterior, posterior,* and *septal fascicles*. The bundle branches and fascicles further divide into the specialized conduction system known as the *Purkinje network*, which rapidly activates the ventricular myocardium uniformly from endocardium to epicardium and from apex to base to produce an effective stroke volume from both ventricles. Simultaneous right and left ventricular activation results in a narrow QRS complex. In some people, an *accessory pathway* known as the *bundle of Kent* (not shown in figure 30.1) bypasses the AV node and directly connects atrial muscle to ventricular muscle, causing early ventricular activation. This developmental anomaly, called *preexcitation* or the *Wolff–Parkinson–White syndrome*, is frequently associated with rapid cardiac arrhythmias. In addition to the bundle of Kent, there may be other accessory pathways in and around the AV junction permitting preexcitation of the ventricles. These pathways, known either as *James fibers* or *Mahaim fibers*, connect atrial or AV nodal tissue to fascicles of the ventricular conduction system and provide the anatomic substrate for supraventricular tachycardias (24).

Features of Normal and Abnormal Impulse Formation and Conduction

An operational framework for conceptualizing disturbances in rhythm and conduction is shown in figure 30.2. Aspects of impulse formation include site of origin, rate, regularity, and mode of onset. In addition to the primary pacemaker in the SA node, electrical impulses may originate early in the cardiac cycle from active foci or late in the cardiac cycle from passive escape pacemakers elsewhere in the heart. Premature impulses occur as single or multiple sequential beats from isolated or multifocal sites of origin in the atria (premature atrial complexes or PACs), in the AV junction (PJCs), or in the ventricles (PVCs). Passive *escape beats* originate in latent pacemaker cells in the AV junction or ventricles as a protective measure when the primary pacemaker in the SA node fails to maintain an adequate heart rate or when heart block prevents supraventricular impulses from activating the ventricles at an adequate rate. Escape beats and rhythms from the AV junction occur at rates from 40 to 60 beats/min, whereas those from the ventricles occur more slowly, 30 to 50 beats/min. Active or *accelerated junctional* or *ventricular rhythms* are usually the result of an abnormal perturbation such as ischemia, electrolyte abnormalities, or mechanical force (e.g., myocardial stretch) and tend to overtake or usurp the normal sinus rhythm. Finally, a variety of rapid rhythms, known as *tachycardias,* can originate in the atria or AV junction (*supraventricular*) and in the ventricles. An important aspect of accurately identifying a tachycardia is determining whether the rhythm is regular or irregular and whether it originates in the atria or the ventricles.

Also illustrated in figure 30.2 are the characteristics of electrical conduction. Depending on the site of origin, impulses may travel forward (antegrade), backward (retrograde), or both directions. For example, premature or escape beats originating in the AV junction may activate the ventricles (antegrade) and the atria (retrograde) at the same time. On the ECG, the antegrade activation results in the QRS complex, and the retrograde activation results in a retrograde

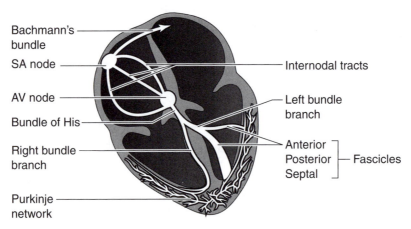

FIGURE 30.1 The cardiac electrical system.

P wave. Similarly, impulses originating in the ventricles may transmit backward through the AV junction, resulting in retrograde P waves. Understanding impulse formation and conduction greatly enhances the clinician's ability to recognize the ECG aspects of cardiac arrhythmias and conduction abnormalities. Common conduction abnormalities are shown in figure 30.3. Conduction abnormalities in the AV junction are divided into three degrees as illustrated in figure 30.4, *a-d*. In *first-degree AV block* (figure 30.4*a*), every P wave is followed by a QRS complex but AV conduction is abnormally slow, resulting in a prolonged PR interval (>0.2 s). In *second-degree AV block*, there is intermittent failure of AV conduction such that some P waves conduct to the ventricles and some do not. The two types of second-degree AV block are named after the individuals who first described them. *Wenckebach*, or *type I*, second-degree AV block (figure 30.4*b*) usually occurs in the AV node and is characterized by progressive

lengthening of the PR interval until a P wave fails to conduct (arrow). *Mobitz II*, or *type II*, second-degree AV block (figure 30.4*c*) is characterized by fixed PR intervals until conduction failure occurs (arrow). Whereas type I AV block is usually in the AV node, type II AV block often occurs in one of the bundle branches in the setting of preexisting block of the opposite bundle. The QRS complex is usually wide. For example, in a patient with right bundle-branch block, intermittent failure of the left bundle will result in a Mobitz II second-degree AV block. Type II AV block is sometimes located in the bundle of His, and the QRS may be narrow. In third-degree AV block (figure 30.4*d*), there is complete failure of AV conduction and the ventricles are activated by slow escape rhythms originating in the bundle of His or ventricular pacemaker cells. Independently occurring rhythms in the atria and ventricles, known as *AV dissociation*, occur when separate sites of impulse formation activate the atria and ventricles.

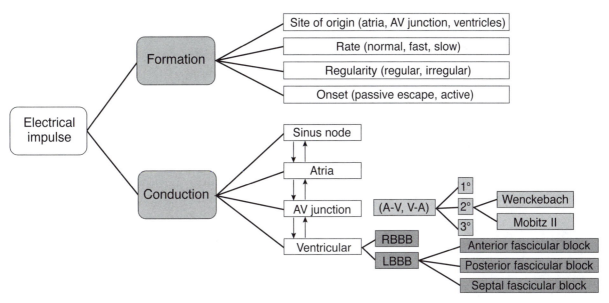

FIGURE 30.2 Impulse formation and impulse conduction.

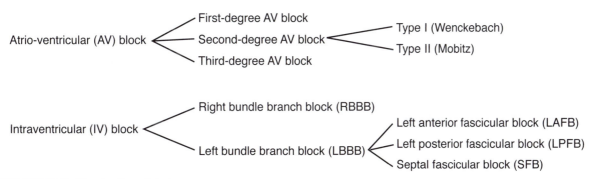

FIGURE 30.3 Conduction disturbances.

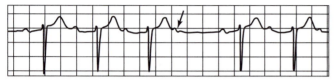

a First-degree AV block

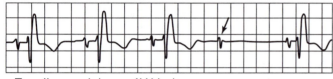

b Type I second-degree AV block (Wenckebach)

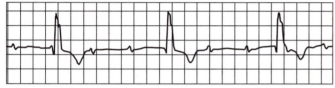

c Type II second-degree AV block

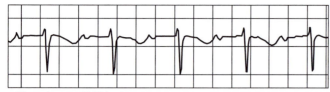

d Third-degree AV block with ventricular escape rhythm

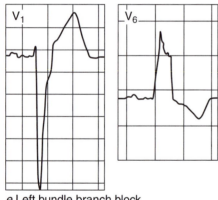

e Left bundle branch block

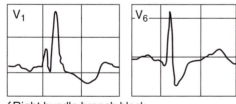

f Right bundle branch block

FIGURE 30.4 AV and IV conduction abnormalities.

Ventricular conduction abnormalities typically are located within the bundle branches and fascicles. These disorders may occur in the absence of clinical heart disease or may be associated with a variety of degen-erative processes involving ventricular conduction and contractile tissues. When a particular bundle branch fails, the ventricles are activated sequentially rather than simultaneously. Activation begins in the ventricle with the intact bundle branch and subsequently moves into the ventricle with the blocked bundle branch. This results in a widened QRS complex ($\geq$0.12 s). Sample ECG tracings of *left bundle-branch block (LBBB)* and *right bundle-branch block (RBBB)* in leads V1 and V6 are illustrated in figure 30.4, *e* and *f*.

ECG Aspects of Cardiac Arrhythmias

Cardiac arrhythmias are generally categorized into two major categories: supraventricular and ventricu-lar. The following sections describe the ECG aspects of both categories beginning with supraventricular arrhythmias. Pertinent clinical implications are also discussed.

Supraventricular Arrhythmias

The term *supraventricular* refers to rhythms originating above the bifurcation of the bundle of His (figure 30.1). Figure 30.5 lists the active and passive supraventricular arrhythmias. Sample ECG tracings of common supra-ventricular arrhythmias as seen in lead V1 are shown in figure 30.6. PACs and PJCs (figure 30.6, *a-d*) have three possible outcomes on their way to the ventricles. The most common outcome is normal activation of both ventricles, resulting in a narrow QRS complex similar to the sinus beats (figure 30.6*a*, arrow). PACs earlier in the cycle may find a bundle branch or fascicle refractory and temporarily unable to conduct. The resultant QRS complex will have the morphology of bundle branch or fascicular block, referred to as *aberration*. Figure 30.6*b* shows a PAC (arrow) with RBBB aberration; figure 30.6*c* shows two PACs (arrows) with LBBB aberration. Finally, a very early PAC (figure 30.6*d*, arrow) may find the AV junction refractory and unable to conduct the ventricles. These *nonconducted* PACs may be difficult to recognize because the P waves are often hidden in the T wave of the preceding beat. A close look at other T waves in the same lead will often help identify the hidden premature P wave.

Atrial fibrillation is recognized by the absence of P waves and irregularly spaced QRS complexes. Atrial activity may be identified by either coarse or fine undulations of the ECG baseline. The ventricular rate is determined by the state of AV conduction and may be

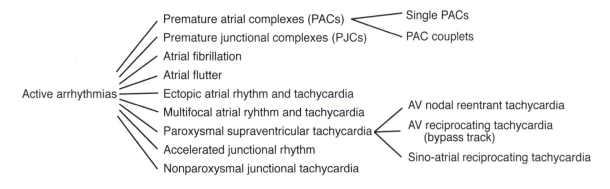

FIGURE 30.5 The active and passive supraventricular arrhythmias.

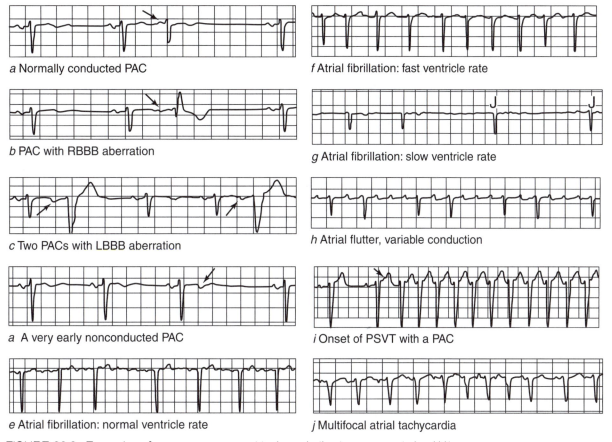

a Normally conducted PAC

b PAC with RBBB aberration

c Two PACs with LBBB aberration

a A very early nonconducted PAC

e Atrial fibrillation: normal ventricle rate

f Atrial fibrillation: fast ventricle rate

g Atrial fibrillation: slow ventricle rate

h Atrial flutter, variable conduction

i Onset of PSVT with a PAC

j Multifocal atrial tachycardia

FIGURE 30.6 Examples of common supraventricular arrhythmias as seen in lead V1.

normal (figure 30.6*e*), fast (figure 30.6*f*), or slow (figure 30.6*g*). When the ventricular rate gets too slow, escape pacemakers from the AV junction (labeled *J* in figure 30.6*g*) or the ventricles may take over. Escape beats occur at a specific rate depending on the location of the latent pacemaker. In atrial fibrillation, escape beats are recognized by regularly occurring QRS complexes at a slow heart rate.

Atrial flutter is characterized by regular flutter waves occurring at approximately 300 beats/min. New-onset atrial flutter usually conducts with 2:1 AV block, resulting in a ventricular rate of approximately 150 beats/min. In figure 30.6*h*, atrial flutter alternates between 2:1 and 4:1 AV conduction. Depending on the particular ECG lead, atrial flutter waves may be easy or difficult to recognize. The best leads on the 12-lead

ECG are usually leads II, III, and aVF, where a *sawtooth* appearance is often seen.

The onset of paroxysmal supraventricular tachycardia (PSVT) is illustrated in figure 30.6*i*. The arrow indicates an early PAC that initiates the tachycardia. In most cases, the location of the tachycardia circuit is in the AV junction using two pathways, one for antegrade and the other for retrograde conduction. This is called *AV nodal reentrant tachycardia*. This tachycardia starts abruptly, usually with a PAC or PVC, and is maintained by the different electrical properties of the two AV pathways. Any perturbation that delays conduction in one of the pathways, such as using vagal maneuvers or AV-slowing drugs (e.g., adenosine), can break the circuit and terminate the arrhythmia. People with Wolff–Parkinson–White syndrome and other preexcitation syndromes are also prone to PSVT where one pathway (usually antegrade) is the AV junction and the other (usually retrograde) is the accessory pathway. This is called *atrioventricular reciprocating tachycardia*.

Finally, *multifocal atrial tachycardia* is illustrated in figure 30.6*j*. This uncommon tachycardia is usually seen in people who are seriously ill with an intense sympathetic or catecholamine response to hypoxia, infection, or other metabolic derangements. The ECG is characterized by P waves of varying morphology and an irregular tachycardia somewhat similar to atrial fibrillation.

Ventricular Arrhythmias

Figure 30.7 lists the various types of ventricular arrhythmias, and examples are illustrated in figure 30.8 as they might appear in lead V1. The ventricular origin of PVCs and ventricular tachycardia can usually be derived from the morphology and spatial orientation of the QRS complex. PVCs, shown in figure 30.8, *a-d*, include left ventricular PVCs (figure 30.8*a*), right ventricular PVCs (figure 30.8*b*), multifocal PVCs (figure

30.8*c*), and PVC couplets (figure 30.8*d*). Two examples of ventricular tachycardia are illustrated in figure 30.8, *e* and *f*, one from the left ventricle (figure 30.8*e*) and one from the right ventricle (figure 30.8*f*). In figure 30.8*f*, AV dissociation is identified by independent P waves (arrows), supraventricular captures *(C)*, and *fusion beats (F)*. A fusion beat is a QRS complex resulting from two simultaneous activation fronts in the ventricles, one of which is usually the normal activation sequence coming from the AV junction. An example of an accelerated ventricular rhythm is seen in figure 30.8*g* beginning with the third QRS complex, and AV dissociation is also present during the short run. Figure 30.8*h* shows an example of a polymorphic ventricular tachycardia, called *torsades de pointes* (described in detail later), seen in a patient with the long QT syndrome.

Differential Diagnosis of Wide QRS Beats

Wide QRS complexes that occur as premature beats, accelerated rhythms, or tachycardias are often difficult ECG diagnostic challenges. Wide QRS complexes may either be supraventricular with bundle-branch block aberration or ventricular in origin. An accurate diagnosis is critical because ventricular rhythms are usually serious arrhythmias, especially in the setting of advanced heart disease. Important clues to the correct diagnosis can be derived from analysis of the QRS morphology seen especially in lead V1 or a monitored lead simulating lead V1 (9). In figure 30.9, diagrams of up-going or positive QRS complexes are illustrated. A triphasic QRS with rsR' components (figure 30.9, 1 and 2) is most likely supraventricular in origin with RBBB aberration. A notched (or slurred) QRS with the notch following the peak of the QRS (figure 30.9, 4) is almost certain to be from the left ventricle. If the notch (or slur) precedes the peak of the QRS (figure 30.9, 3), however, it can be either supraventricular with RBBB aberration or ventricular in origin. Finally, if the QRS has an initial q

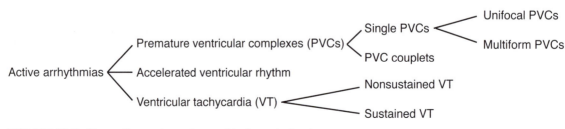

FIGURE 30.7 The active and passive ventricular arrhythmias.

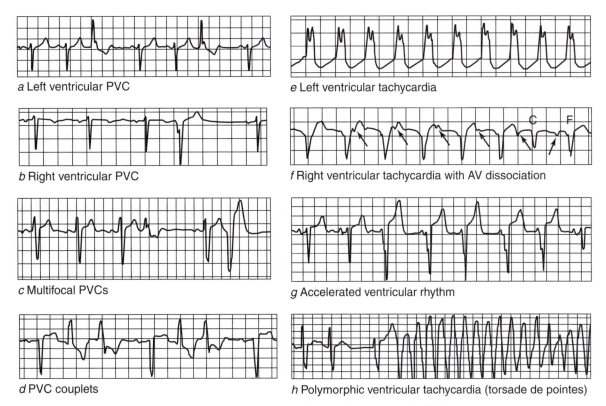

a Left ventricular PVC

b Right ventricular PVC

c Multifocal PVCs

d PVC couplets

e Left ventricular tachycardia

f Right ventricular tachycardia with AV dissociation

g Accelerated ventricular rhythm

h Polymorphic ventricular tachycardia (torsade de pointes)

FIGURE 30.8   Examples of ventricular arrhythmias as they might appear in lead V1.

Analyze QRS morphology in V1;
is the QRS mostly up-going (positive)?

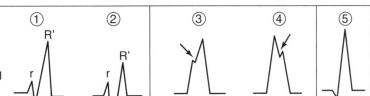

1. RBBB aberrancy
2. RBBB aberrancy
3. Either (50:50)
4. LV-ectopy

5. LV-ectopy, *except* if previous
   AS-MI or normal variant QS
   complex in lead V1 (consider
   RBBB aberrancy)

FIGURE 30.9   Aberrancy versus ventricular ectopy: up-going QRS morphologies.

wave followed by a tall R wave (figure 30.9, 5), it is most likely ventricular in origin. In a patient with a previous anteroseptal MI, a wide QRS with a qR pattern in lead V1 may be supraventricular with RBBB aberration.

If the wide QRS in question is down-going or negative, specific morphologic clues can help to differentiate supraventricular beats with LBBB aberrancy from right ventricular ectopy (figure 30.10) (9). In LBBB,

the initial r wave, if present, is narrow and the large S wave that follows moves rapidly to its nadir (figure 30.10, 1), also seen in figure 30.4*e*. Any one of three features (figure 30.10, 2) is very suggestive of right ventricular ectopy: a wide or fat r wave, a notch or slur on the downstroke of the S wave, or a delay of ≥0.06 s from QRS onset to the nadir of the S wave (figure 30.8, *b* and *f*).

Analyze QRS morphology in V1 or V2;
is the QRS mostly down-going (negative)?

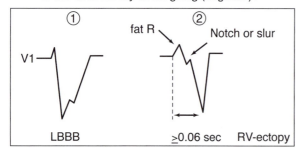

FIGURE 30.10 Aberrancy versus ventricular ectopy: down-going QRS morphologies.

Clinical Recognition and Diagnostic Tools

Cardiac arrhythmias and conduction disturbances may exist in a silent state only to be detected during routine examinations and ECG studies. Symptoms, when present, may include benign palpitations, lightheadedness, and chest discomfort or more serious complications including syncope and sudden death. Catastrophic events are generally seen in people with advanced heart disease, although it is possible for such events to occur in asymptomatic people without structural heart abnormalities. Paradoxically, people with the most annoying palpitations often have no evidence of heart disease, whereas heart patients with more serious arrhythmias may be unaware of the underlying electrical disturbance.

The electrocardiogram is usually the initial diagnostic tool. The resting 12-lead ECG is sufficient to detect bundle-branch and fascicular blocks but may not detect transient or provocable rhythm or conduction disturbances. Therefore, periodic monitoring may be required. If symptoms are frequent enough to occur within a single 24-hr period, ambulatory (*Holter*) ECG monitoring is recommended. A continuous ECG recording device is worn for 24 hr, and the occurrence of symptoms is documented in a diary. The ECG data are analyzed off-line, and abnormalities, if present, are correlated with symptoms. Alternatively, when symptoms are less frequent, the patient can wear an event recorder for several weeks and use the telephone to transmit ECG data associated with symptoms to the clinical ECG station. If symptoms are associated with exercise, an exercise ECG test may be the appropriate diagnostic tool. Exercise testing may also be used in these individuals to assess the safety of exercise and to determine a safe heart rate range for training

purposes. Finally, more serious heart rhythms and conduction disturbances may require evaluation and treatment in the cardiac catheterization laboratory using sophisticated mapping, stimulation, and ablation methodologies.

Treatment Considerations

Decisions regarding the treatment of cardiac arrhythmias and conduction disturbances often depend on the clinical circumstances under which they occur. In the absence of clinically manifest heart disease or disabling symptoms, many electrical abnormalities can be managed conservatively with periodic follow-up and simple reassurance. Elimination of environmental or behavioral precipitating factors helps to prevent benign premature beats that can be annoying. These include caffeine, alcohol, tobacco, and over-the-counter cold medications containing pseudoephedrine or other stimulants. Also, exercising in adverse weather conditions or exposure to environmental pollutants can cause cardiac arrhythmias. If reassurance and environmental modifications are unsuccessful in relieving symptoms of benign arrhythmias, a trial of β-blocker therapy can be considered.

More serious atrial and ventricular arrhythmias can be approached in a systematic way: eliminating environmental stimulants, using various pharmacological agents, and, when necessary, incorporating sophisticated nonpharmacological catheter and device-based therapies. The following discussion focuses on evaluation and treatment of two common age- and disease-related arrhythmias: atrial fibrillation and ventricular tachyarrhythmias. Both disorders are frequent concerns of health professionals working in cardiac rehabilitation and exercise training facilities.

Atrial Fibrillation

Atrial fibrillation (AF) is the most common sustained supraventricular arrhythmia experienced by adults (16). The prevalence increases with age—from less than 0.2% in those younger than 55 to 10% or more in those older than 85 (16). AF can occur in the absence of underlying diseases of the heart or other organ systems (called "lone AF"). Several predisposing risk factors and conditions increase the likelihood developing AF.

Risk Factors

Age

Emotional stress

Exercise

Left atrial size

Tobacco

Alcohol

Medications

PACs

Febrile condition

Anemia

Sleep apnea

Obesity

Conditions

Hypertension

Coronary heart disease

Mitral valve disease

Sick sinus syndrome

Congenital heart disease

Pericarditis

Cardiac tumors

Lung disease

Central nervous system disease

Thyrotoxicosis

Four clinical subtypes of AF have been described (13). New-onset or *first-detected* AF is the first AF that the patient or clinician notices and is typically short lasting and self-terminating. Recurrent episodes are classified as *paroxysmal* AF if self-terminating or *persistent* AF if not self-terminating. Most paroxysmal episodes of AF terminate within a few days. Persistent AF requires pharmacological or electrical cardioversion to restore sinus rhythm. The fourth subtype is long-lasting or *permanent* AF and is not amenable to cardioversion. This classification pertains to AF episodes lasting at least 30 s that are not secondary to a known precipitating event like acute myocardial infarction or recent cardiac surgery. Over time, recurrent episodes of AF progress to permanent AF attributable to electrical and anatomic remodeling of the atria.

In managing AF, the first consideration is whether cardioversion should be attempted to return to sinus rhythm. Recent evidence suggests that many patients with persistent or permanent AF who are not experiencing significant symptoms can be managed with a rate-control strategy using drugs that slow AV conduction (8, 20, 35). Recent guidelines recommend resting heart rates of 60 to 80 beats/min and exercise heart rates no greater than 115 beats/min (13). In patients with AF, and particularly in elderly adults, the adequacy of rate control during physical activity must be determined to avoid excessive tachycardia. A combination of digoxin with a calcium channel blocker (diltiazem or verapamil) or a β-blocker (e.g., metoprolol, atenolol) is often needed to maintain heart rate below 115 beats/min during activity and minimize the likelihood of permanent myocardial damage. Monitoring heart rates during exercise in clients with AF is especially important in cardiac rehabilitation and adult fitness facilities.

New-onset AF usually does not require urgent intervention unless it is associated with a rapid heart rate and is accompanied by severe symptoms of heart failure, hypotension, angina pectoris, or acute myocardial infarction (29). Electrical cardioversion is the treatment of choice under these life-threatening circumstances. Patients with new-onset AF who are tolerating the arrhythmia can be managed more conservatively with heart rate–slowing medications plus appropriate considerations for stroke prevention (described subsequently). Pharmacologic cardioversion using propafenone, flecainide, or ibutilide can be performed in a clinic or emergency room (29). Oral propafenone, flecainide, or amiodarone is usually required to maintain sinus rhythm after successful cardioversion.

For younger and physically active patients with symptomatic AF, an intervention to restore sinus rhythm is preferable to heart-rate control. Electrical or pharmacological cardioversion is generally recommended, along with continued antiarrhythmic drug therapy using propafenone, flecainide, or amiodarone to maintain sinus rhythm. As an alternative to continuous antiarrhythmic drug therapy, a "pill-in-the-pocket" approach has been described for low-risk patients with recurrent AF using self-administered single-dose flecainide or propafenone (1).

Regardless of whether a rate-control or a rhythm-control strategy is chosen, attention must be given to preventing ischemic stroke and systemic embolism. Various algorithms based on age and risk factors have been proposed for reducing the incidence of stroke in patients with nonvalvular AF (13, 15). Risk factors for embolic events include history of hypertension, poor left ventricular function, diabetes mellitus, rheumatic heart disease, prosthetic heart valve, and history of stroke, transient attack, or systemic embolus. Aspirin therapy (325 mg/day) is recommended for those younger than 65 and without risk factors. For patients between ages 65 and 75 who have no risk factors, either aspirin or adjusted-dose warfarin (international normalized ratio 2.0-3.0) is recommended. Patients older than 75 generally should receive warfarin therapy unless they have increased risk of bleeding complications. Unless contraindicated, patients with risk factors should receive warfarin therapy regardless of age.

Patients with prosthetic heart valves need to achieve an international normalized ratio of 2.5 to 3.5. Additional therapeutic options for prevention of thromboembolism will likely emerge from newer agents that are under investigation.

Recently, the possibility of a permanent cure for AF using catheter or surgical ablation techniques has been described for patients with paroxysmal and persistent AF (28). The rationale for this approach stems from the observation that episodes of AF primarily arise from ectopic pacemaker activity originating in the orifices of the pulmonary veins (19). In this approach, circumferential and linear ablation lesions isolate the four pulmonary veins from the rest of the left atrium and prevent the onset of AF. Preliminary results from this technique suggest a lower recurrence rate compared with antiarrhythmic drug therapy as well as improved quality of life, morbidity, and mortality (2, 30). This new technique is rapidly evolving and is expected to take a prominent role in the management of AF.

Ventricular Tachyarrhythmias

Ventricular tachycardia (VT) and ventricular fibrillation (VF) are potentially the most serious and life-threatening arrhythmias among people with or without structural heart disease. VT is usually defined as three or more consecutive PVCs at rates greater than 115 beats/min. Subcategories of VT include *sustained* VT, defined as ongoing VT lasting at least 30 s or any VT that is associated with hemodynamic instability; *nonsustained* VT, defined as an episode of three or more consecutive PVCs lasting up to 30 s and not associated with hemodynamic compromise; *monomorphic* VT, VT for which all the QRS complexes in a given lead look similar; and *polymorphic* VT, VT for which the QRS complexes vary in shape from beat to beat. A unique form of polymorphic VT is *torsades de pointes* (figure 30.8*h*), the characteristic arrhythmia in the long QT syndromes. In this form of VT, the QRS complexes gradually rotate in polarity around the baseline. From an electrophysiologic perspective, VT can be caused by a reentrant circuit, an automatic pacemaker focus, or by triggered automaticity related to early or delayed afterdepolarizations (21).

Treatment decisions are usually based on the presence of specific disease characteristics or risk factors for sudden cardiac death and arrhythmia-related symptoms. In the absence of structural heart abnormalities, ventricular arrhythmias including PVCs and nonsustained VT are usually benign. Elimination of proarrhythmic environmental factors such as caffeine, sympathomimetic agents, nicotine, emotional stressors,

and sudden strenuous physical exertion often reduces arrhythmic events and symptoms. A trial of β-blocker therapy may be warranted in people with persistent arrhythmia following environmental and behavioral modification. Reassuring the patient that these arrhythmias are likely benign will often reduce the anxiety associated with having arrhythmia.

Ventricular arrhythmias are often seen during routine exercise testing of people with and without clinically manifest heart disease. Infrequent arrhythmias are generally benign, especially in people with normal left ventricular function. However, in a population of 29,244 adults referred for diagnostic symptom-limited exercise testing, frequent ventricular ectopy during the recovery period following peak exercise was significantly associated with a 1.5-fold increase risk of death during 5 years of follow-up (12). In this study, frequent ventricular ectopy was defined as 7 or more PVCs per minute, PVC couplets, nonsustained or sustained VT, ventricular fibrillation, or torsades de pointes. Interestingly, ventricular ectopy occurring only during exercise was not associated with increased mortality risk. The investigators hypothesized that blunted reactivation of vagal tone after exercise contributed to the adverse outcomes.

A unique form of ventricular tachycardia called monomorphic right ventricular outflow track (RVOT) tachycardia has been observed in otherwise healthy individuals and usually is not associated with adverse outcomes (6). Originating in the RVOT, this tachycardia is catecholamine sensitive and is initiated by surges in sympathetic stimulation, as occur during exercise. The primary ECG findings are left bundle-branch block morphology in the precordial leads and an inferior axis in the frontal plane leads. Salvos of nonsustained VT are more common than sustained VT. When evaluating individuals with RVOT tachycardia, clinicians must rule out more serious structural heart abnormalities including *arrhythmogenic right ventricular dysplasia*, which is associated with an increased incidence of exercise-related sudden cardiac death and heart failure (32). Noninvasive imaging studies and the signal-averaged ECG are useful modalities for excluding arrhythmogenic right ventricular dysplasia and other occult heart diseases. Treatment considerations in RVOT tachycardia depend on the frequency of arrhythmic events and the presence of symptoms. In the absence of structural heart abnormalities, patient reassurance may be the initial approach if episodes are infrequent and not symptomatic. Drugs including β-blockers, verapamil, and diltiazem may be effective in eliminating symptomatic arrhythmias. For more intractable arrhythmias and symptoms, intracardiac ablation therapy has been successful in eliminating the arrhythmia (25).

Many forms of heart disease are complicated by ventricular arrhythmias. VT and VF are common events during the early minutes of acute myocardial infarction (MI) and may be benign as long as basic and advanced cardiac life support is initiated quickly. In contrast, ventricular arrhythmias occurring later in the course of an acute MI or following hospital discharge for MI are often the result of severe left ventricular dysfunction and may contribute to adverse outcomes, including sudden cardiac death. Because of the potential seriousness of these arrhythmias, ECG monitoring in post-MI patients is recommended during phase II cardiac rehabilitation programs. Studies have shown that post-MI patients with ejection fractions less than 35% have better outcomes with implantable cardiac defibrillators (ICDs) than with antiarrhythmic drugs alone (26). Similar recommendations for ICD therapy apply to the growing population with chronic congestive heart failure, among whom the incidence of sudden death is high (3).

Intracardiac Devices: Pacemakers and Defibrillators

Cardiac pacing with artificial pacemakers has evolved over the past 50 years from simple fixed-rate ventricular pacing to complex multichamber, rate-adaptive, programmable devices that are often combined with antitachycardia and defibrillator functions. Greater complexity of these devices has broadened their clinical application to a wide variety of disturbances of cardiac rhythm, conduction, and function. The American College of Cardiology, the American Heart Association, and the North American Society of Pacing and Electrophysiology have summarized current recommendations and guidelines for using cardiac pacemakers and antiarrhythmic devices (17). Health care professionals working in cardiac rehabilitation or other exercise

testing and training facilities need to be familiar with these devices to ensure that appropriate safeguards are in place during exercise activities.

Pacemaker and defibrillator units are generally implanted under the skin of the upper left chest with the lead wires inserted through the left cephalic and subclavian veins and into the myocardium of the right atrium and right ventricle. An additional lead for biventricular pacing can be placed in a similar fashion through the right atrium and then into the coronary sinus and into the left ventricular myocardium. Expected battery life depends on the complexity of the pacemaker and defibrillator and generally ranges from 5 to 10 years. Patients with these devices are followed closely in pacemaker clinics, where sophisticated testing equipment is used to interrogate and program the various parameters and functions of the unit.

A standardized five-letter code for classifying pacemakers developed by North American Society of Pacing and Electrophysiology and the British Pacing and Electrophysiology Group is shown in figure 30.11 (4). The first two letters of the code define the chambers being paced and sensed (*A* for atria, *V* for ventricles, and *D* for both); the third letter characterizes the response to a sensed event (*I* if the sensed event inhibits discharge of the pacemaker; *T* if the response to a sensed event triggers a pacemaker discharge); the fourth letter indicates the presence or absence of rate modulation (*R* for rate modulation or *O* for no modulation); and the fifth letter describes multisite pacing (*A* for biatrial pacing, *V* for biventricular pacing, *D* for both, *O* for none). The first three letters of the code often are used alone when rate modulation and multisite pacing are not device functions.

Figure 30.12*a* shows right atrial pacing (AOO); note that a pacing stimulus artifact (arrow) precedes each P wave. Figure 30.12, *b* and *c*, provides examples of dual-chamber or AV sequential pacing (arrows point to pacing artifacts). Atrial triggered ventricular pacing (DDD) is when the patient's own P wave is sensed and triggers the ventricular pacemaker after

1	2	3	4	5
Chamber(s) paced	**Chamber(s) sensed**	**Sensed response**	**Rate modulation**	**Multisite pacing**
A = atrium	O = none	O = none	O = none	O = none
V = ventricle	A = atrium	T = triggered	R = rate modulation	A = atrium
D = dual A & V	V = ventricle	I = inhibited		V = ventricle
	D = dual A & V	D = dual T & I		D = dual

FIGURE 30.11 Pacemaker coding functions and nomenclature.

allowing a reasonable interval for atrial contraction to contribute to ventricular filling (figure 30.12*b*). Both atria and ventricles are paced sequentially in the example illustrated in figure 30.12*c*. Ventricular demand pacing (VVI) is illustrated in figure 30.12*d*. In this example, the patient has a slow sinus rhythm that intermittently captures the ventricles *(C)* which, in turn, inhibit the pacemaker. The ventricular pacemaker only fires (arrow) when there is a predefined pause in the rhythm.

Pacemakers are usually indicated when there is marked slowing in heart rate attributable to sinus node dysfunction or heart block conditions in the AV junction or bundle-branch system (17). The simplest and least expensive pacemaker is the VVI or ventricular demand pacemaker with a single right ventricle electrode that has both pacing and sensing functions. This pacemaker often is used in elderly patients to protect against bradyarrhythmias attributable to sinus node dysfunction or AV heart block (figure 30.12*d*). The disadvantage of this pacemaker is that it lacks rate modulation and atrioventricular synchrony. It is most appropriate in patients with chronic atrial arrhythmias to prevent symptomatic bradycardia. For more active

people, in whom rate modulation is needed, a VVIR pacemaker allows for better rate adjustments during physical activity. Rate adjustments are usually made by sensing body motion, vibration, or minute ventilation.

For patients with sinus node dysfunction, but normal AV conduction, a simple atrial demand pacemaker with or without rate adjustment (AAI or AAIR) can be used (figure 30.12*a*). If there is concern about possible AV conduction abnormalities at any point, a dual-chamber pacemaker is preferred (DDD or DDDR; figure 30.12, *b* and *c*). Modern dual-chamber pacemakers can switch modes to avoid rapid heart rates in the face of sustained atrial arrhythmias.

Synchronized biventricular pacing has been found to improve function, symptoms, and survival in patients with chronic congestive heart failure who have a low ejection fraction (<35%) and prolonged QRS duration (>130 ms) (5). In this regard, greater improvements in cardiac output and function occur with simultaneous pacing of the right and left ventricles than with the sequential ventricular activation that occurs in bundle-branch block. This is particularly relevant in patients with LBBB, where late activation of the left ventricle

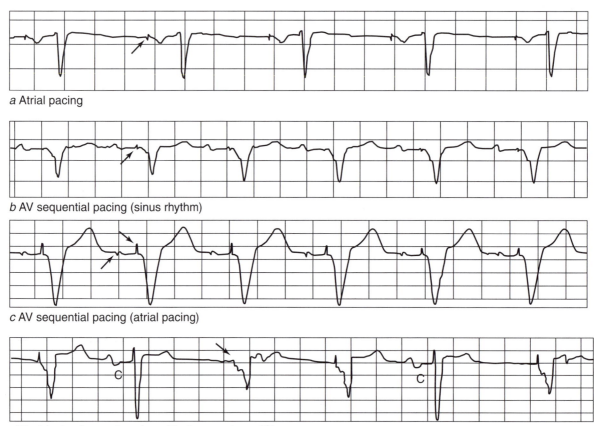

a Atrial pacing

b AV sequential pacing (sinus rhythm)

c AV sequential pacing (atrial pacing)

d Ventricular demand pacing with sinus captures (C)

FIGURE 30.12 ECG in pacemaker rhythms.

by the right ventricular activation wave front results in compromised left ventricular diastolic filling attributable to late closure of the aortic valve and delayed opening of the mitral valve (18).

Indications for intracardiac defibrillators have evolved considerably since they were introduced more than 20 years ago (17). The intracardiac defibrillator (ICD) has antitachycardia functions that can be used to terminate ventricular tachycardia by overdrive pacing. Initially, these devices were used only in high-risk people who already had experienced a cardiac arrest or life-threatening arrhythmia (e.g., for secondary prevention). Recent evidence suggests that the prophylactic insertion of an ICD in post-MI or idiopathic cardiomyopathy patients with poor left ventricular function (ejection fraction <30%) can improve function and clinical outcomes (3, 26). Greater use of ICD devices increases the likelihood that health care providers will encounter these patients in settings of exercise testing, training, and rehabilitation. Thus, both patients and clinicians must know the heart rate limits above which antitachycardia pacing is programmed to begin. Unexpected discharge of an ICD during exercise testing has been reported (23) and may be particularly distressing to both patient and exercise personnel.

Considerations Relevant to Exercise Training and Testing

The cardiovascular and functional benefits of regular physical activity and exercise training are well established (11, 27). Authorities agree that people with and without clinically manifest cardiovascular disease should be encouraged to lead active lifestyles (11, 27). The potential for exercise-induced hemodynamic instability and catastrophic events in people with arrhythmias may be disconcerting to exercise and medical professionals. Nevertheless, given the increasing number of elderly people in our society, evaluation and management of individuals with arrhythmias are becoming routine in a variety of health care and wellness settings.

The usefulness of exercise testing as a clinical tool for evaluating people with benign and malignant arrhythmias as well as for monitoring the effectiveness of antiarrhythmic therapies is becoming established and has been extensively reviewed elsewhere (2, 11, 14, 22, 31, 37). Neural, metabolic, and mechanical changes in the heart during graded exercise exposure may create a proarrhythmic environment. Exercise testing may unmask arrhythmias that go undetected during activities of daily living, particularly in sedentary individuals. Exercise testing is often used to evaluate the hemodynamic, chronotropic, and functional significance of arrhythmias and antiarrhythmic therapies. It is also used to evaluate the effectiveness of pharmacological rate control in AF and to titrate additional drugs or adjust pacing devices to achieve desired heart rate responses during physical exertion in AF patients. Exercise testing may be particularly useful in evaluating the effectiveness of antiarrhythmic medication in individuals with adrenergic-dependent rhythm disturbances. The prognostic value of exercise test–induced arrhythmia is not fully understood, but available prospective data suggest that the prognostic value is greatest in people with existing structural heart disease and left ventricular dysfunction and in those with complex compared with simple ectopy.

Exercise testing in people with arrhythmia generally is seen to be safe, with untoward events occurring most often in patients with advanced heart disease or a history of severe malignant arrhythmia or aborted sudden cardiac death. Current guidelines list tachyarrhythmias, bradyarrhythmias, and high-degree AV block as relative contraindications for exercise testing, whereas uncontrolled symptomatic and hemodynamically limiting arrhythmia is an absolute contraindication (11, 14). The occurrence of arrhythmia and conduction disturbances other than sustained VT is considered a relative indication for terminating an exercise test. Adequate emergency procedures and equipment for cardioversion and resuscitation, and direct physician supervision of tests that involve high-risk patients, will minimize fatal and long-standing morbid events.

Implantable devices are often used for cardiac pacing and for automatic cardioversion from ventricular arrhythmia in people with rhythm and conduction abnormalities. Exercise testing of patients with implantable cardiac defibrillators (ICDs) warrants particular consideration to avoid inappropriate defibrillator discharges (22, 23, 31). Many implantable devices have both pacing and defibrillating functions, and most of these devices recognize and respond to rate rather than rhythm patterns. Thus, the exercise testing staff must know whether the device is programmed for variable pacing to accommodate the positive chronotropic demand of graded exercise and must know the rate threshold at which the device has been programmed to discharge a defibrillator shock. This is particularly relevant in young or exercise-trained people who receive an ICD and present for clinical evaluation with well-preserved functional capacity (23). Deactivation of the ICD prior to the exercise test will avoid inappropriate shocks during the test but also will render the patient unprotected from malignant arrhythmia during the testing period.

Specifics of the exercise test must be considered. People with left ventricular dysfunction or chronic heart failure and some elderly patients may have marked sign- or symptom-limited exercise intolerance and low functional capacity, which may result in an insufficient exercise duration to provoke an arrhythmia in a diagnostic setting. Conversely, young patients may have higher functional levels, but the onset of arrhythmia in these individuals may be sudden and unexpected. Therefore, exercise protocols with short stage durations (1-2 min) and small workload increments ($\leq$1 MET) should be used, examples of which are the modified Naughton and the Balke treadmill protocols (11). A prolonged cool-down period is recommended for people with rhythm disturbances, particularly those who are adrenergic dependent. In many instances, the presence of arrhythmia or the use of certain drug therapies may confound the use of a percentage of age-predicted maximal heart rate as a test end point. Certain drugs (e.g., digoxin, amiodarone), specific conduction disturbances (e.g., LBBB), or the presence of AV-sequential pacing limits the diagnostic significance of exercise-induced ST-T wave depression. Therefore, volitional exhaustion or the occurrence of symptoms may serve as a test end point.

Exercise Programming Considerations

Individuals with rhythm and conduction disturbances can achieve meaningful improvements in functional capacity from exercise training (2, 22, 31). The resulting physiological adaptations are likely associated with lower chronic disease risk factors and enhanced functional independence (11, 33), which may be particularly important in arrhythmia patients with comorbid conditions such as diabetes, hypertension, left ventricular dysfunction, or heart failure. Endurance exercise training improves hemodynamic responses and thus lowers myocardial oxygen demand at a given level of exertion, which reduces the risk of myocardial infarction and associated arrhythmia in patients with myocardial ischemia. Improved sympathetic responsiveness during exercise also may result in heart rate responses during physical exertion that override ectopic foci and eliminate ectopic beats during exercise and for a period of time thereafter. Physical activity and exercise training are contraindicated primarily in those with severe symptomatic and hemodynamically unstable arrhythmias or heart failure.

Most people with well-controlled arrhythmias, particularly those who are sedentary or insufficiently active or who have low functional capacity, will benefit from accumulating at least 30 min of moderate-intensity physical activity on 5 or more days of the week (11, 27). Physical activity sessions of at least 10 min duration can be undertaken throughout the day to meet the targeted total of at least 30 min/day. Moderate intensity is defined as 40% to 60% of maximal oxygen uptake or 55% to 70% of maximal heart rate (11). The use of heart rate to determine activity intensity may be inappropriate in individuals with arrhythmia; therefore, a perceived exertion of approximately 12 to 15 on a 6- to 20-point Borg scale should be targeted once the person is comfortable in rating his or her level of physical exertion (11). Activities such as brisk walking and bicycling, stair stepping, or other large-muscle dynamic activities are recommended. Muscular strengthening activities may be required to improve physical functioning beyond the effects of aerobic activity. Performing 1 to 2 sets of 12 to 15 repetitions with low resistance (50-70% maximal voluntary contraction) for major upper- and lower-body muscle groups once or twice a week is recommended (11). Consultation with an exercise specialist is highly recommended before beginning a resistance exercise program. An adequate warm-up period is required prior to both aerobic and resistance activity. This might include a combination of calisthenics, walking, or bicycling of gradually increasing intensity until appreciable increases in heart rate, perceived exertion, breathing rate, and body temperature have been achieved. Similarly, a cool-down period should follow the primary activity program and include a gradual decline in activity intensity to achieve a heart rate or perceived exertion close to resting levels. Physical activity should be terminated with the occurrence of excessive light-headedness, blurred vision, chest discomfort, or palpitations. The occurrence of these symptoms during or after activity should be immediately reported to one's health care provider.

People with rhythm and conduction abnormalities who are otherwise asymptomatic and medically stable can safely participate in unsupervised physical activity. High-risk individuals with malignant arrhythmia, poorly controlled atrial fibrillation, or coexisting severe but stable left ventricular dysfunction should be on continuous ECG telemetry during exercise and for a brief period thereafter. Although referral to cardiac rehabilitation programs might seem appropriate for these individuals, Medicare will not reimburse programs for this purpose.

Summary

Cardiac arrhythmias and conduction disorders are frequent concerns among health care professionals working with athletes, sedentary and active individuals, and patients with cardiovascular disorders. This chapter reviewed important aspects of electrocardiographic recognition, evaluation strategies, and treatment considerations relevant to exercise testing and training. Evaluation and treatment of cardiac rhythm and conduction disorders continue to evolve as new drugs and devices become available. Clinicians working in exercise-related fields must keep abreast of new developments in these areas.

Peripheral Arterial Disease

Kerry J. Stewart, EdD

Peripheral arterial disease is a manifestation of systemic atherosclerosis. Although a peripheral artery is any blood artery outside of the heart, such as the carotid or renal arteries, the term *peripheral arterial disease (PAD)* most commonly refers to the gradual and progressive narrowing of arterial vessels in the lower limbs. The term PAD has been used interchangeably with *peripheral vascular disease (PVD)*, although this use is incorrect. PVD is a broader term for the group of diseases that affect arteries, veins, and the lymphatic system of the body except for the vessels of the heart. PAD is a form of PVD but is more specifically the disease that causes narrowing of the arteries to the legs because of plaque deposits and stiffening of the artery walls.

As many as 10 million people in the United States have PAD, and the prevalence is greater than 10% in people older than 60 years (5). People at the greatest risk for developing PAD are described in Overview of Peripheral Arterial Disease.

The mismatch of oxygen delivery and metabolic demand during physical activity causes ischemia and often results in claudication, the primary symptom of PAD. Claudication is walking-induced pain in one or both legs that does not go away with continued walking and is relieved by rest. Similar to ischemia that causes chest pain, or angina pectoris, claudication is the angina of the legs. The term *claudication* traces back to the Roman emperor Claudius, who walked with a limp. Although estimates vary, claudication symptoms are present in less than half of persons affected with PAD (1). Why some people with PAD do not have claudication is not entirely clear, but some possibilities are that these patients (a) do not walk far or fast enough to induce muscle ischemic symptoms because of comorbidities such as pulmonary disease or arthritis; (b) have neuropathies that deaden nerve endings in the legs; (c) have atypical symptoms unrecognized as intermittent claudication; (d) fail to mention their symptoms to their physician; or (e) have sufficient collateral arterial channels to allow them to tolerate arterial obstruction in larger arteries (1). It is not uncommon for clinicians to attribute leg pain to sciatica, arthritis, poor muscle strength, or aging. However, normal aging should not cause PAD and claudication. Some of the common signs and symptoms of PAD are listed in Overview of Peripheral Arterial Disease on page 310. The extent to which a person has some or all of these signs or symptoms will depend on the severity of the disease.

For patients with claudication, the initial treatment is focused on reducing the symptoms that cause functional impairment and a poor quality of

Address correspondence concerning this chapter to Kerry J. Stewart, John Hopkins Bayview Medical Center, 4940 Eastern Ave, Baltimore, MD 21224-2734. E-mail: kstewart@jhmi.edu

Overview of Peripheral Arterial Disease

People at risk for developing PAD have the following characteristics:

- Age less than 50 with diabetes and one atherosclerosis risk factor
- Age 50 to 69 with diabetes and a history of smoking
- Age 70 or older
- History of coronary artery, renal, or carotid disease

Common signs and symptoms of PAD include the following:

- Exertional leg pain, fatigue, aching, or numbness most commonly in the calf but also in the buttock, thigh, or foot. Symptoms are relieved by resting.
- Slowly healing or nonhealing wounds of the legs or feet
- Coolness of the toes and feet
- Loss of leg hair
- Pain at rest, particularly when elevating the legs
- Gangrene

The presence of these symptoms will depend on the severity of the disease.

life. Extreme presentations of PAD include rest pain, tissue loss, or gangrene; these limb-threatening manifestations of PAD are collectively termed *critical limb ischemia*. Regardless of symptoms, it is critical to treat the underlying systemic atherosclerosis because of the high risk for cardiovascular ischemic events in these patients (12, 25). This chapter is concerned primarily with exercise training for claudication because there is considerable evidence to support the use of exercise in the management of this debilitating symptom. It is presumed that patients with asymptomatic PAD would also benefit from exercise training, although there is a lack of research studies with which specific recommendations or guidelines can be formulated.

Assessing the Peripheral Circulation

Proper diagnosis of PAD is important to prevent progression and relieve symptoms. The initial assessment of PAD begins with a thorough medical history and physical examination. Palpation of peripheral pulses should be a routine component of the physical exam and should include assessment of the femoral, popliteal, and pedal vessels. However, pulse assessment has a high degree of interobserver variability. In contrast, the ankle–brachial index (ABI) is a reproducible and reasonably accurate noninvasive method to detect PAD and determine disease severity. The ABI is the ratio of ankle to arm systolic blood pressure and is readily obtainable with blood pressure cuffs and a Doppler device. A pencil-size Doppler probe is used, because the curved and uneven anatomy of the foot makes it difficult to detect the pulse reliably with a stethoscope. The normal range of ABI values is between 0.91 and 1.30. The interpretation of ABI values is shown in table 31.1.

An ABI >1.30 suggests a noncompressible, calcified vessel. Among persons with a high cardiovascular disease risk factor profile, a simple ABI measurement can identify a substantial number of patients with previously unrecognized PAD (15). Although the primary responsibility for diagnosing PAD lies with the personal health care provider, some cardiac rehabilitation and clinical exercise physiology programs have initiated ABI testing as part of their initial evaluation because many of their clients are at high risk for PAD.

Ankle systolic blood pressure and ABI are often further reduced after exercise because blood flow is shunted into the proximal leg musculature at the expense of the periphery and distal circulation in the

TABLE 31.1 Interpretation of the Ankle–Brachial Index (ABI)

ABI	Interpretation
0.90-1.30	Normal
0.70-0.89	Mild
0.40-0.69	Moderate
≤0.40	Severe
>1.30	Noncompressible vessels

leg. Although serial measurements of ABI are used to assess progression in disease severity, an increase in leg blood flow is not a common response to exercise training (27). Therefore, ABI is not useful for assessing the efficacy of exercise interventions.

Besides noting an abnormal ABI and the classic symptom of claudication, clinicians should be aware of other symptoms of PAD. These include decreased warmth or color of the extremity; loss of hair on the legs, feet, and toes; skin lesions; ulcers or wounds that do not heal; impaired balance when standing on both feet; reduced walking velocity and abnormal gait; increased time to arise from a chair; low hip abduction force; reduced leg strength; poor nail health; and absence of pedal or posterior tibial pulses.

If the ABI is abnormal or the patient has worsening symptoms, other tests may be recommended. Among the available diagnostic methods are the following:

■ Doppler and ultrasound (duplex) imaging is a noninvasive method for visualizing the artery with sound waves and measuring blood flow in an artery to determine the severity of blockages.

■ Computed tomographic angiography is a noninvasive test that uses an X ray to provide high-resolution images of the arteries in the legs and can be used to evaluate arteries in the abdomen, pelvis, and legs. This test is particularly useful in patients with pacemakers or stents.

■ Magnetic resonance angiography is a noninvasive imaging test that uses high-strength magnetic fields instead of an X ray to provide images of the blood vessels.

■ Angiography of the blood vessels can also be used, particularly if the clinical evaluation suggests that the patient may require an invasive intervention such as leg bypass surgery, angioplasty, or stent placement. As occurs with a cardiac angiogram, a contrast agent is injected into the leg artery, and X rays are taken to reveal any blockages that may be present.

Other diagnostic methods include pulse volume recording, segmental blood pressure measurement, postocclusive reactive hyperemic blood flow, transcutaneous oximetry, near-infrared spectroscopy, and exercise testing, which are discussed later in this chapter.

Effects on Exercise Tolerance

Because of impaired walking ability, many patients with claudication experience considerable difficulty in carrying out routine daily activities. To avoid leg discomfort, patients with claudication will alter their gait and decrease their ambulatory pace and distance, often reducing their daily physical activity and maximal oxygen uptake as much as 50% compared with healthy subjects of similar age. Lack of muscle strength in the legs may also contribute to a decline in functional performance in patients with PAD (20). Many affected patients are so deconditioned because of physical inactivity that they become housebound or dependent on others (10). Patients with PAD and intermittent claudication often have coronary artery disease, diabetes, and other comorbid medical problems. Smoking adversely affects exercise capacity in patients with PAD, whereas the presence of coronary artery disease, diabetes, and other medical problems has a modest impact on exercise capacity (17). The modest impact of comorbid medical conditions on walking ability in patients with PAD reflects the overwhelming limitation in ambulatory function attributable to the claudication pain. Nevertheless, in one study, patients with PAD and diabetes had poorer lower-extremity function than those with PAD alone (6). This difference in functioning was largely explained by diabetes-associated neuropathy, differences in exertional leg symptoms, and greater cardiovascular disease in patients with diabetes.

Therapeutic Strategies

The natural history of PAD is defined by symptoms and ischemic events that occur in the affected limb or as a result of systemic atherosclerosis in other vascular territories. Nearly three fourths of patients with claudication will continue to have stable exertional symptoms during the 5 years after diagnosis (32). For the remaining patients, approximately 16% will develop worsening claudication or more severe limb ischemia. Rapidly worsening PAD is unusual, and the lifetime need for lower-extremity revascularization is relatively low (7%), as is the risk of limb amputation (4%). More important, patients have an associated 20% to 30% 5-year mortality and morbidity rate from coronary and cerebrovascular ischemic events (myocardial infarction and stroke) once claudication develops. Therefore, in addition to treating the symptoms of claudication, PAD rehabilitation must decrease cardiovascular disease risk factors. The strongest risk factors for the development of PAD are advancing age, tobacco use, diabetes mellitus, hypertension, lipid abnormalities, and hyperhomocysteinemia. Reviews of cardiovascular disease risk factors and potential therapies for patients with PAD have been published (12, 25). All patients with PAD, regardless of severity of symptoms, should undergo risk factor modification and receive antiplatelet therapy. Recommendations for risk modification include the following:

- Smoking cessation
- LDL cholesterol <100 mg/dL
- Glycosylated hemoglobin <7.0%
- Blood pressure <130/85
- Angiotensin-converting enzyme inhibition
- Antiplatelet therapy with aspirin or clopidogrel

PAD exercise rehabilitation should be considered a first-line therapeutic modality for most patients with claudication (28). Patients with claudication who are unable to attend an exercise rehabilitation program, do not tolerate treadmill-based training, or who are unresponsive to exercise therapy may benefit from medical therapy. The two FDA-approved pharmacologic therapies for the treatment of claudication are cilostazol (Pletal, Otsuka Pharmaceuticals, Inc., and Pharmacia & Upjohn) and pentoxifylline (Trental, Aventis). Cilostazol has been shown to be efficacious in improving both pain-free and maximal treadmill walking distance when compared with placebo in several studies. Conversely, pentoxifylline appears to have a limited beneficial effect on walking ability. It is unknown whether exercise combined with pharmacotherapy would produce beneficial additive or synergistic effects beyond the use of either therapy alone.

Invasive Therapies for Claudication

For patients who are markedly incapacitated by their exercise limitation and for those with limb-threatening ischemia, invasive intervention may be appropriate. The availability of percutaneous treatments, including balloon angioplasty, atherectomy, and stents, has expanded the interventional options for physicians treating patients with PAD. These techniques have been promoted as safe, cost-effective, reliable, and durable alternatives to conventional vascular surgical procedures, and they have been offered to many patients with mild degrees of ischemia who would not meet conventional criteria for surgical intervention. However, few prospective, randomized, clinical trials have fully evaluated the long-term efficacy of these therapies in terms of vessel patency and recurrence of symptoms. In selecting a surgical intervention for a specific patient, the physician must balance the chances

for procedural success, associated cardiovascular risk, and expected durability of the therapy. Some of the same complications that occur with coronary artery revascularization may also affect patients with peripheral artery revascularization. For example, similar to coronary stents, peripheral stents can become surrounded by scar tissue, which can result in restenosis in some patients. Drug-eluting stents, which are commonly used in coronary artery angioplasties, may soon be available for leg artery stenting. Exercise therapy also plays a role in patients who have undergone limb revascularization. In one study, the combination of exercise and limb revascularization was more effective in improving symptom-free walking distance than either intervention alone (19).

Effects of Exercise Training

Prospective studies have demonstrated a benefit of exercise training in patients with claudication (9, 18, 24, 30). Most patients studied had mild to moderate claudication. Less is known about the clinical benefits of exercise in patients with asymptomatic PAD or critical leg ischemia. Although exercise-induced improvements in walking ability are well established, the magnitude of the response to training has been variable across studies. Such variability may be explained by differences among studies in the intensity, duration, and frequency of exercise and the methods for measuring exercise capacity. One meta-analysis (9) that examined both nonrandomized and randomized trials of exercise training showed that pain-free walking time improved by an average of 180% and maximal walking time increased by 120% in claudication patients who underwent exercise training. The exercise parameters associated with the greatest improvements in walking ability are summarized in table 31.2. A meta-analysis from the Cochrane Collaboration (18) that considered only randomized controlled trials concluded that exercise improved maximal walking ability by an average of 150% (range 74-230%).

Exercise-induced improvements in walking ability translate to increases in routine daily activity. In one uncontrolled study (7), 6 months of exercise training improved treadmill walking ability and resulted in a 31% increase in routine daily activity as measured by accelerometry. Self-reported physical activity increased by 62%. Controlled studies have also shown higher levels of routine daily activity in patients with claudication after exercise training (27). In a prospective, randomized controlled trial of elderly patients limited

TABLE 31.2   Exercise Training Parameters and Their Values Associated With the Greatest Improvements in Walking Distance

Exercise parameter	Values
Intensity	Moderate or greater pain while walking
Duration	>30 min per session
Frequency	≥3 times per week
Mode	Walking
Length	>6 months
Type	Supervised

by claudication (30), 12 weeks of exercise training improved the time to onset of pain by 88%, time to maximal pain by 70%, and 6-min walk distance by 21%. These functional gains translated into marked increases in perceptions of health-related quality of life, indicating that these patients were more functionally independent. Such increases in physical activity, if associated with improvements in cardiovascular risk factors, might also reduce the risk of adverse cardiovascular events, thereby potentially improving the poor prognosis for survival in this population.

The time course of the response to a program of exercise has not been fully established. Exercise-induced clinical benefits have been observed as early as 4 weeks and have been observed to continue to accrue after 6 months of participation (11). Gardner and colleagues (8) reported that improvements in walking ability after 6 months of supervised exercise rehabilitation 3 times per week were sustained when patients continued to participate in an exercise maintenance program for an additional 12 months. In a prospective nonrandomized study (33), patients who followed clinical instructions to walk and not to smoke showed an increase in maximal walking distance throughout treatment. Follow-up ranged from 3 months to 4 years. The mean monthly increase achieved in the first 6 months was substantially greater than that after 6 months. Notably, patients who adhered to exercise training but continued to smoke exhibited an increase in their walking capacity in the first 6 months; however, after 6 months, the effect of treatment was null.

Recommendations for Exercise Testing

Because patients with claudication commonly have concomitant clinical or occult coronary artery disease, hypertension, and diabetes, they may experience adverse cardiovascular and physiological responses during exercise training. Although serious adverse events have been rare in clinical practice and research studies, it is recommended that treadmill exercise testing with 12-lead electrocardiographic monitoring be performed before a patient begins an exercise program so that ischemic symptoms, ST-T wave changes, or arrhythmias may be identified (28). These patients will, by definition, have claudication-limited exercise and may not achieve an adequate heart rate response to reveal cardiovascular electrocardiographic abnormalities or symptoms. Nevertheless, the findings from the exercise test can be used to determine that there are no untoward cardiovascular responses at the exercise level reached. The exercise test also provides information about claudication thresholds and heart rate and blood pressure responses that the clinician can use to develop an exercise prescription.

The treadmill test protocol should be progressive, with gradual increments in grade (10, 13). Such gradual increases in exercise intensity allow clinicians to classify the walking distances of patients according to their disease severity. Common treadmill protocols for PAD patients use a fixed walking speed of 2 mph at 0% grade, with gradual increases in grade of either 2.0% every 2 min or 3.5% every 3 min. The measurements most often used to evaluate functional capacity are distance or time to initial pain and distance or time to maximal tolerated pain.

To evaluate cardiovascular responses with exercise when treadmill walking is limited, clinicians can assign bicycle ergometry as an alternative modality. Cycling reduces the muscular work of the calves, placing more emphasis on the muscles of the thighs. Unfortunately, bicycle ergometer testing may also be limited because of the deconditioned status of these muscles. For these reasons, pharmacological stress testing may be the best modality for diagnostic evaluation of cardiovascular responses to increased myocardial demand.

Other useful measures of function capacity are the 6-min walk and measures of gait, balance, flexibility, and lower-body strength. Evaluation of functional status using validated questionnaires is also a useful adjunct to exercise treadmill testing. These questionnaires can provide an objective measure of clinical improvement resulting from participation in PAD rehabilitation. Some of the available questionnaires are briefly described next.

- The Walking Impairment Questionnaire (WIQ) is a disease-specific questionnaire that assesses the ability of the patient with claudication to walk in terms of distance, speed, stair-climbing ability, and claudication severity (27). This questionnaire correlates well with treadmill walking distance and is sensitive to changes in functional capacity.

- The Medical Outcomes Study Short Form (MOS SF-36) is a non-disease-specific questionnaire that assesses domains of physical and mental health, including physical functioning, role limitations attributable to physical and emotional problems, bodily pain, social functioning, general mental health, vitality, and general health perceptions (31).

- The PAD Quality of Life Questionnaire (PADQL) is a PAD-specific questionnaire designed to reveal difficulties with diagnosis and management of claudication, limitations in physical functioning and social functioning, symptom experience, compromise of self, uncertainty, and adaptation (29).

Recommendations for Exercise Prescription

Walking is the most effective exercise for reducing claudication symptoms and improving functional capacity. Regardless of the specific mechanism for benefit, the stimulus for the adaptive responses to exercise training in patients with claudication is the ischemia that occurs in the legs while walking.

Exercise training is performed on a treadmill with the initial work rate set to a speed and grade that elicits claudication symptoms within 3 to 5 min. To reach the appropriate pain level, the patient should be instructed to reach a pain scale rating of 3 or 4 out of 5 during the walking phase of the workout.

The patient then stops walking for a brief period of standing or sitting rest to permit symptoms to resolve. The exercise–rest–exercise pattern (also known as interval training) should be repeated throughout the exercise session. The initial duration will usually include 35 min of intermittent walking, which is increased by 5 min each session until a total of 50 min of intermittent walking can be accomplished. The work rate should be increased by changes in treadmill speed or grade (or both) if the patient is able to walk for 8 to 10 min without moderate claudication pain.

Treadmill or track walking should be performed at least 3 times per week initially. As the patient adapts to exercise and experiences less postexercise muscle soreness, the frequency should be increased to 5 times per week or even daily.

As functional capacity improves with exercise training and higher heart rates and blood pressure are attained, central cardiac responses may assume greater importance and angina may be revealed. This response may require reevaluation of cardiovascular status and modification of medical management and the exercise prescription.

Other Forms of Exercise

Resistance training is usually recommended for people with other manifestations of cardiovascular disease because of its beneficial effects on strength and endurance, cardiovascular function, metabolism, coronary risk factors, and psychosocial well-being. Many patients with claudication also have reduced muscle mass (20) and a lack of muscle strength and endurance, which exacerbate their physical impairment. However, in patients with claudication, resistance training does not appear to directly improve walking ability; rather, walking itself is most effective in increasing claudication-limited walking capacity (14, 27). Patients with claudication can perform resistance training as tolerated for general fitness and well-being, but it should be adjunctive to a walking program.

Because patients with claudication pain are limited in both walking speed and duration, the benefits of walking exercise may be insufficient to yield a cardiovascular training effect (4). For this reason, other modalities of exercise may be required to supplement walking to attain cardiovascular benefits from exercise. Exercise on a stationary cycle is less likely to cause claudication and may be a useful adjunct modality. However, many patients will be limited in the amount of work they can perform on a cycle because of deconditioning of their leg muscles. Polestriding is walking with poles and uses the muscles of the upper and lower body in a continuous movement similar to cross-country skiing but without the skis. This exercise modality increases the total exercising muscle mass and may allow for increased perfusion to the leg muscles because of the longer period of time the leg muscles are relaxed between each stride (4). As such, patients may experience a delayed onset of claudication pain permitting them to sustain a higher walking intensity and longer duration. After 6 months in a supervised moderate-intensity interval training program with walking poles, patients with claudication increased their walking time and oxygen uptake and also decreased their systolic blood pressure, heart rate, and rate pressure product at given submaximal work rates on a treadmill test. Patients also increased their health-related quality of life as measured by the MOS SF-36 to a degree that was comparable to that of other patients undergoing traditional walking. Although these results using polestriding show benefit, the lack of a direct comparison with traditional walking precludes a definitive conclusion that it can be used as a substitute for walking without poles.

The use of a stair stepper versus treadmill training was examined in a study of 12 patients with claudication (16). After 12 weeks, mean exercise time before the onset of claudication pain increased, but greater improvements were seen on the specific training apparatus. In other words, treadmill training resulted in improvement in treadmill exercise performance with less improvement noted when tested on the stair stepper, and vice versa. Although small, these results suggest potential value of stair stepping as a supplement to walking.

Given the available data, walking remains the central component of an exercise program for claudication. The use of other modalities, including upper-arm exercise, may be useful in some patients who would benefit from reaching higher exercise work rates to attain the full benefits of cardiovascular conditioning. Of note, some patients who reach higher heart rates, either by increasing their walking capacity or by using other exercise modalities, may begin to experience angina, which was not evident at lower-exercise intensities. Key Features of the Exercise Prescription for Claudication below summarizes exercise recommendations.

▪ Key Features of the Exercise Prescription for Claudication

- The patient should walk fast enough or increase treadmill grade to reach moderate-intensity pain within 3 to 5 min, and then rest until the pain resolves.

- The patient should repeat this pattern of walking and resting for a total of 35 min initially and progress to 50 min of walking by adding 5 min each week, as tolerated.

- Walking consistently improves claudication symptoms.

- The patient should increase work rate if moderate pain is not reached.

- Cycling, upper-body, or other exercises can be used for cardiovascular conditioning if target heart rate cannot be reached with walking, but these exercises are generally done in addition to and not as a substitute for walking.

- Resistance training is recommended for general conditioning if tolerated but is done in addition to and not as a substitute for walking.

In addition to following these recommendations, patients should enroll in a medically supervised exercise program with electrocardiographic, heart rate, blood pressure, and blood glucose monitoring. Such a program has the following advantages over unsupervised programs:

- Supervision increases the likelihood that the exercise will be carried out.

- Because the patient may be resistant to waking with pain on their own, the work rate can be monitored to ensure that claudication pain provides a stimulus as the patients improve their walking ability.

- Supervision is important as patients increase their walking ability and reach higher heart rate and blood pressure levels because cardiac signs and symptoms could appear.

- Electrocardiographic monitoring is advised for the initial sessions and additional monitoring is determined by clinical responses.

- Blood glucose levels can be monitored in patients with diabetes.

It is prudent to routinely monitor the initial exercise sessions to assess cardiac responses. Individual clinical responses then would determine the need for monitoring in subsequent sessions. Center-based programs (26) are generally superior to home-based programs at improving distance walked and time to claudication pain at up to 6 months (2). A key advantage of a center-based program is that specific advice about exercise can be provided. Almost half of patients with intermittent claudication do not exercise, and lack of advice and supervision is cited as an important barrier to exercise (13). There is no evidence to support the efficacy of telling a patient to "go home and walk," which is the most typical exercise prescription for claudication offered by health care providers. Another advantage of a supervised program is that patients are often reluctant to push themselves during walking because of ischemic pain. Many patients need to be reassured that moderate pain in their legs is the stimulus for improvement and that the small risk of damage to their skeletal muscles is outweighed by the overall benefits of the exercise program. A supervised program ensures that patients receive a standardized exercise stimulus in a safe environment (23, 24, 26).

Although a supervised program is recommended, there is a role for a home-based program. In one study, successful outcomes such as increased walking time, improved functional ability, and enhanced quality of life were achieved among patients who continue to exercise an average of 48 months after completing a formal 12-week program (22). The attained benefits compare favorably with those of surgical interventions, without the risk of surgical complications. Still, only 44% of patients maintained an adequate level of exercise. There are too few studies to formulate specific recommendations regarding long-term efficacy and adherence when comparing home-based programs and center-based programs. The availability of center-based exercise programs specifically for patients is also limited. Fortunately, many cardiac rehabilitation exercise programs can accommodate patients with claudication, providing an environment conducive for the lifestyle change that underlies long-term compliance to exercise and risk factor modification. A CPT code (Current Procedural Terminology 93668) was published by the American Medical Association in January 2001. Despite the strong scientific basis for PAD rehabilitation, the mere existence of such a code has not yet resulted in widespread health care insurance payment for such services.

Comparisons With Exercise for Patients With Coronary Artery Disease

Coronary artery disease (CAD) and peripheral artery disease are manifestations of atherosclerosis, and many patients have both conditions. However, there are distinct differences in the approach to exercise training for PAD and CAD. Patients with PAD often remain at the same level of walking impairment for several years. Because the symptoms remain stable, the exercise goals are to relieve symptoms, reduce CAD risk factors, improve functional status, and increase walking ability. In contrast, patients with CAD typically have spontaneous recovery after a myocardial infarction, coronary artery bypass graft surgery, or percutaneous revascularization procedures. Cardiac rehabilitation exercise programs that begin soon after a cardiac event are focused on recovery from the acute event, avoiding deconditioning, improving cardiovascular and muscle fitness, and modifying risk factors. In many patients with CAD, there are few symptoms with exercise because of revascularization or cardiac medications. Another key difference is that patients with PAD need to walk at an intensity that produces a moderate degree of leg pain in order to gain benefit. In contrast, patients with CAD who experience chest pain and other ischemic symptoms need to stop their exercise or use nitroglycerine as appropriate. Although ischemia may also be a stimulus for structural and functional adaptations in the heart (21), cardiac ischemia markedly increases the risk of life-threatening arrhythmias and myocardial damage that may also affect the heart's pumping ability. For these reasons, chest pain is a contraindication to exercise training. These differences in the approach to the patient with PAD compared with patients with CAD are summarized in table 31.3.

Mechanisms for Benefit With Exercise Training

The beneficial effects of exercise for reducing symptoms of claudication may be explained by several mechanisms. These changes, which have been reviewed extensively elsewhere (7), include improvements in skeletal muscle metabolism, endothelial vasodilator function, blood viscosity, oxygen extraction by the working muscles, and inflammatory responses.

TABLE 31.3 Peripheral Artery Disease (PAD) Versus Coronary Artery Disease (CAD) Exercise Programs

PAD	CAD
Patients will often remain at the same level of functional ability for many years.	Patients typically have spontaneous recovery from an acute cardiac event.
Exercise goals are to relieve claudication symptoms, improve functional status, increase walking ability, and modify cardiac risk factors.	Early cardiac rehabilitation avoids deconditioning, improves recovery from an acute event, improves cardiovascular and muscle fitness, and modifies cardiac risk factors through lifestyle change.
Walking with leg pain is needed to stimulate beneficial adaptations in the leg muscles.	Chest pain and other myocardial ischemia symptoms are contraindications to exercise.

Exercise training also increases walking economy, which results from reductions in claudication pain leading to an improved walking gait. The improvement in biomechanical walking efficiency reduces the amount of oxygen required by the muscles at the same work rate after training. Mechanisms for which there is inconsistent and limited evidence to account for the substantial increases in function and reductions in symptoms with exercise training are increases in blood flow to the muscles through collateral blood vessels or a redistribution of blood away from inactive to active muscles (7).

Although not studied specifically, it would be expected that patients with claudication would also accrue cardiovascular and metabolic benefits by participation in a program of walking, especially if performed regularly. In patients with other manifestations of cardiovascular disease, regular exercise promotes moderate losses in body weight and reductions in abdominal obesity, decreases in blood pressure and serum triglycerides, increases in high-density lipoprotein cholesterol, and improvements in insulin sensitivity and glucose homeostasis.

Foot Care

Proper foot care is essential to reduce the risks of developing foot complications and limb loss. The combination of PAD and diabetes-related peripheral neuropathy, which is common in patients with PAD, deadens the sensation in the feet and leads to a high incidence of foot problems. These patients are prone to nonhealing blisters, wounds, and foot ulcers that can become infected; in severe PAD, gangrene can develop leading to amputation. Proper shoes and socks are required during exercise training sessions and for all other activities to protect the foot from pressure and shear stress. Keeping the feet clean will help to prevent soft tissue damage. Patients should be encouraged to inspect their feet daily because associated neuropathies will prevent them from feeling any sore or blisters. If foot ulcers are not healing, a patient should discontinue walking and may need complete bed rest. Patients need to trim their toenails carefully. Patients should see their physician or podiatrist if they experience discomfort or notice any wounds, blisters, or ulcers on their feet.

Summary

Exercise is an effective primary treatment for most patients with claudication, the key symptom of PAD. Studies have consistently shown that exercise training reduces claudication symptoms, improves quality of life, and increases walking ability. Along with exercise training, aggressive cardiovascular disease risk factor treatment is necessary, given that PAD markedly increases the risk of cardiovascular disease morbidity and mortality. An advantage of exercise training is that in addition to improving walking ability, it reduces blood pressure, improves lipid profile, reduces obesity, and enhances glycemic control in patients with concomitant diabetes. Supervised treadmill programs are most effective for increasing walking performance and decreasing claudication pain severity. Other forms of exercise like cycling and resistance training may improve cardiovascular health and increase muscle strength but are not a substitute for walking for specifically treating claudication. Despite its proven efficacy, exercise training has not been widely used as a primary therapeutic choice for PAD. Many patients and health care providers are unaware that exercise rehabilitation carries multiple benefits and can be a mainstay of therapy for most patients with claudication. Because patients need to walk with pain to gain benefit, many patients find it difficult to adhere to their exercise prescription, particularly when exercise is not supervised. A challenge for health professionals is to promote PAD awareness among health care providers and their patients and to develop programs that offer state-of-the-art PAD exercise rehabilitation services.

CHAPTER 32

Chronic Heart Failure

Steven J. Keteyian, PhD

Daniel E. Forman, MD

Heart failure (HF) is a complex clinical syndrome with an equally complex pathophysiology that has widespread impact on a variety of cells, tissues, organs, and organ systems. Whereas HF is commonly defined in terms of impaired heart pumping function (i.e., a heart that is unable to meet the body's needs with normal intracardiac chamber pressures), ultimately the impact of the disorder goes well beyond the heart. Systemic manifestations are an important part of HF pathophysiology, including a constellation of effects that are integral to notorious HF morbidity and mortality. In this chapter, we present an overview of the epidemiology, pathophysiology, and treatment of HF, emphasizing the systemic effects of the disease and the relevance of rehabilitation on this cardiac problem. We also describe the use of exercise training to modify HF-related cardiac and peripheral manifestations.

Epidemiology

Unlike other cardiovascular diseases such as acute myocardial infarction (MI), HF is increasing in the United States in terms of both prevalence and incidence. An estimated 5 million Americans suffer from HF, including more than 1 million people with New York Heart Association (NYHA) class III-IV symptoms (1). About 500,000 new cases occur each year, with the incidence rate for this disorder expected to increase over the next 30 years as the population ages and interventions for MI, sudden death, and other heart diseases enable

more adults to survive into their senior years. HF is the most common reason for hospitalizations in people 65 years of age and older and directly contributes to 250,000 deaths annually. The 5-year mortality rate for a person newly diagnosed with HF in the United States is 45% (23).

Beyond its mortality impact, HF is associated with devastating effects on quality of life, including diminished functional capacity as well as increased dyspnea, falls, frailty, and depression. The economic burden imposed by HF is staggering, totaling more than US$28 billion annually in the United States.

Pathophysiology

Whereas HF is often defined in terms of impaired heart pumping function, this definition falls short of describing the fundamentally systemic nature of the condition (19). Specifically, even though a reduced cardiac output is a key trigger, intrinsic cardiac decline leads to subsequent deterioration throughout the body (figure 32.1).

A wide range of circumstances can lead to the initial cardiac injury of HF. Among leading etiologies of systolic injury in the United States are MI and end-stage hypertension. Infection, toxins, and autoimmune injury

Address correspondence concerning this chapter to Steven J. Keteyian, 6525 Second Avenue, Detroit, MI 48202. E-mail: sketeyi1@hfhs.org

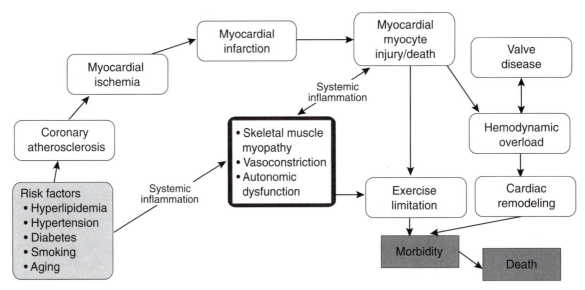

FIGURE 32.1 Central and peripheral physiologic abnormalities attributable to chronic heart failure due to systolic dysfunction.

are also common. Irrespective of etiology, once cardiac output declines, a generally homogeneous cascade of physiological sequelae ensues, with progressive impairment both in the heart and systemically.

Cardiac dilation is common as myocytes initially stretch to facilitate greater pumping efficiency. However, progressive heart dilation ultimately leads to worsening valvular regurgitation, arrhythmia, and further pumping deterioration.

Systemic effects of HF are even more complex. Neurohormonal responses include elevated levels of serum renin, angiotensin, and noradrenaline. Initially, these endogenous peptides provide benefit, augmenting intravascular volume (blood volume) and vascular tone (to compensate for low cardiac output) and improving cardiac inotropicity and lusitropicity (ventricular contraction and relaxation, respectively). Ultimately, however, these neurohormonal peptides accelerate damage. Systemic effects include skeletal muscle myocyte apoptosis, with weakening and inefficiency leading to functional limitations and dyspnea.

Impaired vasodilation leads to a greater likelihood of demand ischemia and high afterload stress. Fluid accumulations increase intracardiac pressures, which cause high cardiac work demands and added susceptibility to arrhythmias. More fundamentally, diminished cardiac output leads to a pervasive catabolic state. Endogenous noradrenaline and angiotensin II combine with tumor necrosis factor-α, interleukin-1β, and reduced insulin-like growth factor-1 to impose an elevated state of oxidation stress and progressively jeopardize cellular function and viability in the heart as well as in tissue beds throughout the body (26).

Signs and symptoms of HF vary depending on the phase of the disease course. Whereas intrinsic heart weakening may lead to changes in the cardiac exam with the new onset of a gallop or murmur, symptoms such as shortness of breath, fatigability, and functional limitation often have little correlation to pump function and relate more to systemic effects such as muscle wasting and increased vascular impedance. Thus, although the management of HF once focused exclusively on pump performance, HF is now considered a disorder whereby the peripheral effects of the disease are so debilitating that they warrant a treatment strategy that focuses on skeletal muscle development (17, 28).

Another dimension of complexity regarding HF is that HF can also occur in the context of preserved systolic heart function. In contrast to the common conception of HF as a weakly squeezing heart, so-called "HF with normal ejection fraction" identifies a heart that pumps adequately but cannot fill sufficiently to sustain normal cardiac output (i.e., diastolic impairment). Such a condition is especially common when a heart develops wall stiffening attributable to hypertension, ischemia, diabetes, or an infiltrative process that hinders ventricular filling. Coincident central vascular stiffening is also typical, which compounds ventricular afterload pressures and further impedes diastolic filling. In addition, disease- and age-related changes in myocyte mitochondrial function also bring about ventricular filling abnormalities (i.e., declining capacity to synthesize requisite fuel for cellular relaxation leads to impaired diastolic function and associated propensity to HF). HF with normal ejection fraction is especially common among older adults with hypertension or coronary heart disease, a population that is growing in prevalence as more adults survive into their senior years (32).

Diagnosis

This brief overview of the pathophysiology of HF is intended to convey the systemic intricacy of the disease and the challenge associated with developing a single diagnostic algorithm for a disease process that includes a wide range of signs and symptoms. Diagnostic criteria of HF are now based on a staged classification system (17):

- Stage A distinguishes people who are at risk for developing HF (i.e., those with risk factors such as hypertension, coronary artery disease, diabetes, or family history of cardiomyopathy) but still have normal cardiac anatomy and function.

- Stage B pertains to those who have structural heart disease but remain asymptomatic.

- Stage C refers to those who have structural disease and are intermittently symptomatic.

- Stage D refers to those who have structural heart disease, are symptomatic all the time, and require specialized interventions.

Not only do these diagnostic criteria extend HF diagnosis to a much larger group of adults, they also link risk with disease, thereby mandating therapy very early to interrupt an otherwise inexorable pathophysiological demise. Juxtaposed with the newer HF classification based on stages remains the familiar and often used NYHA functional classification system of HF. This index pertains to HF patients in stage C and D and provides a related measure of functional capacity, ranging from patients with structural heart disease and pumping abnormalities with no functional limitations or symptoms (NYHA class I) to those with severe functional limitations and marked symptoms even at rest (NYHA class IV).

Among the noninvasive tools that are often used to assess cardiac function are echocardiography and serum assessment of brain natriuretic peptide (BNP). Echocardiography provides a convenient, noninvasive means to safely view and quantify systolic and diastolic performance. More recently, technical enhancements have facilitated load-independent echocardiographic assessment of diastolic function using Doppler tissue imaging (18). This is quickly becoming a standard tool to recognize and treat HF in patients with a normal ejection fraction.

Serum BNP is a peptide that is synthesized in excess when a heart is stretched by mechanical and pressure overload. Elevated BNP (>100 pg/mL) can be used as a sensitive index of decompensated HF, even when other clinical signs are nebulous (25). Serum BNP can, for example, distinguish dyspnea from HF versus pulmonary disease, a particularly useful tool in patients whose physical examination is nonspecific (3) or in those people with poor echocardiographic images.

Despite their utility, neither echocardiography, BNP, nor other assessments of cardiac function quantify the full scope of HF as a disease that has both cardiac and systemic impact. However, assessment of exercise capacity stands out as the one important exception, whereby functional capacity is measured in terms of maximal oxygen consumption (peak $\dot{V}O_2$ or related measurements of breathing efficiency) (figure 32.2). Measuring $\dot{V}O_2$ during a cardiopulmonary test is one of the most reliable and reproducible means to assess integrated body function. For example, peak $\dot{V}O_2$ is routinely used as a key index to identify HF patients who are likely to benefit from heart transplant. Likewise, a cardiopulmonary exercise test can be used to assess the relative progression of HF or the benefits of therapy to mitigate such progression (7).

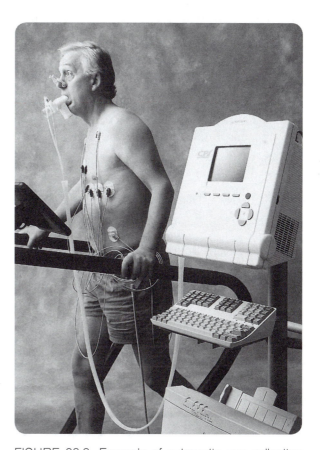

FIGURE 32.2 Example of automatic gas collection system to assess expired air during cardiopulmonary exercise testing.

Courtesy of Medical Graphics Corporation

Management

Whereas HF therapy once focused predominantly on pumping concerns, these goals are conspicuously inadequate for this complex disease process. Therapeutic objectives have shifted to prioritize pharmacological and nonpharmacological modalities that interrupt insidious HF pathophysiology and help reduce mortality. Among the top pharmacological priorities for medical management are angiotensin converting enzyme (ACE) inhibitors and β-adrenergic blocking agents (figure 32.3), both of which attenuate progression of asymptomatic disease and the harmful effects of advanced HF, intervene in the neurohormonal aspects of HF pathophysiology, and carry significant survival benefits. Similarly, aldosterone-blocking medications (e.g., spironolactone, eplerenone) have also been demonstrated to reduce mortality of HF patients, but only in those with more advanced disease. Other medications, including digoxin and thiazide diuretics (e.g., hydrochlorothiazide), loop diuretics (e.g., furosemide), and a more potent variant of thiazides called metolazone, are still often used for HF patients. However, their applications must be tailored to the symptoms and circumstances of each patient, because a standardized patient regimen does not exist. In addition, these agents do not confer life-prolonging benefits.

Recent therapeutic advances have emphasized the benefits of device therapy. Cardiac resynchronization therapy (biventricular pacing), implantable defibrillators, and combined technology devices have all been heavily emphasized in the literature (2, 6). Biventricular pacing is indicated for patients with low ejection fraction and widened QRS waveforms, but the benefits of this treatment to modify maladaptive ventricular remodeling and improve function and quality of life are leading to broader applications. The benefits of implantable defibrillators are well documented for patients with dilated hearts with low ejection fractions, particularly as a means to reduce mortality that results from the common occurrence of ventricular arrhythmias.

Surgical interventions that are already well proven to benefit selected patients with HF include revascularization for ischemic HF and repair of valvular flow abnormalities. Certainly, ischemic HF patients should be considered for revascularization unless there is specific reason to omit this therapy. Moreover, complete revascularization through surgery is often more beneficial than partial revascularization using percutaneous catheter techniques, particularly in context of low ejection fraction. Surgery also affords opportunity to repair valvular flow abnormalities. In addition to these treatments, patients with HF may benefit from exercise training (28).

Many prototypical HF symptoms relate to systemic abnormalities that accompany the disease, and regular rehabilitation can lead to clinical gains and systemic improvements, even when cardiac pumping dysfunction is irremediable.

Exercise Management

The systemic effect of regular exercise on so many tissues and organ systems makes exercise training uniquely qualified to affect this disorder. Specifically,

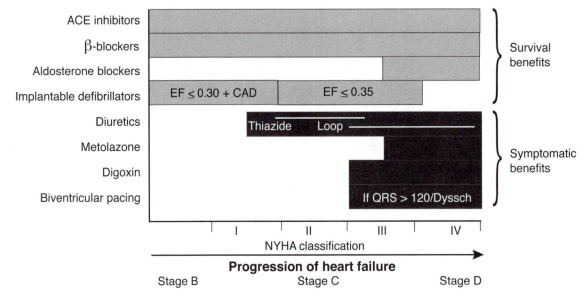

FIGURE 32.3 Device and pharmacotherapy of systolic heart failure. ACE = angiotensin-converting enzyme; EF = ejection fraction; CAD = coronary artery disease; NYHA = New York Heart Association.

regular exercise training mediates autonomic function, cardiac function, skeletal muscle histology and chemistry, immune function, and exercise tolerance (22). What is not adequately tested or clearly understood is to what extent, if any, exercise training improves clinical outcomes (i.e., survival and hospitalizations).

Fortunately, a multisite, randomized clinical trial is now underway to evaluate the clinical effectiveness of exercise training in patients with chronic HF. Called HF-ACTION (A Controlled Trial Investigating Outcomes of Exercise TraiNing), this trial is due to report its findings in 2008. HF-ACTION evaluates whether regular, supervised exercise that is followed by home-based exercise training influences clinical outcomes and quality of life and does so in a cost-effective manner.

Although one might think that the marked reductions in exercise tolerance common in HF and the systemic nature of the disorder would require alterations when prescribing exercise in these patients, major modification of the exercise prescription is rarely

the case. In fact, the prescription of exercise in these patients is more similar to that used in people with normal systolic function than it is different.

In the only consensus scientific statement on this topic to date, one is reminded that "agreement on a universal exercise prescription for this population does not exist" (28, p. 1219). However, many single-site clinical trials show generally similar benefits with relatively similar methods.

Concerning eligibility criteria, most prior trials involved NYHA class II or III patients and an ejection fraction less than 35%. And as of late, the percentage of patients in clinical exercise trials on ACE inhibitors and β-adrenergic blockade is increasing. Prior to exercise training, all sedentary patients with heart failure should be evaluated by a physician or physician extender to screen for any cardiac or noncardiac contraindications to exercise (see Relative and Absolute Contraindications to Exercise in Patients with Heart Failure below).

■ Relative and Absolute Contraindications to Exercise in Patients With Heart Failure

Relative contraindications

- 1.5 to 2.0 kg increase in body mass over previous 3 to 5 days
- Concurrent continuous or intermittent dobutamine therapy
- Abnormal increase or decrease of blood pressure with exercise
- New York Heart Association Functional class IV
- Complex ventricular arrhythmia at rest or appearing with exertion
- Supine resting heart rate ≥100 beats/min
- Preexisting comorbidity or behavior disorder
- Implantable cardiac defibrillator with heart rate limit set below the target heart rate for training
- Extension of myocardial infarction resulting in left ventricular dysfunction within the previous 4 weeks

Absolute contraindications

- Signs or symptoms of worsening or unstable heart failure over previous 2 to 4 days
- As defined by existing evidence-based guidelines, abnormal blood pressure, early ischemic changes, or unexpected life-threatening arrhythmia
- Uncontrolled metabolic disorder (e.g., hypothyroidism, diabetes)
- Acute systemic illness or fever
- Recent embolism or thrombophlebitis
- Active pericarditis or myocarditis
- Third-degree heart block without pacemaker
- Significant uncorrected valvular disease except mitral regurgitation attributable to HF-related left ventricular dilatation

Adapted, by permission, from J. Ehrman et al., 2003, *Clinical Exercise Physiology* (Champaign, IL: Human Kinetics), 271.

Table 32.1 summarizes the modality, frequency, intensity, and duration of exercise used in selected randomized trials conducted over the last 10 years. In reviewing these trials, one can summarize that the exercise prescription to improve peak $\dot{V}O_2$ (aerobic or cardiorespiratory fitness) is as follows: a gross motor activity such as walking or biking performed for 30 to 40 min on 3 to 5 days per week and at an intensity that falls near ventilatory anaerobic threshold or in the range of 60% to 75% of peak $\dot{V}O_2$ or heart rate reserve. This exercise guideline provides a target dose, in that it is sometimes prudent to start previously inactive patients at a lower work rate and in a supervised exercise setting. Some data now suggest that aerobic interval training is also very effective in reversing the exercise intolerance characteristic of patients with heart failure (31).

Although the majority of all trials conducted to date have used cardiorespiratory activities to improve function and exercise tolerance, some studies have investigated resistance training only and combined aerobic and resistance training regimens (9, 10, 29). These and

TABLE 32.1 Review of Selected Exercise Training Trials

Authors	Training intensity	Training duration, min	Training mode	Training frequency, days/week	Peak $\dot{V}O_2$, ml·kg^{-1}·min^{-1} (before/after)
Belardinelli et al. (4)	60% of peak $\dot{V}O_2$	40	Bike	2-3	T: 15.7/19.9 C: 15.2/16.0
Braith et al. (5)	40-70% of peak $\dot{V}O_2$	30-45	Walk	3	T: 12.8/12.0 C: 13.0/16.3
Curnier et al. (8)	HR at anaerobic threshold	30	Bike	5-6	+BB: 15.6/19.0* −BB: 13.8/16.2*
Forissier et al. (12)	HR at anaerobic threshold	30-70	Bike	7	+BB: 20.0/23.4 −BB: 18.1/21.2
Giannuzzi et al. (13)	60% of peak $\dot{V}O_2$	30-60	Bike, walk	3-7	T: 13.8/16.2 C: 13.8/13.7
Hambrecht et al. (16)	70% of peak $\dot{V}O_2$	≥40	Bike	7	T: 17.5/23.3 C: 17.9/17.9
Keteyian et al. (20)	70-80% of peak $\dot{V}O_2$	33	Bike, walk, row	3	T: 16.1/18.4 C: 14.6/15.3
Keteyian et al. (21)	70-80% of peak $\dot{V}O_2$	30	Bike, walk, row	3	T: 16.3/18.6 C: —/—
Linke et al. (24)	70% of peak $\dot{V}O_2$	60	Bike ergometer	6	T: 16.0/19.4 C: 16.9/16.3
McKelvie et al. (27)	60-70% peak HR	30	Bike, arm ergometer, resistance training	3	T: 13.8/15.7 C: 14.2/14.5
Roveda et al. (30)	HR at anaerobic threshold	25-40	Bike	3	T: 14.8/20.6 C: 16.6/17.5

HR = heart rate; $\dot{V}O_2$ = volume of oxygen consumed; T = treatment, before/after training; C = control, before/after training; +BB and −BB = both groups underwent exercise training, taking and not taking a β-adrenergic blocking agent, respectively.

*$\dot{V}O_2$ at ventilatory threshold before and after exercise training (peak $\dot{V}O_2$ not reported).

other similar trials indicate that lift intensity should start at 50% to 60% of 1RM, with the patient starting with one set of 10 to 12 repetitions and progressing to one set of 15 repetitions. The specific exercises should address the individual needs of the patient but will likely include all of the major muscle groups. As patients improve, lift load should be increased 5% to 10%.

Exercise and Rehabilitation Outcomes

Randomized controlled trials using aerobic exercise in patients with HF attributable to systolic dysfunction indicate that exercise capacity, as measured by peak $\dot{V}O_2$, improves 15% to 25% (table 32.1). However, most of these trials were performed with fewer than 50% of the subjects taking a β-adrenergic blocking agent. That said, two of the trials in table 32.1 are randomized trials in which patients were taking a β-adrenergic blocking agent (8, 12). In each of these two trials, the increase in $\dot{V}O_2$ was quite similar to the increase in $\dot{V}O_2$ observed in patients not taking a similar agent. The mechanisms responsible for the increases in exercise capacity are many, given that abnormalities in central transport, nutritive blood flow to the active skeletal muscles, and skeletal muscle function all contribute to exercise intolerance.

Health and physiologic improvements with exercise include less chronotropic incompetence (for patients not taking β-blockers) (20); modest improvements (8-15%) in stroke volume and cardiac output (figure 32.4) (15); slight improvement in left ventricular ejection fraction and left ventricular end-diastolic size (figure 32.5) (13); partial normalization of endothelial function (24); partial reversal of abnormalities in sympathetic function (23); partial reversal of abnormalities in skeletal muscle including increases in mitochondrial volume density, the enzymes involved with aerobic metabolism, and the percentage of myosin heavy chain I isoforms (16, 21); muscle-specific improvement in inflammatory state (14); improvements in ventilatory efficiency; and improved quality of life. Increases in skeletal muscle strength and endurance also occur when moderate and progressive resistance training are part of the treatment plan (9, 10, 29).

As mentioned, no large-scale trials have evaluated safety and clinical outcomes. Belardinelli and colleagues (4) conducted a 1-year trial involving 99 subjects and showed that 14 months of exercise training lowered subsequent all-cause cardiac event rate (relative risk = 0.33) (figure 32.6). A meta-analysis (11) showed similar findings; whereas the 12-month EXERT trial showed no difference (27). Given the widespread and increas-

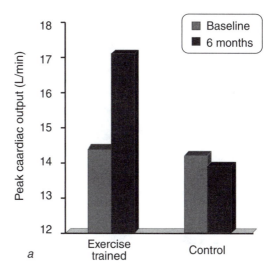

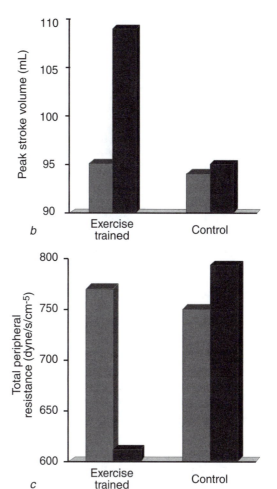

FIGURE 32.4 *(a)* Cardiac output, *(b)* stroke volume, and *(c)* total systemic peripheral resistance at baseline and 6 months in exercise trained subjects and controls. Adapted from Hambrecht et al. 2000.

ing prevalence of HF and the potential for exercise to affect this disorder, the results of the HF-ACTION trial are important.

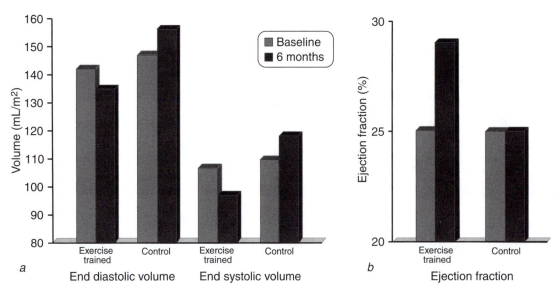

FIGURE 32.5 Change in left ventricular function and remodeling in patients with HF undergoing exercise training and controls. Adapted from Giannuzzi et al. 2003.

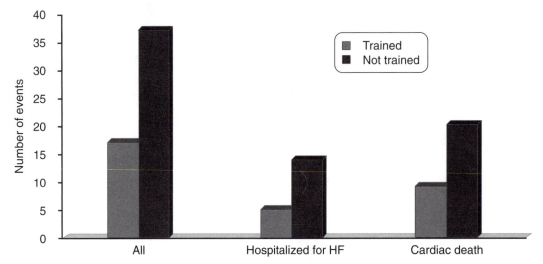

FIGURE 32.6 Cardiac events according to study group (trained, n = 50; not trained, n = 49) and type of event. Adapted from Belardinelli et al. (4).

Summary

Just 15 to 20 years ago, patients with chronic heart failure were told by their doctor to avoid exercise or moderate to vigorous exertion for fear that the exercise itself might worsen heart function and disease-related morbidity. However, during this same period dozens of well-conducted single-site controlled exercise trials demonstrated that regular moderate exercise not only does not worsen the disease state but indeed can reverse exercise intolerance, improve the pathophysiology, and possibly improve clinical outcomes and quality of life. More research is needed in these and other areas before exercise training is incorporated into the future revisions of evidence-based clinical guidelines directed at optimizing the care of patients with chronic heart failure.

CHAPTER 33

Cardiac Transplant

Ray W. Squires, PhD

Richard J. Rodeheffer, MD

The first successful human heart transplant was performed by Christian Barnard in Cape Town, South Africa, in 1967 (1). Although the patient lived only 18 days, the resulting publicity and enthusiasm spurred a number of surgical centers to perform the operation. Long-term survival was poor, and the procedure did not enjoy widespread application during the 1960s and 1970s. Developments at Stanford University, including improved techniques for preservation of the donor organ, the transvenous right ventricular endomyocardial biopsy technique for early detection of acute rejection, a grading scale for rejection, and the introduction of the powerful immunosuppressant cyclosporine in the 1980s, resulted in marked improvement in survival (29). These important advances, and eventual insurance funding of the operation and aftercare in the United States, made the procedure an attractive treatment for patients with terminal heart failure.

The Registry of the International Society for Heart and Lung Transplantation's 2004 report contained 66,353 heart transplantations and 3,049 heart-lung transplantations performed worldwide over the years (7). There are approximately 140 heart transplant centers in the United States and 10 in Canada. The age range of heart transplant recipients is from newborn to the eighth decade of life. For adults, the average age at transplant is 51 ± 12 years. The average age of the donors is 31 ± 13 years.

Approximately 90% of patients who require transplantation suffer from coronary heart disease (ischemic left ventricular dysfunction, 45%) or idiopathic dilated cardiomyopathy (46%) (38). Additional diseases, conditions, and treatments resulting in terminal heart failure include hypertension, valvular heart disease, myocarditis, alcohol abuse, chemotherapy, acquired immunodeficiency syndrome, complex congenital heart disease, infiltrative diseases of the myocardium (amyloidosis, hemachromatosis), and peripartum (31). Almost 70% of transplant candidates require pre-transplant hospitalization, 47% on inotropic support and 18% with ventricular assist devices (38).

The waiting time for an organ depends on blood type and the degree of medical urgency. Unfortunately, the number of potential candidates for heart transplantation greatly exceeds the available supply of donor organs.

Orthotopic transplantation is the usual surgical technique, which involves excision of the recipient's

Correspondence concerning this chapter should be addressed to Ray W. Squires, Division of Cardiovascular Diseases and Internal Medicine, Mayo Clinic, 200 First Street SW, Rochester, MN 55905. E-mail: squires.ray@mayo.edu diseased heart and anastomosis of the donor heart to the great vessels and atria of the recipient (31). Rarely, in the circumstances of excessive pulmonary vascular resistance with severe pulmonary hypertension or a marked donor–recipient body weight mismatch, a heterotopic or "piggyback" transplant may be used. With this procedure, the recipient's diseased heart is left intact and the donor heart is sewn in parallel to the existing heart. This procedure results in the unique electrocardiographic appearance of two separate QRS complexes on the electrocardiogram.

For patients with end-stage heart failure, cardiac transplantation is the accepted form of definitive treatment, carrying 1-year and 5-year survival rates of approximately 83% and 68%, respectively (38). The annual mortality through 14 years of follow-up is 4% per year. Early mortality (first year after transplantation) is most commonly attributable to graft failure, acute rejection, and infection. Late mortality (5 or more years after transplant) is usually a result of cardiac allograft vasculopathy, malignancy, or infection.

The goals of cardiac transplantation are improved survival, reduced symptoms, and increased exercise capacity. After recovery from surgery, most patients report a reasonably favorable quality of life (9). Many patients return to work, school, or their usual avocational activities, although exercise capacity generally remains below average, as discussed later in the chapter. However, because of immunosuppressant medications and other transplant-related factors, patients are prone to develop serious medical problems. Table 33.1 lists the prevalence of common medical problems observed in cardiac transplant recipients.

TABLE 33.1   Cumulative Prevalence of Medical Problems in Survivors Within 7 Years of Cardiac Transplantation

Condition	Prevalence, %
Hypertension	97
Hyperlipidemia	89
Allograft vasculopathy	43
Renal dysfunction	36
Diabetes mellitus	35
Malignancy	24

Data from Taylor et al. 2003.

Rejection

Rejection of the transplanted heart is a major cause of hospitalization and death in the first year after surgery (20). There are four types of rejection: hyperacute, acute cellular, acute humoral (vascular), and chronic.

Hyperacute rejection occurs shortly after surgery and is caused by preformed antibodies to the donor heart (20). This type of rejection results in acute inflammatory infiltration with vessel necrosis of the transplanted organ and patient death. Fortunately, with immunologic matching of donor and recipient, hyperacute rejection is rare.

Acute cellular rejection is most common during the first 6 months after transplantation and is attributable to T-lymphocyte and macrophage infiltration of the myocardium (20). The diagnosis is made using routine, periodic transvenous endomyocardial biopsy of the right ventricle. If acute cellular rejection is not treated promptly, myocardial injury and necrosis may occur. Based on tissue sample analysis, acute cellular rejection is graded from mild to severe, as shown in table 33.2. The treatment of acute cellular rejection involves additional immunosuppressants and may require hospitalization. Severe acute rejection, resulting in substantial myocyte necrosis and fibrosis, may produce left ventricular dysfunction and heart failure (31).

Acute humoral (vascular) rejection occurs within days to weeks of transplantation and is relatively rare (20). Initiated by antibodies, the process may impair coronary vasodilatory reserve, resulting in ventricular dysfunction. Diagnosis is made by identifying immunoglobulins or complement in the vessels of the graft using biopsy material.

Chronic rejection, also called cardiac allograft vasculopathy or accelerated graft coronary artery disease, occurs months to years after transplantation (20). Chronic rejection is the major limiting factor in long-term survival after cardiac transplantation. Cardiac allograft vasculopathy is present in 43% of heart transplant recipients at 7 years (38). The disease is an unusually accelerated form of coronary disease affecting epicardial and intramyocardial coronary arteries and veins (39). The pathophysiology is incompletely understood but is thought to be associated with repetitive immunologic endothelial injury, ischemia–perfusion injury, viral infection, immunosuppressant medications, and traditional coronary risk factors, such as dyslipidemia, insulin resistance, and hypertension. The lesions usually diffusely involve the entire vessel, although focal obstructive lesions are sometimes seen. This disease process occurs in pediatric and adult recipients with equal regularity. Annual coronary angiography

TABLE 33.2 Standardized Cardiac Biopsy Acute Rejection Grading Scale

Grade	Findings
0	No rejection
1	Mild rejection
1A	Focal infiltrate without necrosis
1B	Diffuse, sparse infiltrate, no necrosis
2	Moderate rejection, one focus with aggressive infiltration or myocyte damage
3	Moderate rejection
3A	Multifocal aggressive infiltrates or myocyte damage
3B	Diffuse inflammatory process with necrosis
4	Severe rejection, diffuse aggressive polymorphous infiltrates with necrosis

Adapted, by permission, from R.W. Squires, 1990, "Cardiac rehabilitation issues for heart transplantation patients," *Journal of Cardiopulmonary Rehabilitation* 10:159-168.

is performed in most patients to detect the disease. Because of the diffuse nature of the typical lesions, retransplantation is the most common treatment. In patients with discrete, focal lesions, revascularization, either catheter-based or coronary bypass graft surgery, may be effective.

Medications

Cardiac transplant recipients require unique medications to tolerate the donor organ. Immunosuppressants, hydroxymethylglutaryl coenzyme A reductase inhibitors, and fibric acid derivatives are the common types of medications used in transplant patients.

Immunosuppressants

Immunosuppressant medications are given to prevent acute rejection of the donor heart (31). Maintenance drugs generally include combination therapy with a calcineurin inhibitor (cyclosporine or tacrolimus), an antiproliferative agent (azathioprine or mycophenolate mofetil), and a steroid (prednisone) (20). These powerful drugs enable the patient to tolerate the donor heart but carry several common side effects. For example, cyclosporine may result in renal dysfunction, has general vasopressor effects, and may cause skeletal muscle cramping. Prednisone, in the dose range used in transplantation, is particularly bothersome. It alters body fat distribution with resultant truncal obesity and a "moon-faced" appearance for many patients. Prednisone may also cause mood swings as well as skeletal muscle atrophy and weakness, osteoporosis, and dyslipidemia. During the first 1 to 2 years after transplantation, an attempt is usually made to taper and stop prednisone. Table 33.3 lists the common immunosuppressants and their side effects.

TABLE 33.3 Common Immunosuppressant Drugs and Associated Side Effects

Drug (brand name)	Potential common side effects
Cyclosporine (Gengraf, Neoral, Sandimmune)	Renal dysfunction, tremor, hypertension, hirsutism, gum hyperplasia, muscle cramps, acne
Azathioprine (Imuran)	Nausea and vomiting, leukopenia, thrombocytopenia, anemia
Prednisone	Muscle atrophy and weakness, hypertension, fluid retention, osteoporosis, asceptic necrosis of bone, "moon-face" appearance, truncal obesity, increased insulin resistance, cataracts, glaucoma, mood swings, personality change, insomnia, peptic ulcer disease
Tacrolimus (Prograf)	Tremor, headache, diarrhea, hypertension, nausea, renal dysfunction
Mycophenolate mofetil (Cellcept)	Diarrhea, leukopenia, sepsis, vomiting, infection, edema

Hydroxymethylglutaryl Coenzyme A Reductase Inhibitors (Statins) and Fibric Acid Derivatives

Statin medications (such as pravastatin and simvastatin) and fibric acid derivatives (such as gemfibrozil) may slow progression of accelerated graft coronary disease and improve survival (36, 40). In addition, statins have been shown to reduce the incidence of acute rejection and improve left ventricular function (10, 41). These benefits appear to be independent of these drugs' effects in improving the blood lipid profile.

Common Nonrejection Medical Problems

Unfortunately, many potential nonrejection medical conditions may affect cardiac transplant recipients. The following are the most frequent types of problems encountered by these patients.

■ *Infection and malignancy.* Immunosuppressed transplant recipients are at a higher risk of opportunistic infections and malignancy than the general population of patients with cardiovascular diseases. During the first several weeks after surgery, pulmonary bacterial infections are common (21). Late after transplantation, viral, bacterial, and fungal infections pose a threat. Special precautions should be taken to minimize the chances of exposure to persons with active infections. Patients are encouraged to wear a surgical mask and gloves as an infection barrier in public places, particularly during the first 3 months after surgery. Malignancy risk is substantial for transplant patients. At 7 years after surgery, the incidence of malignancy (primarily skin cancers) is 24% (38).

■ *Hypertension.* Hypertension is common after transplantation, affecting ≥95% of patients at 7 years (38). The extremely high prevalence is thought to be attributable to the use of calcineurin inhibitors and their adverse affects on renal function (21). Use of combination antihypertensive drug therapy is often required. Blood pressure after transplantation is usually sensitive to the dietary sodium load.

■ *Obesity.* Weight gain and obesity after cardiac transplantation are common. In a cohort of 95 patients at our institution, body mass index (BMI) averaged 28 ± 1 kg/m² at the time of surgery (19). The average increase in BMI and body weight by the first anniversary after transplantation was 2.1 ± 3.6 kg/m² and 6.3 ± 8.7 kg, respectively. Corticosteroid use plays a major role in posttransplant weight gain.

■ *Dyslipidemia.* Blood lipid abnormalities after cardiac transplantation are almost as universal as is hypertension (19). Immunosuppressants, diuretics prescribed for the treatment of hypertension, and renal insufficiency contribute to the problem. Statin medications are effective in treating dyslipidemia in these patients, although the risk of rhabdomyolysis is increased with concurrent statin and calcineurin inhibitor use.

■ *Diabetes.* Diabetes is common after transplant and is present in 35% of patients at 7 years (38). Pretransplant diabetes, glucocorticoid and calcineurin inhibitor use, and obesity contribute to the high prevalence of the disease (21). Diabetes is associated with a poorer long-term survival in cardiac transplant recipients.

■ *Chronic renal insufficiency.* Renal insufficiency, defined as creatinine levels >2 mg/dL, is a common side effect of calcineurin inhibitors (21). Fortunately, less than 10% of transplant recipients develop end-stage renal disease.

■ *Osteoporosis.* Advanced heart failure is associated with osteopenia and osteoporosis before transplantation. Glucocorticoid use after transplantation results in additional loss of bone mineral. Osteoporosis resulting in vertebral fractures is common in heart transplant recipients, affecting up to 30% of patients (21).

■ *Depression.* Depression has been reported in approximately 25% of heart transplant recipients at 1 to 3 years after surgery (21). Therefore, many of these patients take antidepressant medications.

Psychological Factors

The psychological response to the transplant process is understandably intense for most patients (16). During the period of waiting for the operation after acceptance as a transplant candidate, emotions range from relief and happiness to anxiety (indefinite waiting time, lack of absolute assurance that the transplant will occur) and thoughts of death. Patients who require continuous hospitalization while waiting for an organ may find the environment supportive or merely tedious and boring. Immediately after transplantation, patients are usually relieved at the prospects of a longer, higher-quality life.

As the period of convalescence continues, patients must adjust to the tedium of medical appointments and procedures. As previously discussed, the immunosuppressant prednisone may cause mood swings and personality change. The first episode of acute rejection may heighten feelings of anxiety and transient depression. As the recovery from surgery progresses and the degree of medical surveillance decreases, patients generally shift their attention from transplant-related activities to becoming more independent, assuming family roles, and resuming occupational and avocational pursuits. The adjustment to life after transplantation requires months, and the 1-year anniversary is an important milestone in this process. Most patients are able to return to productive and meaningful lives.

Responses to Exercise

The responses of heart transplant recipients to acute exercise are unique and are related, in part, to the following factors (23, 31):

- With harvesting of the donor organ, the transplanted heart is surgically denervated and receives no direct efferent input from the autonomic nervous system and provides no direct afferent signals to the central nervous system. Months after transplantation, some patients demonstrate signs of partial cardiac reinnervation. This is discussed later in this chapter.

- During organ harvesting and with transplantation, the donor heart has experienced ischemic time and reperfusion.

- There is no intact pericardium.

- Diastolic dysfunction (elevated filling pressures at rest and with exercise) is common. Reasons for abnormal diastolic function include hypertension (common after transplant), acute rejection episodes resulting in myocardial scarring and fibrosis, and allograft vasculopathy.

- Abnormal skeletal muscle histology and energy metabolism, developed during the course of chronic heart failure, may continue after transplantation.

- Peripheral and coronary vasodilatory capacity may be impaired, attributable, in part, to endothelial dysfunction.

Heart Rate and Exercise

Because the donor heart loses parasympathetic innervation with transplantation, heart rate at rest is elevated, at approximately 95 to 115 beats/min, and represents the inherent rate of depolarization of the sinoatrial node (32). With graded exercise, the heart rate typically does not increase during the first several minutes (delayed increase), which is followed by a gradual increase with peak heart rates slightly lower than normal (approximately 150 beats/min) attributable to sympathetic nervous system denervation. Many patients achieve their highest exercise heart rate during the first few minutes of recovery from exercise, rather than at the point of maximal exercise intensity. Heart rate may remain near peak values for several minutes during recovery before gradually returning to resting levels (delayed decrease). The chronotropic reserve (the difference between the maximal and resting heart rates) is less than normal. Regulation of heart rate during exercise is dependent on circulating catecholamines. Figure 33.1 shows the heart rate response to graded exercise of the same patient 1 year before and 3 months after orthotopic transplantation.

With orthotopic cardiac transplantation, it is possible that the sinoatrial (SA) node of the recipient's heart is left intact. The depolarization wave from the SA node generally does not cross the suture line in the right atrium, but the ECG may show two distinct p waves (one from the recipient and one from the donor SA nodes).

Blood, Intracardiac, and Vascular Pressures

Blood pressure at rest is mildly elevated in heart transplant patients, even though most patients receive antihypertensive medications. During exercise, blood pressure generally increases appropriately, although peak exercise blood pressure is slightly lower than expected for normal persons (14). Vascular resistance is elevated, as are intracardiac and pulmonary vascular pressures (particularly right-sided pressures) (11).

Left Ventricular Function

For most heart transplant patients, left ventricular ejection fraction is normal at rest and during exercise (11). However, as mentioned previously, left ventricular diastolic function is often impaired, as evidenced by an elevated filling pressure for a given end-diastolic volume. This impairment results in a below-normal increase in stroke volume during exercise. The impaired increase in stroke volume, coupled with the below-normal heart rate reserve, results in an impaired exercise cardiac output.

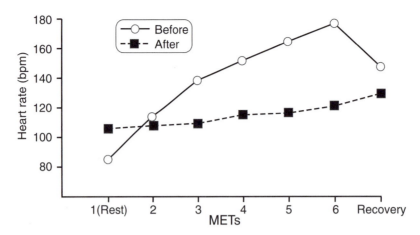

FIGURE 33.1 Heart rates measured during graded exercise in the same patient 1 year before and 3 months after orthotopic cardiac transplantation. Note the elevated resting heart rate and the delayed increase in heart rate during exercise after transplantation consistent with complete denervation. METs = metabolic equivalents.

Adapted, by permission, from R.W. Squires, 1990, "Cardiac rehabilitation issues for heart transplantation patients," *Journal of Cardiopulmonary Rehabilitation* 10:159-168.

Exercise Cardiac Output

With the onset of exercise, cardiac output in transplant recipients with complete cardiac denervation increases attributable to augmentation of stroke volume via the Frank–Starling mechanism. Later, increased heart rate also contributes to augmentation of cardiac output (28). Left ventricular end-diastolic volume index increases to a greater extent, relative to controls, during exercise in transplant patients and results in an enhanced Frank–Starling effect. However, at rest and during exercise, the cardiac index is lower for transplant recipients than for normal persons.

Skeletal Muscle Structure and Biochemistry

During the clinical course of chronic heart failure, several skeletal muscle structural and biochemical abnormalities develop:

- Reduced aerobic metabolic enzyme activity
- Lower capillary density
- Endothelial dysfunction with impaired vasodilation during exercise
- Conversion of some slow-twitch motor units to fast-twitch motor units with greater reliance on anaerobic than aerobic energy production

These abnormalities generally persist after transplantation, with partial improvement after several months for some patients (17, 37).

Pulmonary Function and Arterial Oxygenation

The efficiency of pulmonary ventilation during exercise is below normal during at least the first several months after transplantation, illustrated by an elevation in the ratio of minute ventilation to carbon dioxide production (the ventilatory equivalent for CO_2, $\dot{V}_E/VCO_2$) (31). This excess ventilation results in a heightened sense of shortness of breath during exercise. The normal increase in tidal volume during exercise is blunted, probably as a result of respiratory muscle weakness, deconditioning, and the effects of corticosteroid medications (3). Alveolar gas diffusion impairment is present in approximately 40% of patients. However, arterial oxygen saturation at rest and during exercise is normal for most patients (34). Azathioprine may cause anemia in some patients, resulting in a reduced arterial oxygen content (31).

Oxygen Extraction by Exercising Skeletal Muscle

Extraction of oxygen from the arterial blood by metabolically active body tissues, as indicated by the arterial–mixed venous oxygen difference, is normal at rest after transplantation. However, during exercise the arterial–mixed venous oxygen difference does not increase in a normal manner and reflects abnormalities with both the delivery of capillary blood to the exercising skeletal muscle and impairment of the oxidative capacity of the muscle (11).

Oxygen Uptake Kinetics, Peak Exercise $\dot{V}O_2$

With the onset of exercise, the rate of increase in $\dot{V}O_2$ (oxygen uptake kinetics) is slower than normal as a result of both an impaired increase in cardiac output and a diminished oxidative capacity of the skeletal muscle (reduced arterial–mixed venous oxygen difference) (25). Oxygen uptake is generally lower for a given cycle ergometer power output during graded exercise testing after transplantation compared with controls, consistent with slower $\dot{V}O_2$ kinetics.

Because of the dual abnormalities of an impaired exercise cardiac output and a reduced arterial–mixed venous oxygen difference described above, peak exercise oxygen uptake (peak $\dot{V}O_2$) is usually below normal for transplant patients. In a series of 95 patients with a mean age of 49 years who performed a cardiopulmonary exercise test approximately 1 year after transplantation, the mean peak $\dot{V}O_2$ was 20 ml·kg^{-1}·min^{-1} (62% of age- and gender-predicted value) (26). Marked variability in response was evident, with a range for peak $\dot{V}O_2$ of 11 to 38 ml·kg^{-1}·min^{-1} (39-110% of age- and gender-predicted value). Selected, highly trained transplant patients may achieve even higher values:

- Mean peak $\dot{V}O_2$ of 40 ml·kg^{-1}·min^{-1} in 14 men (mean age 43 years) with highest value of 54 ml·kg^{-1}·min^{-1} (27)
- Mean peak $\dot{V}O_2$ of 45 ml·kg^{-1}·min^{-1} in 12 men (mean age 47 years) (28)

There are additional, interesting abnormal exercise physiology findings in cardiac transplant recipients. The most common abnormalities include these:

- Increased resting heart rate
- Delayed heart rate increase at onset of exercise
- Blunted maximal heart rate
- Delayed return of heart rate to resting level after cessation of exercise
- Reduced heart rate reserve
- Increased exercise left ventricular end-diastolic pressure (diastolic dysfunction)
- Increased exercise pulmonary artery pressure, pulmonary capillary wedge pressure, right atrial pressure
- Increased left ventricular end-systolic and end-diastolic volume indexes
- Impaired increase in stroke volume during exercise

- Reduced exercise cardiac output
- Decreased exercise arterial–mixed venous oxygen difference
- Slowed oxygen uptake kinetics during exercise
- Decreased maximal oxygen uptake
- Reduced maximal power output during exercise testing
- Decreased ventilatory anaerobic threshold
- Increased exercise ventilatory equivalents for oxygen and carbon dioxide

Partial Cardiac Reinnervation

Occasionally, a heart transplant patient with graft vessel disease resulting in myocardial ischemia will report typical anginal symptoms, suggesting at least partial afferent cardiac reinnervation (13). It also appears that partial cardiac sympathetic efferent reinnervation occurs in many patients during the first several months to years after surgery. The evidence for this statement is based on neurochemical evaluation of autonomic nervous system activity in the heart and the observation of improved responsiveness of the heart rate during exercise (13).

The heart rate reserve (also called chronotropic response), defined as the difference between the heart rate at rest and the highest value during maximal exercise, increases during the first 6 weeks after surgery in many patients. In a subset of patients, the heart rate reserve increases further over the next 6 to 12 months. A more rapid decline in heart rate from peak exercise to baseline is observed in some patients at 1 to 2 years after transplantation.

Heart rate responsiveness to maximal graded exercise was assessed in a group of 95 transplant recipients at 1 year after surgery (35). Partial normalization of the heart rate response to exercise was defined as an increase in heart rate for each minute of graded exercise, maximal heart rate occurring at peak exercise, and a decrease in heart rate during each minute of recovery. By this definition, 32 subjects (33.7%) exhibited partial normalization of the heart rate response. Maximal heart rate was higher (147 vs. 134 beats/min, $p < .008$) and exercise test duration was longer (8.2 vs. 7.2 min, $p < .05$), although peak $\dot{V}O_2$ was similar (20.9 vs. 19.4 ml·kg^{-1}·min^{-1}, p not significant). Figure 33.2 shows the heart rate responses to graded exercise for the same patient at 3 and 12 months after transplantation. Note the typical denervated response at 3 months and the partially normalized response at 12 months.

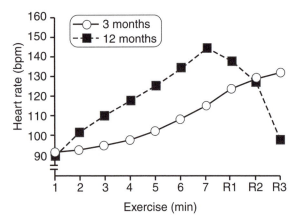

FIGURE 33.2 Heart rate responses to graded exercise in the same patient at 3 months and 12 months after cardiac transplantation demonstrating both denervation (at 3 months) and partial reinnervation (at 12 months). R1 = minute one of recovery after exercise; R2 = minute two of recovery after exercise; R3 = minute three of recovery after exercise.

Reprinted, by permission, from R.W. Squires, 2002, "Partial normalization of the heart rate response to exercise after cardiac transplantation: Frequency and relationship to exercise capacity," *Mayo Clinic Proceedings* 77:1295-1300.

Graded Exercise Testing

Exercise testing after cardiac transplantation is helpful in determining the exercise capacity, prescribing exercise training, and counseling patients regarding the timing of return to work or school or resumption of avocational pursuits. The ECG of transplant recipients commonly demonstrates right bundle-branch block and nonspecific repolarization abnormalities. The sensitivity of the exercise ECG in detecting the presence of accelerated graft coronary disease is poor (<25%) unless combined with myocardial imaging (5).

Because of the healing and recovery process after surgery and the usual deconditioned state prior to surgery, it is best to wait 6 to 8 weeks after surgery before performing graded exercise testing to maximal effort. For patients with more complicated postoperative courses, an even longer period of recovery is recommended before performance of an exercise test.

Treadmill or cycle ergometer protocols, with continuous exercise (2 or 3 min stages), or ramp tests may be used. The initial exercise intensity should be approximately 2 METs, with 1 to 2 MET increments in intensity per stage (5). Continuous multilead ECG monitoring with blood pressure measurement and Borg perceived exertion ratings for each stage is recommended. For precise determination of aerobic capacity and the ventilatory anaerobic threshold, direct measurement of $\dot{V}O_2$ and associated variables is highly desirable. The end points of the graded exercise test should be maximal effort (symptom-limited maximum) or standard signs of exertional intolerance (6).

In our laboratory, we prefer to use the treadmill, with a beginning speed of 2.0 mph at 0% grade. We use 2 min stages with a 1 to 2 MET increase in intensity per stage and an active recovery period of 3 min duration. For a group of 17 cardiac transplant recipients who participated in our supervised, 3 session/week exercise program of 6 to 8 weeks duration and underwent graded treadmill exercise testing at the end of the program (less than 3 months after surgery), the following responses (means ± SD) were reported (4):

■ Resting heart rate: 101 ± 12 beats/min

■ Resting systolic/diastolic blood pressure: 126 ± 8/86 ± 8 mmHg

■ Exercise test duration: 7.5 ± 1.1 min

■ Peak exercise heart rate: 132 ± 24 beats/min

■ Peak $\dot{V}O_2$: 19 ± 4 ml·kg^{-1}·min^{-1}

Responses to Exercise Training

Cardiac transplant recipients are excellent candidates for progressive exercise training for several reasons:

■ Pretransplant syndrome of chronic heart failure with poor exercise capacity attributable to central and peripheral circulatory abnormalities as well as skeletal muscle pathology

■ Deconditioning and the healing process with open-heart surgery similar to that observed with coronary or valvular surgery

■ Posttransplant use of corticosteroid medications with resultant skeletal muscle atrophy and weakness

Aerobic Exercise Training

The literature contains several reports demonstrating the benefits of aerobic exercise training for patients after cardiac transplantation (12, 15, 26, 33). Transplant recipients generally respond to training in a similar fashion to other cardiac patients. Peak $\dot{V}O_2$ improves by an average of 24% after 2 to 6 months of training. Exercise training improves mitochondrial oxidative capacity but apparently does not increase skeletal muscle capillary density as it does in healthy subjects (18). Potential additional benefits of regular exercise for transplant recipients include the following:

- Improved submaximal exercise endurance
- Increased peak treadmill exercise workload or peak cycle power output
- Increased maximal heart rate
- Decreased exercise heart rate at the same absolute submaximal workload
- Increased ventilatory (anaerobic) threshold
- Decreased submaximal exercise minute ventilation
- Reduced exercise ventilatory equivalent for CO_2
- Lessened symptoms of fatigue and dyspnea
- Reduced rest and submaximal exercise systolic and diastolic blood pressure
- Decreased peak exercise diastolic blood pressure
- Reduced submaximal exercise ratings of perceived exertion
- Improved psychosocial function
- Increased lean body mass
- Reduced body fat mass
- Increased bone mineral content

The first study of exercise training after cardiac transplantation was published in 1983 and included only two subjects in a case presentation format (33). After a 6-week period of training, ratings of perceived exertion and systolic blood pressure were consistently lower for all submaximal exercise intensities as evidenced by pre- and posttraining graded exercise test results.

Early investigations were limited to fewer than 20 subjects. The first large study was that of Niset and colleagues in 1988 (26), who studied 62 patients after orthotopic transplantation at approximately 1 month after surgery and again at the 1-year anniversary. Patients were instructed in exercise training principles and were started in a supervised program. No control group was used. A precise description of the exercise prescriptions and patient compliance to the program was not provided. Directly measured peak $\dot{V}O_2$ increased by 33% ($p < .01$).

In 1988, Kavanagh and associates (12) reported the results of a 16-month exercise training program in 36 transplant recipients (no control group). Exercise training (walk–jog) began approximately 7 months after surgery and was carefully supervised. Patients demonstrated many benefits after training, including an average 27% increase in peak $\dot{V}O_2$.

Some of the limitations of these earlier investigations were overcome in a 6-month study reported in 1999 by Kobashigawa and colleagues (15). Twenty-seven transplant patients were randomized to an exercise or control group early after surgery. The exercise group underwent supervised training (aerobic and strengthening exercises), whereas the control group performed an unstructured home walking program. Peak $\dot{V}O_2$ improved more in the supervised training group (+4.4 vs. +1.9 ml·kg^{-1}·min^{-1}, $p < .01$). There were no differences between the two groups for number of episodes of acute rejection or infection. Thus, supervised training programs appear to improve fitness to a greater extent than less structured approaches.

Daida and colleagues (4) compared aerobic exercise capacity in transplant and coronary bypass surgery patients at the completion of phase II cardiac rehabilitation (approximately 3 months after surgery) and at 1 year after surgery. At the end of phase II, both groups were similar in peak $\dot{V}O_2$. However, the coronary bypass surgery patients demonstrated a greater further improvement in fitness over the first year after surgery and were substantially more fit than the transplant recipients (+6 ml·kg^{-1}·min^{-1} in peak $\dot{V}O_2$). Most transplant recipients apparently do not respond to traditional long-term training as well as do patients after coronary bypass surgery. Novel approaches to training, such as interval high-intensity training and longer-duration or higher-frequency training, need further evaluation in these unique patients.

As mentioned previously, some patients after cardiac transplantation may develop outstanding aerobic fitness (2-3 times the usual age and gender average peak $\dot{V}O_2$ for transplant recipients), although they appear to be a small minority. Twelve men (average age of 47 years) who trained for 2 years, undertaking 7 to 20 hr/week of jogging or cycling, achieved an average peak $\dot{V}O_2$ of 45 ml·kg^{-1}·min^{-1} (30). Another study of 14 male transplant patients (average age 43 years) who competed in a 600 km relay running race reported an average peak $\dot{V}O_2$ of 42 (range 32-54 ml·kg^{-1}·min^{-1}) (30).

Resistance Exercise

Most cardiac transplant patients require prednisone, at least during the first several months after surgery, for immunosuppression. Skeletal muscle atrophy and weakness are common side effects related to prednisone. Resistance exercise training partially reverses corticosteroid-related myopathy and improves skeletal muscle strength. Horber and associates (8) found definite evidence of skeletal muscle wasting and weakness in the lower extremities of renal transplant patients who received prednisone. Fifty days of isokinetic strength training substantially increased muscle mass and strength in these patients. In addition, strength training has been shown to improve bone density and to reduce the potential development of osteoporosis (also caused by prednisone) in cardiac transplant recipients (2).

Effect of Exercise Training on Immune Function and Longevity

An obvious and important question concerning exercise training in immunosuppressed cardiac transplant recipients regards the effect of training on immune function. Traditional, moderate training does not increase or decrease the number or severity of episodes of acute rejection (15). In addition, training does not require changes in immunosuppressant dosage or treatment. Infection risk is not changed by exercise training. There are no data regarding the effect of exercise training on survival after cardiac transplantation.

Exercise Programming Suggestions

Exercise for heart transplant patients may begin before surgery. Cardiopulmonary exercise testing and subsequent pretransplant exercise training are routinely performed in patients who are able to perform exercise. Posttransplant exercise training may begin in the hospital soon after surgery and can continue indefinitely after hospital dismissal.

Pretransplant Graded Exercise Testing and Training

As part of the evaluation process for transplantation, ambulatory patients undergo cardiopulmonary exercise testing. Peak $\dot{V}O_2$ is a powerful prognostic indicator: Patients with an aerobic capacity of 14 ml·kg^{-1}·min^{-1} (4 METs) or less experience a markedly reduced 1-year survival, independent of left ventricular ejection fraction (22).

The results of the exercise test can be used to develop an exercise prescription for the patient with the goal of maintaining or even improving cardiorespiratory fitness while waiting for a donor organ. Ideally, the exercise program should be carried out under medical supervision, although many patients have performed home-based, independent exercise successfully. The exercise prescription follows the same guidelines used for other patients with chronic heart failure, as described in chapter 32.

Early Mobilization and Inpatient Exercise Training

After surgery, patients are extubated expeditiously, usually within 24 hr. Passive range-of-motion exercises for both the upper and lower extremities, sitting up in a chair, and slow ambulation may begin and progress gradually after extubation (24). Walking or cycle ergometry may be increased in duration to 20 to 30 min, as tolerated. Exercise intensity is guided using the Borg perceived exertion scale ratings of 11 (fairly light) to 13 (somewhat hard), keeping the respiratory rate below 30 breaths/min and arterial oxygen saturation greater than 90%. Exercise frequency is 2 to 3 sessions per day (31). Patients whose postoperative courses are uncomplicated remain hospitalized for 7 to 10 days.

During inpatient rehabilitation, as well as during the outpatient phases, episodes of acute rejection of a moderate or greater severity may require alteration of the exercise plan. If the rejection episode is graded as moderate, activity may be continued at the current level but should not progress until the rejection has been adequately treated. Severe acute rejection necessitates suspension of all physical activity with the exception of passive range-of-motion exercises.

Outpatient Exercise Training

Cardiac transplant recipients may enter an outpatient cardiac rehabilitation program as soon as they are dismissed from the hospital (31). Patients are generally required by the transplant team to remain near the transplant center for close follow-up for approximately 3 months. Ideally, patients should exercise both in a supervised environment (3 sessions per week) and independently (3 or more sessions per week).

Continuous monitoring of the ECG during the first few supervised exercise sessions is standard practice, although many weeks of ECG-monitored exercise is seldom useful. It is not necessary to perform graded exercise testing before beginning the outpatient exercise program. Performance of a 6-min walk is helpful in assessing functional capacity, however. Graded exercise testing should be performed 6 to 8 weeks after surgery for a patient without complicated recoveries, when the patient has recovered sufficiently from surgery so that the clinician can assess the cardiopulmonary responses to exercise and to refine the exercise prescription.

Exercise prescription for cardiac transplant patients is similar to methods used with patients who have undergone coronary bypass, coronary valve, or other cardiothoracic surgery. The one exception is that a target heart rate is not used unless the patient exhibits a partially normalized heart rate response to exercise, as discussed previously. The typical denervated heart increases in rate slowly during submaximal exercise, and the heart rate may either drift gradually higher during steady-state exercise or plateau after several minutes (32). Borg perceived exertion scale ratings of 12 to 14 (somewhat hard) may be used to prescribe exercise intensity (31). The exercise prescription should include standard warm-up and cool-down activities and a gradual increase in aerobic exercise duration to 30 to 60 mins, with a frequency of 4 to 6 sessions per week. Typical modes of aerobic exercise used during the early outpatient recovery period include walking outdoors (or at shopping centers or schools), treadmill walking, cycle ergometry, and stair climbing.

Because of the sternal incision, special emphasis on upper-extremity active range-of-motion exercises is required. At approximately 6 weeks after surgery, when sternal healing is nearly completed, rowing, arm cranking, combination arm–leg ergometry, outdoor cycling, hiking, jogging, and swimming (and other water-based exercise) become additional options, depending on the patient's fitness level. Sports such as tennis and golf may be performed as early as 6 weeks after surgery if patient fitness is adequate (5 METs or greater) and sternal healing is nearly complete.

Skeletal muscle weakness in cardiac transplant recipients is very common and is related to the following factors:

- Skeletal muscle atrophy attributable to advanced heart failure
- Pretransplant deconditioning
- Corticosteroid use posttransplant as part of the immunosuppressant regimen

Muscle strengthening exercises should be incorporated into the exercise program to counteract these factors. For the first 6 weeks after surgery, bilateral arm lifting is restricted to less than 10 lb (4.5 kg) to avoid sternal nonunion. During this early stage of rehabilitation, light hand weights are an excellent method of introducing resistance exercise. After at least 6 weeks of healing, patients may be started on standard weight machines, emphasizing moderate resistance, 10 to 20 slow repetitions per set, 1 to 3 sets of exercises for the major muscle groups, with a frequency of 2 or 3 sessions per week (14, 31). We recommend Borg perceived exertion scale ratings of 12 to 14 to gauge the intensity of lifting. Strength gains of 50% or greater

commonly occur after 8 weeks of strength training in these patients. Performing the strengthening exercises immediately following the aerobic portion of the exercise prescription (after the cool-down) is recommended. Because cardiac transplant recipients are likely to require antihypertensive medications, periodic blood pressure measurement during both aerobic and strengthening exercise is recommended.

The transplant team and the primary health care provider should consistently encourage the transplant recipient to continue a lifelong exercise program. Patients should continue a supervised exercise program indefinitely, exercise independently, or use a combination of supervised and unsupervised exercise. We recommend annual graded exercise tests with revision of the exercise prescription as necessary.

Summary

Cardiac transplantation is an attractive treatment for patients with terminal heart failure. One-year survival after surgery exceeds 80% in most centers. Unfortunately, the number of candidates for cardiac transplantation greatly exceeds the available supply of donor organs. Heart transplant recipients have unique characteristics, including risks of acute and chronic organ rejection, the need for lifelong immunosuppressant medications, multiple potential nonrejection medical problems, and unique responses to exercise.

The transplanted heart is surgically denervated, and the autonomic nervous system does not directly affect cardiac performance during exercise. The heart rate response to graded exercise is decidedly abnormal. The heart rate does not increase during the first few minutes of exercise, slowly rises thereafter, and may remain near peak values for several minutes after cessation of exercise. At 1 year after transplantation, aerobic exercise capacity averages 60% to 70% of age and sex norms, although some transplant recipients may achieve superior fitness with aggressive exercise training. At 1 year after surgery, approximately one third of patients have evidence of partial cardiac reinnervation and exhibit a partially normalized heart rate response during exercise.

Both aerobic exercise training and resistance exercise training substantially improve fitness for cardiac transplant recipients. All transplant patients should participate in both inpatient and outpatient cardiac rehabilitation programs. Research is needed to determine the effects of exercise training and aerobic capacity on morbidity and mortality.

CHAPTER 34

Deep Vein Thrombosis

William O. Roberts, MD, MS

Deep vein thrombosis (DVT) is relatively common in both healthy and ill populations and is the third most common cardiovascular disease in the United States. The clinical diagnosis is neither sensitive nor specific, and clinical suspicion must be confirmed by objective testing. In some cases, the first sign of DVT may be cardiovascular collapse or sudden death attributable to pulmonary embolism. DVT is most commonly associated with bed rest, smoking, and inactivity, but athletes and active people are not immune to the problem. In healthy, active people, DVT usually follows travel with prolonged sitting, results from use of the oral contraceptive pill or patch, or is a consequence of either acquired or inherited alterations in hemostatic regulatory proteins. The most common inherited maladies are the factor V Leiden and prothrombin 20210 mutations and can be responsible for venous thrombosis in an otherwise healthy individual. The acquired deficiencies are frequently a consequence of other clinical entities in chronically ill people with cancers, autoimmune syndromes, or diabetes mellitus.

The diagnostic evaluation of DVT requires a clear correlation between clinical probability, diagnostic test selection, and test interpretation. DVT is potentially fatal if untreated and if pulmonary embolism (PE) develops as a complication. PE occurs in more than 250,000 patients each year in the United States and has an 18% to 30% mortality rate. PE is not always detected clinically, and 73% of PE is diagnosed at autopsy. Given the physiology of the anticoagulant protein system, DVT is not common in active people and athletes because of exercise, and regular exercise should be protective. The importance of exercise in treatment of DVT is increasing as the benefits of exercise are shown in clinical studies.

Overview of Clinical Pathophysiology

A DVT is caused by a blood clot formed in a deep vein that is attached to the vein wall and may fully occlude the venous flow. PE develops as a complication of DVT when part of the clot breaks loose from its origin and lodges in the pulmonary circulation, disrupting the lung blood flow and gas exchange. The size and location of the clot will determine the final insult to the person affected by either DVT or PE. The body is in a constant steady state of balancing clotting to repair the system and clot lysis to avoid inappropriate thrombosis that can harm the body. In DVT, the clot is formed in response to a stimulus that inappropriately engages or overengages the clotting system (see figure 34.1). The early clot is soft and compressible, and with aging the clot becomes firm and noncompressible. Clot formation and progression are interrupted by anticoagulation, and lytic drugs destroy any clot that is not fully

Many thanks to Stephan Moll, MD, University of North Carolina, Chapel Hill, NC, for his critical review of this chapter and his suggestions for improvements.

Correspondence concerning this chapter should be addressed to William O. Roberts, Phalen Village Clinic, 1414 Maryland Ave East, St. Paul, MN 55106. E-mail: rober037@tc.umn.edu

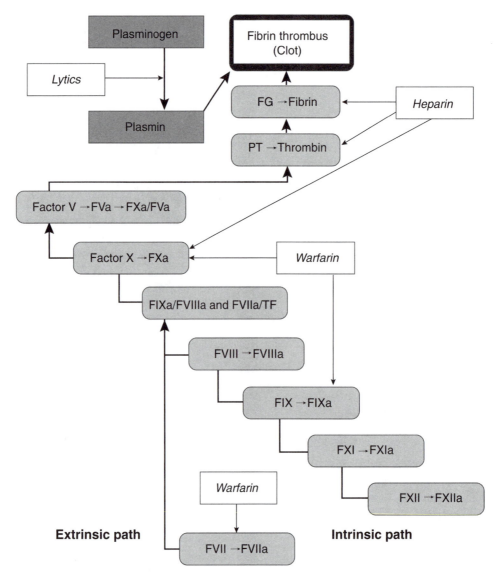

FIGURE 34.1 Clotting cascade and medical interventions. FG = fibrinogen; PT = prothrombin; F = factor (e.g., FVII = factor VII).

organized. The natural history of a clot that is attached to the vein wall is endothelialization in 7 to 10 days. The greatest risk of embolization is in the time period before endothelialization of the clot. Secure adhesion of the clot to the vein wall begins in 1 to 3 weeks. The natural process of clot lysis and vein recanalization occurs in 4 to 6 weeks, although not every clot will fully lyse or recanalize.

Predisposing factors for DVT in active people include dehydration; prolonged standing or squatting; constricting garments; recent surgery; prolonged sitting in bus, car, or plane en route to and from competition; blood doping; and trauma to vein. Although mild to moderate trauma to the extremities is common in active people, DVT rarely forms unless there is some predisposing hereditary factor (see Heredity and Acquired Prothombotic Defects on page 341), prolonged inac-

tivity, underlying occult disease, or hormone-related factor such as use of the oral contraceptive pill or patch, the use of estrogen replacement therapy, or pregnancy. Hospital patients at risk include people who have undergone surgery, women recovering from pregnancy, patients with indwelling central venous catheters, or patients who have undergone trauma with fractures and crush injuries. These high-risk situations are partially a result of a coagulation system that has been activated by the body insult. Several medical conditions carry increased risk for DVT including malignancies, polycythemia vera, essential thrombocytosis, nephritic syndrome, obesity, bacteremia, and heparin-induced thrombocytopenia. Acute myocardial infarction and neurologic diseases with paralysis also increase risk. Stasis from prolonged sitting during airline, car, or bus travel resulting in thrombotic episodes has been referred to as the "economy class syndrome" and puts travelers of all activity levels at risk (6). Periodic leg exercising during flights showed no measurable preventive effects, but it is hypothesized that alterations to the clotting mechanisms produced by long-distance air travel could intensify the risk of DVT in passengers with predisposing risk factors.

Estrogen use is implicated as a risk factor in DVT and poses a risk to both active and inactive people. The link between DVT and the oral contraceptive pill and patch is well known. Several studies have reported an association between hormone replacement therapy (HRT) in postmenopausal women and increased incidence of idiopathic DVT. In women receiving HRT in the Postmenopausal Estrogen/Progestin Interventions study, only baseline fibrinogen varied significantly between those who did and did not have a DVT. Other covariates including age, smoking, body mass index, lipid levels, blood pressure, alcohol, exercise, and prior HRT or oral contraceptive use did not affect this finding. The higher fibrinogen levels may be a marker for coagulopathy that is magnified by exogenous hormones.

■ Heredity and Acquired Prothombotic Defects

The risk of DVT is increased in athletes with the following protein defects, and those who have more than one DVT episode usually require chronic anticoagulation. These proteins are involved in the clotting cascade.

- Factor V Leiden mutation
- Prothrombin mutation G20210A
- Antithrombin deficiency
- Protein C deficiency
- Protein S deficiency
- Antiphospholipid syndrome
  - Lupus anticoagulant
  - Anticardiolipin antibodies
- Homocysteinuria
- Hyperhomocysteinemia
- Elevated factor VII, IX, or XI
- Elevated fibrinogen

Although physical activity can influence the coagulation cascade in several ways, regular exercise has a protective effect for thrombosis (13). Long-term moderate or strenuous physical activity is inversely related to fibrinogen levels. Although data on endurance exercise and the fibrinolytic system are limited, it appears that fibrinolysis increases with persistent endurance activity. Other hemostatic and fibrinolytic parameters are affected by exercise: Factor VII decreases, plasma viscosity decreases, plasminogen activator inhibitor-1 decreases, and tissue-plasminogen activator increases. The effects of chronic exercise on platelet hyperreactivity are unknown. Taken together, these findings indicate that regular exercise should decrease DVT risk in active people. Acute unaccustomed exercise, in contrast, induces transient activation of the coagulation system in healthy subjects. In healthy adults participating in acute intermittent exercise, factor VII levels and plasminogen activator inhibitor-1 remain unchanged, while plasma viscosity and tissue-plasminogen activator are increased and platelet hyperreactivity is static. This set of changes has the potential to transiently increase DVT risk, especially in people with a high-risk profile.

The effects of exercise and catecholamines on platelet reactivity and fibrinolysis are inconsistent in humans. Ikarugi and colleagues (10) used a novel in vitro method to demonstrate that exercise significantly increased shear-induced platelet reactivity, coagulation, and catecholamine levels. The elevation of circulating norepinephrine at levels that are attained during exercise causes platelet hyperreactivity and a platelet-mediated enhanced coagulation (10). This mechanism may link aerobic exercise with thrombotic risk (10). However, physically active people have a lower incidence of circulating thrombocyte aggregate compared with otherwise healthy inactive people (7). Healthy active persons have a significantly higher ($p < .01$) thrombocyte index compared with inactive people (7).

Plasminogen activator (PA) is found in normal subjects after exercise and venous occlusion (4). Exercise to exhaustion is associated with the appearance in plasma of PA in several molecular weight forms, and in one study all forms of tissue plasminogen articulator (tPA) were cleared rapidly after cessation of exercise at exhaustion (4). In the same study, urokinase-type PA activity was identified in pre- and postexercise samples, and qualitatively similar changes in plasma PA were observed after venous occlusion (4). Small quantities of plasmin were generated after strenuous exercise but were not detected in any subjects after venous occlusion (4). Exercise and upright posture produce distinctive alterations in the thrombogenic potential of the blood that may influence the timing of clinical vascular events

(23). Exercise does not increase platelet aggregation to levels beyond that produced by the upright posture, but exercise is associated with a marked increase in fibrinolytic activity (23). This fibrinolytic activity should be thromboprotective.

Venous obstruction and vein wall trauma are also factors in a developing thrombus. Effort thrombosis is a form of axillary-subclavian vein occlusion in young people that is related to anatomic constriction of the subclavian vein by the clavicle and first rib complex (2). This form of DVT is associated with repetitive trauma to the vein resulting in changes in the vein wall that trigger clot formation. The repeated trauma is as important in the genesis of clotting as the anatomic obstruction. Anticoagulation and thrombolytic therapies do not correct the underlying mechanical abnormality, and the clinical outcome is often unsatisfactory unless therapy addresses both the superimposed thrombosis and corrects the constricting mechanism. The anatomic constriction usually affects active people and athletes who do repetitive motions that involve abduction and external rotation of the arm, putting the subclavian vein into a compromised position with respect to the clavicle and first rib.

Effort thrombosis is usually reported in baseball players, swimmers, and gymnasts, but Gorard (9) reported a case of suspected effort thrombosis in an American rules football player following trauma to the leg that shared features of effort thrombosis in the upper extremities. An unpublished case from my practice involved a 20-year-old male recreational snowboarder in good health who had experienced no trauma and developed right leg swelling in the evening after he had pushed himself more than 2 miles with his right leg across the ski area. He presented in clinic the following day with a swollen dusky right thigh and calf (see figure 34.2). The venous Doppler study showed occlusion with DVT and an angiogram showed congenital absence of vena cava. He had no markers for hypercoaguability. His diagnosis was effort thrombosis of the leg caused by restricted venous flow. The possibility of effort thrombosis needs to be considered in active people and athletes presenting with leg injuries and leg swelling, as does the diagnosis of a congenital absence of malformation of the inferior vena cava or pelvic veins (8). A common congenital anatomic variation predisposing to left leg DVT is the May–Thurner syndrome, in which the right common iliac artery presses onto the left common iliac vein, impairing venous return from the right leg and forming a site for DVT formation.

Exercise appears to have both positive and negative effects on the risk of thrombosis. Although acute

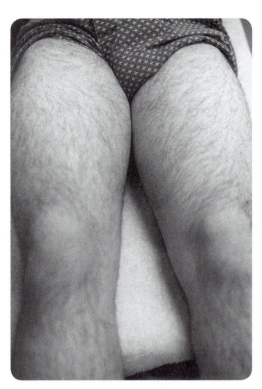

FIGURE 34.2 Swollen right upper leg caused by effort thrombosis in a snowboarder.

unexpected exercise may temporarily increase the risk of thrombosis, regular exercise appears to be protective and is another reason for people to exercise regularly. Repeated trauma to a vein, especially combined with venous flow obstruction, will increase the risk for effort thrombosis in active people who use their arms above shoulder level or who use their legs in a fashion that magnifies the obstruction.

Evaluation of Suspected DVT

The classic DVT presents with a painful swollen leg or arm and localized pain in calf, popliteal space, groin, or axilla. There is often an obvious predisposing factor, a medical history of DVT, a family history of DVT, or a family history of unexplained sudden death. The review of symptoms may suggest an underlying disorder, and it is critical to look for the use of oral contraceptive pills or patch and estrogen supplements, pregnancy, prolonged sitting, repetitive use, or trauma. Physical exam often reveals unilateral distal swelling and edema that are worse with standing or in the dependent position. The veins are sometimes palpable and associated with local inflammation. The arterial pulses are intact. The Homans sign (forced dorsiflexion of the foot leading to calf pain) is not reliable.

The differential diagnosis is listed in table 34.1. In active people, gastrocnemius rupture, subfascial hematoma, and unaccustomed exercise may be the most common confounding conditions. These problems when misdiagnosed as thrombophlebitis result in unnecessary anticoagulation and hemorrhagic complications. However, DVT as a complication following rupture of the medial head of the gastrocnemius muscle has been reported (20). Flare-up of the postthrombotic

syndrome can be difficult to distinguish clinically from a recurrent acute DVT, and imaging studies may be necessary to differentiate the two.

Laboratory parameters can help the clinician diagnose DVT and develop a management plan. The fibrin degradation product, D-dimer, can indicate active thrombosis, and normal levels have a high negative predictive value when the pretest probability for DVT or PE is low (22). The presence of thrombophilias, such as protein C deficiency of antiphospholipid antibody syndrome, may guide decisions on length of anticoagulant therapy.

Diagnostic imaging is required to confirm the DVT. Lower-extremity thrombi that extend into the proximal system into or above the level of the popliteal fossa, termed *proximal DVT*, carry the most risk and require the most aggressive therapy. Venography used to be the most reliable technique to confirm or rule out DVT and is often still considered the gold standard for validation of noninvasive diagnostic methods. However, in clinical practice, venography has almost completely been replaced by the use of Doppler ultrasound technique for lower-extremity evaluation. The first step in evaluation of arm DVT is also Doppler ultrasound, but the proximal veins (axillary, subclavian, brachocephalic and superior vena cava) often cannot be visualized well, particularly in the muscular athlete. CT venography, magnetic resonance venography, and conventional invasive contrast venography are often required to define the extent of thrombosis in the person with arm DVT. Venography may be necessary to show a new intraluminal filling defect in recurrent DVT (18).

Impedance plethysmography is noninvasive and measures changes in electric impedance or resistance attributable to flow variability between patent and obstructed vessels, but it is rarely performed. As already mentioned, ultrasonography with Doppler is a noninvasive imaging procedure that can confirm or rule out the diagnosis of DVT in most patients. More technically sophisticated techniques like compressive real-time B-mode ultrasonography (CUS) and duplex color real-time B-mode Doppler have improved the reliability of these imaging procedures. For negative Doppler ultrasound tests with high clinical suspicion for DVT, two options are available to rule out clinically significant DVT: (a) repeat CUS at day 2 and 8, or (b) perform venography the same day. Same-day venography is the test of choice in negative CUS and high pretest clinical probability. Magnetic resonance imaging has a sensitivity of 87% in the calf and 97% to 100% above knee for DVT and is very useful in pelvic, iliac, and caval thrombosis, but it is time-consuming, expensive, and not widely available.

TABLE 34.1   Differential Diagnosis of Deep Vein Thrombosis

Type of disease	Etiology
Mechanical	Trauma
	Muscle strain
	Gastrocnemius rupture
	Unaccustomed exercise
	Ruptured Baker's cyst
	Malignancy with lymphatic or venous obstruction
	Pregnancy (venous or lymphatic obstruction by uterus)
	Postthrombotic (phlebitic) syndrome
	Paralysis
Circulatory	Congestive heart failure
	Hematoma
	Intramuscular or subfascial hematoma
	Chronic exertional compartment syndrome
	Lymphedema
	Venous insufficiency
Metabolic	Renal disease (nephrotic syndrome)
Inflammatory	Rheumatoid arthritis
	Gout
	Contact dermatitis
	Erythema nodosum
	Superficial thrombophlebitis
Infectious	Cellulitis
	Lymphangitis
	Inguinal abscess

Management of DVT

The goals of DVT management are to alleviate symptoms, halt thrombus progression and recurrence, prevent pulmonary embolism, prevent death from an existing embolus, prevent death and morbidity from recurrent pulmonary embolism, prevent morbidity from recurrent deep vein thrombosis, and prevent postthrombotic syndrome. Postthrombotic syndrome is particularly problematic for active people and athletes.

The cornerstone of DVT management has been anticoagulant therapy using intravenous unfractionated heparin or subcutaneous low molecular weight heparin followed by oral anticoagulant treatment for at least 3 months in people without permanent defects in the coagulation cascade. Heparin along with antithrombin inhibits thrombin, thus inhibiting the conversion of fibrinogen to fibrin (see figure 34.1). Warfarin inhibits the carboxylation and thus the formation of active clotting factors, the vitamin K–dependent coagulation factors (II, VII, IX, X), and proteins C and S. Both medications are intended to stop the progression of clot formation in the acute phase and the formation of new clot in the chronic phase of care.

Acute anticoagulation with unfractionated heparin IV for at least 5 days has been the standard primary therapy, but its effectiveness depends on achieving adequate heparin levels, most importantly during the initial 24 hr, with an activated partial thromboplastin time above a predetermined lower limit. The use of validated dosing protocols for intravenous heparin lessens the likelihood of delayed therapeutic heparinization. Low molecular weight heparin (LMWH) for at least 5 days has been proven to be as effective as unfractionated heparin, yet safer, in the treatment of DVT when administered subcutaneously either once or twice daily. The bioavailability of LMWH is nearly 100%, and it has a longer half-life than unfractionated heparin; in addition, because LMWH is associated with reduced thrombocytopenia and bleeding complications, it offers the opportunity for home therapy (14). LMWH provides predictable anticoagulation and ease of administration with no need for monitoring anticoagulation levels in most patients, enables outpatient therapy in uncomplicated DVT, and makes outpatient treatment possible in at least 75% of patients (16). Both unfractionated heparin and LMWH are continued until the warfarin dose inhibits clotting in the selected therapeutic range as discussed in relation to warfarin therapy. The synthetic pentasaccharide fondaparinux is a drug consisting of the five active sugars also found in unfractionated heparin and in LMWH; by potentiating the effect of antithrombin, synthetic pentasaccharide fondaparinux selectively inhibits factor Xa. Synthetic pentasaccharide fondaparinux can be used as an alternative to LMWH in the acute DVT treatment phase; synthetic pentasaccharide fondaparinux requires once-daily dosing, carries less risk of heparin-induced thrombocytopenia, and does not require monitoring of its anticoagulant effect in most patients.

Thrombolytic therapy is used in the initial management of DVT, and an early diagnosis is essential for effective thrombus dissolution with one of the lytics (streptokinase, urokinase, or alteplase [tPA]). The lytics accelerate the conversion of plasminogen to plasmin and promote fibrinolysis. A local infusion of low-dose streptokinase therapy for clot lysis can be effective in dissolving the clot. Lytics are used more frequently in the treatment of effort thrombosis of the subclavian and related veins than in lower-extremity thrombosis. The use of thrombolytic therapy in axillary-subclavian vein thrombosis has become more routine practice in athletes (15).

The length of warfarin therapy after a DVT depends on the triggering factors and presence or absence of inherited or acquired thrombophilias: (a) 3 months if the DVT was associated with a transient risk factor, such as surgery or major trauma; (b) 6 to 12 months if the DVT was a first event and without triggering factor (idiopathic) (5) or was associated with heterozygous factor V Leiden or heterozygous prothrombin 20210 mutation; (c) at least 12 months, preferably indefinitely, for a spontaneous DVT associated with antiphospholipid antibody syndrome or two or more thrombophilias (such as combined factor V Leiden and prothrombin 20210 mutations); (d) 6 to 12 months and potentially long-term if the DVT was associated with deficiencies of protein C, protein S, or antithrombin; (e) lifelong if there have been recurrent spontaneous thrombotic events. However, the length of warfarin therapy must be decided individually for each case. Recently, additional indicators of a lower risk of recurrent DVT have been identified (female gender, negative D-dimer while on warfarin 3-6 months after the acute DVT, negative D-dimer once off warfarin, absence of residual thrombus on follow-up Doppler ultrasound) that help individualize the assessment of risk of recurrence and help a physician and patient discuss the risk–benefit ratio of continuing or discontinuing warfarin therapy. Finally, other factors need to be considered when discussing the length of warfarin therapy: Did the patient have any bleeding complications? Has the international normalized ratio (INR) been relatively stable, or has it been difficult to keep the INR in the therapeutic range? How has warfarin therapy affected the patient's lifestyle?

Ambulation as tolerated is typically recommended in the acute setting of a DVT (5), with increasing activities of daily living permitted over the first 6 weeks. Bedrest in the acute setting of DVT, although widely recommended in past years, is no longer advised. Leg compression combined with walking is a better alternative to bed rest for the treatment of symptomatic patients with proximal DVT. In one study, patients who were randomized to the compression and walking groups compared with those left at bedrest had less pain, less swelling, greater walking distances, and better life quality (3). Ultrasound revealed less frequent and less pronounced thrombus progression in the exercise and compression groups (3). The role of exercise in the treatment of DVT and in the development or prevention of the postthrombotic syndrome has been insufficiently studied. Thus, no conclusions are possible. However, if postthrombotic syndrome is present, symptoms may slightly worsen with exercise and compression stockings typically do not prevent that worsening (12).

Effort thrombosis is challenging to treat. Effort thrombosis can produce long-term disability from arm swelling and exercise limitation when the vein fails to recanalize or adequate collaterals do not form. Acute treatment consists of heparin administration with consideration of thrombolysis. This can be followed by one of several approaches to decrease the risk of recurrent thrombosis: (a) angioplasty, (b) resection of the stenosed area of the subclavian vein with repair using a patch, (c) surgical bypass, (d) thoracic outlet surgery with first rib resection or fibrous band resection, and (e) long-term warfarin. Good clinical studies on the long-term outcome of these treatment approaches are not available, because publications are often case-series on selected patients with very limited generalizability. An individual decision needs to be made with each patient. Although thoracic outlet surgery can relieve the external compression of the subclavian vein and may allow the person to fully return to daily activities with no recurrence or persistence of symptoms, the low, yet potential risks of the procedure—mainly brachial plexus injury—need to be considered. Although the elimination of venous obstruction appears to minimize the likelihood of severe symptoms of postthrombotic syndrome, many patients do well despite persistent venous occlusion (presumably because of the development of collaterals).

Complications Following DVT

Postthrombotic syndrome (also called postphlebitic syndrome or venous stasis syndrome) following DVT occurs in nearly one third of cases and can be debili-
tating. Postthrombotic syndrome takes the form of a painful swelling and red discoloration of the tissue distal to the DVT site that is associated with poor venous return. This syndrome can be confused with recurrent DVT. Symptoms and signs include heaviness, aching, swelling, throbbing, burning, restless sensation, itching, tingling, and, at its worst, chronic skin ulceration. Graduated compression stockings that are fit to the patient reduce the risk of postthrombotic syndrome after DVT (11) and also seem to relieve the swelling associated with exercise. Postthrombotic syndrome has been considered a risk of exercise following DVT. In a recent study, patients with highest physical activity 1 month after DVT had roughly half the chance of experiencing postthrombotic syndrome during the next 3 months (19). Of the patients who were active prior to DVT, half had returned to their pre-DVT activity level by 4 months (19). For those who are able to exercise, it appears that there is no increase in risk of postthrombotic syndrome from early, regular activity following DVT (12).

A second complication following DVT is bleeding from trauma, either from cuts in the skin or into soft tissue following contusion, while the patient is taking anticoagulant therapy. The risk of trauma and bleeding must be factored into the treatment decisions. A third complication following DVT is significant weight gain and increase in body mass index attributable to inactivity (1). There is greater weight gain in hospitalized patients, but both inpatient and outpatient groups should benefit from increased exercise and dietary limitations for controlling weight during the recovery from DVT.

Exercise Prescription Recommendations and Return to Activity After DVT

The risk of bleeding into the soft tissue requires that athletes and active people restrict contact and collision sports while anticoagulated on warfarin or heparin. Patients employed in occupations or with leisure pursuits that carry a high risk of cuts, contusions, and falls may need to be restricted during the period of anticoagulation following the DVT. At a minimum, these patients need to understand the risks of bleeding associated with the anticoagulant medication before they return to work and must use any available protective clothing and equipment.

There is not a large evidence base to support a universal recommendation for return to fitness exercise, training, or competition after deep vein thrombosis, and each patient must be considered individually. Research indicates that early activity appears to benefit all patients and should be encouraged over the traditional approach of bed rest for a week followed by limited activity for 6 weeks. Unfortunately, the people most affected by DVT are those with other acute and chronic medical problems that may limit their ability to participate in regular exercise. For very active people, there is no standard recommendation for return to activity, and each patient will need an individualized exercise plan. An individualized plan developed for a professional endurance athlete with a DVT in the popliteal space included progressive walking and activities of daily living for weeks 1 to 3, adding swimming (non–weight bearing) in week 4, adding biking (non–impact loading) in week 5, and finally return to running (impact loading) during week 6 (17). The athlete was to wear a support hose and discontinue this progression if there was a return of symptoms. The plan was based on the organization and aging of the clot to decrease the risk of embolism. The athlete accelerated the suggested return-to-training protocol on her own accord and had progressed to running within 3 weeks. She developed a postthrombotic syndrome that she controlled by wearing compression stockings during exercise and prolonged standing; the postthrombotic syndrome resolved within 2 years. The athlete returned to full competition within months of the DVT.

With duplex Doppler ultrasound studies, clots can now be visualized; however, there are insufficient data on whether ultrasound appearance predicts risk of PE, progression of clot, or development of postthrombotic syndrome. Therefore, serial Doppler ultrasounds after an acute clot are not helpful in making a decision on progression of physical exercise. Recent investigations into the postthrombotic syndrome indicate that a more rapid return to higher-level activity may be protective and a majority of people should be able to return to premorbid exercise levels within a month.

Patient Education and Support

Young people and athletes who have been diagnosed with DVT or have a thrombophilia require education about their disorder. Because DVT is mainly a disease of elderly people, young patients and athletes may experience isolation and a lack of support and thus may be unable to interact and exchange thoughts with peers who have experienced a similar disease. A national nonprofit patient advocacy group for people with thrombosis and thrombophilia was founded in 2003, the National Alliance for Thrombosis and Thrombophilia (NATT), which addresses patient and health care provider education on thrombosis as well as support for people with thrombosis. NATT provides education materials through its Web site (14), as well as a regular newsletter and specialized brochures. Another source of patient education materials and support is the Factor V Leiden Thrombophilia Support Page (8) with an associated ListServe (www.fvleiden.org/mailing_list.html).

Summary

Early recognition of DVT allows the option of lytic therapy, and early anticoagulant treatment reduces the risk of pulmonary embolism. With or without lytic therapy, both acute anticoagulation with some form of heparin and long-term anticoagulation with warfarin are indicated for the management of DVT. Early ambulation combined with graduated compression stockings or bandage wraps appears to improve outcome compared with bedrest and can be initiated at diagnosis. Bed rest and limited activity following DVT also contribute to weight gain and problems associated with obesity. Active patients with no obvious reason for DVT should be checked for hypercoaguability, especially if there is a family history or a recurrence of DVT. Length of warfarin therapy needs to be individualized, and clinicians should consider the presence or absence of acquired or inherited thrombophilias. A need for long-term anticoagulation may force changes in lifestyle activities for some active people. Because of a lack of studies, it is not known whether an early return to activity to most noncontact sports has a positive effect, a negative effect, or no effect on the risk of postthrombotic syndrome. However, early return to activity may be beneficial to both the physical and mental health of normally active people and athletes.

Appendix A

Common Medications Used for Cardiovascular Disease[‡]

β-blockers

Use or Condition: Hypertension, angina, arrhythmias including supraventricular tachycardia, and increasing AV block to slow ventricular response in atrial fibrillation, acute myocardial infarction, migraine headaches, anxiety, mandatory as part of therapy for heart failure due to systolic dysfunction

Drug name	Brand name[†]	Drug name	Brand name[†]
Acebutolol **	Sectral **	Nadolol	Corgard
Atenolol	Tenormin	Penbutolol **	Levatol **
Betaxolol	Kerlone	Pindolol **	Visken **
Bisoprolol	Zebeta	Propranolol	Inderal
Esmolol	Brevibloc	Sotalol	Betapace
Metoprolol	Lopressor SR, Toprol XL	Timolol	Blocadren

** β-blockers with intrinsic sympathomimetic activity

β-blockers in Combination with Diuretics

Use or Condition: Hypertension, diuretic, glaucoma

Drug name	Brand name[†]
Atenolol, Chlorthalidone	Tenoretic
Bendroflumethiazide, Nadolol	Corzide
Bisoprolol, Hydrochlorothiazide	Ziac
Metoprolol, Hydrochlorothiazide	Lopressor HCT
Propranolol, Hydrochlorothiazide	Inderide
Timolol, Hydrochlorothiazide	Timolide

α- and β-Adrenergic Blocking Agents

Use or Condition: Hypertension, chronic heart failure, angina

Drug name	Brand name[†]
Carvedilol	Coreg
Labetalol	Normodyne, Trandate

α₁-Adrenergic Blocking Agents

Use or Condition: Hypertension, enlarged prostate

Drug name	Brand name[†]
Cardura	Doxazosin
Flomax	Tamsulosin
Minipress	Prazosin
Terazosin	Hytrin

Central α₂-Agonists and Other Centrally Acting Drugs

Use or Condition: Hypertension

Drug name	Brand name[†]
Clonidine	Catapres, Catapres-TTS patch
Guanfacine	Tenex
Methyldopa	Aldomet
Reserpine	Serpasil

[†]Adapted, by permission, from American College of Sport Medicine, *ACSM's guidelines for exercise testing and prescription*, 8th ed. (Philadelphia, PA: Lippincott, Williams, and Wilkins). (in print)

Central α₂-Agonists in Combination With Diuretics

Use or Condition: Hypertension

Drug name	Brand name†
Methyldopa + hydrochlorothiazide	Aldoril
Reserpine + chlorothiazide	Diupres
Reserpine + hydrochlorothiazide	Hydropres

Nitrates and Nitroglycerin

Use or Condition: Angina, vasodilator in chronic heart failure

Drug name	Brand name†
Amyl nitrite	Amyl Nitrite
Isosorbide mononitrate	Ismo, Imdur, Monoket
Isosorbide dinitrate	Dilatrate, Isordil, Sorbitrate
Nitroglycerin, sublingual	Nitrostat, NitroQuick
Nitroglycerin, translingual	Nitrolingual
Nitroglycerin, transmucosal	Nitrogard
Nitroglycerin, sustained release	Nitrong, Nitrocine, Nitroglyn, Nitro-Bid
Nitroglycerin, transdermal	Minitran, Nitro-Dur, Transderm-Nitro, Deponit, Nitrodisc, Nitro-Derm
Nitroglycerin, topical	Nitro-Bid, Nitrol

Calcium Channel Blockers (Nondihydropyridines)

Use or Condition: Angina, hypertension, increasing AV block to slow ventricular response in atrial fibrillation, paroxysmal supraventricular tachycardia, headache

Drug name	Brand name†
Diltiazem Extended Release	Cardizem CD, Cardizem LA, Dilacor XR, Tiazac
Verapamil Immediate Release	Calan, Isoptin
Verapamil Long-Acting	Calan SR, Isoptin SR
Verapamil Coer 24	Covera HS, Verelan PM

Calcium Channel Blockers (Dihydropyridines)

Use or Condition: Hypertension, angina, neurological deficits after subarachnoid hemorrhage

Drug name	Brand name†
Amlodipine	Norvasc
Felodipine	Plendil
Isradipine	DynaCirc CR
Nicardipine Sustained Release	Cardene SR
Nifedipine Long Acting	Adalat, Procardia XL
Nimodipine	Nimotop
Nisoldipine	Sular

Cardiac Glycosides

Use or Condition: Chronic heart failure in the setting of dilated cardiomyopathy, increasing of AV block to slow ventricular response with atrial fibrillation

Drug name	Brand name†
Digoxin	Lanoxin

Direct Peripheral Vasodilators

Use or Condition: Hypertension, hair loss, vasodilation for heart failure

Drug name	Brand name†
Hydralazine	Apresoline
Minoxidil	Loniten

Angiotensin-Converting Enzyme (ACE) Inhibitors

Use or Condition: Hypertension, coronary artery disease, chronic heart failure due to systolic dysfunction, diabetes, chronic kidney disease, heart attacks, scleroderma, migraines

Drug name	Brand name[†]
Benazepril	Lotensin
Captopril	Capoten
Cilzapril*	Inhibace
Enalapril	Vasotec
Fosinopril	Monopril
Lisinopril	Zestril, Prinivil
Moexipril	Univasc
Perindopril	Aceon
Quinapril	Accupril
Ramipril	Altace
Trandolapril	Mavik

*Available only in Canada

ACE Inhibitors in Combination With Diuretics

Use or Condition: Hypertension, chronic heart failure

Drug name	Brand name[†]
Benazepril + Hydrocholorthiazide	Lotensin
Captopril + Hydrocholorthiazide	Capozide
Enalapril + Hydrocholorthiazide	Vaseretic
Lisinopril + Hydrocholorthiazide	Prinzide, Zestoretic
Moexipril + Hydrocholorthiazide	Uniretic
Quinapril + Hydrocholorthiazide	Accuretic

ACE Inhibitors in Combination With Calcium Channel Blockers

Use or Condition: Hypertension, chronic heart failure, angina

Drug name	Brand name[†]
Benazepril + Amlodipine	Lotrel
Enalapril + Felodipine	Lexxel
Trandolapril + Verapamil	Tarka

Angiotensin II Receptor Antagonists

Use or Condition: Hypertension

Drug name	Brand name[†]
Candesartan	Atacand
Eprosartan	Tevetan
Irbesartan	Avapro
Losartan	Cozaar
Olmesartan	Benicar
Telmisartan	Micardis
Valsartan	Diovan

Angiotensin II Receptor Antagonists in Combination With Diuretics

Use or Condition: Hypertension, chronic heart failure, angina

Drug name	Brand name[†]
Candesartan + hydrochlorothiazide	Atacand HCT
Eprosartan + hydrochlorothiazide	Teveten HCT
Irbesartan + hydrochlorothiazide	Avalide
Losartan + hydrochlorothiazide	Hyzaar
Telmisartan + hydrochlorothiazide	Micardis HCT
Valsartan + hydrochlorothiazide	Diovan HCT

Diuretics

Use or Condition: Edema, chronic heart failure, polycystic ovary syndrome, certain kidney disorders (i.e., kidney stones, diabetes insipidus, female hirsutism, osteoporosis)

Drug name	Brand name[†]
THIAZIDES	
Chlorothiazide	Diuril
Hydrochlorothiazide (HCTZ)	Microzide, Hydrodiuril, Oretic
Indapamide	Lozol
Metolazone	Mykron, Zaroxolyn
Polythiazide	Renese
"LOOP" DIURETICS	
Bumetanide	Bumex
Ethacrynic Acid	Edecrin
Furosemide	Lasix
Torsemide	Demadex
POTASSIUM-SPARING DIURETICS	
Amiloride	Midamor
Triamterene	Dyrenium
ALDOSTERONE RECEPTOR BLOCKERS	
Eplerenone	Inspra
Spironolactone	Aldactone
DIURETIC COMBINED WITH DIURETIC	
Amiloride + hydrochlorothiazide	Moduretic
Triamterene + hydrochlorothiazide	Dyazide, Maxzide

Antiarrhythmic Agents

Use or Condition: Specific for drug but include suppression of atrial fibrillation and maintenance of normal sinus rhythm, serious ventricular arrhythmias in certain clinical settings, increase in AV nodal block to slow ventricular response in atrial fibrillation

Drug name	Brand name[†]
CLASS 1A	
Disopyramide	Norpace
Moricizine	Ethmozine
Procainamide	Pronestyl, Procan SR
Quinidine	Quinora, Quinidex, Quinaglute, Quinalan, Cardioquin
CLASS IB	
Lidocaine	Xylocaine, Xylocard
Mexiletine	Mexitil
Phenytoin	Dilantin
Tocainide	Tonocard
CLASS IC	
Flecainide	Tambocor
Propafenone	Rythmol
CLASS II	
β-Blockers	Refer to Appendix A page 347
CLASS III	
Amiodarone	Cordarone, Pacerone
Bretylium	Bretylol
Sotalol	Betapace
Dofetilide	Tikosyn
CLASS IV	
Calcium channel blockers	Refer to Appendix A page 348

Antilipemic Agents

Use or Condition: Elevated blood cholesterol, low-density lipoproteins, triglycerides, low high-density lipoproteins, and metabolic syndrome

Category	Drug name	Brand name[†]
A	Cholestyramine	Questran, Cholybar, Prevalite
A	Colesevelam	Welchol
A	Colestipol	Colestid
B	Clofibrate	Atromid
B	Fenofibrate	Tricor, Lofibra
B	Gemfibrozil	Lopid
C	Atorvastatin	Lipitor
C	Fluvastatin	Lescol
C	Lovastatin	Mevacor
C	Lovastatin + Niacin	Advicor
C	Pravastatin	Pravachol
C	Rosuvastatin	Crestor
C	Simvastatin	Zocor
D	Atorvastatin + Amlodipine	Caduet
E	Niacin	Niaspan, Nicobid, Slo-Niacin
F	Ezetimibe	Zetia
F	Ezetimibe + Simvasatin	Vytorin

A = Bile Acid Sequestrants, B = Fibric Acid Sequestrants, C = HMG-CoA Reductase Inhibitors, D = HMG-CoA Reductase Inhibitors + Calcium Channel Blocker, E = Nicotinic Acid, F = Cholesterol Absorption Inhibitor

Blood Modifiers (Anticoagulant or Antiplatelet)

Use or Condition: To prevent blood clots, heart attack, stroke, intermittent claudication, or vascular death in patients with established peripheral arterial disease (PAD) or acute ST-segment elevation myocardial infraction. Also, used to reduce aching, tiredness and cramps in hands and feet. Plavix is critical to maintain for one year after percutaneous coronary intervention for drug-eluting stent patency

Drug name	Brand name[†]
Cilostazol	Pletal
Clopidogrel	Plavix
Dipyridamole	Persantine
Pentoxifylline	Trental
Ticlopidine	Ticlid
Warfarin	Coumadin

Respiratory Agents

Steroidal Anti-inflammatory Agents

Use or Condition: Allergy symptoms including sneezing, itching, and runny or stuffed nose, shrink nasal polyps, various skin disorders, asthma

Drug name	Brand name[†]
Beclomethasone	Beclovent, Qvar
Budesonide	Pulmicort
Flunisolide	AeroBid
Fluticasone	Flovent
Fluticasone and salmeterol (β_2 receptor agonist)	Advair Diskus
Triamcinolone	Azmacort

Bronchodilators

Anticholinergics (Acetylcholine Receptor Antagonist)

Use or Condition: To prevent wheezing, shortness of breath, and troubled breathing caused by asthma, chronic bronchitis, emphysema, and other lung diseases

Drug name	Brand name[†]
Ipratropium	Atrovent

Anticholinergics with Sympathomimetics (β_2-Receptor Agonists)

Use or Condition: Chronic obstructive pulmonary lung disease (COPD)

Drug name	Brand name[†]
Ipratropium and Albuterol	Combivent

Sympathomimetics (β_2-Receptor Agonists)

Use or Condition: To prevent wheezing, shortness of breath, and troubled breathing caused by asthma, chronic bronchitis, emphysema, and other lung diseases

Drug name	Brand name[†]
Albuterol	Proventil, Ventolin
Metaproterenol	Alupent
Pirbuterol	Maxair
Salmeterol	Serevent
Salmeterol and Fluticasone (steroid)	Advair
Terbutaline	Brethine

Xanthine Derivatives

Use or Condition: To prevent wheezing, shortness of breath, and troubled breathing caused by asthma, chronic bronchitis, emphysema, and other lung diseases

Drug name	Brand name[†]
Theophylline	Theo-Dur, Uniphyl

Leukotriene Antagonists and Formation Inhibitors

Use or Condition: To prevent wheezing, shortness of breath, and troubled breathing caused by asthma, chronic bronchitis, emphysema, and other lung diseases

Drug name	Brand name[†]
Montelukast	Singulair
Zafirlukast	Accolate
Zileuton	Zyflo

Mast Cell Stabilizers

Use or Condition: To prevent wheezing, shortness of breath, and troubled breathing caused by asthma, chronic bronchitis, emphysema, and other lung diseases

Drug name	Brand name[†]
Cromolyn Inhaled	Intal
Nedocromil	Tilade
Omalizumab	Xolair

Antidiabetic Agents

Biguanides (Decreases hepatic glucose production and intestinal glucose absorption)

Use or Condition: Type 2 or adult onset diabetes

Drug name	Brand name[†]
Metformin	Glucophage, Riomet
Metformin and Glyburide	Glucovance

Glucosidase Inhibitors (Inhibit intestinal glucose absorption)

Use or Condition: Type 2 or adult onset diabetes

Drug name	Brand name[†]
Miglitol	Glyset

Insulins

Use or Condition: Type 1, or sometimes Type 2 or adult onset diabetes

Rapid-acting	Inter-mediate-acting	Inter-mediate- and rapid-acting combination	Long-acting
Humalog	Humulin L	Humalog Mix	Humulin U
Humulin R	Humulin N	Humalog 50/50	Lantus Injection
Novolin R	Iletin II Lente	Humalog 70/30	
Iletin II R	Iletin II NPH	Novolin 70/30	
	Novolin L		
	Nivalin N		

Meglitinides
(Stimulate pancreatic islet β cells)

Use or Condition: Type 2 or adult onset diabetes

Drug name	Brand name†
Nateglinide	Starlix
Repaglinide	Prandin, Gluconorm

Sulfonylureas
(Stimulate pancreatic islet β cells)

Use or Condition: Type 2 or adult onset diabetes

Drug name	Brand name†
Chlorpropamide*	Diabinese
Gliclazide	Diamicron
Glimepiride*	Amaryl
Glipizide*	Glucotrol
Glyburide	DiaBeta, Glynase, Micronase
Tolazamide*	Tolinase
Tolbutamide*	Orinase

* These drugs have been associated with increased cardiovascular mortality.

Thiazolidinediones
(Increase insulin sensitivity)

Use or Condition: Type 2 or adult onset diabetes

Drug name	Brand name†
Pioglitazone	Actos
Rosiglitazone	Avandia

Incretin mimetics (Increase insulin and decrease glucagon secretion)

Use or Condition: Type 2 diabetes

Drug name	Brand name†
Glucagon-like Peptide 1	Byetta

Obesity Management

Appetite Suppressants

Use or Condition: Morbid obesity and metabolic syndrome

Drug name	Brand name†
Sibutramine	Meridia

Lipase Inhibitors

Use or Condition: Morbid obesity and metabolic syndrome

Drug name	Brand name†
Orlistat	Xenical

† Represent selected brands; these are not necessarily all inclusive.

‡Adapted, by permission, from American College of Sport Medicine, *ACSM's guidelines for exercise testing and prescription*, 8th ed. (Philadelphia, PA: Lippincott, Williams, and Wilkins). (in print)

Appendix B

Effects of Medications on Heart Rate, Blood Pressure, the Electrocardiogram (ECG), and Exercise Capacity‡

‡Adapted, by permission, from American College of Sport Medicine, *ACSM's guidelines for exercise testing and prescription*, 8th ed. (Philadelphia, PA: Lippincott, Williams, and Wilkins). (in print)

Medications	Heart rate	Blood pressure	ECG	Exercise capacity
I. β-Blockers (including carvedilol and labetalol)	↓* (R and E)	↓ (R and E)	↓ HR* (R) ↓ ischemia† (E)	↑ in patients with angina; ↓ or ↔ in patients without angina
II. Nitrates	↑ (R) ↑ or ↔ (E)	↓ (R) ↓ or ↔ (E)	↑ HR (R) ↑ or ↔ HR (E) ↓ ischemia† (E)	↑ in patients with angina; ↔ in patients without angina; ↑ or ↔ in patients with chronic heart failure (CHF)
III. Calcium channel blockers				
Amlodipine Felodipine Isradipine Nicardipine Nifedipine Nimodipine Nisoldipine	↑ or ↔ (R and E)	↓ (R and E)	↑ or ↔ HR (R and E) ↓ ischemia† (E)	↑ in patients with angina; ↔ in patients without angina
Diltiazem Verapamil	↓ (R and E)		↓ HR (R and E) ↓ ischemia† (E)	
IV. Digitalis	↓ in patients with atrial fibrillation and possibly CHF Not significantly altered in patients with sinus rhythm	↔ (R and E)	May produce non-specific ST-T wave changes (R) May produce ST segment depression (E)	Improved only in patients with atrial fibrillation or in patients with CHF
V. Diuretics	↔ (R and E)	↔ or ↓ (R and E)	↔ or PVCs (R) May cause PVCs and "false-positive" test results if hypokalemia occurs May cause PVCs if hypomagnesesemia occurs (E)	↔, except possibly in patients with CHF
VI. Vasodilators, nonadrenergic	↑ or ↔ (R and E)	↓ (R and E)	↑ or ↔ HR (R and E)	↔, except ↑ or ↔ in patients with CHF
ACE inhibitors and Angiotensin II receptor blockers	↔ (R and E)	↓ (R and E)	↔ (R and E)	↔, except ↑ or ↔ in patients with CHF
α-Adrenergic blockers	↔ (R and E)	↓ (R and E)	↔ (R and E)	↔
Antiadrenergic agents without selective blockade	↓ or ↔ (R and E)	↓ (R and E)	↓ or ↔ HR (R and E)	↔

(continued)

(continued)

Medications	Heart rate	Blood pressure	ECG	Exercise capacity
VII. Antiarrhythmic agents	All antiarrhythmic agents may cause new or worsened arrhythmias (proarrhythmic effect)			
Class I				
Quinidine	↑ or ↔ (R and E)	↓ or ↔ (R)	↑ or ↔ HR (R)	↔
Disopyramide		↔ (E)	May prolong QRS and QT intervals (R)	
			Quinidine may result in "false-negative" test results (E)	
Procainamide	↔ (R and E)	↔ (R and E)	May prolong QRS and QT intervals (R)	↔
			May result in "false-positive" test results (E)	
Phenytoin				
Tocainide	↔ (R and E)	↔ (R and E)	↔ (R and E)	↔
Mexiletine				
Moricizine	↔ (R and E)	↔ (R and E)	May prolong QRS and QT intervals (R)	↔
			↔ (E)	
Propafenone	↓ (R)	↔ (R and E)	↓ HR (R)	↔
	↓ or ↔ (E)		↓ or ↔ HR (E)	
Class II				
β-Blockers (see I.)				
Class III				
Amiodarone	↓ (R and E)	↔ (R and E)	↓ HR (R)	↔
Sotalol			↔ (E)	
Class IV				
Calcium channel blockers (see III.)				
VIII. Bronchodilators	↔ (R and E)	↔ (R and E)	↔ (R and E)	Bronchodilators ↑ exercise capacity in patients limited by bronchospasm
Anticholinergic agents	↑ or ↔ (R and E)	↔	↑ or ↔ HR	
Xanthine derivatives			May produce PVCs (R and E)	
Sympathomimetic agents	↑ or ↔ (R and E)	↑, ↔, or ↓ (R and E)	↑ or ↔ HR (R and E)	↔
Cromolyn sodium	↔ (R and E)	↔ (R and E)	↔ (R and E)	↔
Steroidal Anti-inflamatory Agents	↔ (R and E)	↔ (R and E)	↔ (R and E)	↔
IX. Antilipemic agents	Clofibrate may provoke arrhythmias, angina in patients with prior myocardial infarction			↔
	Nicotinic acid may ↓ BP			
	All other hyperlipidemic agents have no effect on HR, BP, and ECG			

Medications	Heart Rate	Blood Pressure	ECG	Exercise Capacity
X. Psychotropic medications				
Minor tranquilizers	May ↓ HR and BP by controlling anxiety; no other effects			
Antidepressants	↑ or ↔ (R and E)	↓ or ↔ (R and E)	Variable (R)	
Major tranquilizers	↑ or ↔ (R and E)	↓ or ↔ (R and E)	Variable (R)	
Lithium	↔ (R and E)	↔ (R and E)	May result in T wave changes and arrhythmias (R and E)	
XI. Nicotine	↑ or ↔ (R and E)	↑ (R and E)	↑ or ↔ HR May provoke ischemia, arrhythmias (R and E)	↔, except ↓ or ↔ in patients with angina
XII. Antihistamines	↔ (R and E)	↔ (R and E)	↔ (R and E)	↔
XIII. Cold medications with sympathomimetic agents	Effects similar to those described in sympathomimetic agents, although magnitude of effects is usually smaller			↔
XIV. Thyroid medications Only levothyroxine	↑ (R and E)	↑ HR	May provoke arrhythmias ↑ ischemia (R and E)	↔, unless angina worsened
XV. Alcohol	↔ (R and E)	Chronic use may have role in ↑ BP (R and E)	May provoke arrhythmias (R and E)	↔
XVI. Hypoglycemic agents Insulin and oral agents	↔ (R and E)	↔ (R and E)	↔ (R and E)	↔
XVII. Blood Modifiers (Anticoagulants and Antiplatelets)	↔ (R and E)	↔ (R and E)	↔ (R and E)	↑ or ↔ in patients limited by intermittent claudication (for cilostazol only)
XVIII. Pentoxifylline	↔ (R and E)	↔ (R and E)	↔ (R and E)	↔ in patients limited by intermittent claudication
XIX. Anti-gout medications	↔ (R and E)	↔ (R and E)	↔ (R and E)	↔
XX. Caffeine	Variable effects depending on previous use		May provoke arrhythmias	Variable effects on exercise capacity
XXI. Anorexiants/diet pills	↑ or ↔ (R and E)	↑ or ↔ HR (R and E)	↑ or ↔ HR (R and E)	Increased HR and BP common with norepinephrine re-uptake inhibitors (e.g., sibutramine)

Abbreviations: PVCs = premature ventricular contractions; ↑ = increase; ↔ = no effect; ↓ = decrease; R = rest; E = exercise; HR = heart rate)

*β-Blockers with ISA lower resting HR only slightly.

†May prevent or delay myocardial ischemia (see text).

‡Adapted, by permission, from American College of Sport Medicine, *ACSM's guidelines for exercise testing and prescription*, 8th ed. (Philadelphia, PA: Lippincott, Williams, and Wilkins). (in print)

References

Chapter 1

1. American Association of Cardiovascular and Pulmonary Rehabilitation. *Guidelines for Cardiac Rehabilitation Programs*. Champaign, IL: Human Kinetics; 1991.
2. American Association of Cardiovascular and Pulmonary Rehabilitation Outcomes Committee. *AACVPR Tools Research Guide*. Middleton, WI: American Association of Cardiovascular and Pulmonary Rehabilitation; 1996.
3. American College of Sports Medicine. *Guidelines for Graded Exercise Testing and Prescription*. Philadelphia: Lea & Febiger; 1975.
4. American Heart Association. *Exercise Testing and Training of Apparently Healthy Individuals: A Handbook for Physicians*. New York: American Heart Association; 1972.
5. American Heart Association. *Exercise Testing and Training of Individuals with Heart Disease or at High Risk for Its Development. A Handbook for Physicians*. Dallas: American Heart Association; 1975.
6. Astrand PO, Rhymin I. A monogram for calculation of aerobic capacity (physical fitness) from pulse rate during sub maximal work. *J Appl Physiol* 1954;7:218.
7. Chapman C, Fraser R. Studies on the effect of exercise on cardiovascular functions: cardiovascular responses to exercise in patients with healed myocardial infarction. *Circulation* 1954;9:347-351.
8. Coats AJS, Adamopoulos S, Meyer TE, Conway J, Sleight P. Effects of physical training in chronic heart failure. *Lancet* 1990;335:63-66.
9. Delorme T. Restoration of muscle power by heavy resistance exercises. *J Bone Joint Surg* 1945;27:645-649.
10. Froelicher VF, Pollock ML. Cardiac rehabilitation: a new forum. *J Cardiac Rehabil* 1981;1:11-12.
11. Gottheiner V. Long range strenuous sports training for cardiac reconditioning and rehabilitation. *Am J Cardiol* 1968;22:426-435.
12. Hamm LF, Kavanaugh T, Campbell RC, et al. Timeline for peak improvements during 52 weeks of outpatient cardiac rehabilitation. *J Cardiopulm Rehabil* 2004;24:374-382.
13. Haskell W. Cardiovascular complications during training of cardiac patients. *Circulation* 1978;57:920-924.
14. Heberden W. Pectoris dolor. In: *Commentaries on the History and Cure of Diseases*. London: T. Payne; 1802:362-369.
15. Hellerstein HK, Goldstein E. Rehabilitation of patients with heart disease. *Postgrad Med* 1954;15:265-278.
16. Hilton J. *Rest and Pain*. London: Bell; 1863.
17. Kavanagh T, Mertens DJ, Hamm LF, et al. Prediction of long term prognosis in 12,169 men referred for cardiac rehabilitation. *Circulation* 2002;106:666-671.
18. Kavanagh T, Shephard RJ, Pandit V. Marathon running after myocardial infarction. *JAMA* 1974;229:1602-1605.
19. Kavanagh T, Yacoub M, Mertens DJ, Kennedy J, Campbell RC, Sawyer P. Cardiovascular responses to exercise training after orthotopic cardiac transplantation. *Circulation* 1988;77:162-171.
20. Levine SA, Lown B. Armchair treatment of acute coronary thrombosis. *JAMA* 1952;48:1365-1367.
21. Mathes P, Halhuber MJ. *Controversies in Cardiac Rehabilitation*. New York: Springer-Verlag; 1982.
22. Miller HS, Wilson PK. *Certification: How It Began Thirty Years Ago. American College of Sports Medicine Certified News*. Indianapolis: ACSM; 2003.
23. Mulcahy R, Mickey N. The rehabilitation of patients with coronary heart disease. *Scand J Rehab Med* 1970;2/3:108.
24. Oertel M. Therapie der Krelslaufstorungen. In: Ziemssen J, ed. *Handbuch der allgemeinen therapie*. Leipzig: Vogel; 1875.
25. Pashkow P, Ades PA, Emery CF, et al. Outcome measurement in cardiac and pulmonary rehabilitation. *J Cardiopulm Rehabil* 1995;15:394-405.
26. Schott T. On the treatment of chronic diseases of the heart. *Boston Meg Surg J* 1907;156:623-629.
27. Southard DR, Certo C, Comoss P, et al. Core competencies for cardiac rehabilitation. *J Cardiopul Rehabil* 1994;14:87-92.
28. Stokes, W. *The Diseases of the Heart and the Aorta*. Dublin: Hodges and Smith; 1854.
29. Stone JA, Arthur HM, Canadian Association of Cardiac Rehabilitation. *Canadian Guidelines for Cardiac Rehabilitation and Cardiovascular Disease Prevention*. Winnipeg: CACR; 2004.

30. Taylor RS, Brown A, Ebrahim S, et al. Exercise based rehabilitation for patients with coronary heart disease: systematic review and meta analysis of randomized controlled trials. *Am J Med* 2004;116:682-692.

31. Thomas RJ, Witt BJ, Lopez-Jimenez F, King ML, Squires RW. Quality indicators in cardiovascular care: a case for cardiac rehabilitation. *J Cardiopulm Rehabil* 2005;25:249-256.

32. U.S. Department of Health and Human Services. *Recovering From Heart Problems Through Cardiac Rehabilitation. Cardiac Rehabilitation, Patient Guide*. Washington, DC: U.S. Department of Health and Human Services, Public Health Service, Agency for Health Care Policy and Research, and the National Heart, Lung and Blood Institute (96-0674); October 1995.

33. Vanhees L, McGee HM, Dugmore LD, et al. *The Carinex Survey: Current Guidelines and Practices in Cardiac Rehabilitation within Europe*. Leuven: ACCO; 1999.

34. Wenger NK, Froelicher ES, Smith LK, et al. *Cardiac Rehabilitation. Clinical Practice Guideline, (No. 17)*. Washington, DC: U.S. Department of Health and Human Services, Public Health Service, Agency for Health Care Policy and Research, and the National Heart, Lung and Blood Institute (96-0672); October 1995.

35. Wenger NK, Froelicher ES, Smith LK, et al. *Cardiac Rehabilitation as Secondary Prevention. Clinical Practice Guideline. Quick Reference Guide for Clinician (No. 17)*. Washington, DC: U.S. Department of Health and Human Services, Public Health Services, Agency for Health Care Policy and Research, and the National Heart, Lung and Blood Institute (96-0673); October 1995.

36. Wilson PK, Williams MA, Humphrey R, Hodgkin JE, Lui K. *Contemporary Cardiovascular and Pulmonary Rehabilitation: AACVPR, The First Twenty Years*. Tampa: Faircount LLC; 2005.

37. Zander G. *L'Etablissement deique Medicale Mechanique*. Paris; 1879.

Chapter 2

1. Blair SN, Kohl HW, Paffenbarger RS Jr, et al. Physical fitness and all-cause mortality: a prospective study of healthy men and women. *JAMA* 1989;262:2395-2401.

2. Castelli WP. Cholesterol and lipids in the risk of coronary artery disease—the Framingham heart study. *Can J Cardiol* 1988;4(suppl A):5A-10A.

3. Eaton SB, Konner M, Shostak M. Stone agers in the fast lane: chronic degenerative diseases in evolutionary perspective. *Am J Med* 1988;84:739-749.

4. Flegal KM, Carroll MD, Kuczmarski RJ, Johnson CL. Overweight and obesity in the United States: prevalence and trends, 1960-1994. *Int J Obes* 1988;22:39-47.

5. Greenland P, Knoll MD, Stamler J, et al. Major risk factors as antecedents of fatal and nonfatal coronary heart disease events. *JAMA* 2003;290:891-897.

6. Gregg EW, Cheng YJ, Cadwell BL, et al. Secular trends in cardiovascular disease risk factors according to body mass index in U.S. adults. *JAMA* 2005;293:1868-1874.

7. Grundy SM, Pasternak R, Greenland P, et al. Assessment of cardiovascular risk by use of multiple risk factor assessment equations: a statement for healthcare professionals by the American Heart Association and American College of Cardiology. *Circulation* 1999;100:1481-1492.

8. Hahn RA, Teutsch SM, Rothenberg RB, Marks JS. Excess deaths from nine chronic diseases in the United States, 1986. *JAMA* 1990;264:2654-2659.

9. Ham SA, Yore MM, Fulton JE, Kohl HW. Prevalence of no leisure-time physical activity—35 states and the District of Columbia, 1988-2002. *MMWR* 2004;53:82-86.

10. Hu G, Sarti C, Jousilahti P, et al. Leisure time, occupational, and commuting physical activity and the risk of stroke. *Stroke* 2005;36:1994-1999.

11. Jurca R, LaMonte MJ, Durstine DL. Physical activity and nontraditional CHD risk factors: new pathways for primordial prevention of coronary heart disease. *PCPFS Res Digest* 2005;6:1-8.

12. Kannel WB. Bishop lecture: contribution of the Framingham study to preventive cardiology. *J Am Coll Cardiol* 1990;15:206-211.

13. Khot UM, Khot MB, Bajzer CT, et al. Prevalence of conventional risk factors in patients with coronary heart disease. *JAMA* 2003;290:898-904.

14. Kohl HW III. Physical activity and cardiovascular disease: evidence for a dose response. *Med Sci Sports Exerc* 2001;33:S472-S483.

15. Kruger J, Ham SA, Kohl HW. Trends in leisure-time physical inactivity by age, sex, and race/ethnicity—United States, 1994-2004. *MMWR* 2005;54:991-994.

16. Labarthe DR. *Epidemiology and Prevention of Cardiovascular Diseases*. Gaithersburg, MD: Aspen; 1998.

17. LaMonte MJ, Jurca R, Kampert JB, et al. Exercise tolerance adds prognostic value to the Framingham risk score in asymptomatic women and men. *Circulation* 2005;112(suppl II):II-829.

18. Lauer MS, Froelicher ES, Williams M, Kligfield P. Exercise testing in asymptomatic adults: a statement for professionals from the American Heart Association Council on Clinical Cardiology, Subcommittee on Exercise, Cardiac Rehabilitation, and Prevention. *Circulation* 2005;112:771-776.

19. Lee CD, Folsom AR, Blair SN. Physical activity and stroke risk: a meta-analysis. *Stroke* 2003;34:2475-2482.

20. Lee IM, Sesso HD, Oguma Y, Paffenbarger RS Jr. Relative intensity of physical activity and risk of coronary heart disease. *Circulation* 2003;107:1110-1116.

21. Lloyd-Jones DM, Larson MG, Beiser A, Levy D. Lifetime risk of developing coronary heart disease. *Lancet* 1999;353:89-92.

22. Manson JE, Hu FB, Rich-Edwards JW, et al. A prospective study of walking as compared with vigorous exercise in the prevention of coronary heart disease in women. *N Engl J Med* 1999;341:650-658.

23. Manson JE, Greenland P, LaCroix AZ, et al. Walking compared with vigorous exercise for the prevention of cardiovascular events in women. *N Engl J Med* 2002;347:716-725.

24. McGovern PG, Jacobs DR Jr, Shahar E, et al. Trends in acute coronary heart disease mortality, morbidity, and medical care from 1985-1997: the Minnesota Heart Survey. *Circulation* 2001;104:19-24.

25. National Center for Health Statistics (NCHS). Data-Warehouse. www.cdc.gov/nchs/datawh.htm.

26. Ogden CL, Carroll MD, Curtain LR, et al. Prevalence of overweight and obesity in the United States, 1999-2004. *JAMA* 2006;295:1549-1555.

27. Paffenbarger RS Jr, Hyde RT, Wing AL, et al. The association of changes in physical activity levels and other lifestyle characteristics with mortality among men. *N Engl J Med* 1993;328:538-545.

28. Paffenbarger RS Jr, Hyde RT, Wing AL, Steinmetz CH. A natural history of athleticism and cardiovascular health. *JAMA* 1984;252:491-495.

29. Rosamond WD, Chambless LE, Folsom AR, et al. Trends in the incidence of myocardial infarction and in mortality due to coronary heart disease, 1987-1994. *N Engl J Med* 1998;339:861-867.

30. Seshadri S, Beiser A, Kelly-Hayes M, et al. Lifetime risk of stroke: estimates from the Framingham study. *Stroke* 2006;37:345-350.

31. Stamler J, Stamler R, Neaton JD, et al. Low risk-factor profile and long-term cardiovascular and non-cardiovascular mortality and life expectancy. *JAMA* 1999;282:2012-2018.

32. Tanasescu M, Leitzmann MF, Rimm EB, et al. Exercise type and intensity in relation to coronary heart disease in men. *JAMA* 2002;288:1994-2000.

33. Thom T, Haase N, Rosamond W, et al. 2006. Heart disease and stroke statistics—2006 update. A report from the American Heart Association Statistics Committee and Stroke Statistics Subcommittee. *Circulation* 2006;113:85-151.

34. Thompson PD, Buchner D, Pina IL, et al. Exercise and physical activity in the prevention and treatment of atherosclerotic cardiovascular disease: a statement from the Council on Clinical Cardiology (Subcommittee on Exercise, Rehabilitation, and Prevention) and the Council on Nutrition, Physical Activity, and Metabolism (Subcommittee on Physical Activity). *Circulation* 2003;107:3109-3116.

35. U.S. Department of Health and Human Services. *Physical activity and health: a report of the Surgeon General.* Atlanta, GA: U.S. Department of Health and Human Services, Centers for Disease Control and Prevention, National Center for Chronic Disease Prevention and Health Promotion; 1996.

36. Weller I, Corey P. The impact of excluding non-leisure energy expenditure on the relation between physical activity and mortality in women. *Epidemiology* 1998;9:632-635.

37. Wright JD, Kennedy-Stephenson J, Wang CY, McDowell MA, Johnson CL. Trends in intake of energy and macronutrients—United States, 1971-2000. *MMWR* 2004;53:80-82.

38. Yusuf S, Reddy S, Ounpuu S, Anand S. Global burden of cardiovascular diseases. Part I: general considerations, the epidemiologic transition, risk factors, and impact of urbanization. *Circulation* 2001;104:2764-2753.

Chapter 3

1. Adams F. *The Genuine Works of Hippocrates, Translated From the Greek With a Preliminary Discourse and Annotations.* London: Sydenham Society; 1849.

2. Agency for Health Care Policy and Research. *Clinical Guideline 13: Cardiac Rehabilitation.* Washington, DC: U.S. Dept. of Health and Human Services; 1996.

3. Berryman JW. *Out of Many, One: A History of the American College of Sports Medicine.* Champaign, IL: Human Kinetics; 1995.

4. Blakewell, S. Illustrations from the Wellcome Institute Library: medical gymnastics and the Cyriax collection. *Medical History* 1997;41:487-495.

5. Bouman HD. Delineating the dilemma. *Am J Phys Med* 1967;46:26-31.

6. Durstine JL, Moore GE, eds. *ACSM's Exercise Management in Persons With Chronic Diseases and Disabilities.* 2nd ed. Champaign, IL: Human Kinetics; 2003.

7. Fye WB. *American Cardiology: The History of a Specialty and Its College.* Baltimore: Johns Hopkins University Press; 1996.

8. Heberden W. Some account of a disorder of the breast. *Medical Transactions of the Royal College of Physicians* 1772;2:59-67.

9. Hirt S. Historical bases for therapeutic exercise. *Am J Phys Med* 1967;46:32-38.

10. Kornblueh IH. The future of physical medicine XIII: rehabilitation medicine in a changing world. *Am J Phys Med* 1967;46:1458-1461.

11. Koshland DE Jr. The molecule of the year. *Science* 1992;258:1861.

12. Kraus H. *Principles and Practice of Therapeutic Exercises.* Springfield, IL: Charles C Thomas; 1949.

13. Levine SA, Lown B. "Armchair" treatment of acute coronary thrombosis. *JAMA* 1952;148:1356-1369.

14. Licht S. History. In: *Therapeutic Exercise.* 2nd ed, rev. New Haven, CT: Elizabeth Licht; 1965:426-471.

15. Mallory GK, White PD, Salcedo-Salgar J. The speed of healing on myocardial infarction: a study of the pathologic anatomy in seventy-two cases. *Am Heart J* 1939;18:647-656.

16. Naughton J, Hellerstein HK, eds. *Exercise Testing and Exercise Training in Coronary Heart Disease* (Airlie conference in exercise testing and training of patients). New York: Academic Press; 1973.

17. Osler, W. *The Principles and Practice of Medicine: Designed for the Use of Practitioners and Students of Medicine.* 7th ed. New York: Appleton; 1909.

18. Plato. Translator unknown. The arts in education. In: *The Republic.* Stephanus, 399, circa 360 BC.

19. Saltin B, Blomqvist G, Mitchell JH, Johnson RL Jr, Wildenthal K, Chapman CB. Response to exercise after bed rest and after training: a longitudinal study of adaptive changes in oxygen transport and body composition. *Circulation* 1968;38(5 suppl vii):VII-1-VII-78.

20. White PD, Rusk HA, Williams B, Lee PR. *Rehabilitation of the Cardiovascular Patient.* New York: McGraw-Hill; 1958.

Chapter 4

1. Blackburn H. The concept of risk. In: Pearson TA, Criqui MH, Luepker, RV, et al. eds. *Primer in Preventive Cardiology.* Dallas: American Heart Association; 1994:25-41.

2. Bodenheimer T, Wagner EH, Grumbach K. Improving primary care for patients with chronic disease. *JAMA* 2002;288:1775-1779.

3. Dahlöf B, Sever PS, Poulter NR, et al. Prevention of cardiovascular events with an antihypertensive regimen of amlodipine adding perindopril as required versus atenolol adding bendoflumethiazide as required, in the Anglo-Scandinavian Cardiac Outcomes Trial-Blood Pressure Lowering Arm (ASCOT-BPLA): a multicentre randomized controlled trial. *Lancet* 2005;366:895-906.

4. Elliott WJ, Meyer PM. Incident diabetes in clinical trials of antihypertensive drugs: a network meta-analysis. *Lancet* 2007;369:201-207.

5. Expert Panel on Detection, Evaluation and Treatment of High Blood Cholesterol in Adults. Executive Summary of the Third Report of the Expert Panel on Detection, Evaluation, and Treatment of High Blood Cholesterol (Adult Treatment Panel III). *JAMA* 2001;285:2486-2487.

6. Ford ES, Giles WH, Dietz WH. Prevalence of the metabolic syndrome among US adults. *JAMA* 2002;287:356-359.

7. Greenland P, O'Malley PG. When is a new prediction marker useful? *Arch Intern Med* 2005;165:2454-2456.

8. Grundy SM, Pasternack R, Greenland P, et al. Assessment of cardiovascular risk by use of multiple risk factor assessment equations. *Circulation* 1999;100:1481-1492.

9. Grundy SM, Cleeman JI, Merz CN, et al. Implications of recent clinical trials for the National Cholesterol Education Program Adult Treatment Panel III Guidelines. *Circulation* 2004;110:227-239.

10. Hayden M, Pignone M, Phillips C, et al. Aspirin for the primary prevention of cardiovascular events: a summary of the evidence from the U.S. preventive services task force. *Ann Intern Med* 2002;136:161-172.

11. Hennekens CH, Sacks FM, Tonkin A, et al. Additive benefits of pravastatin and aspirin to decrease risks of cardiovascular disease: randomized and observational comparisons of secondary prevention trials and their meta-analyses. *Arch Intern Med* 2004;164:40-44.

12. Klatsky AL, Armstrong MA, Friedman GD. Alcohol and total mortality. *Ann Intern Med* 1992;117:646-654.

13. Knowler WC, Barrett-Connor E, Fowler SE, et al. Reduction in the incidence of type 2 diabetes with lifestyle intervention or metformin. *N Engl J Med* 2002;346:393-403.

14. MacKay J, Mensah G, Mendis S, et al. *The Atlas of Heart Disease and Stroke.* Geneva, Switzerland: World Health Organization; 2004.

15. Murray DM, Luepker RV, Pirie PL, et al. Systematic risk factor screening and education: a community-wide approach to prevention of coronary heart disease. *Prev Med* 1986;15:661-672.

16. Pearson TA, Mensah GA, Alexander RW, et al. Markers of inflammation and cardiovascular disease: application to clinical and public health practice. *Circulation* 2003;107:499-511.

17. Pearson TA, Jamison DT, Trejo-Gutierrez J. Cardiovascular disease. In: Jamison DT, Mosley WH, Measham AR, Bobadilla JL, eds. *Disease Control Priorities in Developing Countries.* New York: Oxford University Press; 1993:577-594.

18. Pearson TA, Blair SN, Daniels SR, et al. AHA guidelines for primary prevention of cardiovascular disease and stroke: 2002 update. *Circulation* 2002;106:388-391.

19. Pearson TA, New tools for coronary risk assessment: what are their advantages and limitations? *Circulation* 2002;105:886-892.

20. Pepe MS, Janes H, Longton G, et al. Limitations of the odds ratio in gauging the performance of a diagnostic, prognostic and screening marker. *Am J Epidemiol* 2005;159:882-890.

21. The Pooling Project Research Group: Relationship of blood pressure, serum cholesterol, smoking habit, relative weight, and ECG abnormalities to incidence of major coronary events: final report of the Pooling Project. *J. Chronic Dis* 1978;31:201-306.

22. Poulter NR, Wedel H, Dahlöf B, et al. Role of blood pressure and other variables in the differential cardiovascular event rates noted in the Anglo-Scandinavian Cardiac Outcomes Trial-Blood Pressure Lowering Arm (ASCOT-BPLA) *Lancet* 2005;366:907-913.

23. Sacks FM, Svetkey LP, Vollmer WM, et al. From the DASH-Sodium Collaborative Research Group. Effects on blood pressure of reduced dietary sodium and the Dietary Approaches to Stop Hypertension (DASH) diet. *N Engl J Med* 2001;344:3-10.

24. Smith SC Jr, Allen J, Blair SN, et al. AHA/ACC guidelines for secondary prevention for patients with coronary and other atherosclerotic vascular disease: 2006 update. *Circulation* 2006;113:2363-2372.

25. Tuomilehto J, Lindstrom J, Eriksson JG, et al. Prevention of type 2 diabetes mellitus by changes in lifestyle among subjects with impaired glucose tolerance. *N Engl J Med* 2001;344:1343-1350.

26. Wilson PWF, Nam B-H, Pencina M, et al. C-reactive protein and risk of cardiovascular disease in men and women from the Framingham Heart Study. *Arch Int Med* 2005;165:2473-2478.

27. United States Department of Health, Education, and Welfare. *Smoking and Health: Report of the Advisory Committee to the Surgeon General.* Washington, DC: Public Health Service; 1964.

Chapter 5

1. Ades PA, Balady GJ, Berra K. Transforming exercise-based cardiac rehabilitation programs into secondary prevention centers: a national imperative. *J Cardiopulm Rehabil* 2001;21:263-272.

2. American Diabetes Association position statement: standards of medical care in diabetes. *Diabetes Care* 2006;29:S4-S42.

3. Balady G, Ades P, Comoss P, et al. Core components of cardiac rehabilitation/secondary prevention programs: a statement for healthcare professionals from the American Heart Association and the American Association of Cardiovascular and Pulmonary Rehabilitation Writing Group. *J Cardiopulm Rehabil* 2000;20:310-316.

4. Balady G, Ades P, Comoss P, et al. Core components of cardiac rehabilitation/secondary prevention programs: a statement for healthcare professionals from the American Heart Association and the American Association of Cardiovascular and Pulmonary Rehabilitation Writing Group. *Circulation* 2000;102:1069-1073.

5. Chobanian AV, et al. National High Blood Pressure Education Program Coordinating Committee. The seventh report of the Joint National Committee on Prevention, Detection, Evaluation and Treatment of High Blood Pressure: The JNC-7 Report. *Hypertension* 2003;42:1206-1222.

6. Eaton CB, Galliher JM, McBride PE, et al. Family physician's knowledge, beliefs, and self-reported practice patterns regarding hyperlipidemia: a National Research Network (NRN) survey. *J Am Board Fam Med* 2006;19:46-53.

7. Executive summary of the third report of the National Cholesterol Education Program (NCEP) Expert Panel on Detection, Evaluation, and Treatment of High Blood Cholesterol in Adults (Adult Treatment Panel III). *JAMA* 2001;285:2486-2497.

8. Feigenbaum MS, Martin SP, Robertson N, et al. Closing the treatment gap with South Carolina's upstate HeartCare partnership. *Circulation* 2003:108:IV-759.

9. Goff DC Jr, Bertoni AG, Kramer H, et al. Dyslipidemia prevalence, treatment, and control in the Multi-Ethnic Study of Atherosclerosis (MESA): gender, ethnicity, and coronary artery calcium. *Circulation* 2006;113:647-656.

10. Gordon NF, Haskell WL Comprehensive cardiovascular risk reduction in a cardiac rehabilitation setting. *Am J Cardiol* 1997;80:69H-73H.

11. Grundy SM, Cleeman JI, Merz CN, et al. Implications of recent clinical trials for the National Cholesterol Education Program Adult Treatment Panel III Guidelines. *Circulation* 2004;110:227-239.

12. LaBresh KA, Ellrodt AG, Glicklich R. Get with the guidelines for cardiovascular secondary prevention: pilot results. *Arch Intern* 2004;164:203-209.

13. Lear SA, Spinelli JJ, Linden W, et al. The Extensive Lifestyle Management Intervention (ELMI) after cardiac rehabilitation: a 4-year randomized controlled trial. *Am Heart J* 2006;152:333-339.

14. Meis SB, Snow R, LaLonde M, et al. A systematic approach to improve lipids in coronary artery disease patients participating in a cardiac rehabilitation program. *J Cardiopulm Rehabil* 2006;26:355-360.

15. O'Connor GT, Buring JE, Yusus F, et al. An overview of randomized trials of rehabilitation with exercise after myocardial infarction. *Circulation* 1989;80:234-244.

16. Oldridge NB, Guyatt GH, Fischer ME, Rimm AA. Cardiac rehabilitation after myocardial infarction: combined experience of randomized clinical trials. *JAMA.* 1988;260:945-950.

17. Persell SD, Lloyd-Jones DM, Baker DW. Implications of changing national cholesterol education program goals for the treatment and control of hypercholesterolemia. *J Gen Intern Med* 2006;21:171-176.

18. Roumie CL, Elasy TA, Greevy R, et al. Improving blood pressure control through provider education, provider alerts, and patient education: a cluster randomized trial. *Ann Intern Med* 2006;145:165-175.

19. Sanderson BK, Southard D, Oldridge N. AACVPR consensus statement: outcomes evaluation in cardiac rehabilitation/secondary prevention programs. *J Cardiopul Rehabil* 2004;24:68-79.

20. Smith SC, Allen J, Blair SN, et al. AHA/ACC guidelines for secondary prevention for patients with coronary and other atherosclerotic vascular disease: 2006 update. *Circulation* 2006;113:2263-2372.

21. Thom T, Haase N, Rosamond W, et al. AHA heart disease and stroke statistics—2006 update. *Circulation* 2006;113:85-151.

22. Wenger NK, Froelicher ES, Smith LK, et al. *Cardiac Rehabilitation Clinical Practice Guidelines* (AHCPR publication 96-0672). Rockville, MD: Agency for Health Care Policy and Research and the National Heart, Lung, and Blood Institute; October 1995.

Chapter 6

1. Brown MS, Goldstein JL. How LDL receptor influence cholesterol and atherosclerosis. *Sci Am* 1984;251:58-66.

2. Davies MJ. Coronary disease: the pathophysiology of acute coronary syndromes. *Heart* 2000;83:361-366.

3. Davies MJ, Thomas A. Thrombosis and acute coronary-artery lesions in sudden cardiac ischemic death. *N Engl J Med* 1984;310:1137-1140.

4. Dollar AL, Kragel AH, Fernicola DJ, et al. Composition of atherosclerotic plaques in coronary arteries in women <40 years of age with fatal coronary artery disease and implications for plaque reversibility. *Am J Cardiol* 1991;67:1223-1227.

5. Gertz SD, Kragel AH, Kalan JM, et al, and the TIMI investigators. Comparison of coronary and myocardial morphologic findings in patients with and without thrombolytic therapy during fatal first acute myocardial infarction. *Am J Cardiol* 1990;66:904-909.

6. Gertz SD, Malekzadeh S, Dollar AL, et al. Composition of atherosclerotic plaques in the four major epicardial coronary arteries in patients {90 years of age. *Am J Cardiol* 1991;67:1228-1233.

7. Kragel AH, Gertz SD, Roberts WC. Morphologic comparison of frequency and types of acute lesions in the major epicardial coronary arteries in unstable angina pectoris, sudden coronary death and acute myocardial infarction. *J Am Coll Cardiol* 1991;18:801-808.

8. Kragel AH, Reddy SG, Wittes JT, Roberts WC. Morphometric analysis of the composition of coronary arterial plaques in isolated unstable angina pectoris with pain at rest. *Am J Cardiol* 1990;66:562-567.

9. Kragel AH, Roberts WC. Composition of atherosclerotic plaques in the coronary arteries in homozygous familial hypercholesterolemia. *Am Heart J* 1991;121:210-211.

10. Mautner SL, Lin F, Mautner GC, Roberts WC. Comparison in women versus men of composition of atherosclerotic plaques in native coronary arteries and in saphenous veins used at aortocoronary conduits. *J Am Coll Cardiol* 1993;21:1312-1318.

11. Mautner SL, Lin F, Roberts WC. Composition of atherosclerotic plaques in the epicardial coronary arteries in juvenile (type 1) diabetes mellitus. *Am J Cardiol* 1992;70:1264-1268.

12. Mautner SL, Mautner GC, Hunsberger SA, Roberts WC. Comparison of composition of atherosclerotic plaques in saphenous veins used as aortocoronary bypass conduits with plaques in native coronary arteries in the same men. *Am J Cardiol* 1992;70:1380-1387.

13. Mautner GC, Mautner SL, Lin F, et al. Amounts of coronary arterial luminal narrowing and composition of the material causing the narrowing in Buerger's Disease. *Am J Cardiol* 1993;71:486-490.

14. Roberts WC. Atherosclerosis: its cause and its prevention. *Am J Cardiol* 2006;98:1550-1555.

15. Roberts WC. Qualitative and quantitative comparison of amounts of narrowing by atherosclerotic plaques in the major epicardial coronary arteries at necropsy in sudden coronary death, transmural acute myocardial infarction, transmural healed myocardial infarction and unstable angina pectoris. *Am J Cardiol* 1989;64:324-328.

16. Roberts WC, Jones AA. Quantitation of coronary arterial narrowing at necropsy in sudden coronary death: analysis of 31 patients and comparison with 25 control subjects. *Am J Cardiol* 1979;44:39-45.

17. Roberts WC, Jones AA. Quantification of coronary arterial narrowing at necropsy in acute myocardial infarction: analysis and comparison of findings in 27 patients and 22 controls. *Circulation* 1980;61:786-790.

18. Roberts WC, Ko JM, Pearl GJ. Abdominal aortic aneurysm in nonagenarians. *Am J Geriatr Cardiol* 2006;15:319-321.

19. Roberts WC, Ko JM, Pearl GJ. Morphologic features of atherosclerotic plaque in occlusive femoral artery disease treated by endarterectomy. *Am J Geriatr Cardiol* 2008;17:50-52.

20. Roberts WC, Ko JM, Pearl GJ. Relation of weights of intra-aneurysmal thrombi to maximal right-to-left diameters of abdominal aortic aneurysms. *Am J Cardiol* 2006;98:1519-1524.

21. Roberts WC, Kragel AH, Gertz SD, Roberts CS. Coronary arteries in unstable angina pectoris, acute myocardial infarction, and sudden coronary death. *Am Heart J* 1994;127:1588-1593.

22. Roberts WC, Laborde NJ, Pearl GJ. Frequency and extent of media in the internal carotid artery in "endarterectomy" specimens. *Am J Cardiol* 2007;99:990-992.

23. Roberts WC, Turnage TA, Whiddon LL. Quantitative comparison of amounts of cross-sectional area narrowing in coronary endarterectomy specimens in patients having coronary artery bypass grafting to amounts of narrowing in the same artery in patients with fatal coronary artery disease studied at necropsy. *Am J Cardiol* 2007;99:588-592.

24. Roberts WC, Virmani R. Quantification of coronary arterial narrowing in clinically-isolated unstable angina pectoris: an analysis of 22 necropsy patients. *Am J Med* 1979;67:792-799.

25. Virmani R, Kolodgie FD, Burke AP, et al. Lessons from sudden coronary death: a comprehensive morphological classification scheme for atherosclerotic lesions. *Arterioscler Thromb Vasc Biol* 2000;20:1262-1275.

Chapter 7

1. Albert MA, Glynn RJ, Ridker PM. Alcohol consumption and plasma concentration of C-reactive protein. *Circulation* 2003;107:443-447.

2. Albert MA, Glynn RJ, Wolfert RL, Ridker PM. The effect of statin therapy on lipoprotein associated phospholipase A2 levels. *Atherosclerosis* 2005;182:193-198.

3. Apple FS, Wu AH, Mair J, et al. Committee on Standardization of Markers of Cardiac Damage of the IFCC: future biomarkers for detection of ischemia and risk stratification in acute coronary syndrome. *Clin Chem* 2005;51:810-824.

4. Bajaj M, Suraamornkul S, Piper P, et al. Decreased plasma adiponectin concentrations are closely related

to hepatic fat content and hepatic insulin resistance in pioglitazone-treated type 2 diabetic patients. *J Clin Endocrinol Metab* 2004;89:200-206.

5. Baldus S, Heeschen C, Meinertz T, et al. CAPTURE Investigators. Myeloperoxidase serum levels predict risk in patients with acute coronary syndromes. *Circulation* 2003;108:1440-1445.

6. Balkwill FR, Burke F. The cytokine network. *Immunol Today* 1989;10:299-304.

7. Blankenberg S, Barbaux S, Tiret L. Adhesion molecules and atherosclerosis. *Atherosclerosis* 2003;170:191-203.

8. Behm CZ, Lindner JR. Cellular and molecular imaging with targeted contrast ultrasound. *Ultrasound Q* 2006;22:67-72.

9. Blankenberg S, Godefroy T, Poirier O, et al. Athero-Gene investigators. Haplotypes of the caspase-1 gene, plasma caspase-1 levels, and cardiovascular risk. *Circ Res* 2006;99:102-108.

10. Blankenberg S, Rupprecht HJ, Poirier O, et al. Athero-Gene investigators. Plasma concentrations and genetic variation of matrix metalloproteinase 9 and prognosis of patients with cardiovascular disease. *Circulation* 2003;107:1579-1585.

11. Bonaa KH, Njolstad I, Ueland PM, et al. NORVIT Trial investigators. Homocysteine lowering and cardiovascular events after acute myocardial infarction. *N Engl J Med* 2006;354:1578-1588.

12. Boulbou MS, Koukoulis GN, Makri ED, et al. Circulating adhesion molecules in type 2 diabetes mellitus and hypertension. *Int J Cardiol* 2005;98:39-44.

13. Brennan ML, Penn MS, Van Lente F, et al. Prognostic value of myeloperoxidase in patients with chest pain. *N Engl J Med* 2003;349:1595-1604.

14. Cai J, Hatsukami TS, Ferguson MS, et al. In vivo quantitative measurement of intact fibrous cap and lipid-rich necrotic core size in atherosclerotic carotid plaque: comparison of high-resolution, contrast-enhanced magnetic resonance imaging and histology. *Circulation* 2005;112:3437-3444.

15. Cannon CP, Braunwald E, McCabe CH, et al. Pravastatin or Atorvastatin Evaluation and Infection Therapy-Thrombolysis in Myocardial Infarction 22 Investigators. Intensive versus moderate lipid lowering with statins after acute coronary syndromes. *N Engl J Med* 2004;350:1495-1504.

16. Cavusoglu E, Chopra V, Gupta A, et al. Usefulness of the white blood cell count as a predictor of angiographic findings in an unselected population referred for coronary angiography. *Am J Cardiol* 2006;98:1189-1193.

17. Cavusoglu E, Ruwende C, Chopra V, et al. Adiponectin is an independent predictor of all-cause mortality, cardiac mortality, and myocardial infarction in patients presenting with chest pain. *Eur Heart J* 2006;27:2300-2309.

18. Cavusoglu E, Ruwende C, Chopra V, et al. Tissue inhibitor of metalloproteinase-1 (TIMP-1) is an independent predictor of all-cause mortality, cardiac mortality, and

myocardial infarction. *Am Heart J* 2006;151:1101.e1-8.

19. Chen Y, Ke Q, Xiao YF, et al. Cocaine and catecholamines enhance inflammatory cell retention in the coronary circulation of mice by upregulation of adhesion molecules. *Am J Physiol Heart Circ Physiol* 2005;288: H2323-H2331.

20. Cnop M, Havel PJ, Utzschneider KM, et al. Relationship of adiponectin to body fat distribution, insulin sensitivity and plasma lipoproteins: evidence for independent roles of age and sex. *Diabetologia* 2003;46:459-469.

21. Crawford FC, Wood ML, Wilson SE, et al. Cocaine induced inflammatory response in human neuronal progenitor cells. *J Neurochem* 2006;97:662-674.

22. Cunningham KS, Gotlieb AI. The role of shear stress in the pathogenesis of atherosclerosis. *Lab Invest* 2005;85:9-23.

23. Dandona P, Weinstock R, Thusu K, et al. Tumor necrosis factor-α in sera of obese patients: fall with weight loss. *J Clin Endocrinol Metab* 1998;83:2907-2910.

24. Danesh J, Collins R, Appleby P, Peto R. Association of fibrinogen, C-reactive protein, albumin, or leukocyte count with coronary heart disease: meta-analyses of prospective studies. *JAMA* 1998;279:1477-1482.

25. Danesh J, Collins R, Peto R. Lipoprotein(a) and coronary heart disease: meta-analysis of prospective studies. *Circulation* 2000;102:1082-1085.

26. De Martin R, Hoeth M, Hofer-Warbinek R, Schmid JA. The transcription factor NF-κβ and the regulation of vascular cell function. *Arterioscler Thromb Vasc Biol* 2000;20:E83-E88.

27. Dorffel Y, Latsch C, Stuhlmuller B, Schreiber S, et al. Preactivated peripheral blood monocytes in patients with essential hypertension. *Hypertension* 1999;34:113-117.

28. Durga J, van Tits LJ, Schouten EG, et al. Effect of lowering of homocysteine levels on inflammatory markers: a randomized controlled trial. *Arch Intern Med* 2005;165:1388-1394.

29. Dusserre E, Moulin P, Vidal H. Differences in mRNA expression of the proteins secreted by the adipocytes in human subcutaneous and visceral adipose tissues. *Biochim Biophys Acta* 2000;1500:88-96.

30. Elesber AA, Conover CA, Denktas AE, et al. Prognostic value of circulating pregnancy-associated plasma protein levels in patients with chronic stable angina. *Eur Heart J* 2006;27:1678-1684.

31. Ernst E, Resch KL. Fibrinogen as a cardiovascular risk factor: a meta-analysis and review of the literature. *Ann Intern Med* 1993;118:956-963.

32. Field KM. Effect of 3-hydroxy-3-methylglutaryl coenzyme A reductase inhibitors on high-sensitivity C-reactive protein levels. *Pharmacotherapy* 2005;25:1365-1377.

33. Folsom AR, Chambless LE, Ballantyne CM, et al. An assessment of incremental coronary risk prediction

using C-reactive protein and other novel risk markers: the atherosclerosis risk in communities study. *Arch Intern Med* 2006;166:1368-1373.

34. Hammett CJ, Prapavessis H, Baldi JC, et al. Effects of exercise training on 5 inflammatory markers associated with cardiovascular risk. *Am Heart J* 2006;151:367.e7-367.e16.

35. Homocysteine Studies Collaboration. Homocysteine and risk of ischemic heart disease and stroke: a meta-analysis. *JAMA* 2002;288:2015-2022.

36. Iwashima Y, Horio T, Suzuki Y, et al. Adiponectin and inflammatory markers in peripheral arterial occlusive disease. *Atherosclerosis* 2006;188:384-390.

37. Jiang Z, Berceli SA, Pfahnl CL, et al. Wall shear modulation of cytokines in early vein grafts. *J Vasc Surg* 2004;40:345-350.

38. Johnson BD, Kip KE, Marroquin OC, et al. National Heart, Lung, and Blood Institute. Serum amyloid A as a predictor of coronary artery disease and cardiovascular outcome in women: the National Heart, Lung, and Blood Institute-Sponsored Women's Ischemia Syndrome Evaluation (WISE). *Circulation* 2004;109:726-732.

39. Jonasson L, Holm J, Skalli O, et al. Expression of class II transplantation antigen on vascular smooth muscle cells in human atherosclerosis. *J Clin Invest* 1985;76:125-131.

40. Kasapis C, Thompson PD. The effects of physical activity on serum C-reactive protein and inflammatory markers: a systematic review. *J Am Coll Cardiol* 2005;45:1563-1569.

41. Kervinen H, Palosuo T, Manninen V, et al. Joint effects of C-reactive protein and other risk factors on acute coronary events. *Am Heart J* 2001;141:580-585.

42. Koh KK, Han SH, Quon MJ. Inflammatory markers and the metabolic syndrome. *J Am Coll Cardiol* 2005;46:1978-1985.

43. Koenig W, Twardella D, Brenner H, Rothenbacher D. Lipoprotein-associated phospholipase A$_2$ predicts future cardiovascular events in patients with coronary heart disease independently of traditional risk factors, markers of inflammation, renal function, and hemodynamic stress. *Arterioscler Thromb Vasc Biol* 2006;26:1586-1593.

44. Kusuhara M, Isoda K, Ohsuzu F. Interleukin-1 and occlusive arterial diseases. *Cardiovasc Hematol Agents Med Chem* 2006;4:229-235.

45. Libby P. Molecular bases of the acute coronary syndromes. *Circulation* 1995;91:2844-2850.

46. Lindner JR. Evolving applications for contrast ultrasound. *Am J Cardiol* 2002;90:72J-80J.

47. Lindmark E, Diderholm E, Wallentin L, Siegbahn A. Relationship between interleukin 6 and mortality in patients with unstable coronary artery disease: effects of an early invasive or noninvasive strategy. *JAMA* 2001;286:2107-2113.

48. Lobbes MB, Lutgens E, Heeneman S, et al. Is there more than C-reactive protein and fibrinogen? The prognostic value of soluble CD40 ligand, interleukin-6 and oxidized low-density lipoprotein with respect to coronary and cerebral vascular disease. *Atherosclerosis* 2006;187:18-25.

49. Ludvig J, Miner B, Eisenberg MJ. Smoking cessation in patients with coronary artery disease. *Am Heart J* 2005;149:565-572.

50. Lyon CJ, Law RE, Hsueh WA. Minireview: adiposity, inflammation, and atherogenesis. *Endocrinology* 2003;144:2195-2200.

51. Mach F, Schonbeck U, Libby P. CD40 signaling in vascular cells: a key role in atherosclerosis? *Atherosclerosis* 1998;137(suppl):S89-S95.

52. Macphee CH, Nelson J, Zalewski A. Role of lipoprotein-associated phospholipase A$_2$ in atherosclerosis and its potential as a therapeutic target. *Curr Opin Pharmacol* 2006;6:154-161.

53. Madjid M, Awan I, Willerson JT, Casscells SW. Leukocyte count and coronary heart disease: implications for risk assessment. *J Am Coll Cardiol* 2004;44:1945-1956.

54. Madjid M, Naghavi M, Malik BA, et al. Thermal detection of vulnerable plaque. *Am J Cardiol* 2002;90:36L-39L.

55. Malle E, Marsche G, Arnhold J, Davies MJ. Modification of low-density lipoprotein by myeloperoxidase-derived oxidants and reagent hypochlorous acid. *Biochim Biophys Acta* 2006;1761:392-415.

56. Minoretti P, Falcone C, Calcagnino M, et al. Prognostic significance of plasma osteopontin levels in patients with chronic stable angina. *Eur Heart J* 2006;27:802-807.

57. Mintz GS, Painter JA, Pichard AD, et al. Atherosclerosis in angiographically "normal" coronary artery reference segments: an intravascular ultrasound study with clinical correlations. *J Am Coll Cardiol* 1995;25:1479-1485.

58. Mollet NR, Cademartiri F, de Feyter PJ. Non-invasive multislice CT coronary imaging. *Heart* 2005;91:401-407.

59. Muhlestein JB, May HT, Jensen JR, et al. The reduction of inflammatory biomarkers by statin, fibrate, and combination therapy among diabetic patients with mixed dyslipidemia: the DIACOR (Diabetes and Combined Lipid Therapy Regimen) study. *J Am Coll Cardiol* 2006;48:396-401.

60. Nakamura Y, Shimada K, Fukuda D, et al. Implications of plasma concentrations of adiponectin in patients with coronary artery disease. *Heart* 2004;90:528-533.

61. Napoli C, D'Armiento FP, Mancini FP, et al. Fatty streak formation occurs in human fetal aortas and is greatly enhanced by maternal hypercholesterolemia: intimal accumulation of low density lipoprotein and its oxidation precede monocyte recruitment into early atherosclerotic lesions. *J Clin Invest* 1997;100:2680-2690.

62. Nicholls SJ, Tuzcu EM, Sipahi I, et al. Intravascular ultrasound in cardiovascular medicine. *Circulation* 2006;114:e55-e59.

63. Nilsson J. Cytokines and smooth muscle cells in atherosclerosis. *Cardiovasc Res* 1993;27:1184-1190.

64. Nissen SE, Nicholls SJ, Sipahi I, et al, for the ASTEROID investigators. Effect of Very High-Intensity Statin Therapy on Regression of Coronary Atherosclerosis: the ASTEROID trial. *JAMA* 2006;295:1556-1565.

65. Nissen SE, Tuzcu EM, Schoenhagen P, et al. REVERSAL investigators. Effect of intensive compared with moderate lipid-lowering therapy on progression of coronary atherosclerosis: a randomized controlled trial. *JAMA* 2004;291:1071-1078.

66. O'Brien KD, Chait A. Serum amyloid A: the "other" inflammatory protein. *Curr Atheroscler Rep* 2006;8:62-68.

67. O'Leary DH, Polak JF, Kronmal RA, et al. Carotid-artery intima and media thickness as a risk factor for myocardial infarction and stroke in older adults. Cardiovascular Health Study Collaborative Research Group. *N Engl J Med* 1999;340:14-22.

68. Otsuka F, Sugiyama S, Kojima S, et al. Plasma adiponectin levels are associated with coronary lesion complexity in men with coronary artery disease. *J Am Coll Cardiol* 2006;48:1155-1162.

69. Pai JK, Hankinson SE, Thadhani R, et al. Moderate alcohol consumption and lower levels of inflammatory markers in US men and women. *Atherosclerosis* 2006;186:113-120.

70. Pearson TA, Mensah GA, Alexander RW, et al. Centers for Disease Control and Prevention, American Heart Association. Markers of inflammation and cardiovascular disease: application to clinical and public health practice: a statement for healthcare professionals from the Centers for Disease Control and Prevention and the American Heart Association. *Circulation* 2003;107:499-511.

71. Poredos P. Intima-media thickness: indicator of cardiovascular risk and measure of the extent of atherosclerosis. *Vasc Med* 2004;9:46-54.

72. Pickup JC, Crook MA. Is type II diabetes a disease of the innate immune system? *Diabetologica* 1998;41:1241-1248.

73. Pischon T, Girman CJ, Hotamisligil GS, et al. Plasma adiponectin levels and risk of myocardial infarction in men. *JAMA* 2004;291:1730-1737.

74. Pradhan AD, Manson JE, Rifai N, et al. C-reactive protein, interleukin 6, and risk of developing type 2 diabetes mellitus. *JAMA* 2001;286:327-334.

75. Primrose JN, Davies JA, Prentice CR, et al. Reduction in factor VII, fibrinogen and plasminogen activator inhibitor-1 activity after surgical treatment of morbid obesity. *Thromb Haemost* 1992;68:396-399.

76. Ross R. Atherosclerosis—an inflammatory disease. *N Engl J Med* 1999;340:115-126.

77. Ridker PM, Cannon CP, Morrow D, et al. Pravastatin or Atorvastatin Evaluation and Infection Therapy–Thrombolysis in Myocardial Infarction 22 (PROVE IT–TIMI 22) investigators. C-reactive protein levels and outcomes after statin therapy. *N Engl J Med* 2005;352:20-28.

78. Ridker PM, Stampfer MJ, Rifai N. Novel risk factors for systemic atherosclerosis: a comparison of C-reactive protein, fibrinogen, homocysteine, lipoprotein(a), and standard cholesterol screening as predictors of peripheral arterial disease. *JAMA* 2001;285:2481-2485.

79. Rimm EB, Klatsky A, Grobbee D, Stampfer MJ. Review of moderate alcohol consumption and reduced risk of coronary heart disease: is the effect due to beer, wine, or spirits. *BMJ* 1996;312:731-736.

80. Sanguigni V, Pignatelli P, Lenti L, et al. Short-term treatment with atorvastatin reduces platelet CD40 ligand and thrombin generation in hypercholesterolemic patients. *Circulation* 2005;111:412-419.

81. Sattar N, Wannamethee G, Sarwar N, et al. Adiponectin and coronary heart disease: a prospective study and meta-analysis. *Circulation* 2006;114:623-629.

82. Sesso HD, Buring JE, Rifai N, et al. C-reactive protein and the risk of developing hypertension. *JAMA* 2003;290:2945-2951.

83. Shaw LJ, Raggi P, Schisterman E, et al. Prognostic value of cardiac risk factors and coronary artery calcium screening for all-cause mortality. *Radiology* 2003;228:826-833.

84. Sjoholm A, Nystrom T. Inflammation and the etiology of type 2 diabetes. *Diabetes Metab Res Rev* 2006;22:4-10.

85. Smith C, Damas JK, Otterdal K, et al. Increased levels of neutrophil-activating peptide-2 in acute coronary syndromes: possible role of platelet-mediated vascular inflammation. *J Am Coll Cardiol* 2006;48:1591-1599.

86. Stamler J, Wentworth D, Neaton JD. Is relationship between serum cholesterol and risk of premature death from coronary heart disease continuous and graded? Findings in 356,222 primary screenees of the Multiple Risk Factor Intervention Trial (MRFIT). *JAMA* 1986;256:2823-2828.

87. Stefanadis C, Diamantopoulos L, Dernellis J, et al. Heat production of atherosclerotic plaques and inflammation assessed by the acute phase proteins in acute coronary syndromes. *J Mol Cell Cardiol* 2000;32:43-52.

88. Stemme S, Holm J, Hansson GK. T lymphocytes in human atherosclerotic plaques are memory cells expressing CD45RO and the integrin VLA-1. *Arterioscler Thromb* 1992;12:206-211.

89. Tedgui A, Mallat Z. Cytokines in atherosclerosis: pathogenic and regulatory pathways. *Physiol Rev* 2006;86:515-581.

90. The Heart Outcomes Prevention Evaluation (HOPE) 2 Investigators. Homocysteine lowering with folic acid and B vitamins in vascular disease. *N Engl J Med* 2006;354:1567-1577.

91. Thompson SG, Kienast J, Pyke SD, et al. Hemostatic factors and the risk of myocardial infarction or sudden death in patients with angina pectoris. European Concerted Action on Thrombosis and Disabilities Angina Pectoris Study Group. *N Engl J Med* 1995;332:635-641.

92. Tousoulis D, Charakida M, Stefanadis C. Endothelial function and inflammation in coronary artery disease. *Heart* 2006;92:441-444.

93. van de Poll SW, Romer TJ, Puppels GJ, van der Laarse A. Imaging of atherosclerosis: Raman spectroscopy of atherosclerosis. *J Cardiovasc Risk* 2002;9:255-261.

94. van Vark LC, Kardys I, Bleumink GS, et al. Lipoprotein-associated phospholipase A2 activity and risk of heart failure: the Rotterdam Study. *Eur Heart J* 2006;27:2346-2352.

95. Vishnevetsky D, Kiyanista VA, Gandhi PJ. CD40 ligand: a novel target in the fight against cardiovascular disease. *Ann Pharmacother* 2004;38:1500-1508.

96. Willerson JT, Ridker PM. Inflammation as a cardiovascular risk factor. *Circulation* 2003;109(suppl II): II-2–II-10.

97. Wu TC, Leu HB, Lin WT, et al. Plasma matrix metalloproteinase-3 level is an independent prognostic factor in stable coronary artery disease. *Eur J Clin Invest* 2005;35:537-545.

98. Xu Z, Zhao S, Zhou H, Ye H, Li J. Atorvastatin lowers plasma matrix metalloproteinase-9 in patients with acute coronary syndrome. *Clin Chem* 2004;50:750-753.

99. Yuan C, Kerwin WS, Yarnykh VL, et al. MRI of atherosclerosis in clinical trials. *NMR Biomed.* 2006;19:636-654.

100. Zhang R, Brennan ML, Fu X, et al. Association between myeloperoxidase levels and risk of coronary artery disease. *JAMA* 2001;286:2136-2142.

101. Ziccardi P, Nappo F, Giugliano G, et al. Reduction of inflammatory cytokine concentrations and improvement of endothelial functions in obese women after weight loss over one year. *Circulation* 2002;105:804-809.

Chapter 8

1. American College of Sports Medicine. *Guidelines for Exercise Testing and Exercise Prescription.* 7th ed. Baltimore: Lippincott Williams & Wilkins; 2005.

2. American Thoracic Society/American College of Chest Physicians: statement on cardiopulmonary exercise testing. *Am J Respir Crit Care Med* 2003;167:211-277.

3. Armstrong WF, Pellikka PA, Ryan T, et al. Stress echocardiography: recommendations for performance and interpretation of stress echocardiography. *J Am Soc Echocardiogr* 1998;11:97-104.

4. Ashley E, Myers J, Froelicher V. Exercise testing scores as an example of better decisions through science. *Med Sci Sports Exerc* 2002;34:1391-1398.

5. Beckerman J, Wu T, Jones S, Froelicher VF. Exercise test-induced arrhythmias. *Prog Cardiovasc Dis* 2005;47:285-305.

6. Borg GAV. *Borg's Perceived Exertion and Pain Scales.* Champaign, IL: Human Kinetics; 1998.

7. Cerqueira MD. Diagnostic testing strategies for coronary artery disease: special issues related to gender. *Am J Cardiol* 1995;75:52D-60D.

8. Chang JA, Froelicher VF. Clinical and exercise test markers of prognosis in patients with stable coronary artery disease. *Curr Prob Cardiol* 1994;19:533-538.

9. Ehrman JK, Keteyian SJ, Levine AB, et al. Exercise stress tests after cardiac transplantation. *Am J Cardiol* 1993;71:1372-1373.

10. Evans CH, Froelicher VF. Some common abnormal responses to exercise testing: what to do when you see them. *Primary Care* 2001;28:219-231.

11. Franklin BA, Gordon S, Timmis GC, et al. Is direct physician supervision of exercise stress testing routinely necessary? *Chest* 1997;111:262-264.

12. Froelicher VF. *Exercise Test Reporting Aid (EXTRA) Software.* St. Louis: Mosby-Year Book; 1996.

13. Froelicher VF, Myers J. *Exercise and the Heart.* 5th ed. Philadelphia: Saunders; 2006.

14. Gianrossi R, Detrano R, Mulvihill D, et al. Exercise-induced ST depression in the diagnosis of coronary artery disease: a meta-analysis. *Circulation* 1989;80:87-98.

15. Gibbons RJ, Balady GJ, Bricker JT, et al. ACC/AHA 2002 guideline update for exercise testing: a report of the ACC/AHA Task Force on Practice Guidelines (Committee on Exercise Testing). *J Am Coll Cardiol* 2002;40:1531-1540.

16. Gibbons L, Blair SN, Kohl HW, et al. The safety of maximal exercise testing. *Circulation* 1989;80:846-852.

17. Graettinger W, Smith D, Neutel J, et al. Relationship of left ventricular structure to maximal heart rate during exercise. *Chest* 1995;107:341-345.

18. Hambrecht R, Schuler GC, Muth T, et al. Greater diagnostic sensitivity of treadmill versus cycle exercise testing of asymptomatic men with coronary artery disease. *Am J Cardiol* 1992;70:141-146.

19. Herbert DL, Herbert WG. *Legal Aspects of Preventive, Rehabilitative, and Recreational Exercise Programs.* 4th ed. Canton: PRC Publishing; 2002.

20. Iyriboz Y, Hearon CM. Blood pressure measurement at rest and during exercise: controversies, guidelines, and procedures. *J Cardiopulm Rehabil* 1992;12:277-287.

21. Kennedy H, Killip T, Fischer L, et al. The clinical spectrum of coronary artery disease and its surgical and medical management: 1974-1979, the Coronary Artery Surgery Study. *Circulation* 1977;56:756-761.

22. Klocke FJ, Baird MG, Lorell BH, et al. ACC/AHA/ASNC guidelines for the clinical use of cardiac radionuclide imaging—executive summary: a report of the American College of Cardiology/American Heart

Association Task Force on Practice Guidelines. *Circulation* 2003;108:1404-1408.

23. Kotler TS, Diamond GA. Exercise thallium-201 scintigraphy in the diagnosis and prognosis of coronary artery disease. *Ann Intern Med* 1990;113:684-702.

24. Lachterman B, Lehmann KG, Abrahamson D, et al. "Recovery only" ST segment depression and the predictive accuracy of the exercise test. *Ann Intern Med* 1990;112:11-16.

25. Lauer MS. Exercise electrocardiogram testing and prognosis. *Cardiol Clin* 2001;29:401-414.

26. Marconi C, Marzorati M. Exercise after heart transplantation. *Eur J Appl Physiol* 2003;90:250-259.

27. Mark DB. Risk stratification in patients with chest pain. *Primary Care* 2001;28:99-118.

28. Marolf GA, Kuhn A, White RD. Exercise testing in special populations: athletes, women, and the elderly. *Primary Care* 2001;28:55-72.

29. Mason RE, Likar I. A new system of multiple-lead exercise electrocardiography. *Am Heart J* 1966;71:196-205.

30. Morise AP, Diamond GA. Comparison of the sensitivity and specificity of exercise electrocardiography in biased and unbiased populations of men and women. *Am Heart J* 1995;130:741-747.

31. Morris CK, Myers J, Froelicher VF, et al. Nomogram based on metabolic equivalents and age for assessing aerobic exercise capacity in men. *J Am Coll Cardiol* 1994;22:175-182.

32. Myers J. Applications of cardiopulmonary exercise testing in the management of cardiovascular and pulmonary disease. *Int J Sports Med* 2005;26:S49-S55.

33. Myers J. *Essentials of Cardiopulmonary Exercise Testing.* Champaign, IL: Human Kinetics; 1996.

34. Myers J. Optimizing the clinical exercise test: a commentary on the exercise protocol. *Heart Fail Monit* 2004;4:82-89.

35. Myers JN. Perception of chest pain during exercise testing in patients with coronary artery disease. *Med Sci Sports Exerc* 1994;26:1082-1086.

36. Myers J, Buchanan N, Walsh D, et al. Comparison of the ramp versus standard exercise protocols. *J Am Coll Cardiol* 1991;17:1334-1342.

37. Myers J, Walsh D, Buchanan N, et al. Can maximal cardiopulmonary capacity be recognized by a plateau in oxygen uptake? *Chest* 1989;96:1312-1316.

38. Myers J, Voodi L, Umann T, Froelicher VF. A survey of exercise testing: methods, utilization, interpretation, and safety in the VAHCS. *J Cardiopulm Rehabil* 2000;20:251-258.

39. Noakes TD. Maximal oxygen uptake: "classical" versus "contemporary" viewpoints: a rebuttal. *Med Sci Sports Exerc* 1998;30:1381-1398.

40. Philbrick JT, Horowitz R, Feinstein AR. Methodological problems of exercise testing for coronary artery disease: groups, analysis and bias. *Am J Cardiol* 1989;64:1117-1122.

41. Rogers GP, Ayanian JZ, Balady GJ, et al. American College of Cardiology/American Heart Association clinical competence statement on stress testing: a report of the ACC/AHA and American Society of Internal Medicine Task Force on Clinical Competence. *Circulation* 2000;102:1726-1738.

42. Severi S, Picano E, Michelassi C, et al. Diagnostic and prognostic value of dipyridamole echocardiography in patients with suspected coronary artery disease: comparison with exercise electrocardiography. *Circulation* 1994;89:1160-1173.

Chapter 9

1. ACC/AHA guidelines for exercise testing, a report of the American College of Cardiology/American Heart Association task force on practice guidelines (Committee on Exercise Testing). *J Am Coll Cardiol* 1997;30:260-315.

2. American College of Cardiology/American Heart Association. Guidelines update for exercise testing: summary article. *J Am Coll Cardiol* 2002;40:1531-1540.

3. American Heart Association. *Heart and Stroke Statistical Update.* Dallas: American Heart Association; 2005.

4. Amstrong WF. Stress echocardiography: introduction, history, and methods. *Prog Cardiovasc Dis* 1997;39:499-522.

5. Braunwald E, ed. *Heart Disease: A Textbook of Cardiovascular Medicine.* 5th ed. Philadelphia: Saunders; 1997.

6. Brubaker P, Kaminsky L, Whaley M. *Coronary Artery Disease.* Champaign, IL: Human Kinetics; 2002.

7. Dener LL, Gould KL, Goldstein RA, et al. Assessment of coronary artery disease severity by position emission tomography: comparison with quantitative arteriography in 193 patients. *Circulation* 1989;79:825-835.

8. Escolar E, Weigold G, Fuisz A, Weissman, NJ. New imaging techniques for diagnosing coronary disease. *CMAJ* 2006;174:487-495.

9. Fowkes FH, Low FL, Sorin T, Kozak J, on behalf of the AGATHA Investigators. Ankle-brachial index and extent of atherothrombosis in 8891 patients with or at risk of vascular disease: results of the international AGATHA study. *Eur Hear J* 2006;27:1861-1867.

10. Garcia M. Echocardiographic assessment of left ventricular function. *J Nucl Cardiol* 2006;13:280-293.

11. Gianrossi R, Detrano R, Mulvshill D, et al. Exercise induced ST depression in the diagnosis of coronary artery disease: a meta-analysis. *Circulation* 1989;80:87-98.

12. Gibbons RJ, Eckel RH, Jacobs AK, for the Science Advisory and Coordinating Committee. The utilization of cardiac imaging. *Circulation* 2006;113:1715-1716.

13. Goldberg R, Gove J, Alpert JS. Incidence and case fatality rates of acute myocardial infarction (1975-1984): The Worcester Heart Attack Study. *Am Heart J* 1988;115:761-767.

14. Hendel RC, Patel MR, Kramer CM, et al. Appropriateness criteria for cardiac computed tomography and cardiac magnetic resonance imaging. *J Am Coll Cardiol* 2006;48:1475-1497.

15. Kannel W. Prevalence and clinical aspects of unrecognized myocardial infarction and sudden unexpected death. *Circulation* 1987;75(part 2):II4-II5.

16. Marwick TH, ed. *Cardiac Stress Testing and Imaging. A Clinician's Guide.* New York: Churchill Livingstone; 1996.

17. Mieres JH, Shaw LJ. Arai A, et al. Role of noninvasive testing in the clinical evaluation of women with suspected coronary artery disease. *Circulation* 2005;111:682-696.

18. Nesto RW, Kowalchuk GJ. The ischemic cascade: temporal sequence of hemodynamic, electrocardiographic, and symptomatic expression of ischemia. *Am J Cardiol* 1987;57:23C-30C.

19. Nichol G, Walls R, Goldman L, et al. A critical pathway for management of patients with acute chest pain who are at low risk for myocardial ischemia: recommendations and potential impact. *Ann Intern Med* 1997;127:996-1005.

20. O'Rourke RA, Brundage BH, Froelicher VF, et al. ACC/AHA expert consensus document on electron-beam computed tomography for diagnosis and prognosis of coronary artery disease. *Circulation* 2000;102:126-140.

Chapter 10

1. Antman EM, Anbe DT, Armstrong PW, et al. ACC/AHA guidelines for the management of patients with ST-elevation myocardial infarction: a report of the American College of Cardiology/American Heart Association Task Force on Practice Guidelines (Committee to Revise the 1999 Guidelines for the Management of Patients With Acute Myocardial Infarction). *Circulation* 2004;110:e82-e293.

2. Aspirin for the primary prevention of cardiovascular events: recommendations and rationale. US Preventive Services Task Force. *Ann Intern Med* 2002;136:157-160.

3. Bonow RO, Carabello BA, Chatterjee K, et al. ACC/AHA 2006 guidelines for the management of patients with valvular heart disease: a report of the American College of Cardiology/American Heart Association Task Force on Practice Guidelines (Writing Committee to Develop Guidelines for the Management of Patients With Valvular Heart Disease). *Circulation* 2006;114: e84-e231.

4. Chobanian AV, Bakris GL, Black HR, et al. Joint National Committee on Prevention, Detection, Evaluation, and Treatment of High Blood Pressure. National Heart, Lung, and Blood Institute; National High Blood Pressure Education Program Coordinating Committee. *Hypertension* 2003;42:1206-1252.

5. Cook NR, Lee IM, Gaziano JM, et al. Low-dose aspirin in the primary prevention of cancer: the women's health study: a randomized controlled trial. *JAMA* 2005;294:47-55.

6. Cowell SJ, Newby DE, Prescott RJ, et al. A randomized trial of intensive lipid-lowering therapy in calcific aortic stenosis. *N Engl J Med* 2005;352:2389-2397.

7. Dajani AS, Taubert KA, Wilson W, et al. Prevention of bacterial endocarditis—recommendations by the American Heart Association. *Circulation* 1997;96:358-366.

8. Fiore MC, Bailey WC, Cohen SJ, et al. *Treating Tobacco Use and Dependence.* Clinical Practice Guideline. Rockville, MD: U.S. Department of Health and Human Services, Public Health Service; June 2000. www.surgeongeneral.gov/tobacco/treating_tobacco_use.pdf

9. Fuster V, Rydén LE, Cannom DS, et al. ACC/AHA/ESC 2006 guidelines for the management of patients with atrial fibrillation—executive summary: a report of the American College of Cardiology/American Heart Association Task Force on Practice Guidelines and the European Society of Cardiology Committee for Practice Guidelines (Writing Committee to Revise the 2001 Guidelines for the Management of Patients With Atrial Fibrillation). *Circulation* 2006;114:700-752.

10. Grundy SM, Cleeman JI, Bairey Merz CN, et al, for the Coordinating Committee of the National Cholesterol Education Program and Endorsed by the National Heart, Lung, and Blood Institute, American College of Cardiology Foundation, and American Heart Association. Implications of recent clinical trials for the National Cholesterol Education Program Adult Treatment Panel III guidelines. *Circulation* 2004;110:227-239.

11. Hirsch AT, Haskal ZJ, Hertzer NR, et al. ACC/AHA 2005 practice guidelines for the management of patients with peripheral arterial disease (lower extremity, renal, mesenteric, and abdominal aortic): a collaborative report from the American Association for Vascular Surgery/Society for Vascular Surgery, Society for Cardiovascular Angiography and Interventions, Society for Vascular Medicine and Biology, Society of Interventional Radiology, and the ACC/AHA Task Force on Practice Guidelines (Writing Committee to Develop Guidelines for the Management of Patients With Peripheral Arterial Disease). *Circulation* 2006;113: e463-e654.

12. Hunt SA, Abraham WT, Chin MH, et al. ACC/AHA 2005 guideline update for the diagnosis and management of chronic heart failure in the adult: a report of the American College of Cardiology/American Heart Association Task Force on Practice Guidelines (Writing Committee to Update the 2001 Guidelines for the Evaluation and Management of Heart Failure). *Circulation* 2005;112;1825-1852.

13. Krentz AJ, Bailey CJ. Oral antidiabetic agents: current role in type 2 diabetes mellitus. *Drugs* 2005;65:385-411.

14. Lichtenstein AH, Appel LJ, Brands M, et al. Diet and lifestyle recommendations revision 2006: a scientific statement from the American Heart Association Nutrition Committee. *Circulation* 2006;114;82-96.

15. Mosca L, Appel LJ, Benjamin EJ, et al. Evidence-based guidelines for cardiovascular disease prevention in women. *Circulation* 2004;109:672-693.

16. National Cholesterol Education Program (NCEP) Expert Panel on Detection, Evaluation, and Treatment of High Blood Cholesterol in Adults (Adult Treatment Panel III). Third Report of the National Cholesterol Education Program (NCEP) Expert Panel on Detection, Evaluation, and Treatment of High Blood Cholesterol in Adults (Adult Treatment Panel III) final report. *Circulation* 2002;106:3143-3421.

17. National Institute of Diabetes and Digestive and Kidney Diseases. Prescription Medications for the Treatment of Obesity, NIH Publication 04-4191, November 2004. www.win.niddk.nih.gov/publications/PDFs/Prescription meds1104bw.pdf.

18. Pearson TA, Blair SN, Daniels SR, et al. AHA 2002 guidelines for primary prevention of cardiovascular disease and stroke. *Circulation* 2002;106:388-391.

19. Sacco RL, Adams R, Albers G, et al. Guidelines for prevention of stroke in patients with ischemic stroke or transient ischemic attack: a statement for healthcare professionals from the American Heart Association/American Stroke Association Council on Stroke: co-sponsored by the Council on Cardiovascular Radiology and Intervention: The American Academy of Neurology affirms the value of this guideline. *Stroke* 2006;37:577-617.

20. Smith SC, Allen J, Blair SN, et al. AHA/ACC guidelines for secondary prevention for patients with coronary and other atherosclerotic vascular disease: 2006 update. *Circulation* 2006;113:2363-2372.

21. Smith SC Jr, Feldman TE, Hirshfeld JW Jr, et al. ACC/AHA/SCAI 2005 guideline update for percutaneous coronary intervention: a report of the American College of Cardiology/American Heart Association Task Force on Practice Guidelines (ACC/AHA/SCAI Writing Committee to Update the 2001 Guidelines for Percutaneous Coronary Intervention). *J Am Coll Cardiol* 2006;47;e1-121.

22. treatobacco.net: Database and Educational Resource for Treatment of Tobacco Dependence. www.treatobacco.net/home/home.cfm.

Chapter 11

1. Bonow RO, Carabello B, de Leon AC Jr, et al. ACC/AHA guidelines for the management of patients with valvular heart disease: a report of the American College of Cardiology/American Heart Association Task Force on Practice Guidelines (Committee on Management of Patients With Valvular Heart Disease). *Circulation* 1998;98:1949-1984.

2. Cohen JM, Glower DD, Harrison JK, et al. Comparison of balloon valvuloplasty with operative treatment for mitral stenosis. *Ann Thorac Surg* 1993;56:1254-1262.

3. Davies RF, Goldberg AD, Forman S, et al. Asymptomatic Cardiac Ischemia Pilot (ACIP) study two-year follow-up: outcomes of patients randomized to initial strategies of medical therapy versus revascularization. *Circulation* 1997;95:2037-2043.

4. Eagle KA, Guyton RA, Davidoff R, et al. 1999. ACC/AHA guidelines for coronary artery bypass graft surgery: executive summary and recommendations: a report of the American College of Cardiology/American Heart Association Task Force on Practice Guidelines (Committee to Revise the 1991 Guidelines for Coronary Artery Bypass Graft Surgery). *Circulation* 100:1464-1480.

5. English T. Closed mitral valvotomy. In: Wells FC, Shapiro LM, eds. *Mitral Valve Disease*. 2nd ed. London: Butterworths; 1996:107-113.

6. Fischman DL, Leon MB, Baim DS, et al. A randomized comparison of coronary-stent placement and balloon angioplasty in the treatment of coronary artery disease: Stent Restenosis Study investigators. *N Engl J Med* 1994;331:496-501.

7. Folland ED, Hartigan PM, Parisi AF. Percutaneous transluminal coronary angioplasty versus medical therapy for stable angina pectoris: outcomes for patients with double-vessel versus single-vessel coronary artery disease in a Veterans Affairs cooperative randomized trial. *J Am Coll Cardiol* 1997;29:1505-1511.

8. Gillinov AM, Cosgrove DM. Minimally invasive mitral valve surgery: mini-sternotomy with extended transseptal approach. *Semin Thorac Cardiovasc Surg* 1999;11:206-211.

9. Gillinov AM, Cosgrove DM III. Mitral valve repair. In: Cohn LH, Edmunds LH Jr, eds. *Cardiac Surgery in the Adult*. New York: McGraw-Hill; 2003:1013-1030.

10. Gillinov AM, Wierup PN, Blackstone EH, et al. Is repair preferable to replacement for ischemic mitral regurgitation? *J Thorac Cardiovasc Surg* 2001;122:1125-1141.

11. Hartigan PM, Giacomini JC, Folland ED, Parisi AF. Two- to three-year follow-up of patients with single-vessel coronary artery disease randomized to PTCA or medical therapy (results of a VA cooperative study). Veterans Affairs Cooperative Studies Program ACME investigators: angioplasty compared to medicine. *Am J Cardiol* 1998;82:1445-1450.

12. King SB III, Barnhart HX, Kosinski AS, et al. Angioplasty or surgery for multivessel coronary artery disease: comparison of eligible registry and randomized patients in the EAST trial and influence of treatment selections on outcomes: Emory Angioplasty versus Surgery Trial investigators. *Am J Cardiol* 1997;79:1453-1459.

13. Lamb HJ, Beyerbacht HP, de Roos A, et al. Left ventricular remodeling early after aortic valve replacement: differential effects on diastolic function in aortic valve stenosis and aortic regurgitation. *J Am Coll Cardiol* 2002;40:2182-2188.

14. Lindblom D, Lindblom U, Qvist J, Lundstrom H. Long-term relative survival rates after heart valve replacement. *J Am Coll Cardiol* 1990;15:566-573.

15. Lund O, Chandrasekaran V, Grocott-Mason R, et al. Primary aortic valve replacement with allografts over twenty-five years: valve-related and procedure related determinants of outcome. *J Thorac Cardiovasc Surg* 1999;117:77-91.

16. Mihaljevic T, Paul S, Cohn LH, Wechsler A. Pathophysiology of aortic valve disease. In: Cohn LH, Edmunds LH Jr, eds. *Cardiac Surgery in the Adult.* New York: McGraw-Hill; 2003:791-810.

17. Morice MC, Serruys PW, Sousa JE, et al. RAVEL study group: randomized study with the sirolimus-coated Bx velocity balloon-expandable stent in the treatment of patients with de novo native coronary artery lesions: a randomized comparison of a sirolimus-eluting stent with a standard stent for coronary revascularization. *N Engl J Med* 2002;346:1773-1780.

18. Parisi AF, Folland ED, Hartigan P. A comparison of angioplasty with medical therapy in the treatment of single-vessel coronary artery disease: Veterans Affairs ACME investigators. *N Engl J Med* 1992;326:10-16.

19. Passamani E, Davis KB, Gillespie MJ, Killip T. A randomized trial of coronary artery bypass surgery: survival of patients with a low ejection fraction. *N Engl J Med* 1985;312:1665-1671.

20. Pedersen TR, Kjekshus J, Berg K, et al. Scandinavian Simvastatin Survival Study Group: randomized trial of cholesterol lowering in 4444 patients with coronary heart disease: The Scandinavian Simvastatin Survival Study (4S): 1994. *Atheroscler Suppl* 2004;5:81-87.

21. Pitt B, Waters D, Brown WV, et al. Aggressive lipid-lowering therapy compared with angioplasty in stable coronary artery disease: Atorvastatin versus Revascularization Treatment investigators. *N Engl J Med* 1999;341:70-76.

22. Pocock SJ, Henderson RA, Clayton T, Lyman GH, Chamberlain DA. Quality of life after coronary angioplasty or continued medical treatment for angina: three-year follow-up in the RITA-2 trial: Randomized Intervention Treatment of Angina. *J Am Coll Cardiol* 2000;35:907-914.

23. Pocock SJ, Henderson RA, Rickards AF, et al. Meta-analysis of randomized trials comparing coronary angioplasty with bypass surgery. *Lancet* 1995;346:1184-1189.

24. Sellke FW, DiMaio JM, Caplan LR, et al. American Heart Association: comparing on-pump and off-pump coronary artery bypass grafting: numerous studies but few conclusions: a scientific statement from the American Heart Association council on cardiovascular surgery and anesthesia in collaboration with the interdisciplinary working group on quality of care and outcomes research. *Circulation* 2005;111:2858-2864.

25. Society of Thoracic Surgeons National Cardiac Surgery Database. www.sts.org.

26. The TIME investigators. Trial of Invasive versus Medical Therapy in Elderly Patients with Chronic Symptomatic Coronary-Artery Disease (TIME): a randomized trial. *Lancet* 2001;358:951-957.

27. Yusuf S, Zucker D, Peduzzi P, et al. Effect of coronary artery bypass graft surgery on survival: overview of 10-year results from randomised trials by the Coronary Artery Bypass Graft Surgery Trialists Collaboration. *Lancet* 1994;344:563-570.

Chapter 12

1. Anderson JL, Adams CD, Antman EM, et al. ACC/AHA 2007 guidelines for the management of patients with unstable angina/non-ST-elevation myocardial infarction: a report of the American College of Cardiology/American Heart Association Task Force on Practice Guidelines (Writing Committee to Revise the 2002 Guidelines for the Management of Patients With Unstable Angina/Non-ST-Elevation Myocardial Infarction). *J Am Coll Cardiol* 2007;50:e1-e157.

2. Deanfield J, Thaulow E, Warnes C, et al. Management of grown up congenital heart disease. *Eur Heart J* 2003;24:1035-1084.

3. Institute of Medicine. *Exploring the Biological Contributions to Human Health: Does Sex Matter?* National Academy Press: Wahington, DC; 2001.

4. Iung B, Baron G, Butchart EG, et al. A prospective survey of patients with valvular heart disease in Europe: the Euro Heart Survey on Valvular Heart Disease. *Eur Heart J* 2003;24:1231-1243.

5. Iung B, Gohlke-Barwolf G, Tornos P, et al. Recommendations on the management of the asymptomatic patient with valvular heart disease. *Eur Heart J* 2002;23:1252-1266.

6. Jessup M, Pina IL. Is it important to examine gender differences in the epidemiology and outcome of severe heart failure? *J Thorac Cardiovasc Surg* 2004;127:1247-1252.

7. Seventh Report of the Joint National Committee on Prevention, Detection, Evaluation, and Treatment of High Blood Pressure, *Hypertension* 2003;42:1206-1252.

8. Maron BJ. Hypertrophic cardiomyopathy: a systematic review. *JAMA* 2002;287:1308-1320.

9. Mieres JH, Shaw LJ, Arai A, et al. Role of noninvasive testing in the clinical evaluation of women with suspected coronary artery disease: consensus statement from the Cardiac Imaging Committee, Council on Clinical Cardiology, and the Cardiovascular Imaging and Intervention Committee, Council on Cardiovascular Radiology and Intervention, American Heart Association. *Circulation* 2005;111:682-696.

10. Mosca L, Banka CL, Benjamin EJ, et al, for the Expert Panel/Writing Group. Evidence based guidelines for cardiovascular disease prevention in women: 2007 update. *J Am Coll Cardiol* 2007;49:1230-1250.

11. Pina IL. A better survival for women with heart failure? It's not so simple. *J Am Coll Cardiol* 2003;42:2135-2138.

12. Rathore SS, Wang Y, Krumholtz HM. Sex-based differences in the effect of digoxin for the treatment of heart failure. *N Engl J Med* 2002;347:1403-1411.

13. Schweikert RA, Pashkow FJ. Exercise training in special populations: pacemakers and implantable cardioverter-defibrillators. In: Wenger NK, Smith LK, Froelicher ES, Comoss PM, eds. *Cardiac Rehabilitation. A Guide to Practice in the 21st Century.* New York: Marcel Dekker; 1999:163-169.

14. Task Force on the Management of Cardiovascular Diseases During Pregnancy of the European Society of Cardiology. Expert consensus document on management of cardiovascular diseases during pregnancy. *Eur Heart J* 2003;24:761-781.

15. Vaccarino V, Lin Z, Mattera J, et al. Impact of depressive symptoms on the outcome of coronary artery bypass surgery. *J Am Coll Cardiol* 2002;41(suppl 2):529A-530A.

16. Wassertheil-Smoller S, Anderson G, Psaty BM, et al. Hypertension and its treatment in postmenopausal women: baseline data from the Women's Health Initiative. *Hypertension* 2000;36:780-789.

17. Weissman NJ, Panza JA, Tighe JF, Gwynne JT. Natural history of valvular regurgitation 1 year after discontinuation of dexfenfluramine therapy: a randomized, double-blind, placebo-controlled trial. *Ann Intern Med* 2001;134:267-273.

18. Wenger NK. Coronary heart disease: the female heart is vulnerable. *Prog Cardiovasc Dis* 2003;46:199-229

Chapter 13

1. American Association of Cardiovascular and Pulmonary Rehabilitation. Reimbursement. In: *Guidelines for Cardiac Rehabilitation and Secondary Prevention Programs.* 4th ed. Champaign, IL: Human Kinetics; 2004:192.

2. American College of Sports Medicine. *ACSM's Guidelines for Exercise Testing and Prescription.* 6th ed. Baltimore: Lippincott Williams & Wilkins; 2000:69-70.

3. American Medical Association. *Current Procedural Terminology CPT 2005.* Chicago: AMA Press; 2004.

4. Appleby J. Health care tab ready to explode. *USA Today* February 24, 2005:1.

5. Bolus R, Pitts J. Patient satisfaction: the indispensable outcome. *Managed Care Magazine* April 1999;8:24-28.

6. Booth FW, Chakravarthy MV, Corbin CB, Pangrazi RP, Franks D. Cost and consequence of sedentary living: new battleground for an old enemy. *Res Dig* 2002;16:1-8.

7. Booth FW, Gordon SE, Carlson CJ, Hamilton MT. Invited review: waging the war on modern chronic diseases: primary prevention through exercise biology. *J Appl Physiol* 2000;88:774-787.

8. Bush GW, Carter J, Ford GR, et al. *Building a Better Health Care System: Specifications for Reform.* Washington, DC: National Coalition on Health Care; 2004.

9. *Cardiology Preeminence Roundtable. Beyond Four Walls: Cost-Effective Management of Chronic Heart Failure.* Washington, DC: Advisory Board Company; 1994.

10. Centers for Disease Control and Prevention. Effectiveness disease and injury prevention, estimated national spending on prevention—United States, 1998. *MMWR Morbid Mortal Wkly Rep* 1992;41:529-531.

11. Centers for Disease Control and Prevention. Chronic Disease Overview. http://cdc.gov/nccdphp/overview.htm.

12. Centers for Disease Control and Prevention. *CDC Chronic Disease Prevention: The Power of Prevention.* Atlanta, GA: U.S. Department of Health and Human Services; 2003. www.cdc.gov/nccdphp/publications/PowerOfPrevention.

13. Centers for Medicare & Medicaid Services. Proposed Decision Memo for Smoking & Tobacco Use Cessation Counseling (CAG-00241N), December 2004. www.cms.hhs.gov/mcd/viewdraftdecisionmemo.asp?id=130.

14. Centers for Medicare & Medicaid Services. The Chronic Care Improvement Program, May 25, 2004. http://a257.g.akamaitech.net/7/257/2422/14mar20010800/edocket.access.gpo.gov/2004/pdf/04-9127.pdf.

15. DMAA. Disease Management Association of America. www.dmaa.org/phi_definition.asp.

16. Evans M. Good news, bad news: Hospital's net profit margin up, operating margin down. *Modern Healthcare*, November 1, 2004. www.Kellogg.northwestern.edu/news/hits/041101mh.htm.

17. Flegal KM, Carroll MD, Ogden CL, Johnson CL. Prevalence and trends in obesity among US adults. 1999-2000. *JAMA* 2002;288:1723-1727.

18. Hall LK. Creating a discharge destination. Paper presented at: AACVPR National Meeting; October 2002; Charlotte, NC.

19. Halvorson G, cited in Cerne F. The Minnesota model. *Hospitals and Health Networks* June 5, 1994:3-40.

20. Hart AC, Hopkins CA, eds. *ICD-9-CM Professional.* Salt Lake City, UT: Ingenix, SLC; 2004.

21. Hellmich N. Walk the healthy walk. *USA Today* July 10, 2003: Life, Section D. www.usatoday.com/news/health/2003-07-09-america-move-usat_x.htm.

22. Hellmich N. Solace in food no more. *USA Today* March 28, 2005: Life, Section D.

23. House Committee on Ways and Means. Statement of Janet S. Wright, M.D., Testimony Before the Subcommittee on Health of the House Committee on Ways and Means. May 11, 2004. www.gpoaccess.gov/wmhearings/108.html.

24. HPK Group, LLC. The Hospital Financial Dilemma. www.hpk groupllc.com/hospitalcosts.html.

25. Hu FB, Manson JE, Stampfer MJ, et al. Diet, lifestyle, and the risk of type 2 diabetes mellitus in women. *N Engl J Med* 2001;345:790-797.

26. Hu FB, Sigal RJ, Rich-Edwards JW, et al. Walking compared with vigorous physical activity and risk of type 2 diabetes in women: a prospective study. *JAMA* 1999;282:1433-1439.

27. Hu FB, Stampfer MJ, Colditz GA, et al. Physical activity and risk of stroke in women. *JAMA* 2000;283:2961-1967.

28. Kaufman F. *Diabesity*. New York: Bantam; 2005.

29. Kesaniemi YK, Danforth E, Jensen MD, Kipelman PG, Lefebvre P, Reeder BA. Dose-response issues concerning physical activity and health: an evidenced-based symposium. *Med Sci Sports Exerc* 2001;33(6 suppl): S351-s358.

30. National Coalition on Health Care. Facts on Health Insurance Coverage. www.nchc.org/facts/cost.shtml.

31. National Institute of Diabetes and Digestive and Kidney Diseases. Statistics Related to Overweight and Obesity, October 6, 2004. www2.niddk.nih.gov/HealthEducation/HealthNutrit.

32. Pate RR, Pratt M, Blair SN, et al. Physical activity and public health: a recommendation from the Centers for Disease Control and Prevention and the American College of Sports Medicine. *JAMA* 1995;273:402-407.

33. Press Ganey Client Forum. Best Inpatient/Outpatient Practices. www.pressganey.com.

34. Sullivan S, Flynn TJ. The Revolution at Hand. Washington, DC: National Committee for Quality Health Care; 1992:3-65.

35. TriSpan Health Services Intermediary. Outpatient pulmonary rehabilitation services local coverage determination (LCD). Bulletin 2005-75, February 17, 2005, pp 1-17.

36. U.S. Department of Health and Human Services. Prevention Makes Common "Cents," September 2003. www.aspe.hhs.gov/health/prevention/index.shtml.

37. Weatherly LA. The rising cost of health care: strategic and societal considerations for employers, *HR Magazine*, July 2004.

Chapter 14

1. Aldana SG, Whitmer WR, Greenlaw R, et al. Cardiovascular risk reductions associated with aggressive lifestyle modification and cardiac rehabilitation. *Heart Lung* 2003;32:374-382.

2. Banzer JA, Maguire TE, Kennedy CM, O'Malley CJ, Balady GJ. Results of cardiac rehabilitation in patients with diabetes mellitus. *Am J Cardiol* 2004;93:81-84.

3. Billings J, Scherwitz L, Ornish D, Sullivan R. Lifestyle heart trial: comprehensive treatment and group support therapy. In: Allan R, Scheidt S, eds. *Heart and Mind: The Practice of Cardiac Psychology*. Washington DC: American Psychological Association; 1996:233-253.

4. Dansinger ML, Gleason JA, Griffen JL, et al. Comparison of the Atkins, Ornish, Weight Watchers and Zone diets for weight loss and heart disease risk reduction, a randomized trial. *JAMA* 2005;293:43-53.

5. Daubenmier JJ, Weidner G, Sumner M, et al. The contribution of changes in diet, exercise, and stress management to changes in coronary risk in women and men in the Multisite Cardiac Lifestyle Intervention Program. *Ann Behav Med* 2007;33:57-68.

6. *Dr. Dean Ornish Program for Reversing Heart Disease Staff Program Operations Manual*. Sausalito, CA: Preventive Medicine Research Institute; 1993.

7. Gould KL, Ornish D, Scherwitz L, et al. Changes in myocardial perfusion abnormalities by positron emission tomography after long-term intense risk factor modification. *JAMA* 1995;274:894-901.

8. Howard BV, Van Horn L, Hsia J, et al. Low-fat dietary patterns and risk of cardiovascular disease: the Women's Health Initiative Dietary Modification Trial. *JAMA* 2006;295:655-666.

9. Hunninghake DB, Stein EA, Dujovne CA, et al. The efficacy of intensive dietary therapy alone or combined with lovastatin in outpatients with hypercholesterolemia. *N Engl J Med* 1993;328:1213-1219.

10. Koertge J, Weidner G, Elliott-Eller M, et al. Improvement in medical risk factors and quality of life in women and men with coronary artery disease in the Multicenter Lifestyle Demonstration Project. *Am J Cardiol* 2003;91:1316-1322.

11. Lichtenstein AH, Van Horn L. AHA science advisory very low fat diets. *Circulation* 1998;98:935-939.

12. Linden W. Psychological treatments in cardiac rehabilitation: review of rationales and outcomes. *J Psychosom Res* 2000;48:443-454.

13. Merritt-Worden T, Ornish D, Pettengill E. Marked improvement in biomedical and psychosocial cardiac risk factors from a community-based Lifestyle Change Program. *Circulation* 2003;17:IV-758 (abstract).

14. Niebauer J, Hambrecht R, Velich T, et al. Attenuated progression of coronary artery disease after 6 years of multifactorial risk intervention: role of physical exercise. *Circulation* 1997;96:2534-2541.

15. Oldridge NB. Compliance with cardiac rehabilitation services. *J Cardiopulm Rehabil* 1991;11:115-127.

16. Ornish D. Intensive lifestyle changes in the management of coronary heart disease. In: Braunwald E, ed. *Harrison's Advances in Cardiology*. New York: McGraw Hill; 2002:43-52.

17. Ornish D. *Love & Survival: The Scientific Basis for the Healing Power of Intimacy*. New York: HarperCollins; 1998.

18. Ornish DM. Avoiding revascularization with lifestyle changes: The Multicenter Lifestyle Demonstration Project. *Am J Cardiol* 1998;82:72T-76T.

19. Ornish DM. *Dr. Dean Ornish's Program for Reversing Heart Disease*. New York: Random House; 1990.

20. Ornish DM, Brown SE, Scherwitz LW, et al. Can lifestyle changes reverse coronary heart disease? The Lifestyle Heart Trial. *Lancet* 1990;336:129-133.

21. Ornish DM, Scherwitz LW, Billings JH, et al. Intensive lifestyle changes for reversal of coronary heart disease. *JAMA* 1998;280:2001-2007.

22. Ornish DM, Scherwitz LW, Doody RS, et al. Effects of stress management training and dietary changes in treating ischemic heart disease. *JAMA* 1983;249:54-59.

23. Perelson G, Day B, DeVries A, et al. Reduced healthcare costs among cardiac patients making changes in diet and lifestyle: results from three years of claims utilization of patients and matched controls. *Circulation* 2005;111:e311 (abstract).

24. Pischke CR, Weidner G, Elliot-Eller M, et al. Comparison of coronary risk factors and quality of life in coronary artery disease patients with vs. without diabetes mellitus. *Am J Cardiol* 2006;97:1267-1273.

25. Position of the American Dietetic Association and Dietitians of Canada: Vegetarian diets. *J Am Diet Assoc* 2003;103:748-765.

26. Sdringola S, Nakagawa K, Nakagawa Y, et al. Combined intense lifestyle and pharmacologic lipid treatment further reduce coronary events and myocardial perfusion abnormalities compared with usual-care cholesterol-lowering drugs in coronary artery disease. *J Am Coll Cardiol* 2003;41:263-272.

27. St. Joer S, Howard BV, Prewitt P, et al. Dietary protein and weight reduction: a statement for health professionals from the nutrition committee of the council on nutrition, physical, activity and metabolism of the American Heart Association. *Circulation* 2001;104:1869-1874.

28. Sumner MD, Weidner G, Merritt-Worden T, Ornish D. Weight reduction among women and men enrolled in a comprehensive cardiac risk reduction program after 3 and 12 months. *J Cardiopulm Rehabil* 2004;24:348 (abstract).

29. Sumner MD, Weidner G, Merritt-Worden T, Studley J, Marlin R, Ornish D. The effect of comprehensive lifestyle changes on diabetic patients in the Multisite Cardiac Lifestyle Intervention Program (MCLIP). *Psychosom Med* 2005;67:A73 (abstract).

30. Taylor RS, Brown A, Ebrahim S, et al. Exercise-based rehabilitation for patients with coronary heart disease: a systematic review and meta-analysis of randomized controlled trials. *Am J Med* 2004;116:682-692.

31. Yusuf S, Hawken S, Ounpuu S, on behalf of the INTERHEART Study Investigators. Effect of potentially modifiable risk factors associated with myocardial infarction in 52 countries (the INTERHEART study): case-control study. *Lancet* 2004;364:937-952.

Chapter 15

1. Adams V, Lenk K, Linke A, e al. Increase of circulating endothelial progenitor cells in patients with coronary artery disease after exercise induced ischemia. *Arterioscler Thromb Vasc Biol* 2004;24:684-690.

2. American College of Sports Medicine. *ACSM's Guidelines for Exercise Testing and Prescription.* 7th ed. Philadelphia: Lippincott Williams & Wilkins; 2006.

3. Bouchard C, An P, Rice T, et al. Familial aggregation of $\dot{V}O_{2max}$ response to exercise training: results from the HERITAGE Family Study. *J Appl Physiol* 1999;87:1003-1008.

4. Cannon C, Foster C, Porcari JP, Skemp-Arlt KM, Fater DCW, Backes R. The talk test as a measure of exertional ischemia. *Am J Sports Med* 2004;6:52-57.

5. Debusk RF, Stenestrand U, Sheehan M, Haskell WL. Training effects of long versus short bouts of exercise in healthy subjects. *Am J Cardiol* 1990;65:1010-1013.

6. Esteve-Lanno J, Foster C, Seiler S, Lucia A. Impact of training intensity distribution on performance in endurance athletes. *J Strength Cond Res* 2007;21:943-949.

7. Fitz-Clarke JR, Morton RH, Banister EW. Optimizing athletic performance by influence curves. *J Appl Physiol* 1991;71:1151-1158.

8. Foster C, Pollock ML, Anholm JD, et al. Work capacity and left ventricular function during rehabilitation from myocardial revascularization surgery. *Circulation* 1984;69:748-755.

9. Foster C, Thompson NN. Functional translation of exercise responses to recreational activities. *J Cardiopulm Rehabil* 1991;11:373-377.

10. Foster C, Hector LL, Welsh R, Schrager M, Green MA, Snyder AC. Effects of specific versus cross-training on running performance. *Eur J Appl Physiol* 1995;70:367-372.

11. Foster C, Daines E, Hector L, Snyder AC, Welsh R. Athletic performance in relation to training load. *Wisc Med J* 1996;95:370-374.

12. Foster C, Porcari JP. The risks of exercise training. *J Cardiopulm Rehabil* 2001;21:347-352.

13. Foster C, Heimann KM, Esten PL, Brice G, Porcari JP. Differences in perceptions of training by coaches and athletes. *S Afr J Sports Med* 2001;8:3-7.

14. Foster C, Porcari JP. The physiologic basis for the warm-up in therapeutic exercise programs. *Am J Med Sport* 2002;4:158-159.

15. Hansen AK, Fischer CP, Plomgaard P, Andersen JL, Saltin B, Pedersen BK. Skeletal muscle adaptation; training twice every second day vs training once daily. *J Appl Physiol* 2005;98:93-99.

16. Hickson RC, Rosenkoetter MA. Reduced training frequencies and maintenance of increased cardiovascular fitness. *Med Sci Sports Exerc* 1981;13:13-16.

17. Hickson RC, Kanakis C, Davis JR, Moore AM, Rich S. Reduced training duration effects on aerobic power, endurance and cardiac growth. *J Appl Physiol* 1982;53:225-229.

18. Hickson RC, Foster C, Pollock ML, Galassi TM, Rich S. Reduced training intensities and the loss of aerobic power, endurance and cardiac growth. *J Appl Physiol* 1985;58:492-499.

19. Hickson RC, Dvorak BA, Gorostiaga EM, Kurowski TT, Foster C. Potential for strength and endurance training to amplify endurance performance. *J Appl Physiol* 1988;65:2285-2290.

20. Hagoglou A, Foster C, deKoning JJ, Lucia A, Kernozek T, Porcari JP. Effect of warm-up on cycle time trial performance. *Med Sci Sports Exerc* 2005;37:1608-1614.

21. Katch V, Weltman A, Sady S, Freedson P. Validity of the relative percent concept for equating training intensity. *Eur J Appl Physiol* 1978;39:219-227.

22. Le Bris S, Ledermann B, Candau R, Davy JM, Messner-Pellenc P, Le Gallais D. Applying a systems model of training to a patient with coronary artery disease. *Med Sci Sports Exerc* 2004;36:942-948.

23. Meyer K, Samek L, Pinchas A, Baier M, Betz P, Roskamm H. Relationship between ventilatory threshold and onset of ischaemic in ECG during stress testing. *Eur Heart J* 1995;16:623-630.

24. Meyer K, Foster C, Georgakopoulous N, et al. Left ventricular function during interval and steady state exercise in patients with chronic heart failure. *Am J Cardiol* 1998;82:1382-1387.

25. Meyer T, Lucia A, Earnest CP, Kindermann W. A conceptual framework for performance diagnosis and training prescription from submaximal parameters—theory and application. *Int J Sports Med* 2005;26:1-11.

26. Morton RH, Fitz-Clarke JR, Banister EW. Modeling human performance in running. *J Appl Physiol* 1990;69:1171-1177.

27. Pollock ML. How much exercise is enough? *Phys Sportsmed* 1978;6:50-64.

28. Pollock ML, Welsch MA, Graves JE. Exercise prescription for cardiac rehabilitation. In: Pollock ML, Schmidt DH, eds. *Heart Disease and Rehabilitation*. 3rd ed. Champaign, IL: Human Kinetics; 1995:243-276.

29. Quell KJ, Porcari JP, Franklin BA, Foster C, Andreuzzi RA, Anthony RM. Is brisk walking an adequate aerobic training stimulus for cardiac patients? *Chest* 2002;122:1852-1856.

30. Recalde PT, Foster C, Skemp-Arlt KM, et al. The "Talk Test" as a simple marker of ventilatory threshold. *S Afr J Sports Med* 2002;9:5-8.

31. Seiler KS, Kjerland GO. Quantifying training intensity distribution in elite endurance athletes: is there evidence for an "optimal" distribution? *Scand J Med Sci Sports* 2006;16:49-56.

32. Skinner JS, Jaskolski A, Jaskolska A, et al. Age, sex, race initial fitness and response to training: the HERITAGE Family Study. *J Appl Physiol* 2001;90:1770-1776.

33. Swain DP, Franklin BA. $\dot{V}O_2$ reserve and the minimal intensity for improving cardiorespiratory fitness. *Med Sci Sports Exerc* 2002;34:152-157.

34. Turner AP, Cathcart AJ, Parker ME, Butterworth C, Wilson J, Ward SA. Oxygen uptake and muscle desaturation kinetics during intermittent cycling. *Med Sci Sports Exerc* 2006;38:492-503.

35. Voelker SA, Foster C, Porcari JP, Skemp KM, Brice G, Backes R. Relationship between the talk test and ventilatory threshold in cardiac patients. *Clin Exerc Physiol* 2002;4:120-123.

Chapter 16

1. American Association of Cardiovascular and Pulmonary Rehabilitation. *Guidelines for Cardiac Rehabilitation and Secondary Prevention Programs*. 4th ed. Champaign, IL: Human Kinetics; 2003.

2. American College of Sports Medicine. The recommended quantity and quality of exercise for developing and maintaining cardiorespiratory and muscular fitness and flexibility in healthy adults. *Med Sci Sports Exerc* 1998;30:975-991.

3. American College of Sports Medicine. *ACSM's Resource Manual for Guidelines for Exercise Testing and Prescription*. 3rd ed. Baltimore: Williams & Wilkins; 1998;448-455.

4. American College of Sports Medicine. Progression models in resistance training for healthy adults. *Med Sci Sports Exerc* 2002;34:364-380.

5. Banz WJ, Maher MA, Thompson WG, et al. Effects of resistance versus aerobic training on coronary artery disease risk factors. *Exp Biol Med* 2003;228:434-440.

6. Beniamini Y, Rubenstein JJ, Zaichkowsky LD, et al. Effects of high-intensity strength training on quality of life parameters in cardiac rehabilitation patients. *Am J Cardiol* 1997;80:841-846.

7. Borg GAV. Psychophysical bases of perceived exertion. *Med Sci Sports Exerc* 1982;14:377-381.

8. Braith RW, Mills RM, Welsch MA, et al. Resistance training restores BMD in heart transplant recipients. *J Am Coll Cardiol* 1997;28:1471-1477.

9. Braith RW, Welsch MA, Mills RM, et al. Resistance training prevents glucocorticoid-induced myopathy in heart transplant recipients. *Med Sci Sports Exerc* 1998;30:483-489.

10. Carpenter D, Nelson B. Low back strengthening for health, rehabilitation, and injury prevention. *Med Sci Sports Exerc* 1999;31:18-24.

11. Castaneda C, Layne JE, Munoz-Orians L, et al. A randomized controlled trial of resistance exercise training to improve glycemic control in older adults with type 2 diabetes. *Diabetes Care* 2002;25:2335-2341.

12. Chelsey A, MacDougall J, Tarnopolosky M, et al. Changes in human muscle protein synthesis after resistance exercise. *J Appl Physiol* 1992;73:1383-1388.

13. Delagardelle C, Feireisen P, Krecke R, et al. Objective effects of a 6 months' endurance and strength training program in outpatients with congestive heart failure. *Med Sci Sports Exerc* 1999;31:1102-1107.

14. Demichele PD, Pollock ML, Graves JE, et al. Effect of training frequency on the development of isometric torso rotation strength. *Arch Phys Med Rehabil* 1997;27:64-69.

15. Dipietro L. Physical activity, body weight, and adiposity: an epidemiological perspective. In: Holloszy J, ed. *Exercise and Sport Sciences Reviews*. Baltimore, MD: Williams & Wilkins; 1995;275-303.

16. Durstine JL, Haskell WL. Effects of exercise training on plasma lipids and lipoproteins. In: Holloszy J, ed. *Exercise and Sport Sciences Reviews*. Baltimore, MD: Williams & Wilkins; 1994;477-520.

17. Evans WJ. Exercise training guidelines for the elderly. *Med Sci Sports Exerc* 1999;31:12-17.

18. Ewart CK. Psychological effects of resistive weight training: implications for cardiac patients. *Med Sci Sports Exerc* 1989;21:683-688.

19. Feigenbaum MS, Pollock ML. Prescription of resistance training for health and disease. *Med Sci Sports Exerc* 1999;31:38-45.

20. Fleck SJ, Kraemer WJ. *Designing Resistance Training Programs*. 2nd ed. Champaign, IL: Human Kinetics; 1997.

21. Fletcher GF, Balady G, Froelicher VF, et al. Exercise standards: A Statement for Healthcare Professionals From the American Heart Association. *Circulation* 1995;91:580-615.

22. Fluckey JD, Hickey M, Brambrink JK, et al. Effects of resistance exercise on glucose tolerance in normal and glucose-intolerant subjects. *J Appl Physiol* 1994;77:1087-1092.

23. Galvao DA, Taafe DR. Single- vs. multiple-set resistance training: recent developments in the controversy. *J Strength Cond Res* 2004;18:660-667.

24. Garrow JS, Summerbell CD. Meta-analysis: effects of exercise, with or without dieting on the body composition of overweight subjects. *Eur J Clin Nutr* 1995;49:1-10.

25. Ghilarducci LC, Holly RG, Amsterdam EA. Effects of high resistance training in coronary artery disease. *Am J Cardiol* 1989;64:866-870.

26. Goldberg AP. Aerobic and resistive exercise modify risk factors for coronary heart disease. *Med Sci Sports Exerc* 1989;21:669-674.

27. Gordon NF. Hypertension. In: *ACSM's Exercise Management for Persons with Chronic Diseases and Disabilities*. Champaign, IL: Human Kinetics; 1997:59-63.

28. Graves JE, Franklin BA. In: *Resistance Training for Health and Rehabilitation*. Champaign, IL: Human Kinetics; 2001.

29. Haas CJ, Garzarella L, Dehoyas D, et al. Single versus multiple sets and long-term recreational weightlifters. *Med Sci Sports Exerc* 2000;32:235-242.

30. Hare DL, Ryan TM, Selig SE, et al. Resistance exercise training increases muscle strength, endurance, and blood flow in patients with chronic heart failure. *Am J Cardiol* 1999;83:1674-1677.

31. Holloszy JO, Constable CH, Young DA. Activation of glucose transport in muscle by exercise. *Diabetes/ Metabolism Review* 1986;1:409-423.

32. Hunter GR, Bryan DR, Wetzstein CJ, et al. Resistance training and intra-abdominal adipose tissue in older men and women. *Med Sci Sports Exerc* 2002;34:1023-1028.

33. Hurley BF, Hagberg JM, Goldberg AP, et al. Resistive training can reduce coronary risk factors without altering $\dot{V}O_2$max or percent bodyfat. *Med Sci Sports Exerc*. 1988;20:150-154.

34. Kuczmarski RJ, Flegal KM, Campbell SM, et al. The increasing prevalence of overweight among U.S. adults: the National Health and Nutrition Examination Surveys, 1960 to 1991. *JAMA* 1994;272:205-211.

35. Layne JE, Nelson ME. The effect of progressive resistance training on bone density: a review. *Med Sci Sports Exerc* 1999;31:25-30.

36. MacDougall JD, Tuxen D, Sale DG, et al. Arterial blood pressure response to heavy resistance training. *J Appl Physiol* 1985;58:785-790.

37. McCartney N. Acute responses to resistance training and safety. *Med Sci Sports Exerc* 1999;31:31-37.

38. Pollock ML. Prescribing exercise for fitness and adherence. In: Dishman RK, ed. *Exercise Adherence: Its Impact on Public Health*. Champaign, IL: Human Kinetics; 1988:259-282.

39. Pollock ML, Vincent KR. Resistance training for health. *The President's Council on Physical Fitness and Sports Research Digest* December 1996; Series 2, No. 8.

40. Pollock ML, Franklin BA, Balady GJ, et al. Resistance exercise in individuals with and without cardiovascular disease: benefits, rationale, safety, and prescription. *Circulation* 2000;101:828-833.

41. Sale DG. Influence of exercise and training on motor unit activation. In: Pandolf DB, ed. *Exercise and Sport Sciences Reviews*. New York: MacMillan; 1987:95-152.

42. Smutok MA, Reece C, Kokkinos PF, et al. Aerobic versus strength training for risk factor intervention in middle-aged men at high risk for coronary heart disease. *Metabolism* 1993;42:177-184.

43. Spengler D, Bigos S, Martin N, et al. Back injuries in industry: a retrospective study. 1. Overview and cost analysis. *Spine* 1986;11:241-246.

44. Stefanick ML. Exercise and weight control. In: Holloszy J, ed. *Exercise and Sport Sciences Reviews*. Baltimore, MD: Williams & Wilkins; 1993:363-396.

45. Stewart KJ, Mason M, Kelemen MH. Three-year participation in circuit weight training improves muscular strength and self-efficacy in cardiac patients. *J Cardiopulm Rehabil* 1988;8:292-296.

46. Stewart KJ. Resistive training effects on strength and cardiovascular endurance in cardiac and coronary prone patients. *Med Sci Sports Exerc* 1989;21:678-682.

47. Tabata I, Suzuki Y, Fukunaga T, et al. Resistance training affects GLUT-4 content in skeletal muscle of humans after 19 days of head-down bed rest. *J Appl Physiol* 1999;86:909-914.

48. Tanasescu M, Leitzmann RF, Rimm EB, et al. Exercise type and intensity in relation to coronary heart disease in men. *JAMA* 2002;288:1994-2000.

49. U.S. Department of Health and Human Services, Physical Activity and Health. *A Report of the Surgeon General*. Atlanta, GA: U.S. Department of Health and Human Services, Centers for Disease Control and Prevention, National Center for Chronic Disease Prevention and Health Promotion; 1996:22-29.

50. Van Etten LMLA, Verstappen FTJ, Westerterp KR. Effect of body build on weight-training-induced adaptations in body composition and muscular strength. *Med Sci Sports Exerc* 1994;26:515-521.

51. Vincent KR, Braith RW. Resistance exercise and bone turnover in elderly men and women. *Med Sci Sports Exerc* 2002;34:17-23.

52. Wallberg-Henriksson H. Exercise and diabetes mellitus. In: Holloszy J, ed. *Exercise and Sport Sciences Reviews.* Baltimore, MD: Williams & Wilkins; 1992:339-368.

53. Wenger NK, Froelicher ES, Smith LK, et al. *Cardiac Rehabilitation as Secondary Prevention. Clinical Practice Guideline No. 17* (AHCPR publication 96-0672). Rockville, MD: U.S. Department of Health and Human Services, Public Health Service, Agency for Health Care Policy and Research and the National Heart, Lung, and Blood Institute; October 1995.

54. Whaley MH, Kampert JB, Kohl HW, et al. Physical fitness and clustering of risk factors associated with metabolic syndrome. *Med Sci Sports Exerc* 1999;31:287-293.

Chapter 17

1. Alway SE. Force and contractile characteristics after stretch overload in quail anterior latissimus dorsi muscle. *J Appl Physiol* 1994;77:135-141.

2. Amako M, Oda T, Masuoka K, Yokoi H, Campisi P. Effect of static stretching on prevention of injuries for military recruits. *Mil Med* 2003;168:442-446.

3. Bandy WD, Irion JM. The effect of time on static stretch on the flexibility of the hamstring muscles. *Phys Ther* 1994;74:845-852.

4. Bandy WD, Irion JM, Briggler M. The effect of time and frequency of static stretching on flexibility of the hamstring muscles. *Phys Ther* 1997;77:1090-1096.

5. Beaulieu JE. Developing a stretching program. *Phys Sportsmed* 1981;9:59-65.

6. Borms J, van Roy P, Santens J-P, Haentjens A. Optimal duration of static stretching exercises for improvement of coxo-femoral flexibility. *J Sports Sci* 1987;5:39-47.

7. Caro CG, Pedley TJ, Schroter RC, Seed WA. *The Mechanics of the Circulation.* New York: Oxford University Press; 1978.

8. de Vries HA. Prevention of muscular distress after exercise. *Res Quarterly* 1961;32:177-185.

9. Feland JB, Myrer JW, Schulthies SS, Fellingham GW, Measom GW. The effect of duration of stretching of the hamstring muscle group for increasing range of motion in people aged 65 years or older. *Phys Ther* 2001;81:1110-1117.

10. Halbertsma JPK, van Bolhuis AI, Goeken LNH. Sport stretching: effect on passive muscle stiffness of short hamstrings. *Arch Phys Med Rehabil* 1996;77:688-692.

11. Hartig DE, Henderson JM. Increasing hamstring flexibility decreases lower extremity overuse injuries in military basic trainees. *Am J Sports Med* 1999;27:173-176.

12. Henricson AS, Fredriksson K, Persson I, Pereira R, Rostedt Y, Westlin NE. The effect of heat and stretching on the range of hip motion. *J Orthop Sports Phys Ther* 1984;6:110-115.

13. Herbert RD, Gabriel M. Effects of stretching before and after exercising on muscle soreness and risk of injury: systematic review. *Brit Med J* 2002;325:468.

14. Hilyer JC, Brown KC, Sirles AT, Peoples L. A flexibility intervention to reduce the incidence and severity of joint injuries among municipal firefighters. *J Occup Med* 1990;32:631-637.

15. Holmich P, Uhrskou P, Ulnits L, et al. Active physical training for long-standing adductor-related groin pain. *Lancet* 1999;353:439-443.

16. Hubley CL, Kozey JW, Stanish WD. The effects of static stretching exercises and stationary cycling on range of motion at the hip joint. *J Orthop Sports Phys Ther* 1984;6:104-109.

17. Jones KD, Burckhardt CS, Clark SR, Bennett RM, Potempa KM. A randomized controlled trial of muscle strengthening versus flexibility training in fibromyalgia. *J Rheumatol* 2002;29:1041-1048.

18. Lentell G, Hetherington T, Eagan J, Morgan M. The use of thermal agents to influence the effectiveness of a low-load prolonged stretch. *J Orthop Sports Phys Ther* 1992;16:200-207.

19. Magnusson SP, Simonsen EB, Aagaard P, Dyhre-Poulsen P, McHugh MP, Kjaer M. Mechanical and physiological responses to stretching with and without preisometric contraction in human skeletal muscle. *Arch Phys Med Rehabil* 1996;77:373-378.

20. Markos PD. Ipsilateral and contralateral effects of proprioceptive neuromuscular facilitation techniques on hip motion and electromyographic activity. *Phys Ther* 1979;59:1366-1373.

21. McNair PJ, Stanley SN. Effect of passive stretching and jogging on the series elastic muscle stiffness and range of motion of the ankle joint. *Br J Sports Med* 1996;30:313-318.

22. Peters S, Stanley I, Rose M, Kaney S, Salmon P. A randomized controlled trial of group aerobic exercise in primary care patients with persistent, unexplained physical symptoms. *Fam Pract* 2002;19:665-674.

23. Shrier I. Stretching before exercise does not reduce the risk of local muscle injury: a critical review of the clinical and basic science literature. *Clin J Sport Med* 1999;9:221-227.

24. Shrier I. Does stretching improve performance? A systematic and critical review of the literature. *Clin J Sport Med* 2002;14:267-273.

25. Shrier I, Gossal K. Myths and truths of stretching. *Phys Sportsmed* 2000;28:57-63.

26. Taylor BF, Waring CA, Brashear TA. The effects of therapeutic application of heat or cold followed by static stretch on hamstring muscle length. *J Orthop Sports Phys Ther* 1995;21:283-286.

27. Thacker SB, Gilchrist J, Stroup DF, Kimsey CD. The impact of stretching on sports injury risk: a

systematic review of the literature. *Med Sci Sports Exerc* 2004;36:371-378.

28. Wessling KC, DeVane DA, Hylton CR. Effects of static stretch versus static stretch and ultrasound combined on triceps surae muscle extensibility in healthy women. *Phys Ther* 1986;67:674-679.

29. Wiktorsson-Möller M, Öberg BA, Ekstrand J, Gillquist J. Effects of warming up, massage, and stretching on range of motion and muscle strength in the lower extremity. *Am J Sports Med* 1983;11:249-252.

30. Yang S, Alnaqeeb M, Simpson H, Goldspink G. Changes in muscle fibre type, muscle mass and IGF-I gene expression in rabbit skeletal muscle subjected to stretch. *J Anat* 1997;190:613-622.

Chapter 18

1. American Diabetes Association. Nutrition recommendations and interventions for diabetes: a position statement of the American Diabetes Association. *Diabetes Care* 2008;31(suppl 1):S61-S78.

2. Appel LJ, Champagne CM, Harsha DW, et al. Effects of comprehensive lifestyle modification on blood pressure control: main results of the PREMIER clinical trial. *JAMA* 2003;289:2083-2093.

3. Appel LJ, Moore TJ, Obarzanek E, et al. A clinical trial of the effects of dietary patterns on blood pressure. DASH Collaborative Research Group. *N Engl J Med* 1997;336:1117-1124.

4. Appel LJ, Sacks FM, Carey VJ, et al. Effects of protein, monounsaturated fat, and carbohydrate intake on blood pressure and serum lipids: results of the OmniHeart randomized trial. *JAMA* 2005;294(19):2455-64.

5. Burr ML, Fehily AM, Gilbert JF, et al. Effects of changes in fat, fish, and fibre intakes on death and myocardial reinfarction: diet and reinfarction trial (DART). *Lancet* 1989;2:757-761.

6. Chobanian AV, Bakris GL, Black HR, et al. The Seventh Report of the Joint National Committee on Prevention, Detection, Evaluation, and Treatment of High Blood Pressure: the JNC 7 report. *JAMA* 2003;289:2560-2572.

7. de Lorgeril M, Renaud S, Mamelle N, et al. Mediterranean alpha-linolenic acid-rich diet in secondary prevention of coronary heart disease. *Lancet* 1994;343:1454-1459.

8. Dietary Guidelines Advisory Committee D. Report of the Dietary Guidelines Advisory Committee on the Dietary Guidelines for Americans, 2005. Washington, DC: U.S. Government Printing Office; January 2005.

9. Elmer PJ, Obarzanek E, Vollmer WM, et al. Effects of comprehensive lifestyle modification on diet, weight, physical fitness, and blood pressure control: 18-month results of a randomized trial. *Ann Intern Med* 2006;144:485-495.

10. Esposito K, Marfella R, Ciotola M, et al. Effect of a Mediterranean-style diet on endothelial dysfunction and markers of vascular inflammation in the metabolic syndrome: a randomized trial. *JAMA* 2004;292:1440-1446.

11. Fung TT, Willett WC, Stampfer MJ, et al. Dietary patterns and the risk of coronary heart disease in women. *Arch Intern Med* 2001;161:1857-1862.

12. Greenland P, Knoll MD, Stamler J, et al. Major risk factors as antecedents of fatal and nonfatal coronary heart disease events. *JAMA* 2003;290:891-897.

13. Grundy SM, Cleeman JI, Merz CN, et al. Implications of recent clinical trials for the National Cholesterol Education Program Adult Treatment Panel III guidelines. *Circulation* 2004;110:227-239.

14. Grundy SM, Denke MA. Dietary influences on serum lipids and lipoproteins. *J Lipid Res* 1990;31:1149-1172.

15. Hegsted DM, Ausman LM, Johnson JA, et al. Dietary fat and serum lipids: an evaluation of the experimental data. *Am J Clin Nutr* 1993;57:875-883.

16. Hu FB, Rimm EB, Stampfer MJ, et al. Prospective study of major dietary patterns and risk of coronary heart disease in men. *Am J Clin Nutr* 2000;72:912-921.

17. Hu FB, Willett WC. Optimal diets for prevention of coronary heart disease. *JAMA* 2002;288:2569-2578.

18. Institute of Medicine and National Academies of Science. *Dietary Reference Intakes: Energy, Carbohydrates, Fiber, Fat, Fatty Acids, Cholesterol, Protein, and Amino Acids*. Washington, DC: National Academies Press; 2002.

19. Jenkins DJ, Kendall CW, Axelsen M, et al. Viscous and nonviscous fibres, nonabsorbable and low glycaemic index carbohydrates, blood lipids and coronary heart disease. *Curr Opin Lipidol* 2000;11:49-56.

20. Jenkins DJ, Kendall CW, Faulkner D, et al. A dietary portfolio approach to cholesterol reduction: combined effects of plant sterols, vegetable proteins, and viscous fibers in hypercholesterolemia. *Metabolism* 2002;51:1596-1604.

21. Jenkins DJ, Kendall CW, Marchie A, et al. The effect of combining plant sterols, soy protein, viscous fibers, and almonds in treating hypercholesterolemia. *Metabolism* 2003;52:1478-1483.

22. Jenkins DJ, Kendall CW, Marchie A, et al. Effects of a dietary portfolio of cholesterol-lowering foods vs lovastatin on serum lipids and C-reactive protein. *JAMA* 2003;290:502-510.

23. Khot UN, Khot MB, Bajzer CT, et al. Prevalence of conventional risk factors in patients with coronary heart disease. *JAMA* 2003;290:898-904.

24. Knowler WC, Barrett-Connor E, Fowler SE, et al. Reduction in the incidence of type 2 diabetes with lifestyle intervention or metformin. *N Engl J Med* 2002;346:393-403.

25. Lichtenstein AH, Appel LJ, Brands M, et al. Diet and lifestyle recommendations revision 2006: a scientific statement from the American Heart Association Nutrition Committee. *Circulation* 2006 Jul 4;114(1):82-96.

26. Mensink RP. Effects of the individual saturated fatty acids on serum lipids and lipoprotein concentrations. *Am J Clin Nutr* 1993;57:711S-714S.

27. Mensink RP, Katan MB. Effect of dietary fatty acids on serum lipids and lipoproteins: a meta-analysis of 27 trials. *Arterioscler Thromb* 1992;12:911-919.

28. Millen BE, Quatromoni PA, Nam BH, et al. Compliance with expert population-based dietary guidelines and lower odds of carotid atherosclerosis in women: the Framingham nutrition studies. *Am J Clin Nutr* 2005;82:174-180.

29. National Cholesterol and Education Program N. Executive summary of the third report of the National Cholesterol Education Program (NCEP) Expert Panel on Detection, Evaluation, and Treatment of High Blood Cholesterol in Adults (Adult Treatment Panel III). *JAMA* 2001;285(19):2486-97.

30. National Heart, Lung, and Blood Institute. Clinical guidelines on the identification, evaluation, and treatment of overweight and obesity in adults: executive summary. Expert Panel on the Identification, Evaluation, and Treatment of Overweight in Adults. *Am J Clin Nutr* 1998;68:899-917.

31. Ness AR, Hughes J, Elwood PC, et al. The long-term effect of dietary advice in men with coronary disease: follow-up of the Diet and Reinfarction trial (DART). *Eur J Clin Nutr* 2002;56(6):512-18.

32. Obarzanek E, Sacks FM, Vollmer WM, et al. Effects on blood lipids of a blood pressure-lowering diet: the Dietary Approaches to Stop Hypertension (DASH) Trial. *Am J Clin Nutr* 2001;74:80-89.

33. Orchard TJ, Temprosa M, Goldberg R, et al. The effect of metformin and intensive lifestyle intervention on the metabolic syndrome: the Diabetes Prevention Program randomized trial. *Ann Intern Med* 2005;142:611-619.

34. Ornish D, Brown SE, Scherwitz LW, et al. Can lifestyle changes reverse coronary heart disease? The Lifestyle Heart Trial. *Lancet* 1990;336:129-133.

35. Ornish D, Scherwitz LW, Billings JH, et al. Intensive lifestyle changes for reversal of coronary heart disease. *JAMA* 1998;280:2001-2007.

36. Svetkey LP, Harsha DW, Vollmer WM, et al. Premier: a clinical trial of comprehensive lifestyle modification for blood pressure control: rationale, design and baseline characteristics. *Ann Epidemiol* 2003;13:462-471.

37. Svetkey LP, Simons-Morton D, Vollmer WM, et al. Effects of dietary patterns on blood pressure: subgroup analysis of the Dietary Approaches to Stop Hypertension (DASH) randomized clinical trial. *Arch Intern Med* 1999;159:285-293.

38. U.S. Department of Agriculture. *National Nutrient Database for Standard Reference, Release 15.* Washington, DC: USDA; August 2002.

Chapter 19

1. Blanchard BE, Poulin M, Tsongalis GJ, et al. RAAS polymorphisms alter the acute blood pressure response to dynamic exercise. *Eur J Appl Physiol* 2006;97:26-33.

2. Chobanian AV, Bakris GL, Black HR, et al, and the National High Blood Pressure Education Program Coordinating Committee. Seventh Report of the Joint National Committee on Detection, Evaluation, and Treatment of High Blood Pressure. JNC 7—complete version. *Hypertension* 2003;42:1206-1252.

3. Cornelissen VA, Fagard RH. Effect of resistance training on resting blood pressure: a meta-analysis of randomized controlled trials. *J Hypertens* 2005;23:251-259.

4. Ehrman JK, Gordon PM, Visich PS, Keteyian SH, eds. *Clinical Exercise Physiology.* Champaign, IL: Human Kinetics; 2003.

5. Fagard RH. Physical activity in the prevention and treatment of hypertension in the obese. *Med Sci Sports Exerc* 1999;31(suppl):S624-S630.

6. Fagard RH. Exercise characteristics and the blood pressure response to dynamic physical training. *Med Sci Sports Exerc* 2001;33(suppl):S484-s492.

7. Fields LE, Burt VL, Cutler JA, Hughes J, Roccella EJ, Sorlier P. The burden of adult hypertension in the United States 1999 to 2000: a rising tide. *Hypertension* 2004;44:398-404.

8. Fletcher GF, Balady GJ, Amsterdam EA, et al. Exercise standards for testing and training: a statement for healthcare professionals from the American Heart Association. *Circulation* 2001;104:1694-1740.

9. Guidry MA, Blanchard BE, Thompson PD, et al. The influence of short and long duration on the blood pressure response to an acute bout of dynamic exercise. *Am Heart J* 2006;151:1322.e5-12.

10. Halliwill JR. Mechanisms and clinical implications of post-exercise hypotension in humans. *Exerc Sports Sci Rev* 2001;29:65-70.

11. Jakicic JM, Clark K, Coleman E, et al. American College of Sports Medicine. Position stand on appropriate intervention strategies for weight loss and prevention of weight regain for adults. *Med Sci Sports Exerc* 2001;33:2145-2156.

12. Joint National Committee on Detection, Evaluation, and Treatment of High Blood Pressure. The 6th Report of the Joint National Committee on detection, evaluation, and treatment of high blood pressure (JNC VI). *Arch Intern Med* 1997;157:2413-2446.

13. Kelley GA, Kelley KS. Progressive resistance exercise and resting blood pressure: a meta-analysis of randomized controlled trials. *Hypertension* 2000;35:838-843.

14. Kelley GA, Kelley KS, Tran Z. Aerobic exercise and resting blood pressure: a meta-analytic review of randomized, controlled trials. *Prev Cardiol* 2001;4:73-80.

15. Mach C, Foster C, Brice G, Mikat RP, Porcari JP. Effect of exercise duration on postexercise hypotension. *J Cardiopulm Rehabil* 2005;25:366-369.

16. Mason RJ, Broaddus VC, Murray JF, Nadel JA, eds. *Murray and Nadel's Textbook of Respiratory Medicine.* 4th ed. Philadelphia: Saunders; 2005.

17. Mazzeo RS, Cavanagh P, Evans WJ, et al. American College of Sports Medicine position stand: exercise and physical activity for older adults. *Med Sci Sports Exerc* 1998;30:992-1008.

18. Pescatello LS, Franklin D, Fagard R, Farquhar W, Kelly GA, Ray CA. American College of Sports Medicine position stand: exercise and hypertension. *Med Sci Sports Exerc* 2004;36:533-553.

19. Pescatello LS, Guidry MA, Blanchard BE, et al. Exercise intensity alters postexercise hypotension. *J Hypertens* 2004;22:1881-1888.

20. Saltin B, Boushel R, Secher N, Mitchell J, eds. *Exercise and Circulation in Health and Disease.* Champaign, IL: Human Kinetics; 2000.

21. Thompson PD, Buchner D, Pina IL, et al. Exercise and physical activity in the prevention and treatment of atherosclerotic cardiovascular disease: a statement from the Council on Cardiology (Subcommittee on Exercise, Rehabilitation, and Prevention) and the Council on Nutrition, Physical Activity, and Metabolism (Subcommittee on Physical Activity) *Circulation* 2003;107:3109-3116.

22. Wang Y, Wang QJ. The prevalence of prehypertension and hypertension among US adults according to the new Joint National Committee guidelines. *Arch Intern Med* 2004;164:2126-2134.

23. Whaley MH, Brubaker PH, Otto RM, eds. *ACSM's Guidelines for Exercise Testing and Prescription.* 7th ed. Baltimore: Lippincott Williams & Wilkins; 2006.

24. Whelton SP, Chin A, Xin X, He J. Effect of aerobic exercise on blood pressure: a meta-analysis of randomized, controlled trials. *Ann Intern Med* 2002;136:493-503.

25. Zipes DP, Libby P, Bonow RO, Braunwald E, eds. *Braunwald's Heart Disease—A Textbook of Cardiovascular Medicine.* 7th ed. Philadelphia: Saunders; 2005.

Chapter 20

1. Albright A, Franz M, Hornsby G, et al. American College of Sports Medicine position stand: exercise and type 2 diabetes. *Med Sci Sports Exerc* 2000;32:1345-1360.

2. American Diabetes Association. Diagnosis and classification of diabetes mellitus. *Diabetes Care* 2007;30(suppl 1):S42-S47.

3. American Diabetes Association. Standards of medical care in diabetes—2007. *Diabetes Care* 2007;30(suppl 1): S4-S41.

4. American Diabetes Association. Hyperglycemic crises in diabetes. *Diabetes Care* 2004;27(suppl 1):S94-S102.

5. American Diabetes Association. Physical activity/exercise and diabetes. *Diabetes Care* 2004;27(suppl 1):S58-S62.

6. Banzer JA, Maguire TE, Kennedy CM, et al. Results of cardiac rehabilitation in patients with diabetes mellitus. *Am J Cardiol* 2004;93:81-84.

7. Bell DS. Diabetic cardiomyopathy. *Diabetes Care* 2003;26:2949-2951.

8. Centers for Disease Control and Prevention. *National Diabetes Fact Sheet: General Information and National Estimates on Diabetes in the United States, 2005.* Atlanta, GA: U.S. Department of Health and Human Services, Centers for Disease Control and Prevention; 2005.

9. Church TS, Cheng YJ, Earnest CP, et al. Exercise capacity and body composition as predictors of mortality among men with diabetes. *Diabetes Care* 2004;27:83-88.

10. Cryer PE, Davis SN, Shamoon H. Hypoglycemia in diabetes. *Diabetes Care* 2003;26:1902-1912.

11. The Diabetes Control and Complications Trial Research Group. The effect of intensive treatment of diabetes on the development and progression of long-term complications in insulin-dependent diabetes mellitus. *N Engl J Med* 1993;329:977-986.

12. The Diabetes Control and Complications Trial/Epidemiology of Diabetes Interventions and Complications (DCCT/EDIC) Study Research Group. Intensive diabetes treatment and cardiovascular disease in patients with type 1 diabetes. *N Engl J Med* 2005;353:2643-2653.

13. Dimitrios NT, Chalikias GK, Kaski JC. Epidemiology of the diabetic heart. *Coron Artery Dis* 2005;16(suppl 1): S3-S10.

14. Franz MJ, Bantle JP, Beebe CA, et al. Evidence-based nutrition principles and recommendations for the treatment and prevention of diabetes and related complications. *Diabetes Care* 2002;25:148-198.

15. Gan D, ed. *Diabetes Atlas.* 2nd ed. Brussels: International Diabetes Federation; 2003.

16. Gilmer TP, O'Connor PJ, Rush WA, et al. Predictors of health care costs in adults with diabetes. *Diabetes Care* 2003;28:59-64.

17. Grundy SM, Howard B, Smith S, Eckel R, Redburg R, Bonow RO. Prevention Conference VI: Diabetes and Cardiovascular Disease: executive summary: conference proceeding for healthcare professionals from a special writing group of the American Heart Association. *Circulation* 2002;105:2231-2239.

18. Hindmann L, Falko JM, Lalonde M, Snow R, Caulin-Glasser T. Clinical profile and outcomes of diabetic and nondiabetic patients in cardiac rehabilitation. *Am Heart J* 2005;150:1046-1051.

19. Kavanagh T, Mertens DJ, Hamm LF, et al. Peak oxygen intake and cardiac mortality in women referred for cardiac rehabilitation. *J Am Coll Cardiol* 2003;42:2139-2143.

20. Manuel DG, Schulz SF. Health-related quality of life and health-adjusted life expectancy of people with diabetes in Ontario, Canada, 1996-1997. *Diabetes Care* 2004;27:407-414.

21. National Institutes of Diabetes and Digestive and Kidney Diseases. *National Diabetes Statistics Fact Sheet: General Information and National Estimates on Diabetes*

in the United States, 2005. Bethesda, MD: U.S. Department of Health and Human Services, National Institute of Health; 2005.

22. UK Prospective Diabetes Study (UKPDS) Group. Intensive blood-glucose control with sulphonylureas or insulin compared with conventional treatment and risk of complications in patients with type 2 diabetes (UKPDS 33). *Lancet* 1998;352:837-853.

23. Wei M, Gibbons LW, Kampert JB, Nichaman MZ, Blair SN. Low cardiorespiratory fitness and physical inactivity as predictors of mortality in men with type 2 diabetes. *Ann Intern Med* 2000;132:605-611.

24. Wexler DJ, Grant RW, Meigs JB, Nathan DM, Cagliero E. Sex disparities in treatment of cardiac risk factors in patients with type 2 diabetes. *Diabetes Care* 2005;28:514-520.

25. Wild S, Roglic G, Green A, Sicree R, King H. Global prevalence of diabetes: estimates for the year 2000 and projections for 2030. *Diabetes Care* 2004;27:1047-1053.

Chapter 21

1. Buchwald H, Avidor T, Braunwald E, et al. Bariatric surgery: a systematic review and meta-analysis. *JAMA* 2005;293:1724-1737.

2. Call EE, Thun MJ, Petrelli JM, Rodriguez C, Heath CW. Body-mass index and mortality in a prospective cohort of U.S. adults. *N Engl J Med* 1999;341:1097-1105.

3. Duncan JJ, Gordon NF, Scott CB. Women walking for health and fitness: how much is enough? *JAMA* 1991;266:3295-3299.

4. Flechtner-Mors M, Ditschuneit HH, Johnson TD, Suchard MA, Adler G. Metabolic and weight loss effects of long-term dietary intervention in obese patients: four-year results. *Obes Res* 2000;8:399-402.

5. Flegal KM, Carroll MD, Ogden CL, Johnson CL. Prevalence and trends in obesity among US adults, 1999-2000. *JAMA* 2002;288:1723-1727.

6. Gregg EW, Gerzoff RB, Thompson TJ, Williamson DF. Intentional weight loss and death in overweight and obese U.S. adults 35 years of age and older. *Ann Intern Med* 2003;138:383-389.

7. Goldstein DJ. Beneficial health effects of modest weight loss. *Int J Obes Rel Metab Disord* 1992;16:397-415.

8. Haddock CK, Poston WS, Dill PL, Foreyt JP, Ericcson M. Pharmacotherapy for obesity: a quantitative analysis of four decades of published randomized clinical trials. *Int J Obes Rel Metab Disord* 2002;26:262-273.

9. Haluzik M. Adiponectin and its potential in the treatment of obesity, diabetes and insulin resistance. *Curr Opin Investig Drugs* 2005;6:988-993.

10. Heilbronn LK, de Jonge K, Frisard MI, et al. Effect of 6-month calorie restriction on biomarkers of longevity, metabolic adaptation, and oxidative stress in overweight individuals. *JAMA* 2006;295:1539-1548.

11. Hill JO, Wyatt HR, Reed GW, Peters JC. Obesity and the environment: where do we go from here? *Science* 2003;299:853-855.

12. Jakicic JM, Clark K, Coleman E, et al. American College of Sports Medicine position stand: appropriate intervention strategies for weight loss and prevention of weight regain for adults. *Med Sci Sports Exerc* 2001;33:2145-2156.

13. Jakicic JM, Winters C, Lang W, Wing RR. Effects of intermittent exercise and use of home exercise equipment on adherence, weight loss, and fitness in overweight women: a randomized trial. *JAMA* 1999;282:1554-1560.

14. Klem WL, Wing RR, McGuire MT, Seagle HM, Hill JO. A descriptive study of individuals successful at long-term maintenance of substantial weight loss. *Am J Clin Nutr* 1997;66:239-246.

15. Li Z, Maglione M, Tu W, et al. Meta-analysis: pharmacologic treatment of obesity. *Ann Intern Med* 2005;142:532-546.

16. Lin PH, Proschan MA, Bray GA, et al, for the DASH Collaborative Research Group. Estimation of energy requirements in a controlled feeding trial. *Am J Clin Nutr* 2003;77:639-645.

17. Maggard MA, Shugarman LR, Suttorp M, et al. Meta-analysis: surgical treatment of obesity. *Ann Intern Med* 2005;142:547-559.

18. NIH conference: gastrointestinal surgery for severe obesity. Consensus Development Conference Panel. *Ann Intern Med* 1991;115:956-961.

19. National Institutes of Health, National Heart, Lung, and Blood Institute. Clinical guidelines on the identification, evaluation, and treatment of overweight and obesity in adults—the evidence report. *Obes Res* 1998;6(suppl 2):51S-209S. www.nhlbi.nih.gov/guidelines/obesity/ob_home.htm.

20. Ogden CL, Carroll MD, Curtin LT, et al. Prevalence of overweight and obesity in the United States, 1999-2004. *JAMA* 2006;295:1549-1555.

21. Pouliot MC, Despres JP, Lemieux S, et al. Waist circumference and abdominal sagittal diameter: best simple anthropometric indexes of abdominal visceral adipose tissue accumulation and related cardiovascular risk in men and women. *Am J Cardiol* 1994;73:460-468.

22. Report of a Joint FAO/WHO/UNU Expert Consultation. Human Energy Requirements. FAO Food and Nutrition Technical Report Series No. 1. Rome: Food and Agriculture Organization; 2004. www.fao.org/ag/agn/nutrition/requirements_pubs_en.stm.

23. Saris WHM, Blair SN, van Baak MA, et al. How much physical activity is enough to prevent unhealthy weight gain? Outcome of the IASO 1st stock conference and consensus statement. *Obes Rev* 2003;4:101-114.

24. Schoeller DA, Shay K, Kushner RF. How much physical activity is needed to minimize weight gain in previously obese women. *Am J Clin Nutr* 1997;66:551-556.

25. U.S. Department of Health and Human Services. *Physical Activity and Health: A Report of the Surgeon General.* Atlanta, GA: U.S. Department of Health and Human Services, Centers for Disease Control and Prevention, National Center for Chronic Disease Prevention and Health Promotion; 1996.

26. Wadden TA, Butryn ML, Byrne KJ. Efficacy of lifestyle modification for long-term weight control. *Obes Res* 2004;12(suppl):151S-162S.

27. Williamson DF, Thompson TJ, Thun M, Flanders D, Pamuk E, Byers T. Intentional weight loss and mortality among overweight individuals with diabetes. *Diabetes Care* 2000;23(10):1499-1504.

Chapter 22

1. American Heart Association. Cholesterol statistics, November 2, 2006. http://216.185.112.5/presenter.jhtml?identifier=4506.

2. Austin MA, Jansson E, Kaijser L, et al. Hypertriglyceridemia as a cardiovascular risk factor. *Am J Cardiol* 1998;81:7B-12B.

3. Bøsheim E, Knardahl S, Høstmark AT. Short-term effects of exercise on plasma very low density lipoproteins (VLDL) and fatty acids. *Med Sci Sports Exerc* 1999;31:522-530.

4. Crouse S, O'Brien B, Grandjean P, et al. Effects of exercise training and a single session of exercise on lipids and apolipoproteins in hypercholesterolemic men. *J Appl Physiol* 1997;83:2019-2028.

5. Durstine JL, Grandjean P, Cox CA, Thompson PD. Lipids, lipoproteins, and exercise. *J Cardiopulm Rehabil* 2002;22:385-398.

6. Durstine JL, Haskell WL. Effects of exercise training on plasma lipids and lipoproteins. *Exerc Sport Sci Rev* 1994;22:447-521.

7. Expert Panel on Detection, Evaluation, and Treatment of High Blood Cholesterol in Adults. Executive Summary of the Third Report of the National Cholesterol Education Program (NCEP) Expert Panel on Detection, Evaluation, and Treatment of High Blood Cholesterol in Adults (Adult Treatment Panel III). *JAMA* 2001;285:2486-2497.

8. Ferguson M, Alderson N, Trost S, et al. Effects of four different single exercise sessions on lipids, lipoproteins, and lipoprotein lipase. *J Appl Physiol* 1998;85:1169-1174.

9. Fletcher B, Berra K, Ades P, et al. Managing abnormal blood lipids a collaborative approach. *Circulation* 2005;112:3184-3209.

10. Friedewald WT, Levy RI, Fredrickson DS. Estimation of the concentration of low density lipoprotein in plasma without the use of preparative ultracentrifuge. *Clin Chem* 1972;18:499-502.

11. Grandjean PW, Crouse SF, Rohack JJ. Influence of cholesterol status on blood lipid and lipoprotein enzyme responses to aerobic exercise. *J Appl Physiol* 2000;89:472-480.

12. Hagberg JM, Ferrell RE, Katzel LI, et al. Apolipoprotein E genotype and exercise training-induced increases in plasma high-density lipoprotein (HDL)- and HDL$_2$-cholesterol levels in overweight men. *Metabolism* 1999;48:943-945.

13. Halle M, Berg A, König D, et al. Differences in the concentration and composition of low-density lipoprotein subfraction particles between sedentary and trained hypercholesterolemic men. *Metabolism* 1997;46:186-191.

14. Hokanson JE, Austin MA. Plasma triglyceride is a risk factor for cardiovascular disease independent of high-density lipoprotein cholesterol: a meta-analysis of population-based prospective studies. *J Cardiovasc Risk* 1996;3:213-219.

15. Israel RG, Sullivan MJ, Marks RH, et al. Relationship between cardiorespiratory fitness and lipoprotein(a) in men and women. *Med Sci Sports Exerc* 1994;26:425-431.

16. Kane GC, Lipsky JJ. Drug-grapefruit juice interactions. *Mayo Clin Proc* 2000;75:933-942.

17. Kelley GA, Kelley KS, Franklin B. Aerobic exercise and lipids and lipoproteins in patients with cardiovascular disease: a meta-analysis of randomized controlled trials. *J Cardiopulm Rehabil* 2006;26:131-139.

18. Kokkinos PF, Holland JC, Narayan P, et al. Miles run per week and high-density lipoprotein cholesterol levels in healthy, middle-aged men. *Arch Intern Med* 1995;155:415-420.

19. Kraus WE, Houmard JA, Duscha BD, et al. Effects of the amount and intensity of exercise on plasma lipoproteins. *N Engl J Med* 2002;347:1483-1492.

20. Leon AS, Gaskill SE, Rice T, et al. Variability in the response of HDL cholesterol to exercise training in the Heritage Family Study. *Int J Sports Med* 2002;23:1-9.

21. Leon AS, Rice T, Mandel S, et al. Blood lipid response to 20 weeks of supervised exercise in a large biracial population: the Heritage Family Study. *Metabolism* 2000;49:513-520.

22. Levine GN, Keaney JF Jr, Vita JA. Cholesterol reduction in cardiovascular disease. *N Engl J Med* 1995;332:512-521.

23. Petitt DS, Cureton KJ. Effects of prior exercise on postprandial lipemia: a quantitative review. *Metabolism* 2003;52:418-424.

24. St-Amand J, Homme DP, Moorjani S, et al. Apo E polymorphism and the relationships of physical fitness to plasma lipoprotein-lipid levels in men and women. *Med Sci Sports Exerc* 1999;31:692-697.

25. Taimela S, Lehtimaki T, Porkka AVK, et al. The effect of physical activity on serum total and low-density lipoprotein cholesterol concentrations varies with apolipoprotein E phenotype in male children and young adults: the Cardiovascular Risk in Young Finns Study. *Metabolism* 1996;45:797-803.

26. Thompson PD, Clarkson P, Karas RH. Statin-associated myopathy. *JAMA* 2003;289:1681.

27. Thompson PD, Cullinane E, Sady S, et al. Modest changes in high-density lipoprotein concentrations and metabolism with prolonged exercise training. *Circulation* 1988;78:25-34.

28. Thompson PD, Tongalis GJ, Seip RL, et al. Apolipoprotein E genotype and changes in serum lipids and maximal oxygen uptake with exercise training, *Metabolism* 2004;53:193-202.

29. Thompson PD, Yurgalevitch S, Flynn M, et al. Effect of prolonged exercise training without weight loss on high-density lipoprotein metabolism in overweight men. *Metabolism* 1997;46:217-223.

30. Williams PT, Krauss RM, Vranizan KM, et al. Changes in lipoprotein subfractions during diet-induced weight lost in moderately overweight men. *Circulation* 1990;81:1293-1304.

31. Wood PD, Stefanick ML, Williams PT, Haskell WL. The effects on plasma lipoproteins of a prudent weight-reducing diet with or without exercise in overweight men and women. *N Engl J Med* 1991;324:461-466.

32. Ziogas GC, Thomas TR, Harris WS. Exercise training, postprandial hypertriglyceridemia, and LDL subfraction distribution. *Med Sci Sport Exerc* 1997;29:986.

Chapter 23

1. Altman R, Asch E, Bloch D, et al. The American College of Rheumatology criteria for the classification and reporting of osteoarthritis of the knee. *Arthritis Rheum* 1986;29:1039-1049.

2. Arnett FC, Edworthy SM, Bloch DA, et al. The American Rheumatism Association 1987 revised criteria for the classification of rheumatoid arthritis. *Arthritis Rheum* 1988;31:315-324.

3. Baker KR, Nelson ME, Felson DT, Layne JE, Sarno R, Roubenoff R. The efficacy of home based progressive strength training in older adults with knee osteoarthritis: a randomized controlled trial. *J Rheumatol* 2001;28:1655-1665.

4. Centers for Disease Control. Prevalence of arthritis—United States, 1997. *Morbid Mortal Wkly Rep* 2001;50:334-336.

5. Centers for Disease Control. Arthritis related statistics, 2002. www.cdc.gov/arthritis/data_statistics/arthritis_related_statistics.htm#4.

6. Deyle GD, Henderson NE, Matekel RL, Ryder MG, Garber MB, Allison SC. Effectiveness of manual physical therapy and exercise in osteoarthritis of the knee: a randomized, controlled trial. *Ann Intern Med* 2000;132:173-181.

7. Häkkinen A, Sokka T, Hannonen P. A home-based two-year strength training period in early rheumatoid arthritis led to good long-term compliance: a five-year follow-up. *Arthritis Rheum* 2004;51:56-62.

8. Häkkinen A, Sokka T, Kotaniemi A, Hannonen P. A randomized two-year study of the effects of dynamic strength training on muscle strength, disease activity, functional capacity, and bone mineral density in early rheumatoid arthritis. *Arthritis Rheum* 2001;44:515-522.

9. Hawley DJ. Functional ability, health status, and quality of life. In: Robbins L, Burckhardt CS, Hannan MT, DeHoratius RJ, eds. *Clinical Care in the Rheumatic Diseases*. 2nd ed. Atlanta: American College of Rheumatology; 2001:53-60.

10. Hurley MV, Scott DL, Rees J, Newham DJ. Sensorimotor changes and functional performance in patients with knee osteoarthritis. *Ann Rheum Dis* 1997;56:641-648.

11. Maradit-Kremers H, Nicola PJ, Crowson CS, Ballman KV, Gabriel SE. Cardiovascular death in rheumatoid arthritis: a population-based study. *Arthritis Rheum* 2005;52:722-732.

12. Melton-Rogers S, Hunter G, Walter J, Harrison P. Cardiorespiratory responses of patients with rheumatoid arthritis during bicycle riding and running in water. *Phys Ther* 1996;76:1058-1065.

13. Messier SP, Glasser JL, Ettinger WH Jr, Craven TE, Miller ME. Declines in strength and balance in older adults with chronic knee pain: a 30-month longitudinal, observational study. *Arthritis Rheum* 2002;47:141-148.

14. Minor MA, Hewett JE, Webel RR, Anderson SK, Kay DR. Efficacy of physical conditioning exercise in patients with rheumatoid arthritis and osteoarthritis. *Arthritis Rheum* 1989;32:1396-1405.

15. Minor MA, Hewett JE, Webel RR, Dreisinger TE, Kay DR. Exercise tolerance and disease related measures in patients with rheumatoid arthritis and osteoarthritis. *J Rheumatol* 1988;15:905-911.

16. Munneke M, deJong Z, Zwinderman AH, et al. Effect of a high-intensity weight-bearing exercise program on radiologic damage progression of the large joints in subgroups of patients with rheumatoid arthritis. *Arthritis Rheum* 2005;53:410-417.

17. National Heart, Lung, and Blood Institute. The seventh report of the Joint National Committee on Prevention, Detection, Evaluation, and Treatment of High Blood Pressure (NIH Publication No. 04-5230), 2004. www.nhlbi.nih.gov/guidelines/hypertension/jnc7full.pdf.

18. Rolden CA, Chavez J, Wiest PW, Qualls CR, Crawford MH. Aortic root disease and valve disease associated with ankylosing spondylitis. *J Am Col Cardiol* 1998;32:1397-1404.

19. Sharma L, Cahue S, Song J, Hayes K, Pai Y, Dunlop D. Physical functioning over three years in knee osteoarthritis. *Arthritis Rheum* 2003;48:3359-3370.

20. Sharma L, Song J, Felson DT, Cahue S, Samieyeh E, Dunlop DD. The role of knee alignment in disease progression and functional decline in knee osteoarthritis. *JAMA* 2001;286:188-195.

21. Suter E, Herzog W. Does muscle inhibition after knee injury increase the risk of osteoarthritis? *Exerc Sport Sci Rev* 2000;28:15-18.

22. Van den Ende CHM, Vliet Vlieland TPM, Munneke M, Hazes JMW. Dynamic exercise therapy for rheumatoid

arthritis (Cochrane review). In: *The Cochrane Library*, Issue 1. Oxford, UK: Update Software; 2002.

23. Whaley MH, Brubaker PH, Otto RM, eds. *ACSM's Guidelines for Exercise Testing and Prescription*. 7th ed. Philadelphia: Lippincott Williams & Wilkins; 2006.

24. Wolfe F, Smythe HA, Yunus MB, et al. The American College of Rheumatology 1990 criteria for the classification of fibromyalgia. *Arthritis Rheum* 1990;33:160-172.

Chapter 24

1. Allison TG, Farkouh ME, Samrs PA, et al. Management of coronary risk factors by trained nurses versus usual care in patients with unstable angina pectoris (a chest pain evaluation in the emergency room (CHEER) substudy). *Am J Cardiol* 2000;86:133-138.

2. Anisman H, Merali Z. Cytokines, stress and depressive illness: brain-immune interactions. *Ann Med* 2003;35:2-11.

3. Barefoot JC. (1992). Developments in the measurement of hostility. In: Freidman, HS, ed. *Hostility, Coping & Health*. Washington, DC: American Psychological Association; 1992;13-31.

4. Barefoot JC, Dahlstrom WG, Williams RB. Hostility, CHD incidence, and total mortality: a 25-year follow-up study of 255 physicians. *Psychosom Med* 1983;45:59-63.

5. Barefoot JC, Dodge KA, Peterson BL, Dahlstrom G, Williams RB. The Cook–Medley Hostility Scale: item content and ability to predict survival. *Psychosom Med* 1989;51:46-57.

6. Barefoot JC, Larsen S, von der Leith L, Schroll M. Hostility, incidence of acute myocardial infarction, and mortality in a sample of older Danish men and women. *Am J Epidemiol* 1995;142:477-484.

7. Barth J, Schumacher M, Herrmann-Lingen C. Depression as a risk factor for mortality in patients with coronary heart disease: a meta-analysis. *Psychosom Med*. 2004;66:802-813.

8. Beck AT, Steer RA, Brown GK. *Beck Depression Inventory—Second Edition*. San Antonio, TX: Psychological Corp; 1996.

9. Berkman LF, Blumenthal J, Burg M, et al. Effects of treating depression and low perceived social support on clinical events after myocardial infarction: the Enhancing Recovery in Coronary Heart Disease Patients (ENRICHD) Randomized Trial. *JAMA* 2003;289:3106-3116.

10. Black JL, Allison TG, Williams DE, Rummans TA, Gau GT. Effect of intervention for psychological distress on rehospitalization rates in cardiac rehabilitation patients. *Psychosomatics* 1998;39:134-143.

11. Blumenthal JA, Babyak MA, Carney RM, et al. Exercise, depression, and mortality after myocardial infarction in the ENRICHD trial. *Med Sci Sports Exerc* 2004;36:746-755.

12. Blumenthal JA, Babyak MA, Doraiswamy PM, et al. Exercise and pharmacotherapy in the treatment of major depressive disorder. *Psychosom Med* 2007;69:587-596.

13. Blumenthal JA, Babyak MA, Moore KA, et al. Effects of exercise training on older patients with major depression. *Arch Intern Med* 1999;159:2349-2356.

14. Blumenthal JA, Babyak M, Wei J, et al. Usefulness of psychosocial treatment of mental stress-induced myocardial ischemia in men. *Am J Cardiol* 2002;89:164-168.

15. Blumenthal JA, Jiang W, Babyak MA, et al. Stress management and exercise training in cardiac patients with myocardial ischemia: effects on prognosis and evaluation of mechanisms. *Arch Intern Med* 1997;157:2213-2223.

16. Blumenthal JA, Sherwood A, Babyak MA, et al. Effects of exercise and stress management training on markers of cardiovascular risk in patients with ischemic heart disease: a randomized controlled trial. *JAMA* 2005;293:1626-1634.

17. Blumenthal JA, Burg MM, Barefoot J, et al. Social support, type A behavior, and coronary artery disease. *Psychosom Med* 1987;49,331-340.

18. Brummett BH, Babyak MA, Siegler IC, Mark DB, Williams RB, Barefoot JC. Effect of smoking and sedentary behavior on the association between depressive symptoms and mortality from coronary heart disease *Am J Cardiol* 2003;92:529-532.

19. Burell G. Behavior modification after coronary artery bypass graft surgery: effects on cardiac morbidity and mortality. *J Rehabil Sci* 1995;8:39-40.

20. Centers for Disease Control and Prevention. Deaths: leading causes for 2002. *Natl Vital Stat Rep* 2005;53:(17).

21. Chambless DL, Ollendick TH. Empirically supported psychological interventions: controversies and evidence. *Annu Rev Psychol* 2001;52:685-716.

22. Cohen S, Kamarch T, Mermelstein RA. Global Measure of Perceived Stress. *J Health and Soc Beh* 1983;24(4):385-396.

23. Cook WW, Medley DM. Proposed hostility and pharisaic-virtue scales for the MMPI. *J Appl Psychol* 1954;38:414-418.

24. Cowan MJ, Pike KC, Kogan Budzynski H. Psychosocial nursing therapy following sudden cardiac arrest: impact on two-year survival. *Nurs Res* 2001;50:68-76.

25. Davidson KW, Rieckmann N, Rapp MA. Definitions and distinctions among depressive syndromes and symptoms: implications for a better understanding of the depression–cardiovascular disease association. *Psychosom Med* 2005;67(suppl 1):S6-S9.

26. Dusseldorp E, van Elderen T, Maes S, Meulman J, Kraaij V. A meta-analysis of psychoeducational programs for coronary heart disease patients. *Health Psychol* 1999;506-519.

27. First MB, Spitzer RL, Williams JBW, Gibbon M. *Structured Clinical Interview for DSM-IV Axis I Disorders.* American Psychiatric Press, 1996.

28. Frasure-Smith N, Lesperance F, Prince RH, et al. Randomised trial of home-based psychological nursing intervention for patients recovering from myocardial infarction. *Lancet* 1997;350:473–479.

29. Frasure-Smith N, Koszycki D, Swenson JR, et al. Design and rationale for a randomized, controlled trial of interpersonal psychotherapy and citalopram for depression in coronary artery disease (CREATE). *Psychosom Med* 2006;68:87-93.

30. Frasure-Smith N, Lesperance F, Talajic M. Depression following myocardial infarction. Impact on 6-month survival. *JAMA* 1993;270:1819-1825.

31. Frasure-Smith N, Prince R. The ischemic heart disease life stress monitoring program: impact on mortality. *Psychosom Med* 1985;47:431-445.

32. Fridlund B, Hogstedt B, Lidell E, Larsson PA. Recovery after myocardial infarction: effects of a caring rehabilitation programme. *Scand J Caring Sci* 1991;5:23-32.

33. Friedman M, Thoresen CE, Gill JJ, et al. Alteration of type A behavior and its effect on cardiac recurrences in post myocardial infarction patients: summary results of the recurrent coronary prevention project. *Am Heart J* 1986;112:653-665.

34. Glassman AH, O'Connor CM, Califf RM, et al. Sertraline treatment of major depression in patients with acute MI or unstable angina. *JAMA* 2002;288:701-709.

35. Gorman JM, Sloan RP. Heart rate variability in depressive and anxiety disorders: depression as a risk factor for cardiovascular and cerebrovascular disease. *Am Heart J* 2000;140:S77-S83.

36. Gullette EC, Blumenthal JA, Babyak M, et al. Effects of mental stress on myocardial ischemia during daily life. *JAMA* 1997;277:1521-1526.

37. Haines AP, Imeson JD, Meade TW. Phobic anxiety and ischemic heart disease. *BMJ* 1987;295:297-299.

38. Hamilton M. A rating scale for depression. *J Neurol Neurosurg Psychiatry* 1960;23:56-62.

39. Haney TL, Maynard KE, Houseworth SJ, Scherwitz LW, Williams RB, Barefoot JC. Interpersonal hostility assessment technique: description and validation against the criterion of coronary artery disease. *J Pers Assess* 1996;66:386–401.

40. Hofman-Bang C, Lisspers J, Nordlander R, et al. Two-year results of a controlled study of residential rehabilitation for patients treated with percutaneous transluminal coronary angioplasty: a randomized study of a multifactorial programme. *Eur Heart J* 1999;20:1465-1474.

41. Ibrahim MA, Feldman JG, Sultz HA, Stairman MG, Young LJ, Dean D. Management after myocardial infarction: A controlled trial to the effect of group psychotherapy. *Int J Psychiatry Med* 1974;5:253-268.

42. Januzzi JL Jr, Stern TA, Pasternak RC, DeSanctis RW. The influence of anxiety and depression on outcomes of patients with coronary artery disease. *Arch Intern Med* 2000;160:1913-1921.

43. Johnstone A, Goldberg D. Psychiatric screening in general practice. A controlled trial. *Lancet* 1976;i:605-608.

44. Jones DA, West, RR. Psychological rehabilitation after myocardial infarction: multicentre randomised controlled trial. *BMJ* 1996;313:1517-1521.

45. Kaprio J, Koskenvuo M, Rita H. Mortality after bereavement: a prospective study of 95,647 widowed persons. *Am J Public Health* 1987;77:283-287.

46. Kawachi I, Colditz GA, Ascherio A, et al. Prospective study of phobic anxiety and risk of coronary heart disease in men. *Circulation* 1994;89:1992-1997.

47. Kawachi I, Sparrow D, Vokonas PS, Weiss ST. Symptoms of anxiety and risk of coronary heart disease: the Normative Aging Study. *Circulation* 1994;90:2225-2229.

48. Kubzansky LD, Kawachi I, Spiro A III, et al. Is worrying bad for your heart? A prospective study of worry and coronary heart disease in the Normative Aging Study. *Circulation* 1997;95:818-824.

49. Lawlor DA, Hopker SW. The effectiveness of exercise as an intervention in the management of depression: systematic review and meta-regression analysis of randomised controlled trials. *BMJ* 2001;322:763-767.

50. Lett HS, Blumenthal JA, Babyak MA, et al. Depression as a risk factor for coronary artery disease: evidence, mechanisms, and treatment. *Psychosom Med* 2004;66:305-315.

51. Lett HS, Blumenthal JA, Babyak MA, Strauman TJ, Robins C, Sherwood A. Social support and coronary heart disease: epidemiologic evidence and implications for treatment. *Psychosom Med.* In press.

52. Lidell E, Fridlund B. Long-term effects of a comprehensive rehabilitation programme after myocardial infarction. *Scand J Caring Sci* 1996;10:67-74.

53. Linden W. Psychological treatments in cardiac rehabilitation: review of rationales and outcomes. *J Psychosom Res* 2000;48:443-454.

54. Linden W, Stossel C, Maurice J. Psychosocial interventions for patients with coronary artery disease: a meta-analysis. *Arch Intern Med* 1996;156:745-752.

55. Mann DL. Stress-activated cytokines and the heart: from adaptation to maladaptation. *Ann Rev Physiol* 2003;65:81-101.

56. Matthews KA, Glass DC, Rosenman RH, Bortner RW. Competitive drive, pattern A, and coronary heart disease: A further analysis of some data from the Western Collaborative Group Study. *J Chronic Dis* 1977;30:489-498.

57. Matthews KA, Raikkonen K, Sutton-Tyrrell K, Kuller LH. Optimistic attitudes protect against progression of carotid atherosclerosis in healthy middle-aged women. *Psychosom Med* 2004;66:640-644.

58. Mitchell PH, Powell L, Blumenthal J, et al. A Short Social Support Measure for Patients Recovering From

Myocardial Infarction: THE ENRICHD SOCIAL SUPPORT INVENTORY. *J Cardiopulm Rehabil* 2003;23(6):398-403.

59. Musselman DL, Tomer A, Manatunga AK, et al. Exaggerated platelet reactivity in major depression. *Am J Psychiatry* 1996;153:1313-1317.

60. Oldenberg B, Perkins RJ, Andrews G. Controlled trial of psychological intervention in myocardial infarction. *J Consult Clin Psychol* 1985;53:852-859.

61. Porges SW. Cardiac vagal tone: a physiological index of stress. *Neurosci Biobehav* 1995;19:225-233.

62. Radloff LS. The CES-D Scale: A self-report depression scale for research in the general population. *Appl Psychol Meas* 1977;1:385-401.

63. Rahe RH, Ward HW, Hayes V. Brief group therapy in myocardial infarction rehabilitation: three- to four-year follow-up of a controlled trial. *Psychosom Med* 1979;51:229-242.

64. Rees K, Bennett P, West R, Davey SG, Ebrahim S. Psychological interventions for coronary heart disease (review). *Cochrane Library* 2007;4:1-51.

65. Review Panel on Coronary Prone Behavior and Coronary Heart Disease. Coronary prone behavior and coronary heart disease: a critical review. *Circulation* 1981;63:1199-1215.

66. Rosenman RH, Brand RJ, Jenkins CD, Friedman M, Straus R, Wurm M. Coronary heart disease in the Western Collaborative Group Study: final follow-up experience of 8 1/2 years. *JAMA* 1975;233:872-877.

67. Rozanski A, Blumenthal JA, Kaplan J. Impact of psychological factors on the pathogenesis of cardiovascular disease and implications for therapy. *Circulation* 1999;99:2192-2217.

68. Rozanski A, Blumenthal JA, Davidson KW, Saab PG, Kubzansky L. The epidemiology, pathophysiology, and management of psychosocial risk factors in cardiac practice: the emerging field of behavioral cardiology. *J Am Cardiol* 2005;45:637-651.

69. Ruberman W, Weinblatt E, Goldberg JD, Chaudhary BS. Psychosocial influences on mortality after myocardial infarction. *N Engl J Med* 1984;311:552-559.

70. Rugulies R. Depression as a predictor for coronary heart disease: a review and meta-analysis. *Am J Prev Med* 2002;23:51-61.

71. Saint PA, Boissel JP, Leizorovicz A, et al. Comparison of a rehabilitation programme, a counseling programme and usual care after an acute myocardial infarction: results of a long-term randomized trial. *Eur Heart J* 1991;12:612-616.

72. Scheier MF, Carver CS. Optimism, coping, and health: Assessment and implications of generalized outcome expectancies. *Health Psychol* 1985;4:219-247.

73. Scheier MF, Matthews KA, Owens JF, et al. Optimism and rehospitalization after coronary artery bypass graft surgery. *Arch Intern Med* 1999;159:829-835.

74. Seeman TE, Berkman LF. Structural characteristics of social networks and their relationship with social support in the elderly: who provides support. *Soc Sci Med* 1988;26(7):737-49.

75. Smith TW. Hostility and health: current status of a psychosomatic hypothesis. *Health Psychol* 1992;11:139-150.

76. Spielberger, CD. *Manual for the State-Trait Anxiety Inventory.* Palo Alto, CA: Consulting Psychologists Press, 1983.

77. Stern MJ, Gorman PA, Kaslow L. The group counseling vs exercise therapy study: a controlled intervention with subjects following myocardial infarction. *Arch Intern Med* 1983;143:1719-1725.

78. Strike PC, Steptoe A. Behavioral and emotional triggers of acute coronary syndromes: a systematic review and critique. *Psychsom Med* 2005;67:179-186.

79. Taylor CB, Youngblood ME, Catellier D, et al. Effects of antidepressant medication on morbidity and mortality in depressed patients after myocardial infarction. *Arch Gen Psychiatry* 2005;62:792-798.

80. Theorell T, Karasek RA. Current issues relating to psychosocial job strain and cardiovascular disease research. *J Occup Health Psychol* 1996;1:9-26.

81. van Dixhoorn J, Duivenvoorden HJ. Effect of relaxation therapy on cardiac events after myocardial infarction: A 5-year follow-up study. *J Cardiopulm Rehabil* 1999;19(3):178-185.

82. Vermeulen A, Lie KI, Durrer D. Effects of cardiac rehabilitation after myocardial infarction: changes in coronary risk factors and long-term prognosis. *Am Heart J* 1983;105:798-801.

83. Zigelstein RC, Bush DE, Fauerbach JA. Depression, adherence behavior, and coronary disease outcomes. *Arch Intern Med* 1998;158:808-809.

Chapter 25

1. American College of Sports Medicine. *ACSM's Guidelines for Exercise Testing and Prescription.* 7th ed. Whaley MH, Brubaker PH, Otto RM, eds. Philadelphia: Lippincott Williams & Wilkins; 2006.

2. American Heart Association. Heart disease and stroke statistics—2006 update: a report from the American Heart Association Statistics Committee and Stroke Statistics Subcommittee. *Circulation* 2006;113:e85-e151.

3. Adams H, Adams R, Del Zoppo G, et al. AHA/ASA scientific statement: guidelines for the early management of patients with ischemic stroke. 2005 guidelines update. *Stroke* 2005;36:916-923.

4. Adams HP Jr, Bendixen BH, Kappelle LJ, et al. Classification of subtype of acute ischemic stroke: definitions for use in a multicenter clinical trial: TOAST: Trial of Org 10172 in Acute Stroke Treatment. *Stroke* 1993;24:35-41.

5. Adams RJ, Chimowitz MI, Alpert JS, et al. AHA/ASA scientific statement: coronary risk evaluation in patients with transient ischemic attack and ischemic stroke. *Circulation* 2003;108:1278-1290.

6. Fletcher GF, Balady GJ, Amsterdam EA, et al. Exercise standards for testing and training: a statement for healthcare professionals from the American Heart Association. *Circulation* 2001;104:1694-1740.

7. Franklin BF, Gordon NF. *Contemporary Diagnosis and Management in Cardiovascular Exercise*. Newtown, PA: Handbooks in Healthcare; 2005.

8. Goldstein LB, Adams R, Becker K, et al. AHA scientific statement: Primary prevention of ischemic stroke. *Circulation* 2001;103:163-182.

9. Gordon NF, Contractor A, Leighton RF. Resistance training for hypertension and stroke patients. In: *Resistance Training for Health and Rehabilitation*. Graves JE, Franklin BA, eds. Champaign, IL: Human Kinetics; 2001:237-251.

10. Gordon NF, Gulanik M, Costa F, et al. AHA scientific statement: physical activity and exercise recommendations for stroke survivors. *Circulation* 2004;109:2031-2041.

11. *Internal Classification of Functioning, Disability and Health, ICF*. Geneva, Switzerland: World Health Organization; 2001.

12. Latchaw RE, Yonas H, Hunter GJ, et al. AHA scientific statement: guidelines and recommendations for perfusion imaging in cerebral ischemia. *Stroke* 2003;34:1084-1104.

13. Palmer-McLean K, Harbst KB. Stroke and brain injury. In: *ACSM's Exercise Management for Persons With Chronic Diseases and Disabilities*. 2nd ed. Champaign, IL: Human Kinetics; 2003:238-246.

14. Pollock ML, Franklin BA, Balady GJ, et al. Resistance exercise in individuals with and without cardiovascular disease: benefits, rationale, safety, and prescription: an advisory from the American Heart Association. *Circulation* 2001;101:828-833.

15. Sacco RL, Adams R, Albers G, et al. AHA/ASA guideline: guidelines for prevention of stroke in patients with ischemic stroke or transient ischemic attack *Stroke* 2006;37:577-617.

Chapter 26

1. American Heart Association. *Heart Disease and Stroke Statistics—2005 Update*. Dallas, TX: AHA; 2005.

2. Bell-McGinty K, Podell K, Franzen M, Baird AD, Williams M. Standard measures of executive function in predicting instrumental activities of daily living in older adults. *Int J Geriatr Psychiatry* 2002;17:828-834.

3. Clark RE, Brillman J, Davis DA, Lovell MR, Price TR, Magovern GJ. Microemboli during coronary artery bypass grafting: genesis and effect on outcome. *J Thorac Cardiovasc Surg* 1995;109:249-257.

4. Comijs HC, Dik MG, Deeg DJ, Jonker C. The course of cognitive decline in older persons: results from the longitudal aging study in Amsterdam. *Dement Geriatr Cogn Disord* 2004;17:136-142.

5. DeGroot JC, DeLeeuw FE, Oudkerk M, et al. Periventricular cerebral white matter lesions predict rate of cognitive decline. *Ann Neurol* 2002;52:335-341.

6. Dijkstra JB, Strik J, Lousberg R, et al. Atypical cognitive profile in patients with depression after myocardial infarction. *J Affect Disord* 2002;70:181-190.

7. Eguchi K, Kario K, Kazuyuki S. Greater impact of coexistence of hypertension and diabetes on silent cerebral infarcts. *Stroke* 2003;34:2471-2474.

8. Fratiglioni L, Paillard-Borg S, Bengt W. An active and socially integrated lifestyle in late life might protect against dementia. *Lancet Neurol* 2004;3:343.

9. Jellinger KA. Understanding the pathology of vascular cognitive impairment. *J Neurol Sci* 2005;229-230:57-63.

10. Kelly MA. 2005. *Neuropsychological Prediction of Learning and Adherence in Cardiac Rehabilitation* [PhD dissertation, University of Pittsburgh]. http://etd.library.pitt.edu/ETD/available/etd-06152005-192755.

11. Knopman D, Boland LL, Mosley T, et al. Cardiovascular risk factors and cognitive decline in middle-aged adults. *Neurology* 2001;56:42-48.

12. Messier C, Tsiakas M, Gagnon M, Desrochers A, Awad N. Effect of age and glucoregulation on cognitive performance. *Neurobiol Aging* 2003;24:985-1003.

13. Moser DJ, Cohen RA, Clark MM, et al. Neuropsychological functioning among cardiac rehabilitation patients. *J Cardiopulm Rehabil* 1999;19:91-97.

14. Neupert SD, McDonald-Miszczak L. Younger and older adults' delayed recall of medication instructions: the role of cognitive and metacognitive predictors. *Aging Neuropsychol Cogn* 2004;11:428-442.

15. Newman MF, Blumenthal JA, Mark DB. Fixing the heart: must the brain pay the price? *Circulation* 2004;110:3402-3403.

16. Newman MF, Croughwell ND, Blumenthal JA, et al. Predictors of cognitive decline after cardiac operation. *Ann Thorac Surg* 1995;59:1326-1330.

17. Newman MF, Kirchner JL, Phillips-Bute B, et al. Longitudinal assessment of neurocognitive function after coronary-artery bypass surgery. *N Engl J Med* 2001;344:395-402.

18. Rasmusson DX, Rebok GW, Bylsma FW, Brandt J. Effects of three types of memory training in normal elderly. *Aging Neuropsychol Cogn* 1999;6:56-66.

19. Ryan CM. *Cognitive Functioning and Adherence*. Unpublished manuscript, University of Pittsburgh Medical Center; 2000.

20. Selnes OA, Golsborough MA, Borowica LW, Enger C, Quaskey SA, McKhann GM. Determinants of cognitive change after coronary artery bypass surgery: a multifactorial problem. *Ann Thorac Surg* 1999;67:1669-1676.

21. Singh-Manoux A, Britton AR, Marmot M. Vascular disease and cognitive function: evidence from the Whitehall II Study. *J Am Geriatr Soc* 2003;51:1445-1450.

22. Waldstein SR, Brown JR, Maier JJ, Katzel LI. Diagnosis of hypertension and high blood pressure levels negatively affect cognitive function in older adults. *Ann Behav Med* 2005;29:174-180.

23. Waldstein SR, Ryan CM, Polefrone JM, Manuck SB. Neuropsychological performance of young men who vary in familial risk for hypertension. *Psychosom Med* 1994;56:449-456.

Chapter 27

1. American Academy of Sleep Medicine Task Force. Sleep-related breathing disorders in adults: recommendations for syndrome definition and measurement techniques in clinical research. *Sleep* 1999;22:667-689.

2. Bassetti CL. Sleep and stroke. *Semin Neurol* 2005;25:19-32.

3. Doherty LS, Kiely JL, Swan V, McNicholas WT. Long-term effects of nasal continuous positive airway pressure therapy on cardiovascular outcomes in sleep apnea syndrome. *Chest* 2005;127:2076-2084.

4. Gami AS, Pressman G, Caples SM, et al. Association of atrial fibrillation and obstructive sleep apnea. *Circulation* 2004;110:364-367.

5. Giebelhaus V, Strohl KP, Lormes W, Lehmann M, Netzer N. Physical exercise as an adjunct therapy in sleep apnea—an open trial. *Sleep Breath* 2000;4:173-176.

6. Harma, M. Ageing, physical fitness and shiftwork tolerance. *Appl Ergon* 1996;27:25-29.

7. Kawahara S, Akashiba T, Akahoshi T, Horie T. Nasal CPAP improves the quality of life and lessens the depressive symptoms in patients with obstructive sleep apnea syndrome. *Intern Med* 2005;44:422-427.

8. Lin CC, Lin CK, Wu KM, Chou CS. Effect of treatment by nasal CPAP on cardiopulmonary exercise test in obstructive sleep apnea syndrome. *Lung* 2004;182:199-212.

9. Marin JM, Carrizo SJ, Vicente E, Agusti AGN. Long-term cardiovascular outcomes in men with obstructive sleep apnoea-hypopnoea with or without treatment with continuous positive airway pressure: an observational study. *Lancet* 2005;365:1046-1053.

10. Mooe T, Franklin KA, Holmstrom K, Rabben T, Wiklund U. Sleep-disordered breathing and coronary artery disease: long-term prognosis. *Am J Respir Crit Care Med* 2001;164:1910-1913.

11. Norman JF, Von Essen SG, Fuchs RH, McElligott M. Exercise training effect on obstructive sleep apnea syndrome. *Sleep Rev Online* 2000;3:121-129.

12. Parra O, Arboix A, Montserrat JM, Quinto L, Bechich S, Garcia-Eroles L. Sleep-related breathing disorders: impact on mortality of cerebrovascular disease. *Eur Respir J* 2004;24:267-272.

13. Peppard PE, Young T. Exercise and sleep-disordered breathing: an association independent of body habitus. *Sleep* 2004;27:480-484.

14. Peppard PE, Young T, Palta M, Skatrud J. Prospective study of the association between sleep-disordered breathing and hypertension. *N Engl J Med* 2000;342:1378-1384.

15. Phillips B. Sleep-disordered breathing and cardiovascular disease. *Sleep Med Rev* 2005;9:131-140.

16. Phillips B, Kryger MH. Management of obstructive sleep apnea-hypopnea syndrome: overview. In: *Principles and Practice of Sleep Medicine*. Kryger MH, Roth T, Dement WC, eds. Philadelphia: Elsevier Saunders; 2005:1109-1121.

17. Somers VK, Javaheri S. Cardiovascular effects of sleep-related breathing disorders. In: *Principles and Practice of Sleep Medicine*. Kryger MH, Roth T, Dement WC, eds. Philadelphia: Elsevier Saunders; 2005:1180-1191.

18. Stepanski EJ, Wyatt JK. Use of sleep hygiene in the treatment of insomnia. *Sleep Med Rev* 2003;7:215-225.

19. Tryfon S, Stanopoulos I, Dascalopoulou E, Argyropoulou P, Bouros D, Mavrofridis E. Sleep apnea syndrome and diastolic blood pressure elevation during exercise. *Respiration* 2005;71:499-504.

20. Verrier RL, Mittleman MA. Sleep-related cardiac risk. In: *Principles and Practice of Sleep Medicine*. Kryger MH, Roth T, Dement WC, eds. Philadelphia: Elsevier Saunders; 2005:1161-1170.

21. Vgontzas AN, Bixler EO, Chrousos GP. Sleep apnea is a manifestation of the metabolic syndrome. *Sleep Med Rev* 2005;9:211-224.

22. Yaggi HK, Concato J, Kernan WN, Lichtman JH, Brass LM, Mohsenin V. Obstructive sleep apnea as a risk factor for stroke and death. *N Engl J Med* 2005;353:2034-2041.

23. Young T, Palta M, Dempsey J, Skatrud J, Weber S, Badr S. The occurrence of sleep-disordered breathing among middle-aged adults. *N Engl J Med* 1993;328:1230-1235.

24. Young T, Peppard PE, Gottlieb DJ. Epidemiology of obstructive sleep apnea: a population health perspective. *Am J Respir Crit Care Med* 2002;165:1217-1239.

25. Youngstedt SD, Kripke DF. Long sleep and mortality: rationale for sleep restriction. *Sleep Med Rev* 2004;8:159-174.

Chapter 28

1. Aikawa M, Libby P. The vulnerable atherosclerotic plaque: pathogenesis and therapeutic approach. *Cardiovasc Pathol* 2004;13:125-138.

2. Alpert JS, Thygesen K. A call for universal definitions in cardiovascular disease. *Circulation* 2006;114:757-758.

3. Ambrose JA, Fuster V. The risk of coronary occlusion is not proportional to the prior severity of coronary stenosis. *Heart* 1998;79:3-4.

4. American Heart Association Statistics Committee and Stroke Statistics Subcommittee. Heart Disease and Stroke Statistics: 2008 Update. *Circulation* 2008;117:e25-e146.

5. American Diabetes Association. Screening for type 2 diabetes. *Diabetes Care* 2003;26(suppl 1):S21-S24.

6. Antman EM, Anbe DT, Armstrong PW, et al. ACC/AHA guidelines for the management of patients with ST-elevation myocardial infarction—executive summary: a report of the American College of Cardiology/American Heart Association Task Force on Practice Guidelines. *Circulation* 2004;110:588-636.

7. Barnard RJ, MacAlpin R, Kattus AA, Buckberg GD. Ischemic response to sudden strenuous exercise in healthy men. *Circulation* 1973;48:936-942.

8. Cannon CP, Braunwald E, McCabe CH, et al, for the Pravastatin or Atorvastatin Evaluation and Infection Therapy-Thrombolysis in Myocardial Infarction 22 Investigators. Intensive versus moderate lipid lowering with statins after acute coronary syndromes. *N Engl J Med* 2004;350:1495-1504.

9. Centers for Disease Control and Prevention. Cigarette smoking among adults—United States, 2004. *MMWR Morbid Mortal Wkly Rep* 2005;54:1121-1124.

10. Chen ZM, Jiang LX, Chen YP, et al, for the COMMIT (Clopidogrel and Metoprolol in Myocardial Infarction Trial) collaborative group. Addition of clopidogrel to aspirin in 45 852 patients with acute myocardial infarction: randomized placebo-controlled trial. *Lancet* 2005;366:1607-1621.

11. Chobanian AV, Bakris GL, Black HR, et al., for the National Heart, Lung, and Blood Institute Joint National Committee on Prevention, Detection, Evaluation, and Treatment of High Blood Pressure; National High Blood Pressure Education Program Coordinating Committee. The Seventh Report of the Joint National Committee on Prevention, Detection, Evaluation, and Treatment of High Blood Pressure: the JNC 7 report. *JAMA* 2003;289:2560-2572.

12. Chowdhury PS, Franklin BA, Boura JA, et al. Sudden cardiac death after manual or automated snow removal. *Am J Cardiol* 2003;92:833-835.

13. Convertino VA. Effect of orthostatic stress on exercise performance after bed rest: relation to inhospital rehabilitation. *J Cardiac Rehabil* 1983;3:660-663.

14. Dimsdale JE, Hartley H, Guiney T, Ruskin JN, Greenblatt D. Postexercise peril: plasma catecholamines and exercise. *JAMA* 1984;251:630-632.

15. Doll R, Peto R, Boreham J, Sutherland I. Mortality in relation to smoking: 50 years' observation on male British doctors. *BMJ* 2004;328:1519-1533.

16. Dutcher JR, Kahn J, Grines C, Franklin B. Comparison of the left ventricular ejection fraction and exercise capacity as predictors of 2- and 5-year mortality following acute myocardial infarction. *Am J Cardiol* 2007;99:436-441.

17. Eckel RH, Krauss RM, for the AHA Nutrition Committee. American Heart Association call to action: obesity as a major risk factor for coronary heart disease. *Circulation* 1998;97:2099-2100.

18. Emeson EE, Robertson AL Jr. T lymphocytes in aortic and coronary intimas: their potential role in atherogenesis. *Am J Pathol* 1988;130:369-376.

19. Executive Summary of the Third Report of the National Cholesterol Education Program (NCEP) Expert Panel on Detection, Evaluation, and Treatment of High Blood Cholesterol in Adults (Adult Treatment Panel III). *JAMA* 2001;285:2486-2497.

20. Flegal KM, Carroll MD, Ogden CL, Johnson CL. Prevalence and trends in obesity among US adults, 1999-2000. *JAMA* 2002;288:1723-1727.

21. Franklin BA. Cardiovascular events associated with exercise: the risk-protection paradox. *J Cardiopulm Rehabil* 2004;25:189-195.

22. Franklin BA, Gordon NF. *Contemporary Diagnosis and Management in Cardiovascular Exercise.* Newtown, PA: Handbooks in Health Care; 2005.

23. Glagov S, Weisenberg E, Zarins CK, et al. Compensatory enlargement of human atherosclerotic coronary arteries. *N Engl J Med* 1987;316:1371-1375.

24. Gonzales D, Rennard SI, Nides M, et al, for the Varenicline Phase 3 Study Group. Varenicline, an $\alpha4\beta2$ nicotinic acetylcholine receptor partial agonist, vs sustained-release bupropion and placebo for smoking cessation: a randomized controlled trial. *JAMA* 2006;296:47-55.

25. Gurwitz JH, Col NF, Avorn J. The exclusion of the elderly and women from clinical trials in acute myocardial infarction. *JAMA* 1992;268:1417-1422.

26. Haapaniemi S, Franklin BA, Wegner JH, et al. Electrocardiographic responses to deer hunting activities in men with and without coronary artery disease. *Am J Cardiol* 2007;100:175-179.

27. Hoberg E, Schuler G, Kunze B, et al. Silent myocardial ischemia as a potential link between lack of premonitoring symptoms and increased risk of cardiac arrest during physical stress. *Am J Cardiol* 1990;65:583-589.

28. Hoffmann U, Nagurney JT, Moselewski F, et al. Coronary multidetector computed tomography in the assessment of patients with acute chest pain. *Circulation* 2006;114:2251-2260.

29. Kavanagh T, Mertens DJ, Hamm LF, et al. Peak oxygen intake and cardiac mortality in women referred for cardiac rehabilitation. *J Am Coll Cardiol* 2003;42:2139-2143.

30. Kavanagh T, Mertens DJ, Hamm LF, et al. Prediction of long-term prognosis in 12,169 men referred for cardiac rehabilitation. *Circulation* 2002;106:666-671.

31. Kelley GA, Kelley KS, Franklin B. Aerobic exercise and lipids and lipoproteins in patients with cardiovascular disease: a meta-analysis of randomized controlled trials. *J Cardiopulm Rehabil* 2006;26:131-139.

32. Lau J, Antman EM, Jimenez-Silva J, Kupelnick B, Mosteller F, Chalmers TC. Cumulative meta-analysis of therapeutic trials for myocardial infarction. *N Engl J Med* 1992;327:248-254.

33. Leon AS, Norstrom J. Evidence of the role of physical activity and cardiorespiratory fitness in the prevention of coronary heart disease. *Quest* 1995;47:311-319.

34. Libby P. *The Pathogenesis of Atherosclerosis. Harrison's Principles of Internal Medicine.* 16th ed. New York: McGraw-Hill, 2005:1425-1430.

35. Libby P. Current concepts of the pathogenesis of the acute coronary syndromes. *Circulation* 2001;104:365-372.

36. Little WC. Angiographic assessment of the culprit coronary artery lesion before acute myocardial infarction. *Am J Cardiol* 1990;66:44G-47G.

37. McCartney N, McKelvie RS, Martin J, Sale DG, MacDougall JD. Weight-training-induced attenuation of the circulatory response of older males to weight lifting. *J Appl Physiol* 1993;74:1056-1060.

38. McConnell TR, Klinger TA, Garner JK, Laubach CA Jr, Herman CE, Hauck CA. Cardiac rehabilitation without exercise tests for post-myocardial infarction and post-bypass surgery patients. *J Cardiopulm Rehabil* 1998;18:458-463.

39. Melidonis A, Dimopoulos V, Lempidakis E, et al. Angiographic study of coronary artery disease in diabetic patients in comparison with nondiabetic patients. *Angiology* 1999;50:997-1006.

40. Nissen SE, Tsunoda T, Tuzcu EM, et al. Effect of recombinant ApoA-I Milano on coronary atherosclerosis in patients with acute coronary syndromes: a randomized controlled trial. *JAMA* 2003;290:2292-2300.

41. Nissen SE, Tuzcu EM, Schoenhagen P, et al, for the REVERSAL Investigators. Effect of intensive compared with moderate lipid-lowering therapy on progression of coronary atherosclerosis: a randomized controlled trial. *JAMA* 2004;291:1071-1080.

42. Njolstad I, Arnesen E, Lund-Larsen P. Smoking, serum lipids, blood pressure, and sex differences in myocardial infarction: a 12-year follow-up of the Finnmark Study. *Circulation* 1996;93:450-456.

43. O'Connor GT, Buring JE, Yusuf S, et al. An overview of randomized trials of rehabilitation with exercise after myocardial infarction. *Circulation* 1989;80:234-244.

44. Ochoa AB, deJong A, Grayson D, Franklin B, McCullough P. Effect of enhanced external counterpulsation on resting oxygen uptake in patients having previous coronary revascularization and in healthy volunteers. *Am J Cardiol* 2006;98:613-615.

45. Ochoa AB, Franklin BA. Enhanced external counterpulsation therapy: a noninvasive approach to treating heart disease. *Am J Med Sports* 2003;5:194-198.

46. Oldridge NB, Guyatt GH, Fischer ME, Rimm AA. Cardiac rehabilitation after myocardial infarction: combined experience of randomized clinical trials. *JAMA* 1988;260:945-950.

47. Pepine CJ, Abrams J, Marks RG, et al, for the TIDES Investigators. Characteristics of a contemporary population with angina pectoris. *Am J Cardiol* 1994;74:226-231.

48. Pollock ML, Franklin BA, Balady GJ, et al. Resistance exercise in individuals with and without cardiovascular disease: benefits, rationale, safety, and prescription. *Circulation* 2000;101:828-833.

49. Pratt M. Benefits of lifestyle activity vs. structured exercise. *JAMA* 1999;281:375-376.

50. Quell KJ, Porcari JP, Franklin BA, Foster C, Andreuzzi RA, Anthony RM. Is brisk walking an adequate aerobic training stimulus for cardiac patients? *Chest* 2002;122:1852-1856.

51. Rossouw JE, Anderson GL, Prentice RL, et al, for the Writing Group for the Women's Health Initiative Investigators. Risks and benefits of estrogen plus progestin in healthy postmenopausal women: principal results from the Women's Health Initiative randomized controlled trial. *JAMA* 2002;288:321-333.

52. Sivarajan ES, Bruce RA, Almes MJ, et al. In-hospital exercise after myocardial infarction does not improve treadmill performance. *N Engl J Med* 1981;305:357-362.

53. Smith SC Jr, Allen J, Blair SN, et al. AHA/ACC guidelines for secondary prevention for patients with coronary and other atherosclerotic vascular disease: 2006 update. *J Am Coll Cardiol* 2006;47:2130-2139.

54. Stein B, Weintraub WS, Gebhart SP, et al. Influence of diabetes mellitus on early and late outcome after percutaneous transluminal coronary angioplasty. *Circulation* 1995;91:979-989.

55. Strong JP, Malcom GT, McMahan CA, et al. Prevalence and extent of atherosclerosis in adolescents and young adults: implications for prevention from the Pathobiological Determinants of Atherosclerosis in Youth Study. *JAMA* 1999;281:727-735.

56. Swain DP, Franklin BA. Is there a threshold intensity for aerobic training in cardiac patients? *Med Sci Sports Exerc* 2002;34:1071-1075.

57. Swain DP, Franklin BA. Comparison of cardioprotective benefits of vigorous versus moderate intensity aerobic exercise. *Am J Cardiol* 2006;97:141-147.

58. Taylor RS, Brown A, Ebrahim S, et al. Exercise-based rehabilitation for patients with coronary heart disease: systematic review and meta-analysis of randomized controlled trials. *Am J Med* 2004;116:682-692.

59. Taylor RS, Unal B, Critchley JA, Capewell S. Mortality reductions in patients receiving exercise-based cardiac rehabilitation: how much can be attributed to cardiovascular risk factor improvements? *Eur J Cardiovasc Prev Rehabil* 2006;13:369-374.

60. The Tobacco Use and Dependence Clinical Practice Guideline Panel, Staff, and Consortium Representatives. A clinical practice guideline for treating tobacco use and dependence: a US Public Health Service Report. *JAMA* 2000;283:3244-3254.

61. Waller BF, Palumbo PJ, Lie JT, Roberts WC. Status of the coronary arteries at necropsy in diabetes mellitus with onset after age 30 years: analysis of 229 diabetic patients with and without clinical evidence of coronary

heart disease and comparison to 183 control subjects. *Am J Med* 1980;69:498-506.

62. Wenger NK, Froelicher ES, Smith LK, et al. *Cardiac Rehabilitation as Secondary Prevention: Clinical Practice Guideline No. 17* (AHCPR publication no. 96-0672). Rockville, MD: U.S. Department of Health and Human Services, Public Health Service, Agency for Health Care Policy and Research and the National Heart, Lung, and Blood Institute; 1995.

63. Williams PT. Physical fitness and activity as separate heart disease risk factors: a meta-analysis. *Med Sci Sports Exerc* 2001;33:754-761.

64. Willich SN, Maclure M, Mittleman M, Arntz HR, Muller JE. Sudden cardiac death: support for a role of trigging in causation. *Circulation* 1993;87:1442-1450.

Chapter 29

1. *AACVPR Cardiac Rehabilitation Resource Manual.* Champaign, IL: Human Kinetics; 2006.

2. *ACSM's Guidelines for Exercise Testing and Prescription.* 7th ed. Whaley MH, Brubaker PH, Otto RM, eds. Philadelphia: Lippincott Williams & Wilkins; 2005.

3. American Heart Association. 2005. *Heart and Stroke Statistics—Update.* http://circ.ahajournals.org/cgi/reprint/CIRCULATIONAHA.107.187998.

4. Allen K, Dowling R, Fudge T, et al. Transmyocardial revascularization versus medical management: long term follow-up of a randomized, multi-center trial. *Ann Thorac Surg* 2004;77:1228-1234.

5. Allen K, Dowling R, Schuch D, et al. Adjunctive transmyocardial revascularization: five year follow-up of a prospective, randomized trial. *Ann Thorac Surg* 2004;78:458-465.

6. Belardinelli R, Paolini I, Cianci G, et al. Exercise training intervention after coronary angioplasty: the ETICA trial. *J Am Coll Cardiol* 2001;37:1891-1900.

7. Bertand M, Rupprecht H, Urban P, Gershlick A. Double-blind study of the safety of clopidogrel with and without loading dose in combination with aspirin after coronary stenting. *Circulation* 2000;102:624-629.

8. Braunwald E, ed. *Heart Disease: A Textbook of Cardiovascular Medicine.* 5th ed. Philadelphia: Saunders; 1997.

9. Brubaker P, Kaminsky L, Whaley M. *Coronary Artery Disease: Essentials of Prevention and Rehabilitation Programs.* Champaign, IL: Human Kinetics; 2001.

10. Gibbons RJ, Balady GJ, Bricker JT, et al. ACC/AHA 2002 guideline update for exercise testing: summary article: a report of the American College of Cardiology/American Heart Association Task Force on Practice Guidelines. *Circulation* 2002;106:1883-1894.

11. Giuliani ER, Gersh BJ, McGoon MD, Hayes DL, Schaft HV. *Mayo Clinical Practice of Cardiology.* 3rd ed. St. Louis: Mosby; 1996.

12. Hambrecht R, Walther C, Mobius-Winkler S, et al. Percutaneous coronary angioplasty compared with exercise training in patients with stable coronary artery disease. *Circulation* 2004;109:1371-1378.

13. Hedbeck B, Perk J, Hornblad M, et al. Cardiac rehabilitation after coronary bypass surgery: 10-year results on mortality, morbidity and readmission to hospital. *J Cardiovasc Risk* 2001;8:153-158.

14. Henry T, Annex B, McKendall, et al. The VIVA trial: vascular endothelial growth factor in ischemia for vascular angiogenesis. *Circulation* 2003;107:1359-1365.

15. Maseri A, Crea F, Kaski C, Croke T. Mechanisms of angina pectoris in syndrome X. *J Am Coll Cardiol* 1991;17:499-506.

16. Robinson J, Smith B, Maheshwari N, Schrott H. Pleiotropic effects of statins: benefit beyond cholesterol reduction? A meta-regression analysis. *J Am Coll Cardiol* 2005;46:1855-1862.

17. Serruys P, Kutryk M, Ong A. Coronary-artery stents. *N Engl J Med* 2006;345:483-495.

18. Smith S, Blair S, Bonow R, et al. AHA/ACC guidelines for secondary prevention for patients with coronary and other atherosclerotic vascular disease: 2006 update. *J Am Coll Cardiol* 2006;47:2130-2139.

19. Szmitko P, Fedak PW, Weisel RD, et al. Endothelial progenitor cells: new hope for a broken heart. *Circulation* 2003;107:3039-3100.

20. Uren NG, Melin JA, De Bruyne B, Wijns W, Baudhuin T, Camici PG. Relationship between myocardial blood flow and severity of coronary stenosis. *N Engl J Med* 1994;330:1782-1788.

Chapter 30

1. Alboni P, Botto GL, Baldi N, et al. Outpatient treatment of recent-onset atrial fibrillation with the "pill-in-the-pocket" approach. *N Engl J Med* 2004;351:2384-2391.

2. Atwood JE, Myers JN. Atrial fibrillation. In: *ACSM's Exercise Management for Persons With Chronic Disease and Disabilities.* 2nd ed. Durstine JL, Moore G, eds. Champaign, IL: Human Kinetics; 2003:47-51.

3. Bardy GH, Lee KL, Mark DB, et al. Amiodarone or an implantable cardioverter-defibrillator for congestive heart failure. *N Engl J Med* 2005;352:225-237.

4. Bernstein AD, Daubert JC, Fletcher RD, et al. The revised NASPE/BPEG generic code for antibradycardia, adaptive-rate, and multisite pacing. North American Society of Pacing and Electrophysiology/British Pacing and Electrophysiology Group. *Pacing Clin Electrophysiol* 2002;25:260.

5. Bradley DJ, Bradley EA, Baughman KL, et al. Cardiac resynchronization and death from progressive heart failure: a meta-analysis of randomized controlled trials. *JAMA* 2003;289:730-740.

6. Buxton AE, Waxman HL, Marchlinski FE, et al. Right ventricular tachycardia: clinical and electrophysiological characteristics. *Circulation* 1983;68:917-927.

7. Conover MB. *Understanding Electrocardiography.* 8th ed. St. Louis, MO: Mosby; 2002.

8. DeDenus S, Sanoski CA, Carlsson J, et al. Rate vs rhythm control in patients with atrial fibrillation: a meta-analysis. *Arch Intern Med* 2005;165:258-262.

9. Drew BJ, Scheinman MM. Value of electrocardiographic leads MCL1, MCL6 and other selected leads in the diagnosis of wide QRS complex tachycardia. *J Am Coll Cardiol* 1991;18:1025-1033.

10. Dubin D. *Rapid Interpretation of EKGs*. 6th ed. Tampa, FL: Cover; 1991.

11. Fletcher GF, Balady GJ, Amsterdam EA, et al. Exercise standards for testing and training: a statement for healthcare professionals from the American Heart Association. *Circulation* 2001;104:1694-1740.

12. Frolkis JP, Pothier CE, Blackstone EH, et al. Frequent ventricular ectopy after exercise as a predictor of death. *N Engl J Med* 2003;348:781-779.

13. Fuster V, Ryden LE, Asinger RW, et al. ACC/AHA/ESC guidelines for the management of patients with atrial fibrillation: executive summary: a report of the ACC/AHA Task Force on Practice Guidelines and the European Society of Cardiology Committee for Practice Guidelines and Policy Conferences. Developed in collaboration with the North American Society of Pacing and Electrophysiology. *Circulation* 2001;104:2118-2150.

14. Gibbons RJ, Balady GJ, Bricker JT, et al. ACC/AHA 2002 guideline update for exercise testing: a report of the ACC/AHA Task Force on Practice Guidelines (Committee on Exercise Testing). *Circulation* 2002;106:1883-1892.

15. Go AS, Hylek EM, Phillips KA, et al. Implications of stroke risk criteria on anticoagulation decision in nonvalvular atrial fibrillation. The Anticoagulation and Risk Factors in Atrial Fibrillation (ATRIA) Study. *Circulation* 2000;102:11-33.

16. Go AS, Hylek EM, Phillips KA, et al. Prevalence of diagnosed atrial fibrillation in adults: national implications for rhythm management and stroke prevention: the AnTicoagulation and Risk Factors in Atrial Fibrillation (ATRIA) Study. *JAMA* 2001;285:2370-2375.

17. Gregoratos G, Cheitlin MD, Conill A, et al. Guidelines update for implantation of cardiac pacemakers and antiarrhythmia devices: summary article: a report of the American College of Cardiology/American Heart Association Task Force on Practice Guidelines (ACC/AHA/NASPE Committee to Update the 1998 Pacemaker Guidelines). *Circulation* 2002;106:2145.

18. Grines DL, Bashore TM, Boudoulas H, et al. Functional abnormalities in isolated left bundle branch block: the effect of interventricular asynchrony. *Circulation* 1999;79:854-853.

19. Haissaguerre M, Jais P, Shah DC, et al. Spontaneous initiation of atrial fibrillation by ectopic beats originating in the pulmonary veins. *N Engl J Med* 1998;339:659-666.

20. Hohnloser SH, Kuck KH, Lilienthal J, et al. Rhythm or rate control in atrial fibrillation—Pharmacological Intervention in Atrial Fibrillation (PIAF): a randomized trial. *Lancet* 2000;356:1789-1794.

21. Katz AM. *Physiology of the Heart*. 3rd ed. Philadelphia: Lippincott Williams & Wilkins; 2001.

22. Kelly TM. Exercise testing and training of patients with malignant ventricular arrhythmias. *Med Sci Sports Exerc* 1995;28:53-61.

23. LaMonte MJ, Yanowitz FG. ICD discharge during exercise testing. *Med Sci Sports Exerc* 2004;36(5 suppl):S45.

24. Lev M, Fox SM, Bharati S, et al. Mahaim and James fibers as a basis for a unique variety of ventricular pre-excitation. *Am J Cardiol* 1975;36:880-888.

25. Moraday F, Kadish AH, DiCarlo L, et al. Long-term results of catheter ablation of idiopathic right ventricular tachycardia. *Circulation* 1990;82:2093-2099.

26. Moss AJ, Zareba W, Hall WJ, et al. Prophylactic implantation of a defibrillator in patients with myocardial infarction and reduced ejection fraction. *N Engl J Med* 2002;346:877-883.

27. National Institutes of Health. *Physical Activity and Cardiovascular Health: A National Consensus*. Leon AS, ed. Champaign, IL: Human Kinetics; 1997.

28. Oral H, Knight BP, Tada H, et al. Pulmonary vein isolation for paroxysmal and persistent atrial fibrillation. *Circulation* 2002;105:1077-1081.

29. Page RL. Newly diagnosed atrial fibrillation. *N Engl J Med* 2004;351:2408-2416.

30. Pappone D, Rosanio S, Augello G, et al. Mortality, morbidity, and quality of life after circumferential pulmonary vein ablation for atrial fibrillation: outcomes from a controlled nonrandomized long-term study. *J Am Coll Cardiol* 2003;42:185-197.

31. Pashkow FJ, Schweikert RA, Wilkoff BL. Exercise testing and training in patients with malignant arrhythmia. *Exerc Sport Sci Rev* 1997;25:235-269.

32. Thiene G, Nava A, Corrado D, et al. Right ventricular cardiomyopathy and sudden death in young people. *N Engl J Med* 1988;318:129-133.

33. Van Gelder IC, Hagens VE, Bosker HA, et al. A comparison of rate control and rhythm control in patients with recurrent atrial fibrillation. *N Engl J Med* 2002;347:1834-1840.

34. Wagner GS. *Marriott's Practical Electrocardiography*. 11th ed. Philadelphia: Lippincott Williams & Wilkins; 2008.

35. Wyse DG, Waldo AL, DiMarco JP, et al. A comparison of rate control and rhythm control in patients with atrial fibrillation. *N Engl J Med* 2002;347:1825-1833.

36. Yanowitz FG. The Alan E. Lindsay ECG Learning Center in Cyberspace. http://library.med.utah.edu/kw/ecg.

37. Zipes DP, Ackerman MJ, Estes NAM, et al. Task force 7: arrhythmias. *J Am Coll Cardiol* 2005;45:1354-63.

Chapter 31

1. Aronow WS. Management of peripheral arterial disease. *Cardiol Rev* 2005;13:61-68.

2. Ashworth NL, Chad KE, Harrison EL, et al. Home versus center based physical activity programs in

older adults. *Cochrane Database Syst Rev* 2005;(1): CD004017.

3. Bartelink ML, Stoffers HE, Biesheuvel CJ, et al. Walking exercise in patients with intermittent claudication: experience in routine clinical practice. *Br J Gen Pract* 2004;54:196-200.

4. Collins EG, Langbein WE, Orebaugh C, et al. Cardiovascular training effect associated with polestriding exercise in patients with peripheral arterial disease. *J Cardiovasc Nurs* 2005;20:177-185.

5. Criqui, MH. Peripheral arterial disease—epidemiological aspects. *Vasc Med* 2001;6(3 suppl):3-7.

6. Dolan NC, Liu K, Criqui MH, et al. Peripheral artery disease, diabetes, and reduced lower extremity functioning. *Diabetes Care* 2002;25:113-120.

7. Gardner AW, Katzel LI, Sorkin JD, et al. Improved functional outcomes following exercise rehabilitation in patients with intermittent claudication. *J Gerontol A Biol Sci Med Sci* 2000;55:M570-M577.

8. Gardner AW, Katzel LI, Sorkin JD, et al. Effects of long-term exercise rehabilitation on claudication distances in patients with peripheral arterial disease: a randomized controlled trial. *J Cardiopulm Rehabil* 2002;22:192-198.

9. Gardner AW, Poehlman, ET. Exercise rehabilitation programs for the treatment of claudication pain: a meta-analysis. *JAMA* 1995;274:975-980.

10. Gardner AW, Skinner JS, Vaughan NR, et al. Comparison of three progressive exercise protocols in peripheral vascular occlusive disease. *Angiology* 1992;43:661-671.

11. Gibellini R, Fanello M, Bardile AF, et al. Exercise training in intermittent claudication. *Int Angiol* 2000;19:8-13.

12. Hiatt WR. Medical treatment of peripheral arterial disease and claudication. *N Engl J Med* 2001;344:1608-1621.

13. Hiatt WR, Nawaz D, Regensteiner JG, et al. The evaluation of exercise performance in patients with peripheral vascular disease. *J Cardiopulm Rehabil* 1988;12:525-532.

14. Hiatt WR, Wolfel EE, Meier RH, et al. Superiority of treadmill walking exercise versus strength training for patients with peripheral arterial disease: implications for the mechanism of the training response. *Circulation* 1994;90:1866-1874.

15. Hirsch AT, Criqui MH, Treat-Jacobson D, et al. Peripheral arterial disease detection, awareness, and treatment in primary care. *JAMA* 2001;286:1317-1324.

16. Jones PP, Skinner JS, Smith LK, et al. Functional improvements following StairMaster vs. treadmill exercise training for patients with intermittent claudication. *J Cardiopulm Rehabil* 1996;16:47-55.

17. Katzel LI, Sorkin JD, Powell CC, et al. Comorbidities and exercise capacity in older patients with intermittent claudication. *Vasc Med* 2001;6:157-162.

18. Leng, GC, Fowler B, Ernst, E. Exercise for intermittent claudication. *Cochrane Database Syst Rev* 2000;(2): CD000990.

19. Lundgren F, Dahllof AG, Lundholm K, et al. Intermittent claudication—surgical reconstruction or physical training? A prospective randomized trial of treatment efficiency. *Ann Surg* 1989;209:346-355.

20. McDermott MM, Criqui MH, Greenland P, et al. Leg strength in peripheral arterial disease: associations with disease severity and lower-extremity performance. *J Vasc Surg* 2004;39:523-530.

21. McKirnan MD, Bloor CM. Clinical significance of coronary vascular adaptations to exercise training. *Med Sci Sports Exerc* 1994;26:1262-1268.

22. Menard JR, Smith HE, Riebe D, et al. Long-term results of peripheral arterial disease rehabilitation. *J Vasc Surg* 2004;39:1186-1192.

23. Patterson RB, Pinto B, Marcus B, et al. Value of a supervised exercise program for the therapy of arterial claudication. *J Vasc Surg* 1997;25:312-318; discussion 318-319.

24. Regensteiner JG. Exercise in the treatment of claudication: assessment and treatment of functional impairment. *Vasc Med* 1997;2:238-242.

25. Regensteiner JG, Hiatt WR. Current medical therapies for patients with peripheral arterial disease: a critical review. *Am J Med* 2002;112:49-57.

26. Regensteiner JG, Meyer TJ, Krupski WC, et al. Hospital vs home-based exercise rehabilitation for patients with peripheral arterial occlusive disease. *Angiology* 1997;48:291-300.

27. Regensteiner JG, Steiner JF, Hiatt WR. Exercise training improves functional status in patients with peripheral arterial disease. *J Vasc Surg* 1996;23:104-115.

28. Stewart KJ, Hiatt WR, Regensteiner JG, et al. Exercise training for claudication. *N Engl J Med* 2002;347:1941-1951.

29. Treat-Jacobson D, Halverson SL, Ratchford A, et al. A patient-derived perspective of health-related quality of life with peripheral arterial disease. *J Nurs Scholarsh* 2002;34:55-60.

30. Tsai JC, Chan P, Wang CH, et al. The effects of exercise training on walking function and perception of health status in elderly patients with peripheral arterial occlusive disease. *J Intern Med* 2002;252:448-455.

31. Ware JE Jr, Sherbourne CD. The MOS 36-item short-form health survey (SF-36). I. Conceptual framework and item selection. *Med Care* 1992;30:473-483.

32. Weitz JI, Byrne J, Clagett GP, et al. Diagnosis and treatment of chronic arterial insufficiency of the lower extremities: a critical review. *Circulation* 1996;94:3026-3049.

33. Wolosker N, Nakano L, Rosoky RA, et al. Evaluation of walking capacity over time in 500 patients with intermittent claudication who underwent clinical treatment. *Arch Intern Med* 2003;163:2296-2300.

Chapter 32

1. American Heart Association. *Heart Disease and Stroke Facts, 2006 Update*. Dallas, TX: AHA; 2006.

2. Bardy GH, Lee KL, Mark DB, et al, for the Sudden Cardiac Death in Heart Failure Trial (SCD-HeFT) Investigators. Amiodarone or an implantable cardioverter-defibrillator for congestive heart failure. *N Engl J Med* 2005;352:225-237.

3. Baughman KL. B-type natriuretic peptide—a window to the heart. *N Engl J Med* 2002;347:158-159.

4. Belardinelli R, Georgiou D, Pucaro A. Randomized, controlled trial of long-term moderate exercise training in chronic heart failure. *Circulation* 1999;99:1173-1182.

5. Braith RW, Welsch MA, Feigenbaum MS, Kluess HA, Pepine CJ. Neuroendocrine activation in heart failure is modified by endurance exercise training. *J Am Coll Cardiol* 1999;34:1170-1175.

6. Cleland JG, Daubert JC, Erdmann E, et al. The effect of cardiac resynchronization on morbidity and mortality in heart failure. *N Engl J Med* 2005;352:1539-1549.

7. Corra U, Mezzani A, Bosimini E, Giannuzzi P. Cardiopulmonary exercise testing prognosis in chronic heart failure: a prognosticating algorithm for the individual patient. *Chest* 2004;126:942-950.

8. Curnier D, Galinier M, Pathak A, et al. Rehabilitation of patients with congestive heart failure with or without β-blockade therapy. *J Cardiac Failure* 2001;7:241-248.

9. Delagardelle C, Feiereisen P, Autier P, Shita R, Krecke R, Beissel J. Strength/endurance training versus endurance training in congestive heart failure. *Med Sci Sports Exerc* 2002;34:1868-1872.

10. Delagardelle C, Vaillant M, Lasar Y, Beissel J. Is strength training the more efficient training modality in chronic heart failure? *Med Sci Sports Exerc* 2007;39:1910-1917.

11. ExtTraMATCH Collaborative. Exercise training meta-analysis of trials in patients with chronic heart failure (ExTraMATCH). *Br Med J* 2004;328:189-191.

12. Forissier JF, Vernochet P, Bertrand P, Charbonnier B, Monpere C. Influence of carvedilol on the benefits of physical training in patients with moderate chronic heart failure. *Eur J Heart Fail* 2001;3:335-342.

13. Giannuzzi P, Temporelli PL, Corra U, Tavazzi L. Antiremodeling effect of long-term exercise training in patients with stable chronic heart failure. *Circulation* 2003;108:554-559.

14. Gielen S, Adams V, Mobius-Winkler S, et al. Anti-inflammatory effects of exercise training in the skeletal muscle of patients with chronic heart failure. *J Am Coll Cardiol* 2003;42:861-868.

15. Hambrecht R, Gielen S, Linke A, et al. Effects of exercise training on left ventricular function and peripheral resistance in patients with chronic heart failure. *JAMA* 2000;283:3095-3101.

16. Hambrecht R, Niebauer J, Fiehn E, et al. Physical training in patients with stable chronic heart failure: effects on cardiorespiratory fitness and ultrastructural abnormalities of leg muscles. *J Am Coll Cardiol* 1995;25:1239-1249.

17. Hunt SA, Abraham WT, Chin MH, et al. ACC/AHA 2005 guideline update for the diagnosis and management of chronic heart failure in the adult. A report of the American College of Cardiology/American Heart Association Task Force on Practice Guidelines (Writing Committee to Update the 2001 Guidelines for the Evaluation and Management of Heart Failure). American Heart Association Web site; Feb. 15, 2008. http://circ.ahajournals.org/cgi/reprint/112/12/e154.

18. Isaaz K. Tissue Doppler imaging for the assessment of left ventricular systolic and diastolic functions. *Curr Opin Cardiol* 2002;17:431-442.

19. Jessup M, Brozena S. Heart failure. *N Engl J Med* 2003;348:2007-2018.

20. Keteyian SJ, Brawner CA, Schairer JR, et al. Effects of exercise training on chronotropic incompetence in patients with heart failure. *Am Heart J* 1999;138:233-240.

21. Keteyian SJ, Duscha BD, Brawner CA, et al. Differential effects of exercise training in men and women with chronic heart failure. *Am Heart J* 2003;145:912-918.

22. Keteyian SJ, Spring TJ. Chronic heart failure. In: *Clinical Exercise Physiology*. Ehrman JK, Gordon PM, Visich PS, Keteyian SJ, eds. Champaign, IL: Human Kinetics; 2008:261-280.

23. Levy D, Kenchaiah S, Larson MG, et al. Long-term trends in the incidence of and survival with heart failure. *N Engl J Med* 2002;347:1397-1402.

24. Linke A, Schoene N, Gielen S, et al. Endothelial dysfunction in patients with chronic heart failure: systemic effects of lower-limb exercise training. *J Am Coll Cardiol* 2001;37:392-397.

25. Maisel AS, Krishnaswamy P, Nowak RM. Rapid measurement of B-type natriuretic peptide in the emergency diagnosis of heart failure. *N Engl J Med* 2002;347:161-167

26. Mann DL. Recent insights into the role of tumor necrosis factor in the failing heart. *Heart Fail Rev* 2001;6:71-80.

27. McKelvie RS, Teo KK, Roberts R, et al. Effects of exercise training in patients with heart failure: The Exercise Rehabilitation Trial (EXERT). *Am Heart J* 2002;144:23-30.

28. Pina IL, Apstein CS, Balady GJ, et al. Exercise and heart failure. *Circulation* 2003;107:1210-1225.

29. Pu CT, Johnson MT, Forman DE, et al. Randomized trial of progressive resistance training to counteract the myopathy of chronic heart failure. *J Appl Physiol* 2001;90:2341-2350.

30. Roveda F, Middlekauff HR, Rondon MUPB, et al. The effects of exercise training on sympathetic neural activation in advanced heart failure. *J Am Coll Cardiol* 2003;42:854-860.

31. Wisløff U, Støylen A, Loennechen JP, et al. Superior cardiovascular effect of aerobic interval training versus moderate continuous training in heart failure patients: a randomized study. *Circulation* 2007;115:3086-3094.

32. Zile MR, Baicu CF, Gaasch WH. Diastolic heart failure—abnormalities in active relaxation and passive stiffness of the left ventricle. *N Engl J Med* 2004;350:1953-1959.

Chapter 33

1. Barnard CN. The operation: a human cardiac transplant. An interim report of a successful operation performed at Groote Schuur Hospital, Cape Town. *S Afr Med J* 1967;41:1271-1274.

2. Braith RW, Mills RM, Welsch MA, et al. Resistance exercise training restores bone mineral density in heart transplant recipients. *J Am Coll Cardiol* 1996;28:1471-1477.

3. Brubaker PH, Brozena SC, Morley DL, et al. Exercise-induced ventilatory abnormalities in orthotopic heart transplant patients. *J Heart Lung Transplant* 1997;16:1011-1017.

4. Daida H, Squires RW, Allison TG, et al. Sequential assessment of exercise tolerance in heart transplantation compared with coronary artery bypass surgery after phase II cardiac rehabilitation. *Am J Cardiol* 1996;77:696-700.

5. Ehrman JK, Keteyian SJ, Levine AB, et al. Exercise stress tests after cardiac transplantation. *Am J Cardiol* 1993;71:1372-1373.

6. Gibbons RJ, Balady GJ, Beasley JW, et al. ACC/AHA guidelines for exercise testing: a report of the American College of Cardiology/American Heart Association Task Force on Practice Guidelines (Committee on Exercise Testing). *J Am Coll Cardiol* 1997;30:260-315.

7. Hertz MI, Boucek MM, Deng MC, et al. The registry of the International Society for Heart and Lung Transplantation: introduction to the 2004 annual reports. *J Heart Lung Transplant* 2004;23:789-795.

8. Horber FF, Scheidegger JR, Grunig BF, et al. Evidence that prednisone-induced myopathy is reversed by physical training. *J Clin Endocrinol Metab* 1985;61:83-88.

9. Hummel M, Michauk I, Hetzer R, Fuhrman B. Quality of life after heart and heart-lung transplantation. *Transplant Proc* 2001;33:3546-3548.

10. Jenkins GH, Grieve LA, Yacoub MH, Singer DRJ. Effect of simvastatin on ejection fraction in cardiac transplant recipients. *Am J Cardiol* 1996;78:1453-1456.

11. Kao AC, Van Trigt P, Shaeffer-McCall GS, et al. Central and peripheral limitations to upright exercise in untrained cardiac transplant recipients. *Circulation* 1994;89:2605-2615.

12. Kavanagh T, Yacoub MH, Mertens DJ, et al. Cardiorespiratory responses to exercise training after orthotopic cardiac transplantation. *Circulation* 1988;77:162-171.

13. Kaye DM, Esler M, Kingwell B, et al. Functional and neurochemical evidence for partial cardiac sympathetic reinnervation after cardiac transplantation in humans. *Circulation* 1993;88:1110-1118.

14. Keteyian SJ, Brawner C. Cardiac transplant. In: *American College of Sports Medicine. ACSM's Exercise Management for Persons With Chronic Diseases and Disabilities.* Champaign, IL: Human Kinetics; 1997:54-58.

15. Kobashigawa JA, Leaf DA, Lee N, et al. A controlled trial of exercise rehabilitation after heart transplantation. *N Engl J Med* 1999;340:272-277.

16. Kuhn WF, Davis MH, Lippmann SB. Emotional adjustments to cardiac transplantation. *Gen Hosp Psychiatry* 1988;10:108-113.

17. Lampert E, Mettauer B, Hoppeler H, et al. Structure of skeletal muscle in heart transplant recipients. *J Am Coll Cardiol* 1996;28:980-984.

18. Lampert E, Mettauer B, Hoppeler H, et al. Skeletal muscle response to short endurance training in heart transplantation recipients. *J Am Coll Cardiol* 1998;32:420-426.

19. Leung TC, Ballman KV, Allison TG, et al. Clinical predictors of exercise capacity 1 year after cardiac transplantation. *J Heart Lung Transplant* 2003;22:16-27.

20. Lindenfeld J, Miller GG, Shakar SF, et al. Drug therapy in the heart transplant recipient part 1: cardiac rejection and immunosuppressive drugs. *Circulation* 2004;110:3734-3740.

21. Lindenfeld J, Page II RL, Zolty R, et al. Drug therapy in the heart transplant recipient part III: common medical problems. *Circulation* 2005;111:113-117.

22. Mancini DM, Eisen H, Kussmaul W, et al. Value of peak exercise oxygen consumption for optimal timing of cardiac transplantation in ambulatory patients with heart failure. *Circulation* 1991;83:778-786.

23. Marconi C, Marzorati M. Exercise after heart transplantation. *Eur J Appl Physiol* 2003;90:250-259.

24. McGregor CGA. Cardiac transplantation: Surgical considerations and early postoperative management. *Mayo Clin Proc* 1992;67:577-585.

25. Mettauer B, Zhao QM, Epailly E, et al. VO_2 kinetics reveal a central limitation at the onset of subthreshold exercise in heart transplant recipients. *J Appl Physiol* 2000;88:1228-1238.

26. Niset G, Cousty-Degre C, Degre S. Psychological and physical rehabilitation after heart transplantation: 1 year follow-up. *Cardiology* 1988;75:311-317.

27. Pokan R, Von Duvillard SP, Ludwig J, et al. Effect of high-volume and –intensity endurance training in heart transplant recipients. *Med Sci Sports Exerc* 2004;36:2011-2016.

28. Pope SE, Stinson EB, Daughters GT, et al. Exercise response of the denervated heart in long-term cardiac transplant recipients. *Am J Cardiol* 1980;46:213-218.

29. Rodeheffer RJ, McGregor CGA. The development of cardiac transplantation. *Mayo Clin Proc* 1992;67:480-484.

30. Richard R, Verdier JC, Duvallet A, et al. Chronotropic competence in endurance trained heart transplant recipients: heart rate is not a limiting factor for exercise capacity. *J Am Coll Cardiol* 1999;33:192-197.

31. Squires RW. Cardiac rehabilitation issues for heart transplantation patients. *J Cardiopulmonary Rehabil* 1990;10:159-168.

32. Squires RW. Transplant. In: *Clinical Cardiac Rehabilitation: A Cardiologist's Guide*. 2nd ed. Pashkow FJ, Dafoe WA, eds. Baltimore: Williams & Wilkins; 1999:175-191.

33. Squires RW, Arthur PA, Gau GT, et al. Exercise after cardiac transplantation: a report of two cases. *J Cardiopulmonary Rehabil* 1983;3:570-574.

34. Squires RW, Hoffman CJ, James GA, et al. Arterial oxygen saturation during graded exercise testing after cardiac transplantation. *J Cardiopulmonary Rehabil* 1998;18:348.

35. Squires RW, Leung TC, Cyr NS, et al. Partial normalization of the heart rate response to exercise after cardiac transplantation: frequency and relationship to exercise capacity. *Mayo Clin Proc* 2002;77:1295-1300.

36. Stapleton DD, Mehra MR, Dumas D, et al. Lipid-lowering therapy and long-term survival in heart transplantation. *Am J Cardiol* 1997;80:802-804.

37. Stratton JR, Kemp GJ, Daly RC, et al. Effects of cardiac transplantation on bioenergetic abnormalities of skeletal muscle in congestive heart failure. *Circulation* 1994;89:1624-1631.

38. Taylor DO, Edwards LB, Boucek MM, et al. The registry of the International Society for Heart and Lung Transplantation: twenty-first official adult heart transplant report—2004. *J Heart Lung Transplant* 2003;23:796-803.

39. Weis M, von Scheidt W. Cardiac allograft vasculopathy: a review. *Circulation* 1997;96:2069-2077.

40. Wenke K, Meiser B, Thiery J, et al. Simvastatin reduces graft vessel disease and mortality after heart transplantation: a four-year randomized trial. *Circulation* 1997;96:1398-1402.

41. Wu AH, Ballantyne CM, Short BC, et al. Statin use and risks of death or fatal rejection in the heart transplant lipid registry. *Am J Cardiol* 2005;95:367-372.

Chapter 34

1. Ageno W, Piantanida E, Dentali F, et al. Weight gain after acute deep venous thrombosis: a prospective observational study. *Thromb Res* 2003;109:31-35.

2. Aziz S, Straehley CJ, Whelan TJ. Effort related axillosubclavian vein thrombosis: a new theory of pathogenesis and a plea for direct surgical intervention. *Am J Surg* 1986;152:57-61.

3. Blattler W, Partsch H. Leg compression and ambulation is better than bed rest for the treatment of acute deep venous thrombosis. *Int Angiol* 2003;22:393-400.

4. Booth NA, Walker E, Maughan R, Bennett B. Plasminogen activator in normal subjects after exercise and venous occlusion: t PA circulates as complexes with C1 inhibitor and PAI 1. *Blood* 1987;69:1600-1604.

5. Buller HR, Agnelli G, Hull RD, Hyers TM, Prins MH, Raskob GE. *Chest* 2004;126:401S-428S.

6. Cruickshank JM, Gorlin R, Jennett B. Air travel and thrombotic episodes: the economy class syndrome. *Lancet* 1988;2:497-498.

7. Doskova M, Hrabak P, Puchmayer V, Albrecht V. The effect of physical activity on the incidence of circulating platelet aggregates in healthy persons: the significance for antiaggregating therapy. *Int Angiol* 1991;10:15-18.

8. Factor V Leiden Thrombophilia Support Page. www.fvleiden.org/ask/71.html.

9. Gorard DA. Effort thrombosis in an American football player. *Br J Sports Med* 1990;24:15.

10. Ikarugi H, Taka T, Nakajima S, et al. Norepinephrine, but not epinephrine, enhances platelet reactivity and coagulation after exercise in humans. *J Appl Physiol* 1999;86:133-138.

11. Johnson BF, Manzo RA, Bergelin RO, Strandness DE Jr. The site of residual abnormalities in the leg veins in long term follow up after deep vein thrombosis and their relationship to the development of the post thrombotic syndrome. *Int Angiol* 1996;15:14-19.

12. Kahn SR, Azoulay L, Hirsch A, Haber M, Strulovitch C, Shrier I. Effect of graduated elastic compression stockings on leg symptoms and signs during exercise in patients with deep venous thrombosis: a randomized cross-over trial. *J Thromb Haemostas* 2003;1:494-499.

13. Koenig W, Ernst E. Exercise and thrombosis. *Coron Artery Dis* 2000;11:123-127.

14. National Alliance for Thrombosis and Thrombophilia. www.nattinfo.org/learn.htm.

15. Novak RM, Leikin JB, Duarte B. Use of thrombolytic therapy in axillary subclavian vein thrombosis. *Am J Emerg Med* 1988;6:120-123.

16. Raskob GE. Heparin and low molecular weight heparin for treatment of acute pulmonary embolism. *Curr Opin Pulmon Med* 1999;5:216-221.

17. Roberts WO, Christie DM Jr. Return to training and competition after deep venous calf thrombosis. *Med Sci Sports Exerc* 1992;24:2-5.

18. Rossi R, Agnelli G. Current role of venography in the diagnosis of deep vein thrombosis. *Minerva Cardioangiol* 1998;46:507-514.

19. Shrier I, Kahn SR. Effect of physical activity after recent deep venous thrombosis: a cohort study. *Med Sci Sports Exerc* 2005;37:630-634.

20. Slawski DP. Deep venous thrombosis complicating rupture of the medial head of the gastrocnemius muscle. *J Orthop Trauma* 1994;8:263-264.

21. Thompson Ford JK. Low molecular weight heparin for the treatment of deep vein thrombosis. *Pharmacotherapy* 1998;18:748-758.

22. Wells PS, Anderson DR. Modern approach to diagnosis in patients with suspected deep vein thrombosis. *Haemostasis* 1999;29(suppl S1):10-20.

23. Winther K, Hillegass W, Tofler GH, et al. Effects on platelet aggregation and fibrinolytic activity during upright posture and exercise in healthy men. *Am J Cardiol* 1992;70:1051-1055.

Index

Note: The italicized *f* and *t* following page numbers refer to figures and tables, respectively.

About the Editors

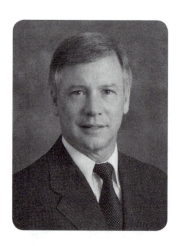

J. Larry Durstine, PhD, is a distinguished professor and chair in the department of exercise science at the University of South Carolina at Columbia. He is also the director of Clinical Exercise Programs.

Dr. Durstine has focused his academic and research career on cardiovascular disease prevention and rehabilitation. He has used his years of experience in cardiovascular rehabilitation programming to mentor both professionals and students in cardiovascular disease prevention and rehabilitation.

A coeditor for *ACSM's Exercise Management for Persons with Chronic Diseases and Disabilities*, Dr. Durstine is a past president of the American College of Sports Medicine (ACSM) and a member of the American Association of Cardiovascular and Pulmonary Rehabilitation (AACVPR). He and his wife, Linda, reside in Columbia. In his free time, Dr. Durstine enjoys home remodeling projects and woodworking. He also enjoys running, water skiing, and snow skiing.

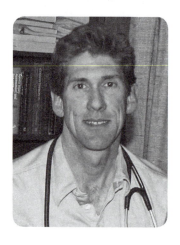

Geoffrey E. Moore, MD, is a founder and director of the Cayuga Center for Healthy Living, a comprehensive lifestyle medicine service based in Ithaca, New York. As an exercise scientist and sports medicine internist, Dr. Moore has developed both clinical and research expertise in basic and applied physiology, chronic medical diseases, musculoskeletal injuries, physiology of exercise intolerance, and lifestyle modification. He has eight years of experience as medical director of cardiac rehabilitation programs and 14 years of basic and applied research focused on mechanisms of exercise intolerance.

Dr. Moore is a coeditor for *ACSM's Exercise Management for Persons With Chronic Diseases and Disabilities*, an ACSM fellow, a member of Health and Science Policy Committee, and the vice chair of the Family Health Issues Committee for the Medical Society of the State of New York. He resides in Ithaca and enjoys windsurfing, running, and cross-country skiing in his free time.

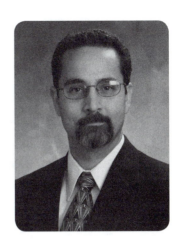

Michael J. LaMonte, PhD, is an assistant professor of epidemiology in the department of social and preventive medicine at the University of Buffalo in New York. Previously, Dr. LaMonte served as the director of epidemiologic research at the Cooper Institute in Dallas, Texas, and director of the Exercise Testing Laboratory at LDS Hospital in Salt Lake City, Utah.

Dr. LaMonte's research has focused on the role of physical activity and functional capacity in the prevention and management of chronic diseases with an emphasis on cardiovascular disease. Additional research interests include the use of noninvasive cardiovascular tests such as exercise testing, electron-beam-computed tomography, carotid artery ultrasound, and arterial reactivity for assessing the structural and functional significance of subclinical cardiovascular disease and its subsequent relationship with clinical cardiovascular disease events.

Dr. LaMonte enjoys spending time with his family, cooking, and watching college sports. When outdoors, he enjoys jogging, snowshoeing, gardening, and tennis.

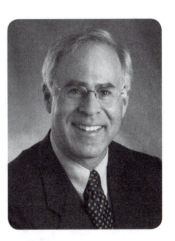

Barry A. Franklin, PhD, is the director of the Cardiac Rehabilitation Program and Exercise Laboratories at the William Beaumont Hospital in Royal Oak, Michigan. In addition, he serves as a professor of physiology in the School of Medicine at Wayne State University in Detroit, Michigan.

During his more than three decades of clinical experience in cardiac rehabilitation, Dr. Franklin has authored over 500 scientific and clinical publications and book chapters and is the coauthor of *Take a Load Off Your Heart* with Joe Piscatella (Workman Publishing). He also serves on the editorial boards of 15 scientific and clinical journals, including the *Journal of Cardiopulmonary Rehabilitation*, *Preventive Cardiology*, *Chest*, *American Journal of Cardiology*, *Medicine and Science in Sports and Exercise*, and the *American Journal of Lifestyle Medicine*.

Dr. Franklin was president of the American Heart Association (AHA), Greater Midwest Affiliate, and vice chair for the AHA Council on Nutrition, Physical Activity, and Metabolism. He is a past president of the American Association of Cardiovascular and Pulmonary Rehabilitation (AACVPR) and American College of Sports Medicine (ACSM) and has also served as editor in chief of *Journal of Cardiopulmonary Rehabilitation* and as an expert panel member for Cardiac Rehabilitation Guidelines, NHLBI/AHCPR. His recognitions include the Award of Meritorious Achievement from the American Heart Association (2006), AACVPR's Michael L. Pollock Excellence in Research Award (2004), and ACSM's Citation Award (2002).

Dr. Franklin and his wife, Linda, live in West Bloomfield, Michigan. Reading for professional development, distance walking, golf, and travel are his favorite leisure pursuits.

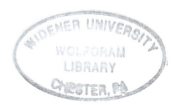

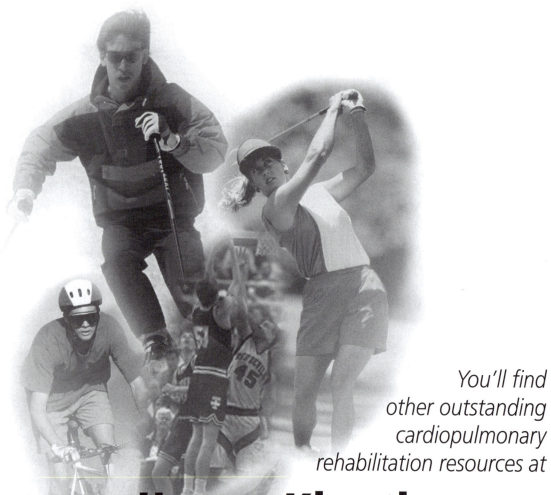

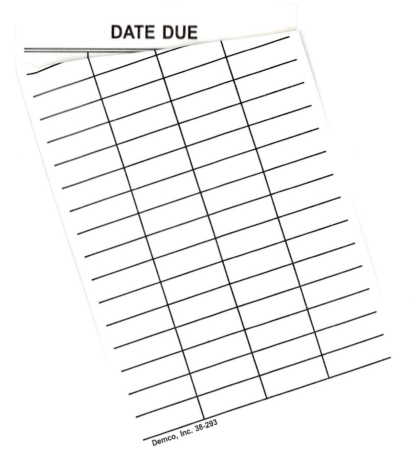

DATE DUE

Demco, Inc. 38-293